VISCOELASTICS
IN
OPHTHALMIC SURGERY

VISCOELASTICS
IN
OPHTHALMIC SURGERY

Lucio Buratto, MD
Pietro Giardini, MD
Roberto Bellucci, MD

Steve A. Arshinoff, MD, FRCSC • Michael Colvard, MD• Eugenio Leite, MD • Simonetta Morselli, MD • Vincenzo Pucci, MD • Robert Stegmann, MD • Manfred Tetz, MD

Illustrations by Massimiliano Crespi

Michael Farbowitz, MD
Editorial Assistants: Katheryn Minette Klein, Diana Bodnar, and Chris Eales

SLACK
INCORPORATED
6900 Grove Road • Thorofare, NJ 08086

Publisher: John H. Bond
Editorial Director: Amy E. Drummond
Assistant Editor: Lauren Biddle Plummer

The procedures and practices described in this book should be implemented in a manner consistent with the professional standards set for the circumstances that apply in each specific situation. Every effort has been made to confirm the accuracy of the information presented and to correctly relate generally accepted practices. The author, editor, and publisher cannot accept responsibility for errors or exclusions or for the outcome of the application of the material presented herein. There is no expressed or implied warranty of this book or information imparted by it.

Care has been taken to ensure that drug selection and dosages are in accordance with currently accepted/recommended practice. Due to continuing research, changes in government policy and regulations, and various effects of drug reactions and interactions, it is recommended that the reader review all materials and literature provided for each drug, especially those that are new or not frequently used.

Any review or mention of specific companies or products is not intended as an endorsement by the author or the publisher.

Viscoelastics in Ophthalmic Surgery is a translated and updated English version of the Italian book *Viscoelastici in Chirurgia Oftalmica* published by CAMO in Milan, Italy.

Published by: SLACK Incorporated
6900 Grove Road
Thorofare, NJ 08086-9447 USA
Telephone: 856-848-1000
Fax: 856-853-5991
World Wide Web: http://www.slackinc.com

Contact SLACK Incorporated for more information about other books in this field or about the availability of our books from distributors outside the United States.

Last digit is print number: 10 9 8 7 6 5 4 3 2 1

CONTENTS

Acknowledgments

On behalf of Pietro Giardini, Roberto Bellucci and myself, I would like to thank all the people that made this book possible.

In particular I would like to thank Michael Colvard and his assistants—through his valuable suggestions and his critical review he made an important contribution to the clarity of the final presentation of this book, ensuring a publication of the very highest standard.

We would also like to thank all the contributors. By their dedicated collaboration and scientific support, they added value to this project and augmented the scientific content.

My most heartfelt thanks go to Peter Slack who made the production of this book possible.

Lucio Buratto, MD

Contributing Authors

Steve A. Arshinoff, MD, FRCSC
Downsview, Ontario

Roberto Carassa, MD
Milan, Italy

Mike P. Holzer, MS
Berlin, Germany

Eugenio Leite, MD, PhD
Coimbra, Portugal

Simonetta Morselli, MD
Verona, Italy

Vincenzo Pucci, MD
Verona, Italy

Robert Stegmann, MD
Pretoria, South Africa

Manfred R. Tetz, MD
Berlin, Germany

Preface

It was the Fall of 1982 when I performed my first cataract operation; I used Healon®. At that time, the product was not commercially available in Italy. I had visited Robert Sinskey around that time and he gave me a vial of the product to try.

After using that first vial I had no doubts that this product would become a fixture of eye surgery in the future, cataract surgery in particular. But that's not all. I was also certain that the future of eye surgery would be a combination of phacoemulsification and intraocular lenses with the continuous and systematic use of Healon® or another viscoelastic substance.

A lot of water has gone under the bridge since then and a large amount of viscoelastic substance has been used in operating rooms around the world. The surgical techniques have changed, evolved, and improved, and many of these improvements have come about due to the continuous use of the viscoelastics.

Viscoelastic substances are now truly important realities in eye surgery, and are used by all surgeons in almost all forms of ocular surgery. These substances are now practically considered surgical instruments. These instruments are essential and irreplaceable, and must be used with care, speed and skill.

Until now, no book has been published that covers these products specifically and indepth. We felt that such a book was missing; and so this publication fills a gap in the international scientific literature.

This book explains the physical properties and chemical features of the viscoelastic substances, it illustrates the clinical indications, it offers a complete and organic description of the most recent operating techniques, and gives a precise description of how the various viscoelastic substances should be used.

With the introduction of viscoelastic substances to surgery, a new form of surgery evolved, as well as a new way of looking at surgery. This book will assist in the understanding of the hows, the whys, and the whens of surgery with viscoelastics.

Understanding how a viscoelastic works, its action mechanism, when, how, and where to use it, the ideal quantity, how the procedure should be approached in terms of the tissue, and knowing in advance the effects of the application are just some of the many important things that form the basis for the correct use of viscoelastics, in order to have optimal completion of the surgical operation.

This book provides full coverage of the topic; it is clear, schematic, and simple. Yet despite its simplicity, it contains all the required information in depth.

The presentation is excellent with numerous drawings and illustrations that clearly demonstrate the use of the viscoelastic substances.

This book will be of particular use to surgeons operating in any branch of eye surgery, but is especially recommended for surgeons specializing in the treatment of cataracts. However, this is not to say that it is of lesser importance for surgeons specialized in vitreoretinal, glaucoma, corneal surgery. In other words, it is the perfect professional handbook for eye surgery in general.

And while the book is directed to all surgeons irrespective of age and experience, it will prove to be of particular interest for our younger, less experienced, colleagues who often find themselves operating alone, in the unenviable position of having to choose the most suitable technique (or they may find themselves in difficulties when faced with complicated cases or eyes which return for further corrective treatment).

In my opinion, this book will provide all its readers with a clear, up-to-date overview of the most recent and efficacious techniques for the most modern viscoelastic substances, including the new viscoadaptive Healon®5.

Lucio Buratto, MD

CHAPTER ONE

Usefulness of Viscoelastic Materials

In recent years, viscoelastic materials have become a predominant element in the performance of ocular surgery. With the help of these materials, ophthalmologists have become accustomed to performing difficult maneuvers, particularly in cataract surgery.

In addition, the development of advanced phacoemulsification techniques has allowed physicians to introduce revolutionary achievements such as topical anesthesia, small sutureless incisions, and soft intraocular lenses (IOLs) into clinical practice. These developments have resulted in a higher rate of functional recovery and have allowed patients improved visual function almost immediately. The advent, development, and diversification of viscoelastic materials have made surgical techniques that otherwise may not have been possible a reality.

The variety and diversity of products available to ophthalmic surgeons enables them to choose the products that best meet the surgical requirements of each individual case. Based on our experience, several considerations are important:

- Surgical stress cannot be precisely quantified. Its extent depends on several elements, including the intervention, ability of the surgeon, features peculiar to each ocular tissue (cornea, iris, macula), difficulty of surgical intervention (nuclear cataract with recent onset, senile total cataract with long history), age of the patient, presence of preoperative complications (cornea guttata, pseudoexfoliation, zonular fragility with phacodonesis, glaucoma, synechiae, miosis, pupillary seclusion), and intraoperative complications (uncontrolled margin of the rhexis, capsular breaking, vitreous loss, detachment of Descemet's membrane, reduction of mydriasis).
- "Intentional" surgical stress, although considered necessary, must be controlled and limited. For instance, it is necessary to open the anterior chamber (AC) (self-sealing corneal incision, sclerocorneal incision, or secondary opening) to perform an anterior capsulotomy (eg, continuous, envelope, can-opener), to remove the nucleus and the cortex, achieve sufficient mydriasis in the presence of synechiae, perform endoocular maneuvers, and center and position the IOL. However, intentional surgical stress must be controlled and limited. In fact, the damage occurring to endothelial cells during extracapsular cataract extraction (ECCE) and phacoemulsification is well-documented. The use of a viscoelastic material allows the surgeon to control the intentional surgical stress necessary for each intraocular maneuver.
- "Accidental" surgical stress may depend on unfavorable preoperative conditions or careless intraocular manipulations that influence the recovery of visual function. Advanced anterior segment microsurgical techniques along with suitable viscoelastic materials conceived for this specific use allow physicians to manage and limit most potential intraoperative complications.

Modern cataract microsurgery relies on the use of viscoelastic materials. Viscoelastic materials are indispensable in the prevention of damage to ocular tissues and are also used as multipurpose tools in all surgical phases. Eisner first put forth the important concept that viscoelastic materials can be used to achieve beneficial surface qualities. From a practical point of view, their use ensures integrity of surfaces and ocular tissues that might be damaged by intentional or accidental contact with surgical tools and devices. Viscoelastics also reduce the aggressive action of infusion fluids and ultrasound on corneal endothelial cells.

Through the use of viscoelastic materials, surgeons are able to employ "space tactics" that create a wide intraocular space inside which the surgeon may perform capsulorhexis, phacoemulsification, irrigation and aspiration, capsular bag stretching, IOL implantation, and all intraocular maneuvers.

As far as intraocular surgical practice is concerned, viscosurgery (a term introduced by Balazs) makes it possible to accomplish procedures and maneuvers that require the performance of space tactics and room strategy by means of viscous materials. The aim of the surgeon can be met by employing both the general and particular properties of viscoelastics.

Important facts about viscoelastics include the following:

- Their general features, such as transparency, purity, nontoxicity, and immobility, determine the degree of biocompatibility and safety when the material is injected in the AC.
- Each viscoelastic material has particular chemical–physical and rheologic features (such as molecular weight and structure) that determine viscosity, elasticity, and pseudoplasticity.
- No two viscoelastics are exactly the same. It is up to the surgeon to assess each individual viscoelastic to optimize its use. In early viscosurgery, all surgical maneuvers were accomplished with the application of only one viscoelastic. Nowadays, multiple viscoelastics can be used during the same surgical procedure.
- Viscoelastics must be considered as true surgical tools rather than simple injectable materials. This is why it is important to know their advantages, drawbacks, and limitations as well as criteria for selection (ie, whether during phacoemulsification an adhesive viscoelastic with lower molecular weight that is more difficult to remove is preferable to a cohesive viscoelastic that is easier to remove and has greater elasticity and pseudoplasticity than the former; which is the most suitable viscoelastic in the presence of a capsular break with or without vitreous loss; and which viscoelastic is best suited for capsular filling in soft IOL implantation).
- The ideal viscoelastic is not yet available. Although it is possible to perform phacoemulsification with only one material, during some phases it would be preferable to use viscoelastics with different qualities more suitable to that specific procedure. For instance, an easily removable viscoelastic is likely to be aspirated or extruded through the AC during fluid infusion, but, if it is a highly pseudoplastic material with high molecular weight, it can be placed precisely and in such an amount that it can be used as a "spatula." If not removed, the viscoelastic will cause severe postoperative intraocular hypertension.
- Viscoelastics currently on the market meet important biocompatibility requirements. Experimental in vivo and in vitro studies continue to disclose new and important properties in addition to already known features.

Chemical, Physical, and Rheologic Features of Viscoelastics

The roles of physical properties such as viscosity, elasticity, adhesiveness, cohesiveness, and pseudoplasticity are fundamental and intrinsic to the effectiveness of the viscoelastic and its ability to create space; separate or stabilize tissues; tamponade fluid leakage from the AC; stop bleeding; and protect endothelial cells from ultrasonic energy, infusion fluid turbulence, and accidental impact with the surface of surgical tools or IOLs. These same qualities may lead the viscoelastic to cause elevated intraocular pressure (IOP) when not removed.

It is up to the surgeon to choose, based on knowledge and experience, which viscoelastic materials should be used in each particular case to achieve the desired outcome. For instance, to ensure hydrodynamic stability of the AC one may choose a highly viscous material with high molecular weight in order to counterbalance the forces extruding the material from the intraocular space. In that case, to employ the highest viscosity from the material, one must exploit the hydrodynamic volume of the nondeformed molecular mass. If extruding forces are pushing, higher molecular weight products (Healon® GV; Pharmacia & Upjohn, Stockholm, Sweden) can be used to attain a stable space. Owing to its weight and high viscosity, the volume of viscoelastic occupying the AC effectively opposes the forces acting to eject it out of the AC. Conversely, if extruding forces are due to turbulence of the irrigation flow during phacoemulsification, a more stable space is achieved with the injection of a more adhesive viscoelastic, such as Viscoat (Alcon; Fort Worth, TX), which has lower viscosity and molecular weight than Healon® GV. Should it be necessary to mobilize tissues, it is better to inject a more fluid, more elastic, and less viscous viscoelastic to achieve "viscomanipulation" without immobilization (ie, Healon®, Provisc [Alcon; Fort Worth, TX], Biolon [Sifi; Lavinaio, Italy]). Highly viscous and elastic viscoelastic materials with very high molecular weight enable physicians to control IOL unfolding inside the capsular bag by counterbalancing the energy emitted by IOL unfolding, with its great elasticity.

The examples mentioned highlight the complexity of rheologic properties of viscoelastics and require the surgeon to acquire a thorough knowledge of viscoelastics to make a correct and safe choice.

The biochemistry of viscoelastics is strictly correlated with safe surgical use. Chemical features form the basis of viscoelastics' optical properties (ie, transparency); their ability to form molecular bonds with ocular tissues; and their ability to act as inert materials that have been purified and are therefore free of particles, nontoxic, apyrogenic, and unable to evoke inflammatory or immunogenic response. The ideal viscoelastic material must have the same osmolality and colloidal osmotic pressure as the cornea and the aqueous humor. Furthermore, viscoelastic materials must be water soluble and removable through biologic means. These chemical aspects determine the basic biocompatibility features of viscoelastics for intraocular use. Rheology, elasticity, and adhesiveness are the result of interactions between the molecular chains of a material that must behave as a viscous fluid and an elastic solid simultaneously.

Chapter Two

Viscoelastic Materials

The use of viscoelastic materials in ocular microsurgery started many years ago. In 1934, Meyer and Palmer were able to isolate hyaluronic acid in the vitreous cortex. In 1958, Balazs was the first to suggest using hyaluronic acid as a possible vitreous substitute in the performance of complicated retinal detachment surgery. In 1972, he accomplished the first intravitreous injection of hyaluronic acid. During a 1979 ocular surgery video symposium held in Cannes, he presented the patent of a viscoelastic material with high molecular weight made of purified hyaluronic acid (Healon®) for use in IOL implantation surgery. Sodium hyaluronate was used in 1977 by Miller to perform experimental IOL implantation in rabbit eyes. In the same year, Fechner used a 1% solution of methylcellulose to maintain the volume of the AC. The technique was to be perfected in the following years, making use of a 2% solution.

The increasing success achieved by viscoelastics in the following years revolutionized ophthalmic surgery. These materials enabled the surgeon to operate in much shorter periods of time. The advantages of such advances are numerous. Viscoelastic materials increase the number of viscosurgery techniques (ie, capsulorhexis, viscoexpression), enhance cataract surgery techniques (ie, senile, congenital, traumatic cataract), and prevent and manage several complications (ie, posterior capsule break, vitreous tamponade). The effectiveness of viscoelastics instigated the passage from ECCE to modern phacoemulsification. Based on this progress, viscoelastic materials also influenced implantation techniques for placing rigid and soft IOLs with small diameters. However, viscosurgery procedures are not limited to cataract surgery. Techniques in viscosurgery have proved indispensable in routinely performed antiglaucomatous filtering surgery, combined surgery, keratoplasty, and anterior vitrectomy.

Viscoelastics are a composite group of surgical tools with chemical, physical, and rheologic features (ie, viscosity, rigidity, elasticity, pseudoplasticity, cohesiveness) that act individually but with a synergistic effect and therefore could be compared with many hand-held tools of the surgeon. The surgeon can use just one of the various functions of viscoelastics as an effective means to separate and join tissues; maintain spaces and divide intraocular structures; and protect ocular surfaces (ie, corneal endothelium, lens capsule, anterior hyaloid) from mechanical shocks and infusion fluids through the effect of chemical bonds on the viscoelastic's surface. The versatility and effectiveness of viscoelastics result in safer ophthalmic surgery.

Over the years, viscoelastics have replaced gas (air) and balanced saline solution (BSS), which provided poor tissue protection and had limited effectiveness in space maintenance. Hyaluronic acid was the first viscoelastic on the market, launched by Pharmacia & Upjohn in 1980 with the trade name Healon®. Its chemical features of viscosity and plasticity should be considered a main reference when comparing more recent molecules.

Relevant Data From the Literature

Hyaluronic acid (Healon®) is the most widely used viscoelastic in operating rooms. It has been compared with other products and studied and assessed in over 400 medical and scientific publications.

Direct comparison of viscoelastic materials is often difficult owing to the lack of uniform and superimposable rheologic data.

The production (homologation) as well as the use of viscoelastics requires nonstop research on biocompatibility, purity, and actual ability to protect the corneal endothelium.

In vivo studies enable the refinement of chemical molecular structures to prevent the viscoelastic from hindering aqueous outflow. A great deal of attention is paid to the interaction of the products' molecules with tissue receptors to ensure the absence of immunogenic and inflammatory reactions trigged by the viscoelastic.

SODIUM HYALURONATE

This polysaccharide molecule of sodium glycuronate and N-acetyl glucosamine contains neither amino acids nor other carbohydrates, but each subunit presents a single negative charge that ensures neutralization of the positive charges normally present on ocular tissues, instruments, and IOL surfaces. Its molecular weight may range from 500,000 to 6 million daltons. It consists of nearly 10,000 disaccharide units. The mean diameter of the molecular chain is 10 mm. The chains forming sodium hyaluronate do not touch one another and small molecules may be present inside the chain molecular structure. Large molecules such as fibrinogen, proteoglycans, and collagen cannot penetrate it.

WHAT IS KNOWN ABOUT SODIUM HYALURONATE?

- High concentrations are present in connective tissue (synovial fluid) as well as in the eye (vitreous cortex, trabeculum). The concentration is low in the aqueous humor and on the corneal endothelial surface. It is also extracted from other sources, such as the umbilical cord, bovine vitreous, and cockscomb.
- In muscles and the skeleton, sodium hyaluronate acts as a lubricant and is involved in shock-absorbing mechanisms.
- Sodium hyaluronate has a function in the wound repair processes as it does not interfere with the movement of fibroblasts and epithelial cells.
- Sodium hyaluronate is produced by plastic membranes and then released in the extracellular matrix.
- Sodium hyaluronate influences interaction and growth of cells as well as their mobility. In vitro it has been shown to inhibit the growth and release of prostaglandins by macrophages during phagocytosis processes.
- In vivo studies have produced evidence of the presence of receptors on corneal endothelium (hyaluronic acid binding sites) in humans, rats, monkeys, and rabbits.

The use of hyaluronic acid (Healon®) in the performance of ocular surgery is by no means the introduction of a foreign material with antigenic ability, because it is a natural component commonly present in human tissues.

In fluids, particularly in the aqueous humor, hyaluronic acid usually takes up a large hydrodynamic volume owing to its winding structure. It is compact but not preordained, which gives it a peculiar "spongy" feature.

The double-helix architecture structuring the arrangement of chains is the basis of the molecule's viscoelasticity and pseudoplasticity. In high concentrations, the molecule organizes its constituent chains in a complicated tridimensional arrangement. Therefore, the viscosity of a material is linked to the sodium hyaluronate concentration (a fivefold increase in concentration means a thousandfold greater viscosity) and its molecular weight (length of the molecular chain). In the specific case of Healon®, it has been observed that elasticity is a more predominant aspect than viscosity. This is evident in the low concentration and flow. In practice, it can be easily injected through a 30-gauge (G) cannula and, after passing through the needle, is able to recover high viscosity and its original shape.

Its chemical structure does not differ with the source; however, the molecular weight changes according to the origin of the material. Early production of sodium hyaluronate was extremely problematic. The main difficulty was in obtaining a material with satisfactory purity and high molecular weight. Furthermore, the first hyaluronic acid solutions trigged severe inflammatory processes in the vitreous, which occurred a few days after injection due to an endotoxic and nonimmunogenic process. Impurities in the material were thought to be the cause of this reaction.

Modern production of a pure, biocompatible sodium hyaluronate preparation free from foreign bodies that can cause inflammatory response and with high molecular weight and optimal concentration is rather expensive. The inflammatory potential of Healon® is tested in each parcel of the material by studies on monkey eyes (owl monkey eye test).

Hyaluronic acid is produced by using a variety of different sources. For instance, Healon® and Healon® GV are made with cockscomb-derived hyaluronic acid, which is sterilized directly in vials. Other companies manufacture viscoelastic materials such as IAL (Fidia Oftal) and Vitrax (Allergan, Irvine, Calif) using the same source, but a different sterilization process. Other production chains, such as Provisc, Biolon, and Amvisc Plus, are based on bacterial fermentation of streptococci cultures. This process uses tissue cultures that can be obtained through continuous or en block fermentation. In the latter, cells are at different stages of their life cycle and, therefore, present different metabolic conditions that determine both the production and destruction of part of the hyaluronic acid. This causes a rapid turnover of cellular walls containing undesired materials such as lipoproteic acids. Conversely, continuous fermentation minimizes cell degradation and favors the production of substances with different molecular weight while changing the conditions of growth in bacterial cultures.

Once injected in the AC, hyaluronic acid is removed following the aqueous humor pathway through the natural transtrabecular outflow. Studies performed on guinea pigs by a group of medical biochemistry researchers from the Biomedical Center of Uppsala in Sweden, in collaboration with Pharmacia & Upjohn, demonstrated that sodium hyaluronate, suitably dyed with radioactive means, is not metabolized in ocular tissues but in the liver (>90%), spleen, and marrow, where significant tropism was evident involving lymph cells.

HYDROXYPROPYLMETHYLCELLULOSE

In 1977, Fechner introduced methylcellulose 1% solution, which was later increased to 2%. Originally employed for its ability to cover and lubricate with low surface tension, this material is now used more for its viscoadhesiveness than for its viscoelasticity because it is not likely to show particular elasticity. Therefore, it requires a larger cannular diameter and higher pressure for injection than Healon®.

Methylcellulose, from which hydroxypropylmethylcellulose (HPMC) is derived, is commonly used as a lubricating material (Methocel) during diagnostic lens application and as an additive in foods. Unlike hyaluronic acid, HPMC is not a material present in the human or animal body, but is a component of vegetal fibers such as cotton and wood. It is a polymer of cellulose (methylcellulose) whose chemical base is a D-glucose molecule chain linked with B-glycosidic bonds. It is produced by extracting cellulose paste that is processed first by sodium hydroxide to obtain alkaline cellulose and then by methylic radicals. The addition of hydroxypropyl groups in lateral chains increases the hydrophilic factor of the material. The large dimensions of the chains result in its poor ability to rotate around the central axis. The molecule also has a certain rigidity which in a solution means poorer elasticity and ability to absorb shocks.

HPMC is produced at 2% concentration by Storz ophthalmics (Occucoat), Ciba in Marcon, Italy (Hymecel), and Adatomed by Chiron Vision Corporation in Claremont, Calif (Adatocel). Manufactured by Vision Biology, Cellugel is a 2.2% solution of modified HPMC.

OCCUCOAT

Occucoat is the first material produced with a high-purified molecule that is biocompatible with ocular tissues. In particular, it develops a small contact angle and less superficial tension with the polymethylmethacrylate (PMMA) surface of IOLs. However, owing to its low molecular weight (86,000 d) and poor viscosity (4,000 cps) it does not provide sufficient pseudoplasticity, and exhibits:

- poor ability to maintain the AC in the presence of high vitreous pressure
- difficult removal
- good coatability of surfaces in tissues, instruments, and IOLs owing to viscoadherence
- reduced transparency
- storage at room temperature and availability
- possible autoclave sterilization
- low cost

CHONDROITIN SULFATE

Chondroitin sulfate is the main polysaccharide component of cartilaginous connective tissues. In the eye, it is present in the cornea. Similar to hyaluronic acid, it can also be found in the extracellular matrix of humans. It is contained in other connective tissues such as vitreous and syovial fluid. The main source of chondroitin sulfate is shark fin cartilage. In nature, it is not present as a free material, but in the form of a protein–polysaccharide molecule component, ie, proteoglycan.

Chondroitin sulfate and hyaluronic acid have similar chemical structures and comparable physical properties. Both are composed of disaccharide units. More precisely, they share a glycuronic acid molecule, which in chondroitin sulfate is bound to N-acetyl-galactosamine, whereas in hyaluronic acid it is bound to N-acetyl-glucosamine. Contrary to hyaluronic acid, chondroitin sulfate has a sulfate group on its molecular chain and a double negative charge that permits it to neutralize the positive charges normally present on ocular tissues and surgical instruments. This chemical characteristic also results in better coatability.

In the literature there are several examples of chondroitin sulfate used in solutions with different concentrations. Some characteristics are listed in the following.

Characteristics of Chondroitin Sulfate in Solutions With Different Concentrations

Molecular weight about 20,000 d with a molecular chain length of 50 nm is small in comparison to the length of the hyaluronic acid molecule (Healon®: 10,000 nm).

In 20% solution, chondroitin sulfate shows good coatability, but low viscosity rate ineffective to maintain space or separate tissues. In 50% solution, chondroitin sulfate has a higher viscosity rate, but possesses hyperosmolality that causes endothelial dehydration and cell loss.

Viscoat

Viscoat is a viscoelastic with a mixture of 4% chondroitin sulfate and 3% hyaluronic acid (1:3 ratio). The sodium hyaluronate used in this preparation is derived from bacterial fermentation. This combination of two similar polymers results in a compound with 600,000 d molecular weight and average high viscosity of 50,000 cps.

The characteristics of Viscoat provide sufficient space maintenance and proper viscomanipulation of tissues, good injectability, good coatability on the corneal endothelium as a consequence of the negative charge present on molecular surface, increased protection from vibrations during phacoemulsification, decreased transparency due to uneven interface between Viscoat and the aqueous humor, and greater adhesion to surfaces that results in less cohesiveness of the molecule when aspirating Viscoat, which is removed en bloc.

Polyacrylamide

Polyacrylamide is a synthetic polymer with a high molecular weight. It is derived from acrylamide, which consists of carbon organized like fatty acid, carotenoids, and natural rubber.

As a single element, acrylamide monomer is toxic, whereas when it is added to a long chain with a polymerization process it has evidenced physiologic features compatible with intraocular application. In aqueous solution, it behaves like hydrophilic gel, with high molecular weight (1,000,000 d), high viscosity (40,000 cps), and good coatability. It also produces a smaller contact angle on surfaces.

Manufactured by Optical Radiation Corporation, Orcolon consists of this macromolecule and has shown good elasticity and pseudoplasticity. It is stored at room temperature and can be easily injected through a 27-G cannula. After injection in the AC, it remains in the aqueous humor for several hours and is completely metabolized in the spleen and liver after some weeks.

Although it has been tested and approved by many studies as a safe viscoelastic, it was withdrawn from the market in 1991 after contamination inside the syringe due to insoluble microgels, which triggered intraocular pressure (IOP) elevation and uveitis in the 15,000 patients treated with this material.

Collagene

Collagene is a viscoelastic material consisting of Type IV collagen that is extracted from human placenta. Unlike Types I, II, or III, Type IV collagen contains no fibrils. Manufactured by DomiLens under Chiron Vison Corp. in Claremont, California with the trade name Collagel at 1.4% concentration, it has a molecular weight exceeding 2,000,000 d and viscosity equal to 500,000 cps at low shear rate.

Some scientists (including Arshinoff) have pointed out that rheologic properties of Collagel change significantly with temperature. In particular, a remarkable decrease in viscosity has been observed when the temperature is raised from 25 to 37 °C. Along with the advantages of this highly elastic and rigid material, its extreme sensitivity to temperature and drop in viscosity and elasticity due to increasing shear rate must also be considered. Furthermore, some studies reported instances of turbidity caused by material that came into contact with BSS.

Collagel has been withdrawn from the market as a consequence of the increasing concern about human immunodeficiency virus (HIV) transmission with products derived from human tissues.

CHAPTER THREE

Rheologic and Physical Properties

The laws regulating the behavior of a viscoelastic at rest and while flowing must be considered as the basis of modern viscosurgery, as different materials have rheologic features that are suitable for specific tasks and applications.

VISCOSITY

Viscosity is the resistance encountered by the particles of a body while sliding with respect to one another (internal friction) that is evident in the occurrence of more or less superficial tensions according to the nature of the body.

Dynamic viscosity, normally indicated with n (absolute viscosity), is the relationship between any one of the tangent efforts caused by the internal friction of a material and the corresponding flow speed. n Is measured in poise, which is equal to 1 dyne/sec/cmq. The coefficient is 1 poise when the force that should be applied to 1 cmq of fluid stratum to make it move at the constant speed of 1 cm/sec with respect to another parallel stratum lying at 1 cm is equal to 1 dyne.

Viscoelastic materials consist of water particles and therefore abide by the same laws; furthermore, their viscosity changes with temperature.

The viscosity of a material also changes according to the speed flow gradient (shear rate) of the material itself. This is the measurement of speed at which two planes shift with respect to one another, measured in reciprocal seconds (Figure 3-1).

The strength of movement per surface unit necessary to provoke shifting between two planes of a material is called shear stress and is measured in dynes/cmq.

FACTS ABOUT VISCOELASTICS

- Fluids that maintain the same viscosity despite variations of shear rate (ie, with maximum and minimum values of shear rate) are called Newtonian fluids (ie, air, BSS and chondroitin sulfate).
- Fluids that change viscosity with different flow rates are called non–Newtonian fluids. In particular, viscosity decreases according to the increase in shifting speed (ie, high shear rate values). This is when a viscoelastic material loses its viscosity to become more fluid (Figure 3-2).

The viscosity of a material depends on molecular weight (molecular chain length, size of the molecule); concentration of the material; temperature; and solvent used in water solution. A viscoelastic material with high molecular weight due to a long molecular chain shows high viscosity at 0 shear rate (maximum viscosity) while at rest (Figure 3-3). This property of viscoelastics enables the surgeon to create and maintain wide, stable spaces in proportion to the weight and viscosity of the material in question.

The minimum viscosity of high molecular weight material is reached at high shear rate values. The movement of the viscoelastic during injection in the AC depends on the concentration of the material itself and determines the limit of injectability through a cannula (Figure 3-4).

High viscosity rate values can be reached by starting with a molecule with average molecular weight (1 million daltons) and then increasing the material in question by 4% (40 mg/mL). However, a viscoelastic with this concentration cannot be used because it would provide too high of a colloidal–osmotic pressure (Figure 3-5).

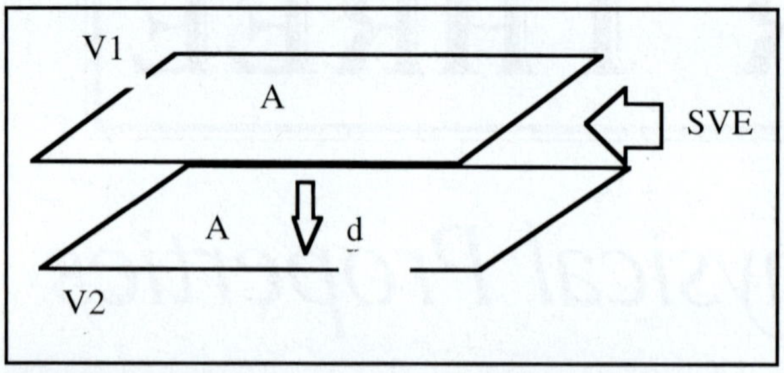

Figure 3-1. The concept of shear rate. Two parallel planes with the same area (A) are separated by a certain distance (d) and move in the same direction at different speeds. The speed gradient is the measure of speed that the planes move with respect to one another and is defined in reciprocal seconds. The force per area unit required to produce the shearing action is defined as shear rate stress and its measure unit is the dyne. Viscosity (poise) = shear stress/shear rate.

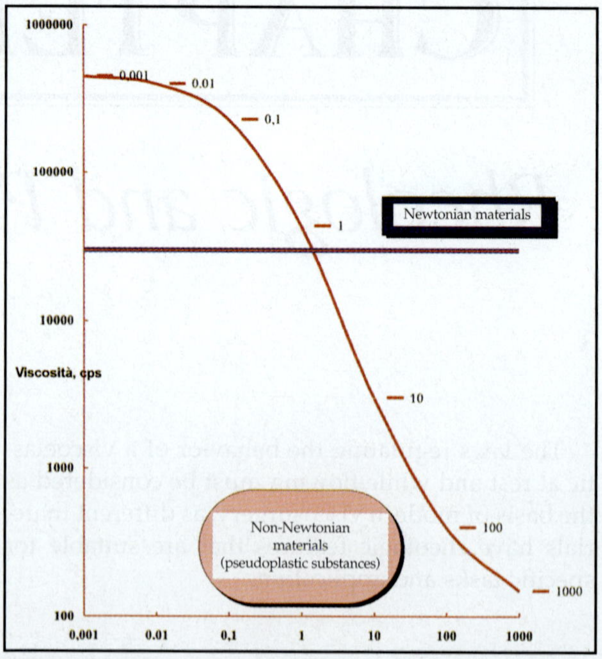

Figure 3-2. Pseudoplastic solutions. Non-Newtonian materials have a viscosity that decreases as shear rate increases. A stiff curve indicates pseudoplasticity. Conversely, Newtonian materials such as water have a constant viscosity.

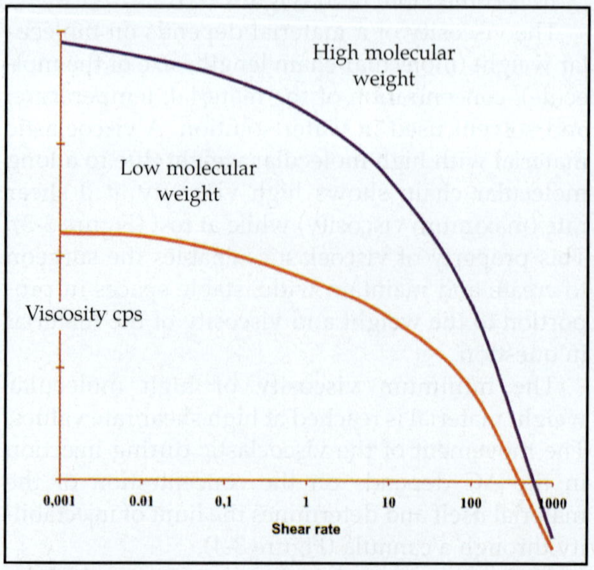

Figure 3-3. The curves represent two materials at the same concentration with different molecular weights. Maximum viscosity, at low shear rate, depends on the shape and length of molecular chains (molecular weight). Minimum viscosity depends on the molecular concentration of the solution (high shear rate value).

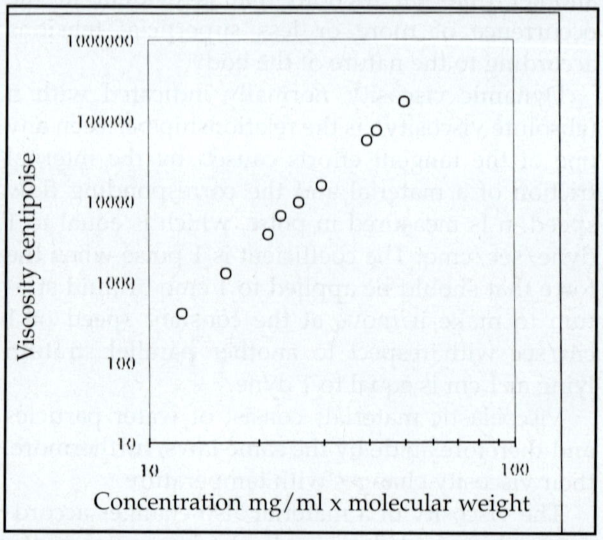

Figure 3-4. The viscosity of hyaluronic acid at 0 shear rate is a function of the material's concentration multiplied by its molecular weight (x axis). The caption shows how viscosity increases with increased concentration and molecular weight.

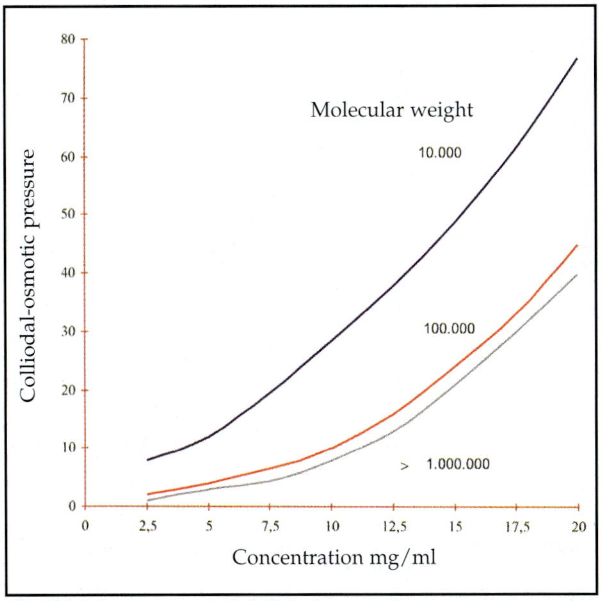

Figure 3-5. Colloidal–osmotic pressure of hyaluronate solutions is a function of the concentration and molecular weight. The pressure rapidly rises when the concentration increases, but becomes independent of the molecular weight at high weights (greater than 100,000). For intraocular applications, hyaluronate must have a concentration equal to at least 10 mg/mL.

If one increases the viscosity of a material by increasing the length of the macromolecular chain, one has a higher maximum viscosity without affecting concentration and injectability, depending on minimum viscosity.

Maximum viscosity of a material at 0 shear rate determines its stabilizing effect. Medium viscosity at medium shear rate produces the mobilizing effect. The least viscosity at high shear rate measures the ease of injection of the material (Figure 3-6).

PSEUDOPLASTICITY

The viscosity of a viscoelastic is a function of its shear rate. In other words, shifting ability, which depends on internal friction, is determined by a reduction of viscosity as a consequence of deformation of molecular chains.

When the flow rate of a material is high its viscosity is lowest. Pseudoplasticity is the ability of a material to pass from a situation of high viscosity and stiffness, prior to being injected, to a fluid state with low viscosity during which internal frictions decrease and the material flows.

This is a basic feature of polysaccharide molecules (Healon® GV, Healon®, Amvisc, Provisc) in that it determines the ability of these materials to keep space and be injected. With a shear rate increase the polysaccharide chains line up following the direction of the flow and viscosity decreases. This phenomenon occurs not only while the material is passing through a cannula, but also during movements of surgical instruments inside the viscoelastic solution (Figure 3-7).

In a Cartesian plane, where the abscissa depicts the degree of shear rate (reciprocal seconds) and ordinate viscosity values are expressed in poises, the curve of pseudoplasticity is inclined according to the dynamic behavior of viscosity with flow change. The steeper the curve, the more material flows and thus the decrease in viscosity is greater (Figure 3-8). Although a steep curve indicates easy flowing of the viscoelastic through a cannula, it also permits maneuvers such as irrigation and phacoemulsification to thrust the material out of the AC. This applies in the cases of Healon® GV, Healon®, IAL-F, IAL, Provisc, Biolon, and Amvisc. Viscoelastics (Viscoat, Vitrax, Occucoat) with a less steep pseudoplasticity curve are less likely to flow and, therefore, require a larger cannular lumen for injection; however, they effectively maintain contact with the aqueous and tissues during turbulence owing to surgical maneuvers.

Based on our experience and that of our colleagues, we have concluded that Healon® GV, Healon®, Biolon, Provisc, and Amvisc can be injected through a 30-G cannula, whereas Viscoat requires a 27-G cannula and HPMC (Occucoat) needs a 25 to 23-G cannula. It is more difficult to start and maintain injection with HPMC than it is with other viscoelastics.

Pseudoplasticity is a mandatory feature of viscoelastic materials. The different viscosities a material may reach while changing its rheologic state from viscous to fluid enable the surgeon to perform several intraocular maneuvers. Taking into account the viscosurgical tactics mentioned by Eisner in Tactics of Surface, Space and Tissues, it is evident that to keep a stable hydrodynamic space in the AC, the viscoelastic must be either viscous enough or

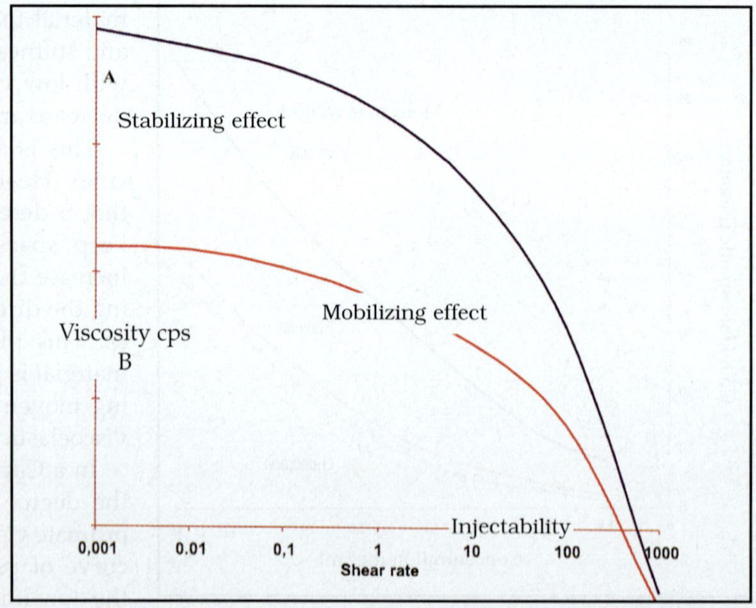

Figure 3-6. The maximum viscosity of two materials determines their stabilizing effect at low shear rate (top). Mean viscosity at mean shear rate value determines their mobilizing effect (middle). Minimum viscosity at high shear rate defines the limit of injectability through a cannula (bottom). Compared with material B, material A has a mobilizing spatula effect. Both show the same inject-ability.

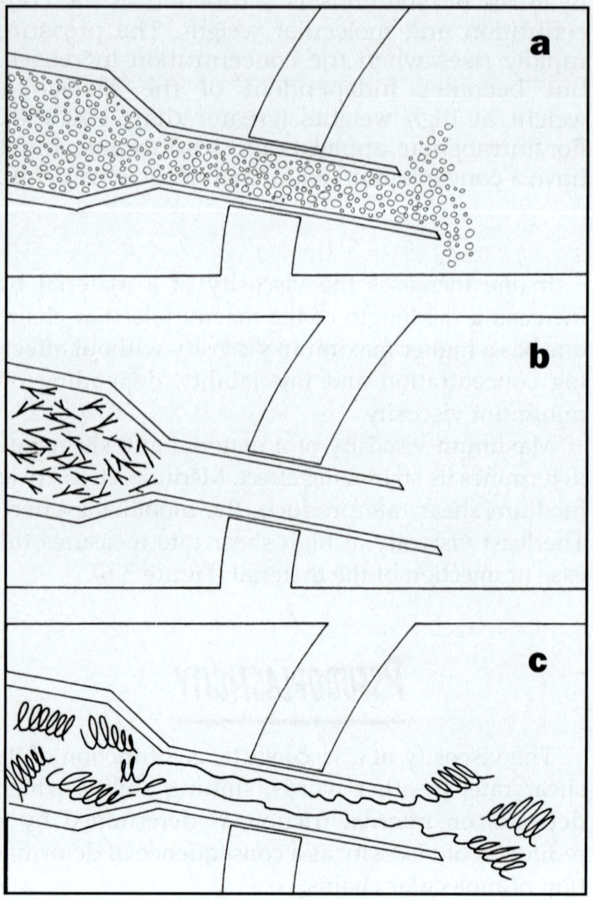

Figure 3-7. Behavior of aqueous (a), viscous (b), and viscoelastic materials. (a) When the lumen of the cannula becomes narrow, the molecules accelerate because the same amount of fluid passes through the cannula in the same amount of time. (b) The relationship between viscosity and lumen caliber may enable or prevent the passage of the viscous material. (c) Molecular chains deform while passing inside the cannula to resume their prior shape when a greater space is available.

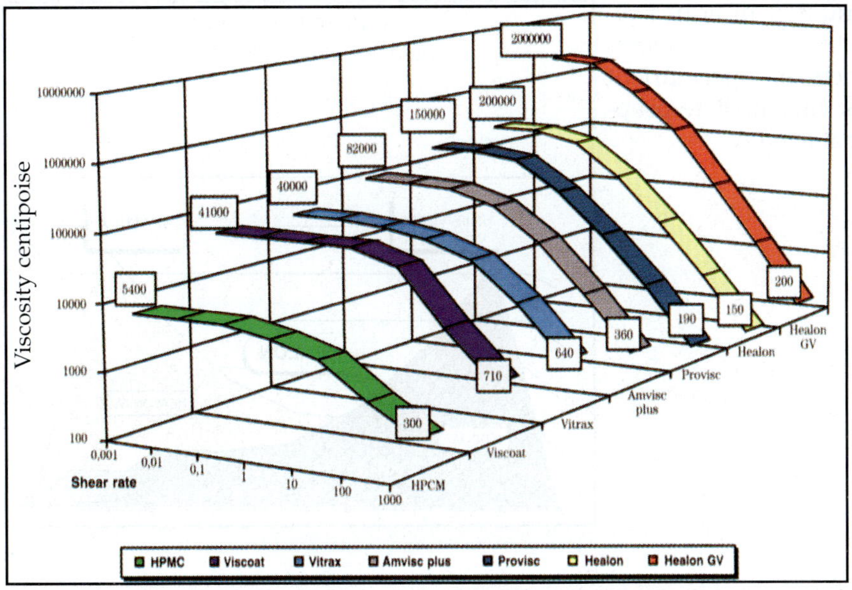

Figure 3-8. Comparison of viscosity curves of viscoelastic materials with changing shear rates.

suitably adherent to oppose the forces that tend to expel it out of the AC (vitreous pressures, infusion fluids). There is no easily injectable viscous material that is able to oppose such forces totally. Materials with elevated coatability such as Viscoat, Vitrax, and methylcellulose, which tend to be more adherent, are able to fulfill such requirements efficiently. Viscoelastics with high molecular weight can counterbalance these forces, but not as well as the aforementioned materials.

Currently, the surgeon can choose a viscoelastic compound with high molecular weight or one with lower molecular weight but greater adhesiveness at high or medium viscosity which at zero flow rate sufficiently opposes the tendency to come out of the AC in the course of viscomanipulations and fluid infusion. As soon as it is injected, it is able to act like a permanent spatula, to immobilize tissues. Simultaneously, the materials with intermediate flow values must show a decrease in viscosity along with an increase of fluidity to enable the operator to accomplish manipulation of tissues (soft or gentle spatula) (Figure 3-9).

Table 3-1 provides a comparison of values referred to viscosity and pseudoplasticity of the main viscoelastics.

ELASTICITY

Elasticity is the tendency of a given viscoelastic to recover its original shape after being compressed or deformed (Figure 3-10).

Long molecular chain molecules (Healon®, Healon® GV, Provisc, Biolon) are more elastic than those with short molecular chains. The mechanical energy applied at low frequency (slow impact) produces irradiation of macromolecules, which slide onto one another, thus determining a viscous movement. This phenomenon is observed during folded soft IOL unfolding.

If a fast impact is applied (high frequency), the chains deform and the mechanical energy is transformed into elasticity. Later, they regain their original shape. An increase in viscosity of a viscoelastic produces an increase in elastic features with a tendency to restore the original volume after deformation (Figure 3-11).

Viscoelasticity is a fundamental characteristic, as it ensures protection from both the energy produced by vibrations during phacoemulsification (high frequency energy) and turbulence caused by irrigation and aspiration. Elasticity and pseudoplasticity are not synonymous, but both features demonstrate how easily a molecule can deform and rearrange its own structure. Elasticity comes into

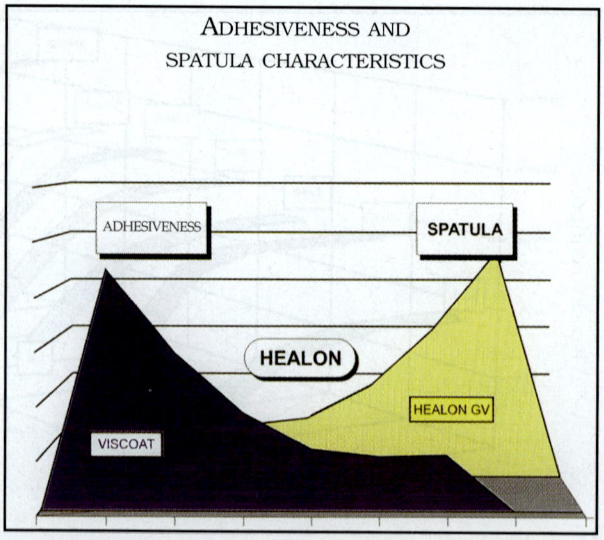

Figure 3-9. Graphic representation of adhesiveness and spatula characteristics. Viscoat shows high adhesiveness. Healon® acts as a permanent and soft spatula. Healon® has intermediate properties between Viscoat and Healon® GV.

Table 3-1.

VISCOSITY AND PSEUDOPLASTICITY OF THE SAME VES

Viscoelastic	Viscosity at 0 Shear Rate (V0)	Viscosity at 1000 Shear Rate 2/sec - 25C°	Viscosity at 1000 Shear Rate (V1000)	Index of Pseudoplasticity V0/V1000
Healon®	>200,000	40,000 - 64,000	150	>1,333
Healon® GV	2,000,00	80,000	200	10,000
Amvisc	100,000	40,000 - 42,000	150	909
Amvisc Plus	102,000	55,000	250	410
Viscoat	41,000	40,000	200	210
Orcolon	35,000	40,000	350	100
Collagel	>2,000,000	n/a	200	>10,000
Occucoat (HPMC)	5,400	4,000	240	23
Vitrax	40,000	n/a	1000	40

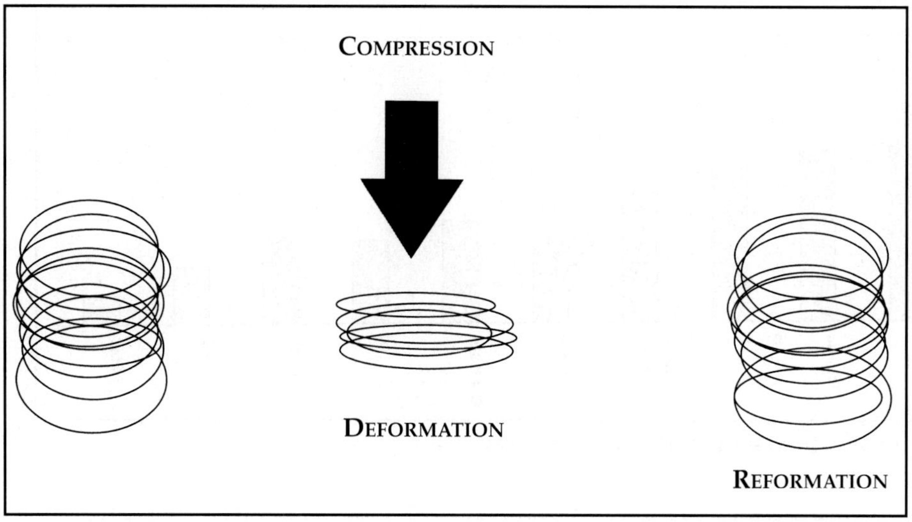

Figure 3-10. The molecule with elasticity gets deformed when stressed by a compression force. It regains its original shape once the compression force has stopped.

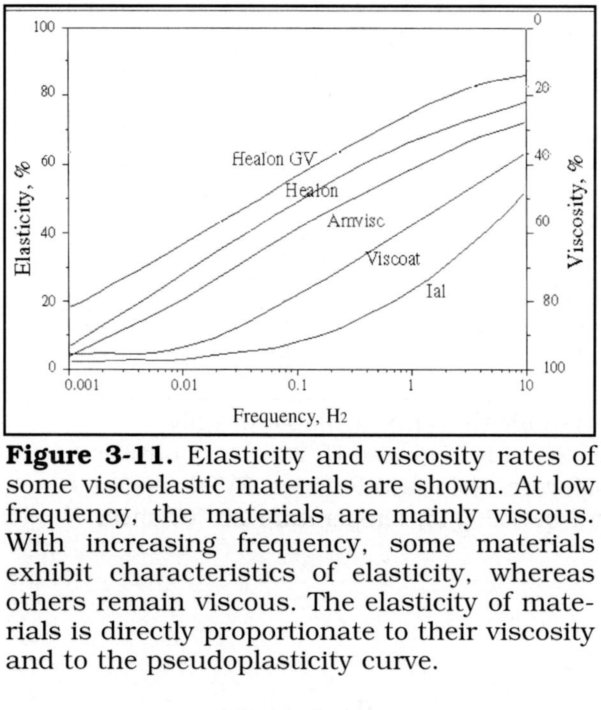

Figure 3-11. Elasticity and viscosity rates of some viscoelastic materials are shown. At low frequency, the materials are mainly viscous. With increasing frequency, some materials exhibit characteristics of elasticity, whereas others remain viscous. The elasticity of materials is directly proportionate to their viscosity and to the pseudoplasticity curve.

play when the viscoelastic material is shifted owing to the effect of surgical maneuvers performed inside it. Pseudoplasticity indicates the ease of deformation in the flow while the material is injected though a cannula. Viscoelasticity, however, must not exceed the viscosity of the material at given shear rate values in the course of surgical procedures (Arshinoff). In fact, if the surgeon uses a highly elastic viscoelastic, it could counterbalance the movements on ocular tissues, acting like a spring that repels the maneuvers accomplished by the surgeon while performing capsulorhexis. For instance, the highly elastic viscoelastic could provoke rolling up of the AC flap.

In Figure 3-12a, we list various viscoelastic materials, ranging from the highest to the lowest elasticity. It should be noted that the order corresponds mostly to the pseudoplastic capacity of the products. Hence, we conclude that both elasticity and pseudoplasticity are dependent on the type of polymer and the length of the molecular chain.

In Figure 3-12b, we assessed some viscoelastic materials based on crossover frequency. High crossover frequency means low elasticity. Crossover frequency is strongly bound to molecular weight. The most elastic product is demonstrated to be Healon® GV (with low crossover frequency); the least elastic material is HPMC (Occucoat) (with high crossover frequency).

COHESIVENESS

Cohesiveness is the extent to which a material can adhere to itself. It is a function of molecular weight and elasticity.

Cohesiveness is proportional to viscosity at zero shear rate. Viscoelastics consisting of long molecules with high molecular weight tend to have high internal cohesiveness and therefore can be easily aspirated and leave the eye en masse.

The materials showing this feature are made of hyaluronic acid with high or very high molecular

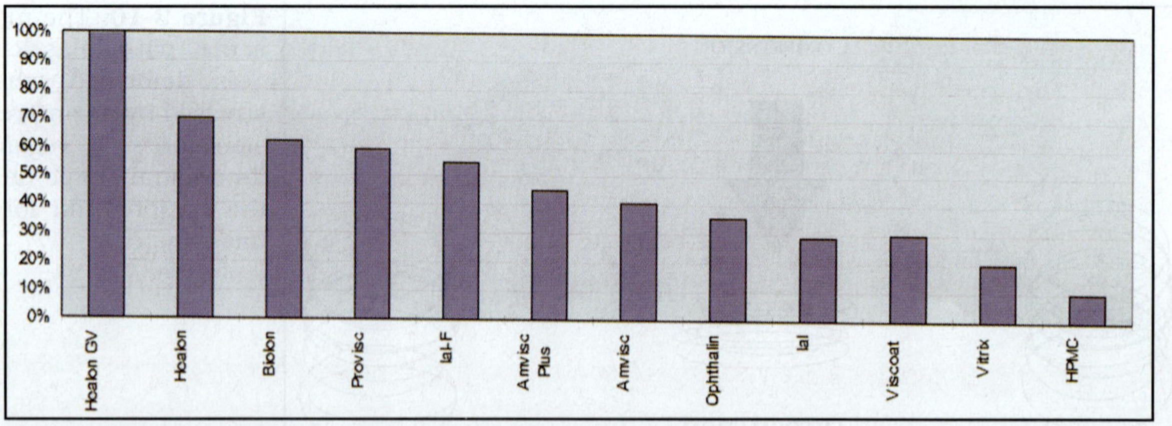

Figure 3-12a. Elasticity of the viscoelastic substances.

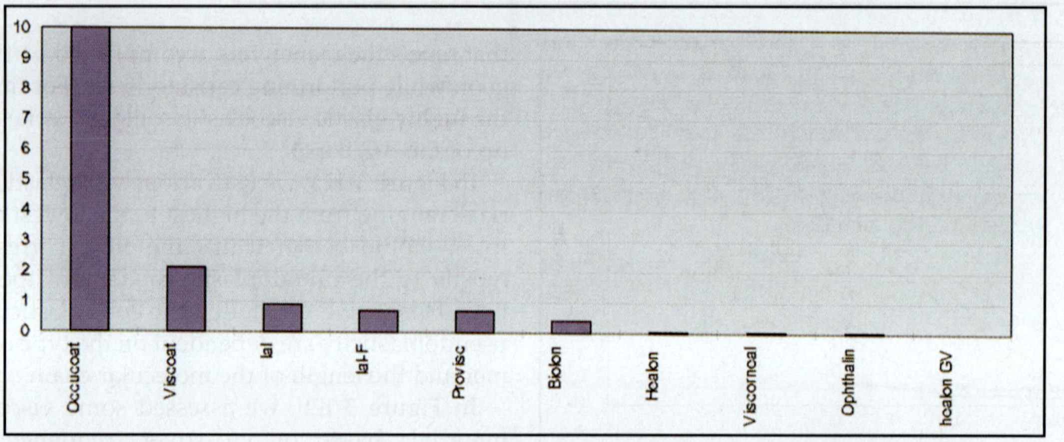

Figure 3-12b. Crossover frequency (Hz-G'+G") for the VES available in Italy. Haake viscosity meter. Measurement head CV20 with Rotovisco RV20; rheocontroller RC20 interface; IBM 750 P-133 computer (software: Rotovisco Rotation RV20 version 2.4). Oscillatory measurements: measurement device Q45, temperature 20 °C, shear rate 0 to 10 Hz.

weight (ie, Healon® GV, Healon®, Biolon, Provisc). On the contrary, materials with short molecular chains and low molecular weight are less cohesive, as they tend to fragment in several parts. This causes them to be more difficult to aspirate (as is the case with Viscoat, HPMC 2%, and Vitrax).

Although the internal cohesiveness of a material is an advantage (for instance, in space maintenance), the material tends to remain inside the eye longer and its mass may cause blockage of the filtering trabeculum. This explains postoperative IOP elevation when too much material is left in the AC.

COATABILITY

Coatability defines the ability of various viscoelastics to adhere to the surface of tissues, instruments, and IOLs.

Coatability or wettability can be measured by assessing surface tension and contact angle; it is the angle formed by the interface of a viscoelastic drop and a plane surface (Figure 3-13). Low superficial tension combined with a very small angle indicates that a viscoelastic material adheres well to a given surface.

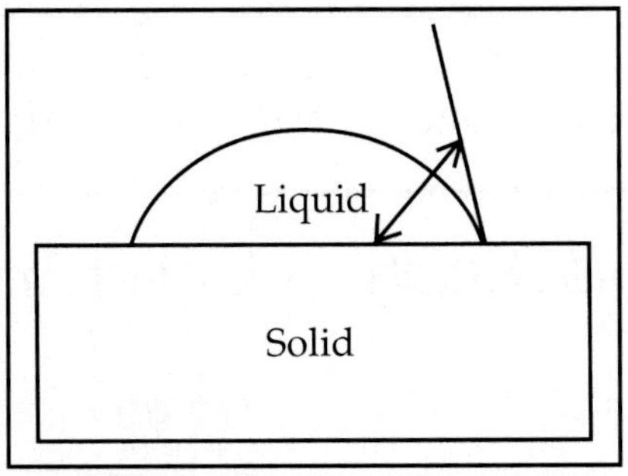

Figure 3-13. Contact angle: the angle formed by the interface between a viscoelastic drop and a flat surface.

Sodium hyaluronate (Healon®) has a contact angle of 60°, whereas Occucoat (HPMC) and Viscoat have angles of 50° and 52°, respectively. These solutions have better coatability.

As previously mentioned, molecules present on the viscoelastic surface that have a greater negative charge (ie, Viscoat) neutralize the positive charges on instruments and tissues more effectively than those with less negative charges. This feature, at least in theory, increases the viscoelastic's ability to adhere to the corneal endothelium, which assures better protection during phacoemulsification and resistance to the irrigation flows that tend to express the viscoelastic in the AC. On the contrary, the low wettability of Healon®, Provisc, and Biolon does not ensure the same adherence to tissues or opposition to expressive forces as Viscoat.

Table 3-2 summarizes some of the main chemical, physical, and rheologic characteristics of the viscoelastic products currently distributed in Italy.

In the columns on the right, the value of contact angle is shown. The most adherent material is HPMC (low contact angle), whereas the least adherent product is Healon® GV (data provided by Fidia Laboratories).

Table 3-2.
PHYSICAL, CHEMICAL, AND RHEOLOGIC FEATURES OF THE SAME VES

Product	Volume (mL)	Viscosity*	Pseudoplasticity	Contact Angle**
Healon®	0.4/0.55/0.85	40,000	++++	78 degrees
Healon® GV	0.55/0.85	60,000	+++++	80 degrees
IAL	2.0/5.0	8,000-10,000	++	75 degrees
IAL-F	1.1	20,000-22,000	+++	73 degrees
Provisc	0.4/0.55/0.85	25,000-28,000	+++	78 degrees
Viscoat	0.5	45,000	+++	72 degrees
Biolon	0.5/1.0	30,000	+++	78 degrees
Ophthalin	0.5	32,000-35,000	++++	78 degrees
Viscorneal	0.55	40.000	++++	78 degrees
Occucoat	1.0	4,000	+	69 degrees

* Expressed in pps and measured at sec-1 (shear rate) and 20 degrees C.
** At 35 degrees C under nitrogen on PMMA

CHAPTER FOUR

The Main Viscoelastic Materials and Their Features

In this chapter, a technical scheme for each viscoelastic material is listed in which the chemical, physical, and rheologic features are indicated along with the individual features of each material (Table 4-1). Also included is a subjective assessment based on the surgical experience of the authors compared with the experience of other cataract and anterior segment surgeons.

Subjective clinical assessment concerns the following surgical steps: AC filling; capsulotomy; phaco maneuvers; expression of the nucleus; irrigation and aspiration; capsular bag filling; IOL insertion; removal of the viscoelastic material; capsular breaks; and special use. Clinical conditions are described as very poor, poor, sufficient, good, or excellent.

HEALON®

Hyaluronic acid was found to be present in the human body many years ago, and it spurred great interest as it was demonstrated in many tissues. Meyer first isolated hyaluronic acid in the vitreous body in 1930. In 1942, Balazs developed a technique to sterilize the viscous solution; in 1970, he collaborated with Pharmacia & Upjohn on an intensive research effort to develop a useful product for ophthalmic surgery.

In 1979, the first attempt was made to replace the vitreous with hyaluronic acid during retinal detachment surgery. Balazs invented the term viscosurgery and patented a purified hyaluronic acid molecule. In 1977, Miller performed the first studies on rabbit eyes, and in 1979, Stegmann demonstrated hyaluronic acid's endothelial protection. In 1980, Pharmacia & Upjohn started manufacturing Healon® (Table 4-2): at present, more than 20 million vials have been produced.

Healon® has been found to be exceedingly safe for use owing to a number of factors. The first is that it is an endogenous compound (a layer of hyaluronic acid is present on endothelial cell surface). In addition, Pharmacia & Upjohn has over 10 years of experience in the purification of biologic materials. The third factor is the sterilization not only of the product but of the packaging during assembly, transportation, and storage. Pharmacia and Upjohn has an outstanding safety record, and there have been no reported cases of intraocular infection associated with the use of Healon® despite millions of vials used during surgery. The manufacturer has designed a special biologic test (the owl monkey test) to ensure that no inflammatory factors are present in the product. Each lot of viscoelastic is tested in monkey eyes according to a strict protocol and no lot is introduced to the market without first passing this test. The pH buffering in the physiologic range (7 to 7.4) also results in high safety.

The well-known effectiveness of Healon® is based on several factors. For one, it is made of sodium hyaluronate with high molecular weight. High molecular weight means a large molecule, whereas low molecular weight indicates smaller molecules. In a sodium hyaluronate 1% solution with high molecular weight, molecules are superimposed and form a very flexible three-dimensional meshwork; this provides high elasticity and viscosity at a low concentration.

From the clinical point of view, high viscosity is an advantage for the surgeon. High viscosity pro-

Table 4-1.
VISCOELASTIC MATERIALS MARKETED IN ITALY

Product	Manufacturer (of raw material)	Composition (million daltons)	Molecular Weight	Source	pH	Osmolality (mOsm/L)
Healon®	Pharmacia (Biomatrix)	1.0% Hyaluronic acid	4.0	Natural	7.0–7.5	302
Healon® GV	Pharmacia (Biomatrix)	1.4% Hyaluronic acid	5.0	Natural	7.0–7.5	302
IAL	Fidia Oftal (Fidia)	1.2% Hyaluronic acid	1.2	Natural	7.2–7.4	300
IAL-F	Fidia Oftal (Fidia)	1.8% Hyaluronic acid	1.2	Natural	7.2–7.4	300
Provisc	Alcon (Genzyme)	1.0% Hyaluronic acid	1.9	Fermentation	7.0–7.5	310
Viscoat	Alcon (Genzyme)	3.0% Hyaluronic acid 4.0% Condroitin sulfate	0.5 0.02	Natural Fermentation	7.0–7.5	325
Biolon	Sifi (General Biotechnology)	1.0% Hyaluronic acid	3.0	Fermentation	7.2–7.4	300
Ophthalin	Ciba Vision (Fermentech)	1.0% Hyaluronic acid	3.6	Fermentation	7.0–7.5	305
Occucoat	Storz	2.0% Hyaluronic acid	0.08	Natural	7.2	285

Table 4-2.
HEALON®

Storage	Refrigeration
Molecular Weight	4.0 M
Concentration	1% Hyaluronic acid
Viscosity at 0 Shear Rate	>200,000
Viscosity at 1000 Shear Rate	150

Features

Injectability	Good through a 27-G cannula owing to high pseudoplasticity
Removability	Very easy owing to cohesiveness inside the molecular chains
Adhesiveness/Coatability	Poor owing to high superficial tension
Space Maintenance	High molecular weight and viscosity ensure good ability to form and keep chamber depth and volume of the capsular bag
Endothelial Protection	Good, owing to maintenance of deep and wide spaces (preventing accidental contact of instruments and implant); low cohesiveness, which enhances shifting of the material on endothelial cells; high pseudoplasticity (favors viscosity drop during movement); and the presence of specific receptors on endothelial surface (hyaluronic acid binding sites)
Tissue Manipulation	Precise and accurate tissue manipulation, as it can be injected through a small cannula (high pseudoplasticity)
Use, Advantages, and Drawbacks	Formation of AC, capsulorhexis, easy advanced phacoemulsification maneuvers, IOL implantation, vitreous body tamponade, removal of synechiae, small pupil surgery, combined phacotrabeculectomy techniques, bleeding cessation, reintervention for IOL extraction
Syringe	0.40–0.55–0.85 mL of product without needle kit, screw piston, 3-year shelf life

vides the ability to move, control, protect, and separate tissues; maintain space; and produce counterpressure.

Healon® also has high elasticity. This is very important in space maintenance and means that molecules can deflect and deform easily and then recover their original shape. Furthermore, Healon® possesses high pseudoplasticity, which means that molecules can stretch when pressed to pass through even small diameter cannulas.

Healon®'s high elasticity provides excellent compression of the material, and from a clinical point of view this results in the ability to absorb shocks and impacts. High molecular weight means that elasticity is achieved at low concentration rate. Low concentration is equal to physiologic colloidal–osmotic pressure, greater safety, and ease of injection and removal.

Healon® (Table 4-2) has a pseudoplasticity index >1333, which, as stated in Chapter 3, is obtained by dividing viscosity at 0 shear rate by the value of viscosity at 1000 shear rate. Alternatively, pseudoplasticity has been described as the ability of the material to change its viscous behavior according to the degree of movement (ie, high viscosity at low shear rate, low viscosity at high shear rate means high pseudoplasticity).

High pseudoplasticity is another element that results in easy injection and removal of Healon®, even through narrow cannulas (27-G). Another useful feature is Healon®'s high cohesiveness based on particular molecular bonds. This results in easy removal of the product, which tends to leave its position en bloc, not in parts, during aspiration. Furthermore, Healon® has excellent transparency.

Based on these characteristics. Healon® is able to:

- Be easily injected
- Provide excellent visibility
- Form and maintain spaces
- Maneuver tissues
- Ease maneuvers with surgical tools
- Keep the shape of formed capsular bag
- Ease IOL implantation
- Keep constant or increase mydriasis
- Favor hemostasis
- Favor nuclear expression (ECCE)
- Ease IOL extraction, when necessary

Healon® is therefore extremely safe, efficient, and versatile, and lacks any major disadvantages. However, the features of Healon® result in three main limitations. Healon® is expensive, can cause postoperative IOP elevation when the material is not removed at the end of surgery, and must be refrigerated. This last limitation is only a problem when surgery is performed in remote areas.

High price is a result of quality control. In our experience, the effect of IOP elevation plays a marginal role, as we believe that any viscoelastic material should always be completely removed from the eye. In addition, features of high cohesiveness and high pseudoplasticity ensure that Healon® is almost always completely removed.

A more controversial issue is the quality of endothelial protection. Pharmacia & Upjohn has demonstrated that Healon®'s protective effect is due to a chemical bond with endothelial cell binding sites (hyaluronic acid binding sites), which persists even many hours after surgery. It is also due to the neutralizing effect that Healon® has on the formation of free radicals that develop during phacoemulsification. Other manufacturers assert the effectiveness of mechanical protection of endothelial cells against compression and shifting (provided by highly adhesive materials only). The persistence of a visible layer of viscoelastic on the corneal endothelium during the entire procedure, as occurs with methylcellulose and chondroitin sulfate, is in their opinion a fundamental aspect of endothelial protection.

Owing to its versatility, Healon® can be employed to perform cataract extraction both with ECCE and phaco techniques, as well as secondary AC IOL implantation. In the presence of positive vitreous pressure not controlled by Healon®, it may be necessary to use viscoelastics with higher molecular weight. Also, in cases of capsular rupture, the surgeon should use materials that have greater adhesiveness or that can be left in the eye if necessary (Viscoat).

HEALON® YELLOW*

Healon® Yellow was designed and manufactured by Pharmacia & Upjohn in an attempt to make Healon® visible. Fluorescein has been added to make the material easier to detect by the surgeon once injected in the AC.

**Healon® Yellow is no longer being manufactured.*

Over time, and with the acceptance of viscoelastic use in routine surgery, surgeons have learned to detect the presence of a viscoelastic, even when the material is transparent and colorless. Because the chemical, physical, and rheologic properties of Healon® Yellow are the same as those of normal Healon®, the material is still useful for educational purposes. It can be used to show young and inexperienced surgeons the correct maneuvers to be performed with a viscoelastic material. Furthermore, Healon® Yellow can be better identified during surgery when a blue filter is placed on the surgery microscope.

Incomplete AC filling and incomplete removal of the material can be easily seen. In cases of capsular rupture, regular Healon® may be indistinguishable from vitreous, whereas the yellow dye of Healon® Yellow makes distinction much easier.

During IOL implantation, the lens can be better appreciated in a dyed viscoelastic and it is possible to assess whether total removal of the material has been accomplished.

HEALON® GV

Healon® GV was originally designed by Pharmacia & Upjohn as a material with high molecular weight and pseudoplasticity that would be able to provide a solution in those occasions when the surgeon must counterbalance high positive pressure or face complicated cases in which permanent tissue immobilization is required. In addition, the material would facilitate advanced maneuvers in anterior segment surgery.

The material has become routinely used in phacoemulsification owing to its pseudoplasticity and high molecular weight. In addition, as phacoemulsification techniques have become more refined, the use of soft foldable IOLs has become common. Healon® GV has become the viscoelastic of choice for soft foldable lens implantation.

The production chain is the same as for Healon®, but differs in higher weight and greater concentration. Viscosity at 0 shear rate (Table 4-3) is much greater in Healon® GV, whereas the values at 1000 shear rate are identical to Healon®. Pseudoplasticity rate is high as well. These features indicate that Healon® GV provides, and even enhances, the same rheologic characteristics that have made Healon® popular worldwide. These characteristics include easy injection of the material, excellent space maintenance, easy performance of advanced instrument maneuvers, stability of the capsular flap during phacoemulsification with a constantly deep AC, and easy removal. When comparing the viscosity of Healon® GV and Viscoat at 0 and 1000 shear rate, it is difficult to find common ground between the two materials. Healon® GV is far more pseudoplastic and its effects as soft spatula and permanent spatula are much greater than those of Viscoat. Phacoemulsification steps such as AC filling, capsulorhexis, capsular bag filling, and IOL implantation are easier with Healon® GV.

Regarding the persistence of the material during surgical procedures, Viscoat stays in the AC longer when compared with the highly pseudoplastic and cohesive Healon® GV. Despite this, Healon® GV has become popular in routine phacoemulsification, particularly in foldable lens implantation.

Studies demonstrating the positive features of Healon® GV have been performed. Space maintenance is much better with Healon® GV than with regular Healon® or other materials. This has been assessed for capsulorhexis performance, after capsular bag filling, and after IOL implantation.

Biometric assessment has demonstrated that the AC formed by Healon® GV is deeper than that achieved with other viscoelastics.

In the chapter on rheologic characteristics (Chapter 3), viscoelastic functions were separated into four groups: 1) superficial function, 2) space function, 3) tissue function, and 4) maneuvering function. The superficial function involves protection of the corneal endothelium. Healon® GV protects the endothelium both mechanically and by binding to hyaluronic acid binding sites present on corneal endothelial cells. Space function is optimized by Healon® GV as it has the highest viscosity at 0 shear rate of any viscoelastic currently available. It is therefore effective in the formation and maintenance of a deep AC when performing maneuvers such as capsulorhexis. Capsular bag opening is largest with this material, which combined with its high elasticity ensures excellent unfolding of the IOL. Tissue functions are ensured by Healon® GV's high molecular weight. This is demonstrated by the widening effect of mydriasis in the presence of a narrow pupil or the need to

Table 4-3.
HEALON® GV

Storage	Refrigeration
Molecular Weight	5 M
Concentration	1.4 % Hyaluronic acid
Viscosity at 0 Shear Rate	>200,000,000
Viscosity at 1000 Shear Rate	200
Features	
Injectability	Very good through a 27-G cannula owing to high pseudoplasticity. Excellent feedback of the pressure necessary for injection.
Removability	The time necessary for complete irrigation and aspiration is identical to that of Healon® (owing to high internal molecular cohesiveness)
Adhesiveness/Coatability	Poorer adhesiveness when compared with Viscoat. Good immobilization of nuclear fragments after cracking or chopping.
Space Maintenance	Better than Healon® owing to higher viscosity at 0 shear rate. Easier to perform capsulorhexis owing to support of the capsular flap. Easier creation of more stable surgical spaces and safer cleavage planes. Provides excellent visibility, better than Viscoat, in the phase of nucleus sculpture.
Endothelial Protection	Effective dampening of compression and friction forces. Presence of specific receptors for hyaluronic acid on the endothelium. Scavenger effect against the formation of free radicals during phacoemulsification
Tissue Manipulation	Better characteristics of soft and permanent spatula than regular Healon®
Use, Advantages, and Drawbacks	Useful for phacoemulsification, foldable IOL implantation, traumatic cataract, secondary implants in phakic and aphakic eyes, combined phacotrabeculectomy, iridoplasty, and IOL extraction
Syringe	0.55–0.85 mL of product in preassembled syringe without needle kit, screw piston, 3-year shelf life

control the vitreous in case of a posterior capsule rupture. Another function is the assurance of instrument maneuvers and IOL insertion. The forceps or the injector must pass through the viscoelastic while it stays in place and does not leak out of the capsular bag or the eye. The viscoelastic must protect tissues while maintaining spaces, be elastic to dampen the unfolding of IOL and loops, and be removed completely from the capsular bag and the AC at the end of surgery.

The elasticity of Healon® GV is ten times higher that that of Healon®: this ensures greater absorption of the mechanical shock due to the unfolding of the IOL, which can unfold quickly and in an uncontrolled fashion.

Soft IOL implantation is made easier by Healon® GV for the following four reasons:

- It ensures control during insertion (very deep AC)
- It ensures control during positioning (space maintenance)
- It ensures control during IOL unfolding (tissue protection and absorption of mechanical shock)
- It ensures control during the performance of all maneuvers (ie, it controls vitreous push, optimizes the performance of capsulorhexis, provides excellent transparency, and protects the endothelium through binding sites and mechanical action)

Healon® GV must be completely removed from the eye. It has been shown that Healon® takes a longer time to be removed completely. Useful tips to remove the material include using high flow and vacuum values and inclining the IOL optic to one side or the other alternately in order to free the viscoelastic material trapped between IOL and capsular bag. The rest of the viscoelastic in the AC can be removed with rotational movements (rock and roll technique).

Healon® GV was originally conceived to cope with the management of difficult situations. In the presence of high positive vitreous pressure, for instance, the material provides resistance to push three times higher than does Healon®.

In cases of capsular rupture, Healon® GV's high molecular weight combined with high viscosity at zero shear rate and permanent spatula effect allow the surgeon better control of the opening through which the vitreous leaks. Anterior vitrectomy is preferably performed with dry technique, without irrigation, as irrigation would hydrate the vitreous, making the vitreous come out more easily through the capsular break. To perform this dry technique the surgeon needs a viscoelastic material like Healon® GV, which is able to keep the vitreous inside its natural space and has its own well-defined morphology, based on high cohesiveness, that enables the surgeon to see the border between the vitreous and the viscoelastic clearly, without adhering to the vitreous. Viscoat also provides excellent control of vitreous in capsular breaks, but is lighter and less viscous at 0 shear rate than Healon® GV. In the face of positive vitreous pressure, these features can be a disadvantage. Viscoat's adhesiveness allows it to stay in place longer while the surgeon performs aspiration and dissects the residual cortex with a thin vitrector or cannula.

Healon® GV is also useful in the management of small pupils. The surgeon must perform a number of maneuvers on eyes treated with chronic miotics or with posterior synechiae secondary to uveitis. These include the following:

- Synechialysis using viscoelastic. Weak adhesions can be broken by the soft spatula effect of Healon® GV. In this case it is fundamental to use an easily injectable, very pseudoplastic and transparent viscoelastic with high molecular weight. Once the synechiae have been removed and the pupil has been enlarged, the permanent spatula effect of the viscoelastic must freeze the pupil in its enlarged state in order to accomplish correct capsulorhexis. The persistence of mydriasis and a deep AC is fundamental.
- Synechialysis using a spatula. Stronger adhesions cannot be broken by the viscoelastic, and the surgeon must use surgical tools (spatula or forceps) to break synechiae. In this case the presence of a deep chamber is mandatory. Very often it is also necessary to use a heavy viscoelastic able to stop bleeding, a common occurrence in these cases (ie, angular synechiae, rubeosis). The ability to sequester the blood far from the area where the surgeon works is a basic condition necessary to continue surgery.
- Stretching of the pupil with hooks
- Removal of fibrotic or hyaline membranes
- Multiple sphyncterotomies
- Mechanical mydriasis, with rigid or flexible aids

All the maneuvers mentioned require good visibility (transparent viscoelastic), hemostasis (permanent spatula effect), deep AC (high viscosity at 0 shear rate), permanent spatula effect on tissues that cannot be freed, possibility to maneuver instruments in the AC (high pseudoplasticity), and the need to dampen impacts that these devices (ie, hooks for mechanical mydriasis) can place on tissues (high elasticity). Healon® GV has the rheologic and physicochemical characteristics to meet such clinical requirements.

In pediatric ophthalmic surgery, which may be difficult owing to very high tissue elasticity, the key to intact capsulorhexis is attainment of the deepest AC possible along with a flat anterior surface of the lens to prevent escape of the capsular flap into the periphery. In these eyes, scleral and corneal rigidity are often very low, high positive vitreous pressure is present due to choroidal congestion, and the iris/lens diaphragm can be pushed forward. A material like Healon® GV enables the surgeon to keep the AC deep while successfully controlling posterior vitreous pressure, and to reposition iris and lens when they tend to come forward. In such cases, iris prolapse occurs very frequently, and Healon® GV acts as a soft spatula to reposition the iris and then as a permanent spatula to keep it in the right position.

A heavy viscoelastic such as Healon® GV is useful in glaucoma surgery, where interventions on the corneoscleral angle, such as goniotomy, are facilitated by the widening of angular recesses achieved with the material. The same is true for corneal surgery (ie, keratoplasty) when the surgeon needs a surgical tool able to counterbalance positive vitreous push, to position the iris tending to come forward, and to protect the donor flap, creating a viscoelastic dome on which the flap can float during suturing.

The chemical, physical, and rheologic characteristics of Healon® GV make it useful for ocular trauma surgery, which is different from case to case. These eyes often have a shallow AC, and it is fundamental to form and maintain a large working space while counterbalancing vitreous pressure. Very frequently the internal anatomy of the eye is altered, and a viscoelastic provided with soft spatula characteristics is very helpful to move and reposition damaged tissues. The vitreous often protrudes and must be pushed back by a suitable viscoelastic.

The iris is occasionally dislocated or extruding and Healon® GV can help reposition it while providing space for pupillostatic or iridodialysis sutures. The surgeon is frequently faced with blood clots or fibrin adherent to ocular structures or intraocular foreign bodies. Healon® GV is able to remove or place these materials in a more favorable position to facilitate removal.

In the presence of bleeding or zonular disinsertion, Healon® GV is helpful to help hemostasis, isolate blood far from the site where the surgeon is working, and counterbalance vitreal protrusion through a zonular dialysis.

In theory, Healon® GV may be useful in the performance of ECCE surgery, as it is very pseudoplastic. The speculation is that, because Healon® has been successfully used to perform ECCE, a material like Healon® GV in which Healon®'s particular features are strengthened should be even better. In our experience, routine use of Healon® GV during ECCE surgery is limited by high cost and the presence of a large incision, which may permit the material to come out in block. It is better to use Healon® GV in advanced extracapsular techniques, such as sutureless manual sections (ie, the procedure suggested by Kansas), or in cases in which maintenance of wide spaces and maneuvers with large instruments must be performed and the risk of contact between nuclear pieces and corneal endothelium must be minimized. In such cases Healon® GV can act as a surgical tool that moves nuclear fragments toward the surgeon and avoids the use of loops or other tools to extract fragments as they are expelled from the eye, carried and pushed by the viscoelastic.

It has been demonstrated that endothelial cell loss in such cases may often be significant, and a viscous tool providing high elasticity and pseudoplasticity is valuable. Performance of the above mentioned techniques is often not the surgeon's first choice. Nevertheless, accidental damage to the phacoemulsificator can occur, and the surgeon who has no other machine available may still operate through a small incision with a sutureless technique to implant a soft foldable lens, provided that he or she has knowledge of nuclear fragmentation manual procedures. In this case, the availability of wide space is mandatory.

Healon® GV is useful in two other uncommon situations: IOL implantation in phakic eyes for the management of high myopia (iris fixation or retroiridal and prelenticular positioning) and IOL extraction.

PROVISC

Provisc (Table 4-4) has been studied and manufactured by Alcon since 1986. It is 1% hyaluronic acid designed for extracapsular cataract surgery or phacoemulsification; in the Duovisc package, it is coupled with Viscoat. One disadvantage of Duovisc is that the surgeon must use two different products to accomplish the same goal when one single product (Healon®) has the same characteristics and can be used for the same purpose. Healon® has been found to protect the corneal endothelium in three ways:

- Mechanical protection (shock absorption owing to its elasticity)
- Biological protection (hyaluronic acid receptors on corneal endothelium)
- Chemical protection–scavenger effect (neutralization of free radicals that are formed during phacoemulsification)

Supporters of Duovisc claim that a single viscoelastic is not able to perform all the functions the surgeon may require, and only the combined use of various viscoelastics with complementary rheologic and chemicophysical characteristics can ensure the most desired effects with the fewest drawbacks.

Table 4-4.
PROVISC

Storage	Refrigeration, in vertical position
Molecular Weight	1.9–2.5 M
Concentration	1% Hyaluronic acid, produced with bacterial fermentation
Viscosity at 0 Shear Rate	>150,000
Viscosity at 1000 Shear Rate	190
Features	
Injectability	Comparable to Healon® owing to high pseudoplasticity, which allows easy insertion through a small diameter cannula
Removability	Similar to Healon® for internal cohesiveness of molecular chains
Adhesiveness/Coatability	Less than Viscoat, similar to Healon®; less control of nuclear fragments
Space Maintenance	Ensures AC depth and stable capsular bag filling; viscosity at 0 shear rate is less than Healon®; suitable for viscoexpression and viscodelineation; good visibility; easy IOL implantation
Endothelial Protection	Good protection; the presence of binding sites on the endothelium or scavenger effect have not been studied with this material
Tissue Manipulation	Useful as soft spatula and similar to Healon®, it is midway between Viscoat (viscoadherent) and Healon® GV (permanent spatula), while possessing high pseudoplasticity
Uses, Advantages, and Drawbacks	Inexpensive; good for extracapsular extraction and tissue manipulation; less biologic control than Healon®
Syringe	0.55–0.85 mL of product in preassembled syringe, 27-G cannula needle kit, 2-year shelf life

Table 4-5 compares the chemicophysical and rheologic features of Provisc and Healon®. These features are almost identical between the two substances, except for the biologic source. Provisc is derived from microbial fermentation, and is very biocompatible, sterile, nonpyrogenic, highly purified, transparent, and buffered between 7 and 7.5 pH.

A rather important disadvantage of Provisc is its method of aseptic sterilization followed by terminal sterilization, which is not accomplished inside the syringe as happens with Healon®.

In monkey eyes, Provisc is drained from the AC in 26 to 30 hours. Studies concerning safety and toxicity have shown that it is not mutagenic. Studies focusing on severe toxicity of the product after subcutaneous, intraperitoneal, and intravenous injection in rats did not demonstrate any pathologic elements. Tissue compatibility has been studied with the acute intramuscular tissue toxicity test, and the outcome exceeded the requisites demanded. This was also true for the passive cutaneous anaphylaxis test, which studied Provisc's immunogenic and sensitizing activity.

The potential complement activation of Provisc was also assessed, and there was no presence of immunogenicity or potential sensitization. No intraocular inflammation was caused by Provisc injection in the AC of rabbits. This aspect was studied in two control groups that were injected with Healon® and buffered phosphate solution: there was no significant difference between the two groups. The test was repeated in monkeys, with AC injection of Provisc and Healon®, and no evidence of significant differences in inflammatory reaction was noted.

Regarding clinical pharmacology, Provisc has been demonstrated to have no pharmacologic

Table 4-5.
PROVISC VERSUS HEALON®

Characteristic	Provisc	Healon®
Viscosity (shear rate; cps)	39,000	40,000
Molecular weight, M	1.9–2.5	4.0
Concentration, %	1	1
pH buffer	Yes, 7.25 ± 0.25	Yes, 7.25 ± 0.25
Osmolality, mOsm/kg	310	302
Luer–Lock syringe	Yes	Yes
Disposable cannula	Yes	Yes
Refrigeration	Yes	Yes
Biologic source	Microbic fermentation	Cockscomb
Syringe capacity, mL	0.4	0.4
	0.55	0.55
	0.85	0.85
		2.0

effect. Its clinical effectiveness is comparable to that of Healon®. Studies on density and morphology of corneal endothelial cells and corneal thickness did not show any significant differences between the two substances.

There are no consistent biologic control tests performed on each lot of Provisc, as is performed on Healon® with the owl monkey test by Pharmacia & Upjohn. This condition and the different sources of production make Healon® preferred over Provisc. Analyses performed at Pharmacia & Upjohn laboratories showed that the molecular weight of Provisc is 2.5 M, and that with 1% concentration the viscosity at 0 shear rate is much lower than that of Healon®. Noticeable differences in molecular weight are also likely to be detected between one lot and another. Furthermore, lower viscosity at zero shear rate is undesirable for the performance of capsulorhexis. In multicenter studies for Provisc approval, nine adverse reactions have been reported: three were corneal decompensations due to previous corneal dystrophy, whereas the other six were attributed to the use of Provisc.

In our clinical experience, the surgical application of Provisc and Healon® is almost identical, with certain important differences as discussed. Provisc is less able to form space than Healon®, but can be removed more easily. The effectiveness and safety of Provisc will be assessed with time and based on the same number of clinical cases studied with Healon®.

The combined use of Provisc and Viscoat during phacoemulsification in cases of posterior capsular rupture and to cope with some complications is very useful. Provisc is excellent in IOL implantation, owing to its good elasticity and pseudoplasticity. It is also excellent for tissue manipulation owing to its soft spatula effect. It is also extremely effective in extracapsular cataract surgery and in the performance of capsulorhexis. By offering Provisc along with Viscoat in one package, Alcon illustrates that the various viscoelastics provide different rheologic characteristics, and for this reason are indicated in some cases but not in others.

VISCOAT

It is important to review some of the physical and chemical features of viscoelastics to appreciate Viscoat (Table 4-6). Fluid viscosity is the ability to resist shifting and is the internal cohesive capacity caused by molecular attraction of the material. Aqueous solutions have low internal molecular cohesion whereas viscous fluids have higher cohe-

Table 4-6.
VISCOAT

Storage	Refrigeration
Molecular Weight	500 K (hyaluronic acid) + 25 K (chondroitin sulfate)
Concentration	3% Hyaluronic acid, 4% chondroitin sulfate
Viscosity at 0 Shear Rate	41,000
Viscosity at 1000 Shear Rate	200
Features	
Injectability	Good injectability through a 27-G cannula, but less than Healon® and Amvisc, which require less force to empty the syringe; it is necessary to inject Viscoat inside itself starting distally and retract the cannula toward the incision to avoid the effect of braid-like shape
Removability	The time required for irrigation/aspiration is 4 to 5 times longer than with Healon® and Healon® GV owing to higher coatability on tissues and IOL posterior surface and less internal cohesiveness
Adhesiveness/Coatability	High on intraocular tissues, implants, and instruments
Space Maintenance	Good, but poorer than other viscoelastics with high molecular weight at 0 shear rate; stays in the eye owing to greater adhesiveness; the maintenance of intraocular volume is proportional to molecular weight
Endothelial Protection	Good protection, but may produce drag forces on the endothelium; no scavenger effect or interaction with hyaluronic acid receptors
Tissue Manipulation	Worse than Healon® owing to poorer pseudoplasticity; better immobilization of nuclear fragments during phacoemulsification
Uses, Advantages, and Disadvantages	Useful in performance of phacoemulsification and management of complications such as capsular breaks and preventing vitreous loss, owing to its adhesiveness; poorer cohesiveness may cause cleavage lines inside the material that result in loss of transparency or trapped air bubbles during phacoemulsification; soft, foldable IOL insertion is more difficult with Viscoat; causes IOP elevation when left in the AC, although less than Healon®
Syringe	0.55 mL of product; preassembled syringe with 27-G screw needle and needle cover; necessary to fill 3/4 of the needle before fixing it to the syringe; vertical storage of the packaging is recommended to avoid incarceration of air bubbles inside the material; 2-year shelf life

sion. Therefore, a greater force will be necessary to move a viscous material. The viscosity of a material is defined as the force one must overcome to move it divided by the movement speed (viscosity shear stress/shear rate).

Viscous (Newtonian) materials maintain the same viscosity independent of friction speed. Non–Newtonian fluids are very viscous at rest and move more fluid with increasing shifting speed (pseudoplasticity). A viscoelastic material is very viscoplastic when it is poorly deformed at rest and greatly deformed when submitted to movement (high viscosity at 0 shear rate, low viscosity at 1000 shear rate). Hyaluronic acid is a non–Newtonian fluid, which means that its viscosity changes according to the speed of shifting. Chondroitin sulfate, on the contrary, is a Newtonian, nonpseudoplastic fluid that has stable viscosity independent of shifting speed. Therefore, the main drawback of hyaluronic acid is that it reacts quickly to movement, thus losing its ability to maintain spaces, as it loses viscosity.

Viscoat consists of a mixture of two-thirds 3% hyaluronic acid and one-third 4% chondroitin sulfate; the combination of materials results in a product that is less viscous at rest and less pseudoplastic owing to the presence of chondroitin sulfate. As a result, its viscosity decreases less quickly with movement and space is maintained for a longer time.

Viscosity at 0 shear rate does not depend on the shape and length of molecules or molecular weight. Nevertheless, a viscoelastic material cannot be assessed by only considering its viscosity at rest. In fact, a material showing higher viscosity at rest and high pseudoplasticity (Healon®) loses viscosity when movement is applied. Healon®, for instance, will easily come out of the cannula (30-G) during injection, but in the same way it will be likely to leave the AC during surgery, as the turbulence of irrigation fluids and vibrations of the phaco tip act to apply motion to the material. Furthermore, the high cohesiveness of the material facilitates its coming out of the eye as a whole. On the contrary, Viscoat requires greater force to be ejected from the cannula (27-G), but can maintain its particular viscosity for a longer period and can therefore maintain spaces and protect tissues.

Elasticity is another basic property of viscoelastics. Healon® is more elastic than Viscoat, and therefore provides greater protection from vibrations and mechanical maneuvers, provided that the material is able to stay in the AC. Viscoat is less elastic owing to the presence of chondroitin sulfate, but can stay in the AC longer owing to its higher adhesiveness.

The long chains particular to viscoelastic materials with high molecular weight (sodium hyaluronate) result in high cohesiveness, whereas materials with short chains and low molecular weight (sodium hyaluronate and chondroitin sulfate) are less cohesive. Highly cohesive materials are easily removed after surgery, and less cohesive materials will require more maneuvers.

Viscoat, like Healon®, is buffered so that its pH ranges between 7 and 7.4.

An important feature of Viscoat is its adhesiveness: if the contact angle between fluid and solid is small, the fluid has greater coatability.

Sodium hyaluronate alone has a large contact angle when compared with sodium hyaluronate with chondroitin sulfate (Viscoat). Therefore, Viscoat demonstrates better coatability of corneal endothelium, IOL, and instruments.

Two active elements coexist in Viscoat to combine the high viscosity of sodium hyaluronate with the excellent adhesiveness of chondroitin sulfate. Both elements are naturally present in human eyes (sodium hyaluronate in vitreous and aqueous humor and chondroitin sulfate in cornea and ocular tissues). The molecules of both materials are bound through hydrogen bonds and the deriving molecule has three negative charges that play a main role in the prevention of endothelial cell loss, as they probably neutralize positive charges on surgical tools.

Hydrogen bonds are labile and, once broken, allow smaller molecules with shorter chain to leave the eye. Sodium hyaluronate is derived from bacterial fermentation of streptococci culture, whereas chondroitin sulfate is obtained by enzymatic extraction from shark fin cartilage. Sterilization is accomplished with ethylene oxide.

Viscoat should be stored vertically so that potential air bubbles are positioned at the end of the syringe. It is also important to follow the manufacturer's directions for mounting the 27-G cannula. At present, no biologic monitoring seems to be performed on Viscoat similar to the controls performed by Pharmacia & Upjohn on Healon® and Healon® GV.

In December 1985, the distribution of Viscoat was halted owing to the presence of high concentrations of phosphate in the buffering solution, followed by reports of calcium precipitates in the cornea after application of Viscoat. In April 1986, the FDA approved the new formulation of the buffer solution, which reduced phosphate concentration to approximately one fourth of the original values. In May 1986, the material was reintroduced to the market. In 1987, about 20,000 syringes were withdrawn because of endotoxins that caused postoperative inflammation. In February 1988, the material was put back on the market.

The following suggestions are useful when Viscoat is used. Avoid excessive AC filling, which may cause capsular blockade. Furthermore, the surgeon should inject the material inside itself to prevent the material from parceling in the injection phase due to its low cohesiveness.

Chondroitin sulfate is the same material used to preserve corneal flaps for implantation (Optisol Chiron 2.5%). Corneas can be safely preserved in this fluid for 2 weeks, whereas hyaluronic acid can keep them for only 24 hours.

Clinical studies have demonstrated that 98% of Viscoat is eliminated in 24 hours, whereas hyaluronic acid requires 6 days for metabolization. In cases where complete removal of Viscoat is difficult owing to its low cohesiveness (ie, secondary implants, capsular breaks, cornea transplantation), small quantities can be left inside the eye as it does not cause a dangerous IOP increase.

A drawback caused by the permanence of viscoelastics during phacoemulsification is the formation of water–viscoelastic cleavage lines that decrease visibility for the surgeon. Also, trapped air bubbles from the irrigation line and cavitational problems may be undesired events.

The issue of corneal endothelial protection is complex. Healon® supporters believe that the hyaluronic acid binding sites concept is the most important factor. Viscoat supporters claim that the adhesiveness of this material provides effective protection from pressure and shifting forces. No good comparative study of endothelial protection between the materials has been performed. In all studies, there were variables of phaco machine setting, nuclear hardness, and phaco technique employed. Some authors compared eyes operated with ECCE techniques with eyes treated with phacoemulsification.

Most surgeons prefer Healon® for capsulorhexis as well as ECCE surgery owing to Healon®'s viscosity at 0 shear rate (five times higher than Viscoat).

Viscoat is less transparent than Healon®; therefore, when capsulorhexis is performed in the presence of poor red reflex, Healon® can be more useful. The same is true for difficult IOL implantation, where the cornea is poorly transparent or the pupil is small and excellent visibility is a crucial element.

Viscoat is an excellent viscoelastic material for phacoemulsification. In particular, its adhesiveness can be useful to minimize trauma of nuclear fragments on corneal endothelium caused by fluid dynamics. On the other hand, the material may be less desirable when high pseudoplasticity is required (ie, injectability, removability, capsulorhexis, IOL implantation in the bag). Recently Alcon has provided the more adhesive and less pseudoplastic material (Viscoat) along with a more pseudoplastic viscoelastic (Provisc). This combined product is called Duovisc, and is a practical example of the combined use of different viscoelastic materials during the same surgical procedure, which enables the surgeon to take advantage of the benefits provided by each one with the fewest drawbacks.

Amvisc and Amvisc Plus

Amvisc and Amvisc Plus (Chiron Vision Corporation, Claremont, Calif)) are very similar viscoelastic materials (Tables 4-7 and 4-8) made of sodium hyaluronate derived from bacterial fermentation. Both show good viscoelasticity and can keep the chamber deep, as well as expand the capsular bag.

Both are supplied in presterilized disposable plastic syringes that have been preassembled in an aseptic environment, a disadvantage when compared with Healon®, which is prepared with the most refined sterilization process among all viscoelastic materials currently used.

The sodium hyaluronate concentration is slightly higher in Amvisc Plus when compared with Amvisc (1.6% versus 1.2%). The declared molecular weight is 1.5 M for Amvisc Plus versus nearly 2.0 M for Amvisc.

Analysis has revealed possible variability of molecular weight and concentration among different lots of both materials. This is probably known to the manufacturer, as the values printed on the explanatory notes in the package (molecular weight greater than 1 M) differ from those reported in the information pamphlet (molecular weight >1.5 M).

Each lot is tested to ensure that no inflammatory factors are present. Both materials are transparent and generally do not trap air bubbles. A disadvantageous aspect is the fact that the solutions are not buffered: in some samples produced by IOLab, the pH values ranged between 6.1 and 6.4. Scientific studies have shown possible structural damage and functional alterations of the corneal endothelium with pH values below 6.8. The manufacturer claims that pH value of the products is stabilized with aqueous humor once the material has been injected in the AC. Product stability is guaranteed for 18 months.

Table 4-7.
AMVISC

Storage	Refrigeration
Molecular Weight	2 M
Concentration	1.2 % Hyaluronic acid (bacterial fermentation)
Viscosity at 0 Shear Rate	40,000
Viscosity at 1000 Shear Rate	240
	Features
Injectability	Good pseudoplasticity favors easy injectability
Removability	Similar to Healon® for internal cohesiveness of molecular chains, it tends to be removed from the AC as a whole mass
Adhesiveness/Coatability	Less than Viscoat, comparable to Healon®
Space Maintenance	Less viscous than Healon® at 0 shear rate; slightly worse in the achievement of a stable intraocular surgical space; good visibility
Endothelial Protection	Good; neither the presence of receptors on the endothelium nor scavenger effect have been studied
Tissue Manipulation	Useful as soft spatula and similar to regular Healon®, it is halfway between Viscoat (viscoadherent) and Healon® GV with high pseudoplasticity
Uses, Advantages, and Drawbacks	Capsular extraction/tissue manipulation; poor control of nuclear fragments due to poor viscoadherence; easy to inject/remove; transparent; comes out during phacoemulsification
Syringe	0.5–0.8 mL in plastic syringe; 27-G cannula needle, 2-year shelf life

Table 4-8.
AMVISC PLUS

Storage	Refrigeration
Molecular Weight	1.5 M
Concentration	1.6% Hyaluronic acid (bacterial fermentation)
Viscosity at 0 Shear Rate	55,000
Viscosity at 1000 Shear Rate	360
	Features
Injectability	Good through a 27-G cannula
Removability	More difficult to remove than Healon®,but easier than Viscoat; the molecular chain length of Amvisc Plus is between that of Healon® and Viscoat
Adhesiveness/Coatability	Amvisc Plus is less adhesive than Viscoat, which is more cohesive, but more adhesive than Amvisc, Provisc, and Healon®
Space Maintenance	This product does not have the same ability to maintain intraocular volume as Healon®, as it does not have comparable viscosity at 0 shear rate; it cannot ensure stability of spaces as well as other more viscous material (ie, Healon® GV)
Endothelial Protection	High and comparable to Amvisc
Tissue Manipulation	Amvisc Plus does not have comparable high viscosity qualities to Healon® GV; it has soft spatula characteristics similar to Amvisc; Amvisc Plus has greater viscosity than Amvisc and a higher concentration of Hyaluronic acid
Uses, Advantages, and Disadvantages	Useful in phacoemulsification and ECCE; coatability is not enough to stop fragments of nucleus and cortex; easy to inject, provides good viscosity, remains in the AC during phacoemulsification; easily seen, difficult to remove
Syringe	0.5–0.8 mL of product in plastic syringe with 27-G needle; 18 months shelf life

From the clinical point of view, the two materials are used differently based on their chemical and physical characteristics. Amvisc Plus has molecular chains of intermediate length, and therefore provides medium cohesiveness and remains in the AC longer during phaco procedures, but requires longer time for complete removal. Amvisc has lower concentration and greater cohesiveness. Its high cohesiveness eases injectability and removal; nevertheless, owing to the same feature, it tends to leave the AC prematurely during phacoemulsification, similar to Healon®.

The philosophy leading to the production of Amvisc Plus was to create a viscoelastic that is cohesive and dispersive at the same time. It is known that cohesive products are highly viscous, able to form space, but on the other hand are likely to come out during phacoemulsification. On the contrary, adhesive products form a smaller space, but do not leave the eye with irrigation fluids. Cohesive products have long molecular chains, whereas adhesive products have short molecular chains. Long chains make the product highly cohesive easy to remove as a whole. On the other hand, short molecular chains result in poor cohesiveness and make removal difficult.

Therefore, a product like Amvisc Plus, which has intermediate molecular length and cohesiveness, remains in the AC long enough to provide mechanical protection for corneal endothelial cells. This material possesses good viscosity, ability to form space, and transparency. Thus, it is useful in the performance of capsulorhexis and other maneuvers inside the AC. During phacoemulsification, Amvisc Plus leaves the AC only partially, and remains to protect corneal endothelium. Its viscosity is sufficient to open and stretch the capsular bag and ensure safe IOL implantation. Removal is much more difficult when compared with Healon®, but easier to remove than Viscoat. This viscoelastic can therefore link products with greater cohesiveness, like Healon® and Healon® GV, and more dispersive materials like Viscoat and Vitrax.

Comparative studies on postoperative IOP demonstrated an advantage of Amvisc and Amvisc Plus as related to Healon® and Viscoat: shorter molecular chains helped the outflow through trabecular meshwork. The longer chains and greater cohesiveness of Healon® and the greater coatability of Viscoat can contribute to postoperative IOP elevation.

The fact that viscoelastic tends to be removed at the end of surgery is of basic importance. A more cohesive viscoelastic, when left inside the eye, causes greater IOP increase; however, it is also known that high cohesiveness means easy, complete, and quick removal. Conversely, more adhesive materials (Viscoat, HPMC 2%), when left inside the eye, cause less IOP elevation, but are often almost impossible to remove completely. We believe, therefore, that it is preferable to manage a more cohesive material at the end of surgery, as it can be removed more easily and completely.

HYDROXYPROPYLMETHYLCELLULOSE 2%

OCCUCOAT, HYMECEL, CELLUGEL, AND ADATOCEL

Hydroxypropylmethylcellulose was the first viscoadherent material used in ocular surgery (1977). It was initially used for lubricating endoocular prostheses and for the application of contact glasses for gonioscopy. It is present in nature (wood, cotton), but not in the human body.

HPMC consists of long glucose molecular chains where hydrogens have been replaced by methoxy-hydroxypropyl chains, thus increasing hydrophilia. No intraocular adverse reactions have been observed following use of HPMC. Occucoat (Table 4-9) is probably the best-known product of this material: Occucoat was initially registered in the United States under the names Viscolon and Cellucoat (1987).

HPMC consists of a synthetic material of methylcellulose 2% solution derived from purified cellulose pulp. This solution is first refined by solubilizing peptides and then sterilized by autoclave.

Hymecel (Table 4-10) and Adatocel consist of the same material; Cellugel (Table 4-11) is made of a synthetic carbohydrate polymer, which has demonstrated severe inflammatory activity during the owl monkey test. This product has not been approved by the FDA.

Unlike hyaluronic acid products derived from bacterial fermentation or animals, methylcellulose cannot be considered as a viscoelastic material. In fact, although its molecular weight is >80,000 daltons, its viscosity is 5600 cps at 0 shear rate and 240 at 1000 shear rate.

Table 4-9. OCCUCOAT	
Storage	No refrigeration required, protection from light
Molecular Weight	86 K
Concentration	1 Hydroxypropylmethylcellulose 2% (HPMC)
Viscosity at 0 Shear Rate	5400
Viscosity at 1000 Shear Rate	240
Features	
Injectability	Due to viscoadhesion and poor pseudoplasticity, injection is more difficult than with hyaluronic acid; it is hard to control the force applied and get true manual "feedback"
Removability	Irrigation/aspiration times are longer as a consequence of less cohesion between molecules of the product
Adhesiveness/Coatability	Low surface tension and smaller contact angle than hyaluronic acid results in greater coatability of ocular structures and IOL surface
Space Maintenance	Less effective than hyaluronic acid due to no pseudoplasticity; when deformed, the material is unlikely to recover its original shape
Endothelial Protection	The properties of viscoadhesion are thought to result in protection against pressure and shifting forces. Compared to hyaluronic acid, it does not possess receptors on the endothelial surface and has no scavenger effect against free radicals during phacoemulsification; nevertheless, several studies show the effectiveness of HPMC in endothelial protection
Tissue Manipulation	Excessive force must be applied to achieve gradual shifting and placing of the material; therefore tissue manipulation is limited
Uses, Advantages, and Disadvantages	Occucoat costs less than viscoelastics of animal origin; visibility is poorer when compared with other viscoelastics; air bubbles are likely to be trapped inside HPMC; no biologic mechanism eliminates the product intraocularly; nuclear fragments or cortex may be "incarcerated" in the material during phaco
Syringe	1 mL of product in three-section syringe to be assembled, with 27-G cannula needle kit; advisable to fill needle with BSS to prevent formation of air bubbles; 1-year shelf life

The main advantages of this material are low cost, ability to store at environment temperature, and a large amount of product provided in the syringe (Occucoat 1 mL; Hymecel 2 mL; Adatocel 2.25 mL; Cellugel 1.5 mL).

The interesting feature of this material is its viscoadhesion, despite low molecular weight and absent viscosity.

The small contact angle and low surface tension have proved to be useful to ensure adhesion to instruments, tissues, and implants.

When compared with the contact angle of materials made of hyaluronic acid of different molecular weights, HPMC has the best wettability for PMMA surfaces. Due to the smaller size of its molecular chains, 97% of this is eliminated through the trabecular meshwork 24 hours after injection in the AC.

Studies performed by Storz on postoperative IOP when HPMC is intentionally left in the AC showed a temporary pressure increase that requires no pressure-reducing medications. Nevertheless, complete removal of the product after surgery is recommended.

This study contrasts the work of Chumbley et al, who demonstrated a remarkable IOP increase 24 hours following surgery when HPMC has not been removed. Features of this material that provide endothelial protection from shifting or contact forces include high adhesion to endothelial surface and good biocompatibility with no presence of intraocular inflammatory reactions. Clinical studies using an endothelial cells abrasion test (Glasser) did

Table 4-10.
HYMECEL

Storage	Room temperature
Molecular weight	86,000 Daltons
Concentration	2% HPMC
Viscosity at 0 shear rate	4000
Viscosity at 1000 shear rate	300
	Features
Injectability	Difficult to accomplish through a thin cannula (25-G is in the kit provided) due to problems with the piston, which brings air in when not kept under pressure
Removability	Viscoadhesive product, requires longer times than cohesive materials for removal
Adhesiveness	High coatability on implants and instrument surfaces, similar to Occucoat, Adatocel, and Cellugel
Space Maintenance	This is proportional to molecular weight and high viscosity; Hymecel has molecular weight 45 times lower than Healon® whereas viscosity at 0 shear rate is 15 times lower. Space maintenance is therefore remarkably less than that of Healon®
Endothelial Protection	Protection is theoretically equal to Healon®, although some studies report higher and lower values; because HPMC is a vegetable material, neither receptors on the endothelial surface nor scavenger effect have been demonstrated
Tissue Manipulation	This material does not have a soft spatula effect, and the material is less manageable than Healon®, which is far more pseudoplastic
Uses, Advantages, and Disadvantages	Hymecel is viscoadherent and not viscoelastic; it remains in the anterior chamber, does not keep space, and is not suitable for advanced surgery
Syringe	2 mL of product with 25-G cannula-needle; 3 years shelf life

Table 4-11.
CELLUGEL

Storage	Room temperature
Molecular Weight	100 K
Concentration	2% modified HPMC
Viscosity at 0 Shear Rate	10,000–25,000
Viscosity at 1000 Shear Rate	500
	Features
Injectability	Difficult through a 27-G cannula; poor feedback with 25-G cannula owing to minimal pseudoplastic features-
Removability	Lower cohesiveness of molecules results in longer irrigation/aspiration times, similar to Occucoat, Hymecel, and Adatocel
Adhesiveness/Coatability	This is high on the surface of implants and instruments, as in Occucoat and Adatocel
Space Maintenance	This is proportional to molecular weight and high viscosity; the molecular weight of Cellugel is 40 times lower than that of Healon, and viscosity at 0 shear rate is 15 times lower. When deformed, the material cannot recover its original shape
Endothelial Protection	All HPMC–based products provide viscoadhesion to endothelial surface, which protects from pressure and shifting forces; the material does not have receptors on the endothelium, nor scavenger effect against the release of free radicals during phaco
Tissue Manipulation	The material has no soft spatula features like Healon or products with analogous chemical or physical properties; its positioning does not occur gradually or through infusion pressure, as with highly pseudoplastic and highly viscous materials
Uses, Advantages, and Disadvantages	Cellugel is a viscoadherent, nonviscoelastic material that is sterilizable and has some permanence in the AC
Syringe	1.5 mL of product with 25-G cannula-needle; 2-year shelf life.

not demonstrate differences in protection provided by HPMC 2% and Healon®, Amvisc, and Viscoat.

Hammer et al conducted a study performing an abrasion test on endothelial surfaces protected by a thin layer of Healon® or HPMC. They showed that HPMC protects the endothelium as effectively as a thick layer of Healon® and better than a thin layer. Studies have shown that wood-pulp derivatives are clinically nontoxic to living tissues.

Tests based on HPMC injection in the AC of rabbit eyes, antibody evocation tests on guinea pigs, and other toxicologic and immunologic tests showed that HPMC is neither pyrogenic nor immunogenic. Furthermore, HPMC is soluble in the aqueous humor and is therefore easier to remove than hyaluronic acid.

Occucoat is marketed as an inexpensive and advanced viscoelastic that is transparent, biocompatible, and comparable to hyaluronic acid for the protection of corneal endothelium and maintenance of AC depth. The manufacturer reports greater effectiveness than Healon® in endothelial protection and space maintenance.

Adatocel and Hymecel are described by the manufacturers as pseudoplastic and elastic viscoelastics made of nontoxic materials that can be diluted in the aqueous humor and therefore easily removed. They are also reportedly able to form an AC volume, stabilize ocular tissues, and protect the corneal endothelium.

The following comments refer to HPMC materials:

- The product is difficult to inject through a small cannula owing to its adhesion and poor pseudoplasticity (5400 cps at 0 shear rate and 300 at 1000 shear rate)
- Under high temperature, the solubility of HPMC drops, causing molecular aggregation and polysaccharide coagulation
- During Occucoat's lifetime, there have been reports of inflammatory reactions and withdrawal of lots for sterility and assembly problems—i.e., 6697 pieces were withdrawn for leakage out of the syringe in 1990, 6478 pieces were withdrawn due to sterility problems in 1991, and 33,189 pieces had assembly problems in 1992. Between 1983 and 1989, there were several reports of inflammation and impurities (Singh, Yamanda, Koster, Pfeiffer), presence of vegetable particles (Rosen), and steady mydriasis following use of HPMC (Tan)

Occucoat is also reportedly indicated for advanced surgical procedures. We believe that the value of Occucoat lies in its convenient price and sufficient surgical performance. Nevertheless, owing to its chemical and physical features, it is not recommended for use in complicated surgery, as Healon® is 75 times more viscous and 500 times more elastic. These properties result in differences in space maintenance and soft and permanent spatula effects. HPMC also comes out of the AC when positive pressure is exerted.

In addition, greater endothelial protection by HPMC has never been proven. Hyaluronic acid can boast a triple mechanism of corneal endothelial protection (hyaluronic acid binding sites, scavenger effect, and mechanical protection).

It has been frequently noticed that HPMC is likely to trap air microbubbles, which may hamper the surgeon's visibility.

When used for phacoemulsification, the properties of HPMC can be summarized as in Table 4-12.

VITRAX

Vitrax (Table 4-14) is a nonpyrogenic sterile viscoelastic solution made of highly purified noninflammatory sodium hyaluronate (3%) diluted in BSS. Vitrax is supplied in a disposable glass syringe, filled with 0.5 or 0.8 mL, with 25-G cannula. Its pH value is 7 to 7.5 and besides sodium hyaluronate the preparation contains sodium, potassium, calcium, and magnesium.

Its molecular weight is 645,000 daltons; viscosity at zero shear rate is equal to 40,000, whereas the value at 1000 shear rate is 640.

The product is to be stored at room temperature (15 to 30 °C), protected from intense light and cold.

Approved by the FDA in August 1989, the preparation was launched at the American Academy of Ophthalmology annual meeting in Fall 1989. The feature specific to Vitrax is a lower endothelial toxicity than Healon® (studies by Bourrie and Genstler). The decreased toxicity is thought to be related to the mixture of sodium hyaluronate and BSS. Additionally, Vitrax contains calcium, magnesium, potassium, citrate, acetate, ions, and electrolytes that are necessary for normal metabolism and cell integrity.

Table 4-12.
PHACOEMULSIFICATION STEPS AND HPMC PROPERTIES

Phaco Step	Property of HPMC
Injectability in Anterior Chamber	Poor, owing to its adhesion; large cannula required
Capsulorhexis	Poor maintenance of space due to low viscosity at low shear rate and low molecular weight
Hydrodissection	Performs well
Phacoemulsification	Good corneal endothelial protection as shown in several studies
Irrigation and Aspiration of Cortical Material	Good protective effect
Capsular bag filling	Not indicated owing to very poor pseudoplasticity and ability to form space
IOL implantation	Useful owing to viscoadhesion to corneal endothelium, IOL, and instruments
Removal	Adhesion makes removal more difficult; the time to remove Healon®, Healon® GV, Viscoat, and Occucoat has been measured, and Healon® and Healon® GV were completely removed in 20 seconds, whereas Viscoat took 3.5 minutes. Occucoat was removed in less than 1 minute

Table 4-13.
SAFETY AND EFFECTIVENESS OF OCCUCOAT VERSUS SODIUM HYALURONATE

Safety Feature	Occucoat	Sodium Hyaluronate
Adverse reactions	0%	0%
Postoperative complications	24.7%	26.8%
Postoperative IOP increase		
> 5 mmHg	26.5%	33.3%
>30 mmHg	3.2%	10.2%
Effectiveness		
Deep AC	99.4%	80.4%
Easier surgery	99.4%	82.1%
Endothelial cell loss	12.1%	10%

Table 4-14.
VITRAX

Storage	Room temperature; protect from light and low temperature
Molecular Weight	645 K
Concentration	3% Hyaluronic acid
Viscosity at 0 Shear Rate	40,000
Viscosity at 1000 Shear Rate	640
Features	
Injectability	Difficult to inject secondary to high viscosity at 1000 shear rate; very large cannula (25-G) is required
Removability	Owing to adhesion to tissue and implants, removal takes longer than with cohesive viscoelastics
Adhesiveness/Coatability	High adhesiveness but lower than Viscoat
Space Maintenance	Less space maintenance than that achieved by other more viscous materials; its low molecular weight hinders this function
Endothelial Protection	The degree of endothelial protection provided by Vitrax is not as well documented as that for Healon®. Vitrax is preserved in a hyperosmolar solution containing calcium and magnesium, which could be harmful to the isoosmolar environment of the aqueous humor and damage the endothelium
Tissue Manipulation	Tissue manipulation is not as effective with Vitrax as with other higher molecular weight materials; poorly adjustable injectability also impedes this function
Uses, Advantages, and Disadvantages	Vitrax is marketed as designed for phacoemulsification; it is more expensive than Healon®; it is likely to trap air bubbles and can be difficult to remove
Syringe	0.5–0.8 mL in preassembled glass syringe; 25-G cannula needle kit; 18-month shelf life

Based on a study conducted by Cobo et al, which relied on the personal impressions of several surgeons comparing Vitrax with other viscoelastics (Healon®, Viscoat, and Amvisc), it has been asserted that visibility, maintenance of AC depth, and permanent spatula effect are almost equal in Vitrax and Healon®, with Vitrax holding a slight advantage. Moreover, Vitrax has greater adhesion. The fact that it is not necessary to refrigerate Vitrax has been touted as a great advantage of this material. Nevertheless, the number of publications concerning Vitrax is limited and Cobo et al's study has limitations. The surgical techniques used in the multicenter study differed and the outcome was often subjectively reported by the surgeons on a 1 to 4 scale.

With a molecular weight six times lower than Healon®, Vitrax does not have enough viscosity (at 0 shear rate the value is five times lower) or pseudoplasticity to achieve good soft spatula performance. In addition, Vitrax has poor injectability (at 1000 shear rate viscosity is four times higher) and removability. Regarding the reported lower toxicity of Vitrax when compared with Healon®, a study by McCulley has demonstrated the opposite result.

Healon®'s strength is its clinical safety, as it has been tested in over 400 studies. Regarding adhesion to tissues and surfaces—specifically, the corneal endothelium—no studies are available comparing the proved triple mechanism of protection particular to Healon® with the protection provided by Vitrax. The observation that Healon® causes a higher IOP rise when compared with Vitrax (increase over 5 mmHg: 37% Healon® versus 24% Vitrax; over 20 mmHg: 35% Healon® versus 28% Vitrax) is reported in one clinical study only, with different techniques and a control group that consists of four different viscoelastic materials.

Among the viscoelastics containing sodium hyaluronate, Vitrax has the lowest molecular weight, the lowest viscosity at 0 shear rate, and the least pseudoplasticity. However, Vitrax is classified as an adhesive material with viscosity, and for this reason it should be grouped with Viscoat (which sometimes has higher adhesion) and Amvisc Plus (which is more viscous and pseudoplastic).

The product does not require refrigeration because its low molecular weight does not require it. As for the observation that Vitrax is the only viscoelastic containing calcium and magnesium, ions essential in the maintenance of endothelial cell metabolism, this aspect is irrelevant with reference to osmotic tolerance, as Healon® is isotonic. Moreover, the calcium contained in Vitrax is not compatible with an irrigation solution containing phosphate (BSS) as the formation of precipitates may occur. In the early development of Healon® calcium was introduced, but later removed as it turned out to be detrimental to cell viability.

Based on its physical and chemical characteristics, Vitrax must be considered as a viscoelastic material with fair ability to maintain spaces, poor pseudoplasticity (it remains in the AC, adheres to the endothelium), and low cohesion that makes removal difficult. Vitrax is a useful material both in the performance of phacoemulsification and ECCE surgery. When the surgeon is faced with complicated cases, a material with better viscosity and pseudoplasticity is recommended. Also, when a more adhesive material is required, other materials are preferred.

Biolon

Recently introduced, Biolon (Table 4-15) consists of 1% hyaluronic acid derived from bacterial fermentation (streptococci), has a molecular weight equal to 3 M daltons, and viscosity 150,000 cps at 0 shear rate. The viscosity value at 1000 shear rate is not indicated, but in our analysis was 180 cps.

Few clinical studies are available about the chemical and physical features of the material and its comparison with other viscoelastics. It is supplied in a preassembled syringe with 27-G cannula needle kit, and the amounts available are 0.5 or 1 mL. It requires refrigeration (like Healon®, Healon® GV, Amvisc, and Amvisc Plus) and its lifetime is 3 years.

Product safety is ensured by a test developed by Bio-Technology General, similar to the owl monkey test, where the material to be tested is inoculated in rat peritoneum. Bio-Technology General declares that the test is as reliable as the owl monkey test used by Pharmacia & Upjohn. At the European Society of Cataract and Refractive Surgery meeting in Innsbruck in September 1993, Colin (France) and Frucht-Perey (Israel) presented two clinical studies comparing Healon® with Biolon and concluded that both products were similar.

Although both products have the same active component (sodium hyaluronate), we believe the materials are not really similar: the source of hyaluronate is different, the production process is different, and quality control, quality assurance, and assessment criteria for admission of the various lots to the market are different. The container for storage is not similar. Data regarding sterilization of the product are not available.

Because there are few studies in the literature regarding Biolon, and the clinical experience has been limited compared to Healon®, more extensive scientific and clinical assessment is necessary. Based on the chemical–physical characteristics of Biolon and limited clinical experience, the product seems to be comparable to Healon® in injectability, space maintenance, protection, and removability.

Collagel

Because there is little published research available regarding Collagel (Table 4-16), assessment of this product is not possible. The product was introduced in 1991, and has undergone many difficulties since then. In France there was a reluctance to use this material secondary to concerns regarding HIV infection in materials derived from human products. In the Netherlands, the product was distributed but not registered, and in Denmark it has not been registered.

IAL

IAL (Table 4-17) consists of 1% hyaluronic acid with molecular weight ranging from 500 to 700 K, 6 to 8 times lighter than Healon®.

Table 4-15.
BIOLON

Storage	Refrigeration
Molecular Weight	3 M
Concentration	Hyaluronic acid 1% (bacterial fermentation)
Viscosity at 0 Shear Rate	150,000
Viscosity at 1000 Shear Rate	NA
Features	
Injectability	Good through a 27-G cannula
Removability	Slightly more difficult than Healon®
Adhesiveness/Coatability	It is a material with medium adhesion, less than Viscoat, and comparable to Healon®
Space Maintenance	Good space maintenance; viscosity at zero shear rate is less than Healon®
Endothelial Protection	No documented ability to bind with endothelial binding receptors (binding sites)
Tissue Manipulation	Useful soft spatula effect, less than that provided by materials with higher pseudoplasticity
Uses, Advantages, and Disadvantages	Biolon is a viscoelastic designed for the performance of phacoemulsification and ECCE surgery and has fair pseudoplasticity and high molecular weight. It is inexpensive and is subject to less biologic control than Healon®; it has been studied in a small number of international publications
Syringe	0.5–1 mL of product in preassembled syringe, 27-G cannula needle kit, 3-year shelf life

Table 4-16.
COLLAGEL

Storage	Refrigeration
Molecular Weight	1 M
Concentration	1.4% Collagen IV (extracted from human placenta)
Viscosity at 0 Shear Rate	2,000,000 at 25 °C–1,500 at 37 °C
Viscosity at 1000 Shear Rate	200 at 25 °C
Features	
Injectability	Not available
Removability	Not available
Adhesiveness/Coatability	Not available
Space Maintenance	Elastic features are more prominent than viscosity; viscosity rapidly changes with increasing temperature: fair at 25 °C, very poor at 37 °C. Surgical volumes are not as stable as hyaluronic acid materials with the same molecular weight. Decreased transparency has been reported when the material has been exposed to BSS
Endothelial Protection	Some studies demonstrate that collagen protects endothelial cells; no endothelial cell receptors have been documented
Tissue Manipulation	Rheologic changes with temperature results in poor soft spatula effect
Uses, Advantages, and Disadvantages	The production of this material has been halted due to concerns regarding HIV infection through human-derived products
Syringe	1 mL

The product's viscosity at 1000 shear rate is comparable to that of Healon®, whereas at 0 shear rate it is 70 times lower. These values imply poor pseudoplasticity compared with other hyaluronic acid products with better rheologic characteristics.

The space maintenance effect, which is a function of the molecular weight and viscosity at zero shear rate, is rather poor, and the product is likely to come out of the AC. Endothelial protection is ineffective, as it is poorly viscous and not viscoadherent.

The greatest advantages of this material are its defects: fluidity and poor adhesiveness make it injectable through narrow cannulas and result in easy removal. Most surgeons find this product easy to manage but with limited surgical utility and tissue manipulation.

IAL was used more frequently in the early days of ocular implant surgery when most of the surgery performed was ECCE and a deep AC was maintained, even with air injection in the AC. As phacoemulsification became more widespread, the use of viscoelastics with high and highest molecular weight (Healon®, Healon® GV) and viscoadherent materials (Viscoat, Vitrax) led to a progressive decrease in the use of IAL.

The limit of IAL is demonstrated by the large quantity of product supplied in the vial (2 to 5 mL). Such a large amount is supplied as the product is likely to come out through surgical incisions during the performance of various maneuvers.

According to the manufacturer, IAL may be left in the eye at the end of surgery owing to its low molecular weight and short molecular chains, which results in partial metabolism in the AC and outflow through the trabeculum. As a result, postoperative IOP is only minimally affected. In our experience, however, all viscoelastic should be removed from the AC at the end of surgery.

Regarding inflammatory reactions induced by the product, Cavaliere showed that the two IAL samples tested in the monkey eye test caused endovitreal precipitates.

With respect to endothelial protection, studies have been performed considering preoperative values and values at 30 days after surgery, but cell density stabilization occurs after at least 3 months.

A further weak point of IAL is the sterilization process, which is performed in an autoclave with the product in vials without Luer-Lok syringes.

IAL-F

The evolution of surgical techniques, both in cataract surgery and in posterior segment surgery, has led to the need for viscoelastic materials with high molecular weight, with strong ability to form space, and that provide good tissue protection. Fidia has introduced a new viscoelastic, IAL-F (Table 4-18), to complement its well-known viscoelastic product IAL.

The advantages of IAL are well known and described previously. It consists of hyaluronic acid, is very well tolerated, has low molecular weight, and shows no distinguished viscosity. Even when not removed at the end of surgery it causes no significant IOP increase. Nevertheless, in the performance of maneuvers where space formation and strong soft and permanent spatula effect are fundamental, the material has limitations.

For this reason, Fidia has produced IAL-F, a viscoelastic material consisting mainly of hyaluronic acid extracted from cockscomb, with a molecular weight equal to 1.2 M. There is a significant difference between IAL-F and Healon®, which has higher molecular weight and more than triple the viscosity at 0 shear rate.

As a result, the surgeon cannot expect the same ability to form space as with Healon®, with poorer soft and permanent spatula effects. Nevertheless, IAL-F is interesting to the ocular surgeon: in fact, viscoelastic materials protect the corneal endothelium not only because they create space, but also because they cover the endothelium in a protective layer. Coatability and consequent protection also depend on the contact angle between fluid and tissues, and therefore on the surface tension of hyaluronic acid solutions. The smaller the contact angle between solution and endothelium, the greater the protective effect of the product.

Hyaluronic acid solutions have a smaller contact angle and therefore better protective effect for the endothelium, and the lower the polymer molecular weight along with the higher concentration, the better protective effect. In this respect, IAL-F (molecular weight 1.2, concentration 1.8%) has turned out to be among the most effective products made of hyaluronic acid on the market.

IAL-F is well tolerated; it consists of a concentrated solution in prefilled syringe, made of a well-defined percentage of hyaluronic acid that is the

Table 4-17.
IAL

Storage	Refrigeration
Molecular Weight	500 K
Concentration	1% Hyaluronic acid extracted from cockscomb
Viscosity at 0 Shear Rate	3300
Viscosity at 1000 Shear Rate	210
	Features
Injectability	Pseudoplasticity and low viscosity result in good injectability
Removability	Easy removal consequent to high fluidity
Adhesiveness/Coatability	Poor coatability due to reduced molecular cohesiveness
Space Maintenance	IAL does not remain in the AC during surgical maneuvers owing to low viscosity
Endothelial Protection	IAL binds to hyaluronic acid binding sites; endothelial protection is not as predictable as with Healon®, due to its lower molecular weight. Few studies have been performed to examine endothelial cell loss; insufficient data are available to assess the effectiveness of the product in postoperative protection
Tissue Manipulation	The product coats tissues, but its soft/permanent spatula effect is poorer than that of viscoelastics with higher molecular weight or concentration
Uses, Advantages, and Disadvantages	IAL is inexpensive and a greater quantity is supplied compared with other viscoelastics; however, as the material tends to come out of the eye, the surgeon must use more material than with the higher molecular weight viscoelastics
Syringe	Glass container with 2 mL (IAL 24) and 5 mL (IAL 60); 2-year shelf life

Table 4-18.
IAL-F

Storage	Refrigeration
Molecular Weight	1.2 M
Concentration	1.8% Hyaluronic acid (derived from cockscomb)
Viscosity at 0 Shear Rate	61,500
Viscosity at 1000 Shear Rate	380
	Features
Injectability	Good injectability through a 27-G cannula owing to good pseudoplasticity
Removability	The product can be removed easily, but the size of the molecules dictates that complete removal is not necessary and the product is well tolerated if left behind
Adhesiveness/Coatability	A high concentration (1.8%) of hyaluronic acid with medium molecular weight (1.2) provides IAL-F with good adhesion and better wettability of tissues and instruments
Space Maintenance	The product exhibits a fair tendency to create and maintain spaces; it does not maintain volumes as well as products with higher molecular weight
Endothelial Protection	IAL-F dampens pressure and friction forces and protects corneal endothelium from the free radicals generated during phaco due to the scavenger effect of hyaluronic
Tissue Manipulation	The product allows good tissue manipulation (soft/permanent spatula effect) due to the relationship between the concentration and molecular weight of hyaluronic acid
Uses, Advantages, and Disadvantages	Useful in ECCE with or without IOL implantation and phaco; also useful in trabeculectomy and corneal surgery; low price; no international clinical reports available
Syringe	1.1 mL in a prefilled syringe without cannula needle kit and with Luer-Lok

same as that used for IAL, a well-known product that has been on the market for some time.

Although it has the same tolerability as IAL, IAL-F ensures greater viscosity and elasticity, although lower than those provided by Healon®.

When compared with IAL, this product is less fluid, but can maintain spaces better, with no occurrence of ocular pressure increase when not removed, a drawback specific to other hyaluronic acid–based materials with higher molecular weight.

Studies performed by Stirpe et al (1992) have shown that IAL-F is effective in extracapsular cataract surgery. The product is also useful in ocular trauma (contusion or perforating trauma), as demonstrated by Dal Fiume et al (1992). It can be successfully used in posterior segment surgery as well, owing to its space-forming features with soft spatula effect, as demonstrated by Reiboldi et al (1992).

In our experience IAL-F demonstrated optimal injectability owing to its good pseudoplasticity and enough ability to form space in routine cases, but still less than that provided by Healon®. Therefore, Healon® and Healon® GV are more useful in difficult cases, where higher viscosity at low shear rate is required.

The contact angle, smaller than that of Healon®, and lower surface tension ensure excellent filling effect and optimal adaptability onto anatomic surfaces. No alterations have been observed in the corneal endothelium, and no inflammatory phenomena have been noted.

Even when not removed at the end of surgery, the product causes minimal IOP increase, and therefore it is useful not only in cataract surgery but in glaucoma and corneal surgery as well.

IAL-F is inexpensive and the amount of product in the syringe is large (1.1 mL).

Table 4-19.
PROPERTIES OF VISCOELASTICS

	SOURCE	PROVIDED BY	MOLECULAR WEIGHT	CONCENTRATION	PH	OSMOLALITY mosm/Kg H_2O
HEALON®	Rooster comb	Pharmacia & Upjohn	4.0 M	1% hyaluronic acid	7.0-7.5	302
HEALON® GV	Rooster comb	Pharmacia & Upjohn	5.0 M	1.4% hyaluronic acid	7.0-7.5	310
AMVISC	Rooster comb	Chiron	1.0 M	1% hyaluronic acid	6.5-7.2	318
AMVISC PLUS	Rooster comb	Chiron	2.0 M	1.6% hyaluronic acid	7.2	340
VISCOAT	Bacterial fermentation (HaNa) Shark fin (chondroitin sulfate)	Alcon	200 K + 25 K	3% hyaluronic acid 4% chondroitin sulfate	7.0-7.5	325
OCCUCOAT	Cellulose paste	Storz	86 K	2% hydroxypropyl methylcellulose	7.2	285
CELLUGEL	Cellulose paste	Vision Biology	100 K	2.2% hydroxypropyl methylcellulose	7.0-7.4	305
MICROVISC	Rooster comb	Domilens	4 M	1.0% hyaluronic acid	7.0-7.5	336
MICROVISC PLUS	Rooster comb	Domilens	5 M	1,4% hyaluronic acid	n.d.	N.D.
BIOLON	Bacterial fermentation	Bio Technology General	3 M	1.0% hyaluronic acid	7.3	340
VITRAX	Rooster comb	Allergan	645 K	3.0% hyaluronic acid	7.0-7.5	310
IAL	Rooster comb	Fidia	500 K	1.0% hyaluronic acid	7.2312	
ADATOCEL	Cellulose paste	Adatomed	86 K	2% hydroxypropyl methylcellulose	6.6	300
PROVISC	Bacterial fermentation	Alcon	1.9/2.5 M	1.1% hyaluronic acid	7.2	310

Table 4-20.
PROPERTIES AND CLINICAL FEATURES OF THE PRINCIPALS VISCOELASTIC PRODUCTS

PRODUCT	COMPOSITION	MOLECULAR	VISCOSITY 0 WEIGHT	VISCOSITY 1000 SHEAR RATE	COHESION SHEAR RATE	ADHESIVENESS	PRESERVATION	PLUS	MINUS
HEALON®	1% hyaluronic acid (rooster combs)	4.0 M	200.000	150	high	low	refrigeration	- excellent biological controls - transparent - easy to use an remove - space maintenance - soft spatula - endothelium protection (HABS)	- may run out of wound during phaco
HEALON® GV	1.4% hyaluronic acid	5.0 M	2.000.000	200	high	low	refrigeration	- high viscosity - optical clarity - space maintenance - easy removal - pediatric/demanding cases - IOL implantation	- may run out of wound during phaco - IOP rise if not removed
VISCOAT	3% hyaluronic acid – bacterial fermentation 4% chondroitin sulfate shark fin	500 K (Ha Na) 25 K (CDS)	41.000	200	low	high	refrigeration (vertical position)	- stays in during phaco - endothelium protection - capsular breaks	- bubbles - difficult to remove - difficult for IOL implantation - difficult to inject
OCCUCOAT HYMECEL CELLUGEL	2% hydroxypropyl methylcellulose (cellulose paste)	86+100 K	5.400 (Occucoat) 4.000 (Hymecel) 10.000/25.000 (Cellugel)	240 (Occucoat) 300 (Hymecel) 500 (Cellugel)	low	high	no refrigeration	- inexpensive - no refrigeration - low cost	- low viscosity - runs out during phaco - bubbles - difficult to implant
PROVISC	1% hyaluronic acid (rooster combs)	1.9/2.5 M	150.000	190	high	low	refrigeration	- low cost - easy to inject and remove - optical clarity - soft spatula	- runs out during phaco
BIOLON	1% hyaluronic acid (fermentation)	3 M	150.000	n.d.	high	low	refrigeration	- low cost - easy to inject and remove - soft spatula - transparent	- runs out during phaco
AMVISC	1% hyaluronic acid (rooster combs)	1.0 M	100.000	240	high	low	refrigeration	- easy to inject and remove - optical clarity - low cost	- runs out during phaco
AMVISC PLUS	1.2% hyaluronic acid (rooster combs)	1.5 M	84.000	360	medium	medium	refrigeration	- easy to inject - stays in - transparent	- difficult to remove
IAL	1.2% hyaluronic acid (rooster combs)	1 M	11.000	210	low	medium	refrigeration	- low cost - easy to inject - transparent	- low space maintenance - runs out
IAL-F	1.8% hyaluronic acid (rooster combs)	1 M	61.500	380	medium	high	refrigeration	- low cost - easy to inject - transparent	- bubbles
VITRAX	3% hyaluronic acid (rooster combs)	645 K	40.000	640	low	high	no refrigeration	- storage - stay in	- transparent - difficult to inject - bubbles - low viscosity

CHAPTER FIVE

Viscoelastic Materials and Corneal Endothelium

Corneal endothelium is a thin layer of nonregenerable cells that ensure dehydration and transparency of the overlying cell layers. Corneal endothelium is the tissue most affected by the performance of intraocular surgery because various factors such as instrument manipulation, cortical and nuclear materials, IOLs, turbulence of irrigation fluids, microbubbles, and free radicals produced by phacoemulsification may cause endothelial cell loss.

To protect the corneal endothelium, viscoelastic materials are used during all intraocular procedures. The features that provide this protection are summarized in the following:

- Endothelial adhesion (coatability)
- Maintenance of the AC
- Shielding against compressive and shifting force (drag force)
- Preservation of endothelial metabolism
  Safe removal at the end of the procedure

Viscoelastic material that is able to cover the endothelium with effective adhesion should provide protection from mechanical forces possibly due to sliding of intraocular implants and instruments on a plane parallel to the endothelial surface. At the same time, no biochemical interaction should be present between the material and the endothelial surface that might prevent viscoelastic removal. Viscoat, consisting of 3% hyaluronic acid and 4% chondroitin sulfate, has a low superficial tension that makes it adherent to intraocular surfaces with excellent coatability, and it is able to resist the forces tending to push it out of the AC. However, Viscoat tends to trap air microbubbles, which can damage the endothelial surface.

On the contrary, viscoelastics with sodium hyaluronate such as Healon® GV, Healon®, Provisc, Amvisc, Amvisc Plus, and Biolon, having high molecular weight, should provide good endothelial protection against the shifting (parallel) and compressive (perpendicular) forces produced by the movement of irrigation fluids during phacoemulsification and irrigation and aspiration of viscoelastic materials. Potential damage to endothelial cells could result from a material with high molecular weight, high viscosity, and internal cohesion, which produces a "shearing" force that affects cells, causing damage due to friction and dragging.

When considering materials with high molecular weight, it is important for the sake of endothelial protection to remember that higher viscosity at 0 shear rate and high pseudoplasticity ensure space maintenance, whereas high elasticity, which opposes vertical compression forces, facilitates quick recovery of the material's original volume as soon as the forces cease to exert pressure.

Contrary to this, the high superficial tension and internal cohesion of all products containing sodium hyaluronate enables the surgeon to remove the material from the AC as a whole, with a greater amount of ease than with more adherent materials such as Viscoat or HPMC. This may be a disadvantage—for instance, in the presence of high flow during phacoemulsification, little viscoelastic is left to protect the endothelium.

Pharmacia & Upjohn (Healon®, Healon® GV) first observed the presence of specific receptors for hyaluronic acid on the endothelial surface (ie, hyaluronic acid binding sites) (Figure 5-1). They also demonstrated that their products are able to neutralize free radicals released during phacoemulsification (scavenger effect). These two important aspects, along with the "mechanical" protection of hyaluronic acid, provide threefold protection for corneal endothelium. This contradicts the theory that viscoadherent materials (Viscoat, 2% HPMC) may provide greater protection, as they can "adhere" and remain in contact with the endothelium longer.

Viscoelastic use in anterior segment surgery involves several fundamental factors that result in endothelial cell protection, many of which do not belong to one single viscoelastic.

ELASTICITY

Elasticity allows the viscoelastic to deform and then recover its original mass. It ensures good defense against the compressive forces exerted vertically on endothelial cells, thus enabling the viscoelastic to "absorb" the shocks generated by vibrations of the phaco tip. There is no unit of measurement currently available for elasticity, but it is closely related to pseudoplasticity: the ability of a viscoelastic to change its own viscosity exponentially while sliding increases as the viscous materials become fluid. High elasticity is a feature particular to materials with high to very high molecular weight (Healon®, Healon® GV, Provisc, Biolon) where long molecular chains are extremely entangled and can better endure shocks. Viscoat, Amvisc Plus, and Vitrax have lower elasticity, and HPMC (Occucoat, Hymecel, Adatocel, and Cellugel) has no elasticity.

If mechanical energy is applied to sodium hyaluronate at low frequency or at slow impact, the solution reacts with viscous motion. High frequency mechanical damage due to phacoemulsification or irrigation flow causes deformation of the molecular chains and the mechanical energy is counterbalanced by elasticity. The higher the hyaluronic acid concentration, the more its molecular chains get entangled and compressed and the higher the viscosity and elasticity of the solution. This results in better endothelial protection from mechanical shocks.

Arshinoff points out that a viscoelastic with greater elasticity than viscosity may become a sort of intraocular spring that could hinder surgical maneuvers. For this reason, the ideal viscoelastic, safe for the endothelium and useful as a surgical tool, should be equally elastic and viscous so that no mutual hindrance can be present.

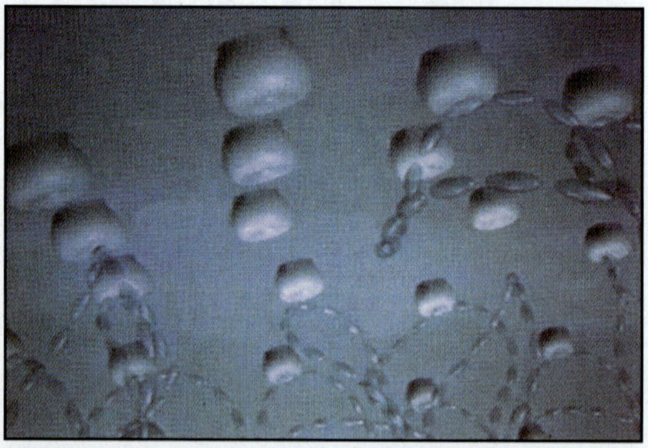

Figure 5-1. Hyaluronic acid binding sites.

COHESIVENESS–ADHESION

Cohesiveness is the tendency of molecules in a material to stick to one another due to their chemical bonds. Hyaluronic acid materials are highly cohesive. Introduced into the AC, these materials are likely to leave the filled space uniformly (en bloc) owing to cohesion between molecular chains. This feature makes aspiration easier.

However, for some products (Healon®, Biolon), this particular aspect of cohesion can harm the corneal endothelium, as premature aspiration could leave part of the internal corneal surface exposed to the mechanical shocks of vibrations and flow. Cohesiveness and pseudoplasticity help ease nuclear expression during ECCE while preventing potential abrasion of the endothelial surface. However, during the subsequent irrigation and aspiration phase, the endothelium is more exposed to BSS flow and therefore more susceptible to damage.

Some materials such as Viscoat, Amvisc Plus, Vitrax, and HPMC show adhesiveness to the endothelial surface, which is the result of low superficial tension. Adhesive materials protect endothelial cells well because of their ability to resist the internal flows produced during phacoemulsification of the nucleus.

Nevertheless, adhesiveness has a potentially harmful implication for the endothelium itself. In fact, longer aspiration time required to remove the whole material may damage the endothelial cells. Moreover, it has been observed that more adhesive materials tend to trap potentially dangerous microbubbles.

VISCOELASTIC MATERIAL BUFFERING– ISO-OSMOLARITY

Buffering and iso-osmolarity provide the viscoelastic with perfect biocompatibility. Buffering of the viscoelastic occurs when pH is equal to 7.0 and may vary slightly according to the material. For instance, Healon®, Healon® GV, and Viscoat have a pH value ranging from 7.0 to 7.5.

Initially, Viscoat and chondroitin sulfate were prepared with higher concentrations of phosphates, which were found to precipitate in the stroma in the form of calcium deposits.

When manufactured by IOLab, Amvisc was distributed in a nonbuffered saline solution. In some stocks, pH value was found to range between 6.1 and 6.4. Should the pH value of the solution turn out to be less than 6.8, morphologic and functional damage can occur in endothelial cells.

Osmolality indicates the solute concentration per solvent unit. The value of intercellular fluid osmolality is 300 mOsmol/Kg. If viscoelastic osmolality, which depends on concentration, is greater than this value, the risk of corneal endothelium dehydration increases. For instance, the 4% osmolarity of chondroitin sulfate present in Viscoat has an osmolality that is 20% too high for the endothelium. Vitrax, which contains 3% hyaluronic acid, is preserved in hyperosmolar solution containing calcium and magnesium. This could be in conflict with the iso-osmolar environment of the aqueous humor toward the endothelial barrier. The values associated with each viscoelastic are shown in the Tables in Chapter 4.

CHEMICAL BONDS–INTRAOCULAR HYALURONATE: COMPARISON WITH VISCOADHERENT MATERIALS

Hyaluronate is naturally present in ocular tissues: sclera, limbus, conjunctival stroma, ciliary body, iris stroma, vitreous, and endothelial surface (Lutjien Drecoll et al 1990). Molander et al (1993) also found hyaluronate in zonular fibers and in the corneal incision (after ECCE in human and rabbit eyes),which he proposed might be a consequence of the healing process of the corneal tissue. Fitzsimmons et al (1991) observed that hyaluronate increased in corneal tissue after excimer laser treatment.

Using synovial cell hyaluronate labeled with tritium and commercial hyaluronate (Healon®) in 1989, Madsen et al demonstrated that:

- Specific protein receptors for hyaluronic acid are present on the surface of corneal endothelial cells (hyaluronic acid binding sites).
- Hyaluronic acid is organized as a layer covering the surface of corneal endothelium.
- The affinity of hyaluronate with receptors is dependent on molecular weight.
- Sodium hyaluronate present on the endothelial surface is removed during surgical maneuvers, but high molecular weight sodium hyaluronate remains.
- After irrigating sodium hyaluronate was injected into the AC of rabbit eyes, the material adhered to the endothelial surface, even after phacoemulsification of the lens.
- A study on corneal endothelium was required to check whether the cells forming the endothelium play a role in catabolism or production of hyaluronic acid.

The study confirmed the results of previous research. Smedsrod (1984) and Laurent (1986) demonstrated that the endothelial cells of hepatic sinusoids have hyaluronic acid receptors on their surfaces.

The interest in corneal endothelial receptors has increased owing to the following factors:

- Comparison of the various viscoelastics available on the market: Those consisting of hyaluronic acid are of animal origin (cockscomb) or derived from bacterial fermentation, whereas mixed solutions (ie, Viscoat–sodium hyaluronate and chondroitin sulfate) and methylcellulose are of vegetal origin.
- Substantial differences in molecular weight among products made of sodium hyaluronate: The heavier the material, the more protection it provides against mechanical and chemical forces.
- Improvement of phacoemulsification technique when compared with extracapsular surgery: Smaller incisions, shorter times of ultrasound delivery provided by nucleofracture maneuvers, and reduced amount and improvement of infusion fluids (BSS Plus) limit endothelial cell loss and corneal thickness much better than does

ECCE. In fact, during ECCE, the main forces damaging the endothelium are the nucleus itself, cortical material, and possible contact of the large-diameter IOL on the surface of the endothelium. Protection of the endothelium is usually accomplished by placing a viscoelastic barrier to protect it from shear forces. Hammer demonstrated experimentally how corneal endothelial protection from friction forces depends on the thickness of the layer of viscoelastic applied.

During phacoemulsification, in addition to friction forces there are also compressive forces released by ultrasound. Furthermore, in a closed intraocular operating field, the amount of fluids is greater and more turbulent against the layer of endogenous sodium hyaluronate, which, under the effect of irrigation, is quickly torn away from the endothelial surface. Injection of sodium hyaluronate restores the AC to its ideal volume and allows endothelial cells to bind with it to establish a chemical barrier able to oppose the forces of friction and compression mentioned. Binding of sodium hyaluronate to the endothelial cells is facilitated by hyaluronic acid binding sites and is proportional to the molecular weight of the material. Pedersen demonstrated that, compared with 2% methylcellulose, hyaluronic acid (Healon®) provides more effective protection of corneal endothelium in eyes on which phacoemulsification of comparable duration was performed owing to the bond between hyaluronic acid binding sites and the molecules of Healon®.

Endothelial cells do not possess receptors for HPMC. The protective action of this material is more limited owing to the absence of chemical interaction with the endothelium. It is effective during ECCE because it achieves results comparable to those of Healon®; however, it is less protective than Healon® during phacoemulsification.

Further confirmation is presented in the work by Fry et al, in which Healon® GV and Healon® were used in standardized ECCE with aspiration times of 20 seconds and the endothelial cell density values were compared 3 months after surgery.

Comparison of Healon® and viscoadherent materials (Viscoat) is interesting in the context of endothelial cell receptors (hyaluronic acid binding sites). Healon® and Healon® GV rely on chemical bonds with endothelial cells to protect them from the turbulence occurring in a closed system during phacoemulsification. In contrast, Viscoat, composed of 4% chondroitin sulfate and 3% hyaluronic acid, is less cohesive and is less likely than Healon® and Healon® GV to leave the AC, as it is more difficult to be aspirated during phaco or irrigation and aspiration. Viscoat adheres better to endothelial cells and protects them longer.

However, Arshinoff pointed out that this beneficial effect can be jeopardized by the longer irrigation and aspiration time required to completely remove Viscoat from the AC. In agreement with Arshinoff, Rafuse compared pre- and postoperative pachymetric values as well as endothelial features such as cell density, polymegathism (variability of cell dimension), pleomorphism (variability of cell shape), mean cell area, mean cell perimeter, and cell shape factor (number of cell sides, length of sides, and subtended angle) in two groups of eyes treated with phacoemulsification. The eyes that received Healon® showed less cell loss than the eyes that received Viscoat. This difference was not statistically significant, however. The eyes that received Healon® demonstrated less polymegathism.

Similarly, Viscoat caused an increase in endothelial cell area and circumference aimed at compensating for greater cell loss. The main aspects emerging from studies where Healon® seemingly provides better endothelial protection than Viscoat depend on different aspiration times of the materials (greater fluid volume is required to remove Viscoat as a whole), different amounts of time and energy needed to accomplish phacoemulsification with two materials that have different rheologic characteristics, and the decreased visibility caused by Viscoat, which would also affect time and energy.

On the contrary, some studies demonstrated better endothelial protection provided by Viscoat when compared with Healon®. Doubt was raised about how effectively chemical bonds between exogenous and endogenous hyaluronic acid protect the endothelium. Many studies demonstrated that air in animal eyes, which was widely used intraoperatively in earlier times, is harmful to endothelial cells.

Beesley et al have pointed out that the accidental presence of air microbubbles on the endothelial surface for 15 minutes caused localized erosion of the cells themselves. In a different study, Craig et al observed the damaging effect of air microbubbles on the corneal endothelium. The authors introduced air into the ACs of cadaver eyes and then performed phacoemulsification in an attempt to assess the action of Healon® and Viscoat. They found a significantly higher rate (4.9%) of endothelial cell loss associated with air microbubbles in the eyes receiving Healon® than in the eyes receiving Viscoat (0.3%) and the control group receiving only air (4.5%). The result seems to be associated with the better endothelial cell protection provided by a viscoadherent material; owing to better adhesion to the endothelium, it is more difficult to remove this material from the AC. The material effectively acts as a barrier between the endothelium and the air microbubbles that are ejected from the phaco tip and moved by fluid turbulence, resulting in a high risk of impact on endothelial cells. Conversely, Healon®, despite the presence of chemical bonds with cell receptors, tends to leave the chamber quickly, as a consequence of its cohesiveness (or internal adhesion of molecules). This allows the microbubbles to move energetically and potentially damage endothelial cells. During phacoemulsification, great care must be taken to prevent accidental introduction of air microbubbles along the infusion line or through the main incision.

Furthermore, it is preferable to use anticavitation tips and sleeves. Glasser demonstrated in animal models that only phacoemulsification caused comparable endothelial damage rates in groups receiving Healon® or Viscoat. Conversely, traumatic IOL insertion caused greater damage in eyes receiving Healon®. In a third of the cases, Viscoat still appeared adherent to the cornea by the end of surgery. Glasser concluded that although Healon® is a good viscoelastic material that effectively protects against compressive forces, it is not as protective against shear forces transmitted on the endothelial surface. In addition, high pseudoplasticity of sodium hyaluronate makes the material leak out of the AC when viscosity decreases due to increased sliding. Viscoat—which contains a Newtonian fluid such as chondroitin sulfate and shows constant viscosity independent of the shear rate—tends to remain in the AC and adherent to the endothelium, even when flow rate values are high. In a later study conducted on animal eyes, Glasser found a statistically insignificant difference in cell loss of eyes submitted to phacoemulsification with Healon®, Viscoat, Occucoat, and Amvisc Plus, even when an IOL was implanted. Nevertheless, cell loss was lower in eyes receiving a viscoadherent material injection (Viscoat, Occucoat).

It must be remembered that viscoadherent materials may trap air bubbles and cortex fragments, thus requiring longer irrigation and aspiration times for complete removal. This is highly harmful to the corneal endothelium.

The demonstrated presence of hyaluronic acid binding sites on the endothelial surface is an advantageous aspect of hyaluronic acid (Healon®). It has also been demonstrated in three different works by Harfstrand, Molander, and Stenevi that the thin layer persisting on the endothelial surface, even after the aspiration of most of the viscoelastic, seems to ensure effective chemical protection. However, the rate of endothelial cell protection depends on the phaco technique used, type of cataract, possible presence of complications (ie, synechiae, poor visibility), and irrigation time and energy.

On the other hand, in particular cases a material with lower molecular weight but greater adhesiveness can better protect from shear forces and the chemical bond of 1% hyaluronic acid on the endothelial surface is not sufficient. Hyaluronic acid with very high molecular weight (Healon® GV) provides a thicker protective layer during phacoemulsification, due to a tougher bond with the corneal endothelium. Nevertheless, it is yet to be proven whether this feature is better or comparable to viscoadhesion provided by other materials that have no chemical cell bonds, but are more difficult to remove from the endothelial surface itself.

The use of different viscoelastics affects cell density, as each material can influence the technique used. In other words, if cell loss evidenced in phacoemulsification interventions in which different viscoelastic materials have been employed is compared, significant differences in the viscoelastic, surgical technique, and aspiration times can be found. The more variables introduced in surgery, the more difficult it is to assess the protective action of a specific viscoelastic on corneal endothelium.

Probst observed that the use of two different materials with comparable viscoadhesive properties, both aspirated in all interventions for nearly 30 seconds, did not affect cell density loss, but cell loss was influenced by the phacoemulsification energy employed.

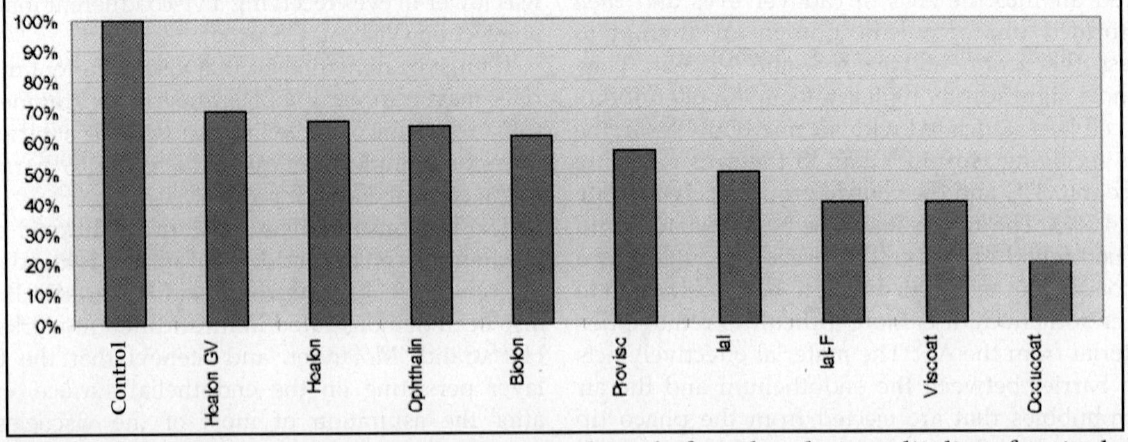

Figure 5-2. Rabbits were held with the treated eye before the photomultiplier of a single photon meter. After administering anesthesia (Ketalar), a limbal incision of 3.0 mm was cut, and the phacoemulsificator (Alcon Universal) was introduced into the AC and operated for 30 seconds with 100% ultrasound power. The emission of photons was measured by the meter. The background assessed before and after each experiment was 230 + 30 cps. The experiments were performed in the dark and each test was repeated three times in each eye. The irrigation medium (BSS) was added with liminol (0.45 mL) and each time the viscoelastic material was under examination (0.05 mL/mL of solution).

SCAVENGER EFFECT

During phacoemulsification, the handpiece tip oscillates as a consequence of ultrasound frequency. The waves produced by ultrasound run in fluids, producing cavitation microbubbles that extend and implode. The consequence is localized energy and high temperature, which results in the onset of free radicals in the AC in an amount proportional to phacoemulsification energy. The production of radicals is essential for cell metabolism, but when they exceed certain levels they can be dangerous to the endothelium. Endothelial damage is caused by free radicals through the hydrogen superoxide pathway.

The molecules able to neutralize free radicals are called scavengers. Sodium hyaluronate is one of the most well-known among these. In two different studies, Shimmura and Holst demonstrated the formation of OH radicals and H atoms during phacoemulsification and evidenced that intraoperative hyaluronic acid and the scavenger radicals present in the irrigation solution greatly contribute to limiting the presence of free radicals and the resulting endothelial damage.

Figure 5-2 depicts the scavenger effect of different viscoelastic materials assessed in rabbit eyes during phacoemulsification (Fidia Labs).

Based on the information presented thus far, it can be concluded that endothelial cell protection depends on the following factors:

- Use of safe viscoelastic materials that have been well tested.
- Short phacoemulsification time with optimal energy level dependent on the type of cataract is ideal.
- Suitable irrigation flows and short times for irrigation and aspiration of the viscoelastic material are beneficial: postoperative hypertension due to residual viscoelastic can be easily managed and is preferable to permanent endothelial damage resulting from excessive amounts of time being spent to remove the material completely from the AC.
- The accidental presence of air bubbles from the infusion line or phaco tip cavitation can damage the endothelium because the bubbles may affect the endothelial surface while being moved by the turbulence present in the closed system or they may be trapped inside viscoadherent materials, which worsens visibility.

- Hyaluronic acid materials with high to very high molecular weight (Healon®, Healon® GV, Provisc, Biolon) have high internal cohesion, bind to the endothelial receptors proportionally to the molecular weight, and are easily aspirated: this limits the aspiration time, but there is also the risk that these materials may leave the AC prematurely.
- Viscoadherent materials (Viscoat, Vitrax) adhere to the endothelium, resist possible expulsion, and provide better protection against friction, but their removal requires long aspiration times.
- Materials with different compositions have different rheologies and may require different phacoemulsification times.
- The transparency of some materials (Viscoat) is poorer: Lower visibility affects the parameters and, above all, times of phacoemulsification.

CHAPTER SIX

Viscoelastic Materials and Intraocular Pressure

The prevailing opinion among anterior segment surgeons historically has been that all viscoelastic materials must be removed from the AC at the end of surgery. In fact, these materials are not metabolized inside the eye and will leave the chamber, while remaining unchanged, through the trabeculum (Figure 6-1). IOP facilitates viscoelastic removal. Moreover, the contractile elements in the trabecular meshwork play a role in the dynamic process of viscoelastic clearance from the AC.

Some experimental models confirm that sodium hyaluronate is partly eliminated through ciliary bodies (Miyauchi et al). Therefore, clearance of viscoelastic materials is not a quick process, but depends on the molecular conformation (different in each material) that is represented by molecular volume, concentration, length of molecular chains, molecular rigidity, and the amount and degree of viscosity.

Viscoelastic materials cause transitory occlusion of the meshwork and postoperative intraocular hypertension. When left in the site or only partly removed from the AC at the end of surgery, the viscoelastic material can cause a temporary pressure increase.

Viscoelastics differ from one another depending on the type of molecules, size of molecules, and length of molecular chains. Each material has a precise molecular weight (molecular dimension, chain length) and typically high values of viscosity (disposition of chain), elasticity (deformability of chains), cohesiveness (intermolecular bound), and adhesiveness (wettability or contact angle). These features define the pseudoplasticity index (the ease of passage from a viscous to a fluid state). A material with very high molecular weight (ie, Healon® GV), consisting of large molecules with long and highly viscous chains (excellent maintenance of space) that adheres poorly to surfaces but is very cohesive (very good ability to be aspirated), may cause obstruction of the meshwork and, therefore, result in a high postoperative pressure increase. The rise in pressure that occurs when Healon® GV is not removed from the AC can be attributed to its high molecular weight.

Molecular weight is dependent on molecular dimensions and length as well as coil positioning of chains. Although Healon® GV has molecular chains that can be easily deformed (high elasticity), it actually behaves like a whole mass that is able to obstruct aqueous humor outflow through the meshwork. Conversely, it can be easily aspirated because it is a very cohesive and pseudoplastic material. Because Healon® GV is likely to be removed as a whole mass from the AC, there is no risk of parcellar aspiration near the filtering structures present in the iris/corneal angle.

Also relevant to Healon® GV–related postoperative hypertension in demanding cases is that in the presence of traumatic cataract (perforation of the anterior capsule, zonular disinsertion), Healon® GV is highly effective because it is able to keep spaces (permanent spatula effect) and manipulate tissue (soft spatula effect). Generally, in such cases, the amount of viscoelastic injected is greater than the amount used in standard phacoemulsification procedures. If it is necessary to keep the chamber formed postoperatively by using viscoelastic, it is best to use viscoelastic products made of hyaluronic acid with lower molecular weight in the final surgical phases to have a more moderate and controlled IOP increase. Furthermore, marked inflammatory reaction, which is always present in these cases, has a tendency to obstruct trabecular pores with fibrin, pigment, and blood cells.

In cases complicated by capsular break and vitreous loss, it is questionable which viscoelastic has a better tamponading effect. Some surgeons prefer a highly concentrated material with high molecular weight (Healon® GV) whereas others prefer a product with less weight and viscosity but high adhesiveness (Viscoat). Postoperative pressure increases are caused equally by Healon® GV and Viscoat depending on the amount of material injected (dose dependent) and the amount that remains in the eye, in addition to surgical damage (inflammatory reaction). It has been observed that the risk of uncontrollable IOP elevation is related to the possible overfilling of the AC that occurs when a viscoelastic is used to maintain AC volume. On the contrary, when good vitreous tamponading is achieved without vitreous loss and the surgeon decides to remove only part of the viscoelastic from the AC, it must be considered that Viscoat adheres strongly to tissues and, therefore, tends to be aspirated en bloc from the meshwork. Because Viscoat has a lower molecular weight and shorter molecular chains than Healon® GV, it can be cleared more easily than Healon® GV and results in a lower postoperative IOP elevation.

IOP elevation consequent to viscoelastic injection is a complicated phenomenon that varies according to the dose injected, the concentration and viscosity of the material, and the amount removed or left in the AC. In addition, the extent of surgical trauma, the presence of inflammatory cells, or a functionally compromised meshwork (glaucoma, repeated intervention) contribute to fluctuations of postoperative pressure elevation that are not always predictable. For this reason, variation of IOP depending on different concentrations of viscoelastic and ease of removal has been studied in experimental models.

Dose-Dependent Hypertension

A 1% sodium hyaluronate solution (Healon®) that takes one third of the aqueous humor volume generally does not cause any significant or harmful

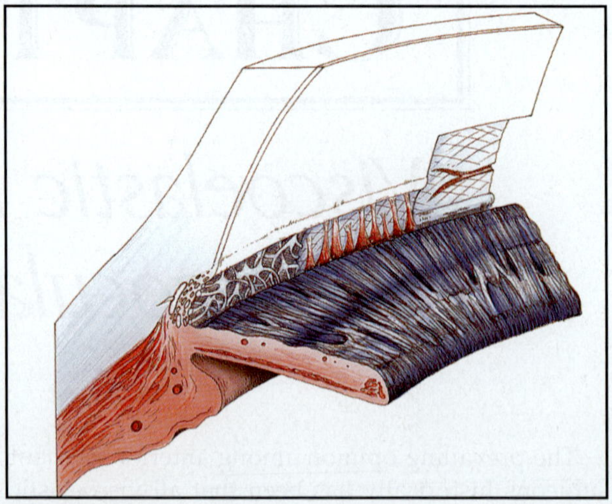

Figure 6-1. These materials are not metabolized inside the eye and will leave the chamber, while remaining unchanged, through the trabeculum.

pressure increase, and when it does, it is transient (peak values are reached 4 to 8 hours after surgery).

Amount of Viscoelastic Removed and its Effect on Pressure Increase

The more cohesive a material (strong intermolecular bound), the more likely it is to leave the AC as a whole mass during the irrigation and aspiration phase. For instance, Healon® GV, Healon®, Provisc, Biolon, Ophtalyn, and Amvisc require similar aspiration times (range 20 to 25 seconds) to be completely cleared. Viscoat, which consists of hyaluronic acid and chondroitin sulfate, and all viscoadherent materials made of 2% methylcellulose, are less cohesive and more adherent to tissues. These latter materials tend to leave the AC in lots and, thus, require a longer irrigation time (2 to 3 minutes) for complete aspiration. It appears that if a surgeon injects equal amounts of different materials (ie, Healon® and Viscoat) and performs removal for 10 seconds, he or she will achieve good clearance for Healon®, but the removal of Viscoat will be incomplete. This results in higher postoperative hypertension in the eye in which

Viscoat was used. The outcome is similar with Healon® GV and Amvisc Plus; the former is highly cohesive and the latter less cohesive and with medium-length molecular chains.

VISCOELASTIC CONCENTRATION AND ITS EFFECT ON PRESSURE INCREASE

Materials with high sodium hyaluronate concentrations are considered adhesive and are difficult to remove. Some examples are Viscoat (3% hyaluronic acid, 4% chondroitin sulfate, low cohesiveness), Amvisc Plus (short molecular chain, 1.6% hyaluronic acid, medium cohesiveness), and Vitrax (3% hyaluronic acid, low cohesiveness). These products require longer irrigation and aspiration times than Healon® GV (1.4% hyaluronic acid), Healon® (1% hyaluronic acid), Provisc (1.1% hyaluronic acid), Biolon (1% hyaluronic acid), and Ophtalyn (1% hyaluronic acid). Early postoperative IOP elevation occurs mostly when more adhesive materials are used with the same irrigation and aspiration times that are used to remove materials with high molecular weight. Therefore, the use of highly adhesive materials requires irrigation times longer than 2 minutes to prevent excessive pressure elevation. Thorough removal of very cohesive viscoelastics with high molecular weight can be achieved with aspiration times of 20 seconds.

THE EFFECT OF MOLECULAR SIZE, VISCOSITY, MOLECULAR WEIGHT, AND CHAIN LENGTH ON PRESSURE INCREASE

Because molecular weight, which defines the viscosity of a material, depends on size of the molecule as well as length of its chains, a product made of highly viscous sodium hyaluronate is barely diluted in water and will quickly pass through the trabecular meshwork. This is why once the viscoelastic is injected in the AC it remains there without causing a sudden IOP elevation. However, if it is not removed at the end of surgery, the material is likely to obstruct the meshwork in the postoperative period, thus causing excessive IOP elevation 4 to 8 hours after surgery. The greater the viscosity (a consequence of molecular size, weight, and chain length), the greater and proportionally higher the IOP elevation. This is due to the longer length of time required by molecules to pass through the trabeculum. In other words, clearance is slower when the molecular weight of the viscoelastic is greater (Table 6-1). For instance, if the same amount of Healon® GV and Viscoat are left in the AC at the end of surgery, the pressure increase in the eye receiving Healon® GV will be higher.

Therefore, we can state some conclusions based on our experience and the cases reported in the literature concerning the use of viscoelastic materials and their ability to affect IOP postoperatively.

- All viscoelastic materials cause postoperative IOP elevation, which peaks 8 hours after surgery. This tends to normalize within 24 to 36 hours postoperatively. When the material is not removed from the AC at the end of the procedure, IOP elevation is high. However, some reports in the international literature described groups who maintained normal IOP levels despite the presence of Viscoat postoperatively. The IOP elevation evidenced in these reports was limited and related to the fact that the molecular chains of Viscoat's sodium hyaluronate are shorter than those of materials with longer chains and higher molecular weight (Healon®). Therefore, Viscoat's clearance is faster. In our experience, both Healon® and Viscoat cause postoperative intraocular hypertension when not removed, and the IOP increase caused by Viscoat is lower. This indicates that viscoelastics having a higher concentration and lower cohesiveness but high adhesiveness (Viscoat, Vitrax) are preferable to materials with high molecular weight when it is necessary to leave a certain volume of viscoelastic in the eye at the end of surgery. Although IOP elevation is evident with these materials, it is limited and more easily controlled with medical therapy in comparison with materials with high molecular weight (Healon® GV, Healon®, Provisc, Biolon).
- In standard phacoemulsification or ECCE, the viscoelastic should be removed at the end of surgery. The surgeon must remember that materials with high molecular weight can be easily removed with short irrigation and aspiration

Table 6-1.
INCREASE IN IOP

	Healon® GV	Healon®	Provisc	Biolon	Amvisc Plus	Amvisc	Vitrax	Viscoat
If left in the AC	↑↑↑↑	↑↑↑	↑↑	↑↑↑	↑↑↑	↑↑↑	↑↑↑	↑↑↑
If removed for 20 minutes	↑	↑	↑	↑	↑↑	↑	↑↑	↑↑
CLEARANCE (TRABECULAR OUTFLOW) BASED ON:								
Concentration and molecular chain length	↑	↑	↑	↑	↑	↑↑	↑↑	↑↑
Molecular weight	↑	↑	↑	↑	↑↑	↑	↑↑↑	↑↑↑

times. This ensures that postoperative IOP is slightly more than preoperative pressure. To achieve the same effect while using materials with greater adhesion and lower molecular weight (ie, Viscoat, Amvisc Plus, Vitrax, and methylcellulose), it is necessary to extend the irrigation and aspiration time needed to remove the viscoelastic at the end of surgery to 2 to 3 minutes. These increased irrigation and aspiration times expose endothelial cells to more prolonged damage.

- Postoperative intraocular pressure can and must be constantly controlled. In our experience and in that cited in the international literature, there have been cases of high postoperative hypertension (from 30 to 50 mmHg) in patients who underwent phacoemulsification or standard ECCE and presented neither risk factors (trauma, repeated surgery, corneal dystrophy, high preoperative IOP, topical–systemic hypotensive treatment) nor intra- or postoperative complications (capsular break, vitreous loss, severe uveitis). In these cases, it is possible to control postoperative hypertension (within 24 to 36 hours) by means of topical therapy (timolol) alone or in addition to systemic treatment (acetazolamide).

INTRAOCULAR HYPERTENSION

Lane et al reported that the most frequent cases of postoperative hypertension (over 35 mmHg and lasting up to 24 hours) were observed in eyes submitted to ECCE from which Viscoat had not been removed. A similar postoperative hypertension rate occurred in eyes from which Occucoat was not removed and IOP rate was only slightly lower in eyes from which Healon® was not removed. The authors found no cases of hypertension that exceeded 35 mmHg in eyes from which Viscoat had been removed. Fry et al found that in patients who underwent ECCE the largest number of hypertension cases over 40 mmHg corresponded to situations when Viscoat was not removed at the end of surgery. In the studies, there were both coincidental data (as stated previously) and contrasting observations (less incidence of high IOP elevation when Healon® was removed). Nevertheless, some generalizations can be elicited from these studies that are consistent with our clinical experience:

- Postoperative hypertension follows the use of all viscoelastics.
- Hypertension reaches peak values between 4 and 24 hours postoperatively, and completely

resolves by 7 days postoperatively.

- Effective and rapid control of endoocular pressure in extreme cases by means of topical and systemic therapy is important.
- In phacoemulsification, we found values of early postoperative hypertension (4 to 24 hours) due to viscoelastic use that are comparable to those of ECCE.

Surgeons have differing opinions about the amount of influence viscoelastics have on IOP. The data reported are frequently incomplete and contradictory. To obtain credible data, it is important that the groups to be compared are homogenous and that the same assessment guidelines are followed. The following is a list of conditions that must be met to asses viscoelastic effect on pressure accurately:

- Postoperative IOP assessment without removal of the viscoelastic
- Postoperative IOP assessment after removal of the viscoelastic
- Change of IOP from preoperative to postoperative values (2, 4, 8, 12 hours)
- Irrigation/aspiration time
- Partial, total, or no removal of the viscoelastic
- Pre- and postoperative medical therapy (ß-blockers, acetazolamide)
- Use of intraoperative myotics (acetylcholine, pilocarpine, carbachol)
- Extent of surgical trauma (nuclear hardness, surgical technique)
- Volume of viscoelastic employed

See Table 6-2 for a form that can be used to assess postoperative hypertension following viscoelastic use.

Table 6-2.
SCHEME FOR POSTOPERATIVE IOP ASSESSMENT FOLLOWING VISCOELASTIC USE

Parameters For IOP Assessment								
Materials:	Healon® GV	Healon®	Provisc	Biolon	Amvisc	Amvisc Plus	Vitrax	Viscoat
Patients								
Preoperative IOP (mean and SD)								
Technique: nuclear hardness								
Volume of viscoelastic employed								
Removal of viscoelastic								
No removal								
Irrigation and Aspiration (seconds)								
With preoperative therapy: ß-blockers, acetazolamide								
Without therapy								
Postoperative IOP Without Therapy (Mean and SD)								
4 hours								
8 hours								
12 hours								
24 hours								
IOP > 35 mmHg								
Postoperative IOP with therapy (mean and SD)								
4 hours								
8 hours								
12 hours								
24 hours								
IOP > 35 mmHg								

CHAPTER SEVEN

Viscosurgery

The term viscosurgery, coined by Balazs, pertains to the use of solutions and gel with viscous, elastic, and pseudoplastic features before, during, or after surgery. Elasticity ensures protection from mechanical shocks and vibrations. Viscosity allows the surgeon to protect and lubricate tissues or isolate some tissues from other ones. Pseudoplasticity enables the material to wrap and can be used to manipulate or support tissues.

Before surgery, viscoelastic materials can form space, whereas during surgery they are useful for support, dissection, and protection of ocular tissues as well as hemostasis. Postoperatively, they keep the space formed by the surgeon and prevent postoperative adhesions.

The ideal viscoelastic material must:

- Be transparent, to provide good visibility for the surgeon during the procedure. Some surgeons prefer a light dyeing of the material to improve its visibility. Nevertheless, owing to the common use of these materials, nearly all surgeons are now able to identify them.
- Be water soluble so when left inside it can leak out of the eye.
- Be easily injected and removed.
- Be able to separate tissues gently (ie, releasing adhesions) without doing harm to the tissues themselves.
- Keep the spaces formed and not scatter during surgical maneuvers.
- Protect tissues from chemical or physical damage.
- Have such pH, osmolarity, and chemical features that neither corneal endothelium nor other ocular structures are damaged by its use.
- Not be allergenic.
- Not cause inflammatory reaction, cataract, or carcinoma.
- Not alter ocular hydrodynamics (at least not permanently).
- Not undergo chemical or physical change while being used.

As mentioned in the chapter on the physicochemical features of viscoelastics (Chapter 3), different features may affect the performance of each product. Therefore, it is useful to remember the following properties:

VISCOSITY/ELASTICITY

- Creates and maintains spaces
- Determines ease of injectability
- Determines postoperative IOP
- Dampens impacts

MOLECULAR WEIGHT

- When high, results in easy removal
- When low, results in low postoperative IOP

PSEUDOPLASTICITY

- When high, results in easy injection
- When high, results in easy IOL implantation

COHESIVENESS:

- When high, results in easy removal
- When high and the material is not removed, results in high postoperative IOP

ADHESIVENESS

- When the contact angle is low there is greater protection of cells and surgical instruments

While performing surgery, the operator can apply a more offensive technique using traditional tools such as forceps, knives, and sutures or take a defensive approach by using viscoelastics. Viscoelastics aim to maintain spaces, create vol-

Table 7-1.
VISCOELASTIC MATERIAL

Preservation of spaces	Formation of volumes	Ability to manipulate	Tissue protection
Stable mydriasis	*Deep AC*	*Capsulorhexis (stability of the flap escaping margin)*	*Corneal endothelium*
IOL implantation	*Stretched capsular bag*	*Synechiae*	*Vitreous hyaloid*
Vitreous tamponade		*Iris tissue*	

umes, and improve manipulation while protecting tissues (Table 7-1).

The surgeon can choose surface or space techniques. Surface techniques protect passive tissue from accidental contact with surgical instruments or implants. This is accomplished by covering the tissue with various agents, such as plastic surfaces or viscous layers. Space techniques provide protection by preserving, creating, or widening spaces between tissues in order to make maneuvers safer.

The viscous materials used to protect tissues from surgical tools or other harmful agents can be used by following two different strategies. Surface techniques are accomplished by coating the whole tissue with the viscoelastic material itself. Space techniques are accomplished by covering the instrument or the IOL to lessen traumatic impact between it and the tissue. The space technique is more comfortable, as it allows the use of a product with fewer side effects; however, it is often less effective than surface techniques.

The use of viscoelastic materials has several indications. Several are mentioned here to demonstrate how these products, once injected in the anterior segment of the eye, can accomplish different functions.

Blockade of Leakage

In this purpose, viscoelastic is used to obstruct passages where intraocular fluids might leak out and to prevent foreign bodies (ie, blood, fluids, lens material) from entering (Figure 7-1).

Soft Spatula

The viscoelastic material can be used to move tissues gently or to shift small foreign bodies toward the surgeon, making them "float" in the material.

Permanent Spatula

Under certain conditions, viscoelastics can freeze tissue flaps, capsular flaps, and small foreign bodies, allowing the surgeon to retrieve them in the most comfortable and safe way possible (Figures 7-2 and 7-3).

Some other examples of viscoelastic use in anterior segment surgery are depicted in Figures 7-4 to 7-12.

Viscoelastic Injection Technique

In the Anterior Chamber

Materials with higher cohesiveness and greater pseudoplasticity are more easily injected and, after coming out of the chamber, restore to their original structure. As far as these materials are concerned, problems with injection inside the AC are far reduced than with less cohesive materials. The material will always appear homogeneous although injected in small, local amounts (Healon®).

The introduction of less pseudoplastic and cohesive materials (Viscoat) is more difficult. The surgeon has to attempt restoring their compact structure by injecting the material inside itself.

It is important to get in the habit of starting to inject the product distal to the site where the cannula is introduced into the eye and continue injecting while retracting the cannula.

The liquids present in the eye are thus pushed out and gradually replaced by the viscoelastic (Figure 7-12).

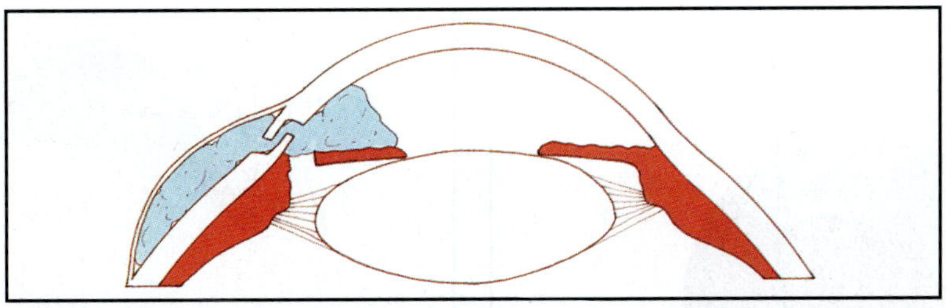

Figure 7-1. Viscoelastics can freeze tissue flaps, capsular flaps, and small foreign bodies, allowing the surgeon to retrieve them in the most comfortable and safe way possible.

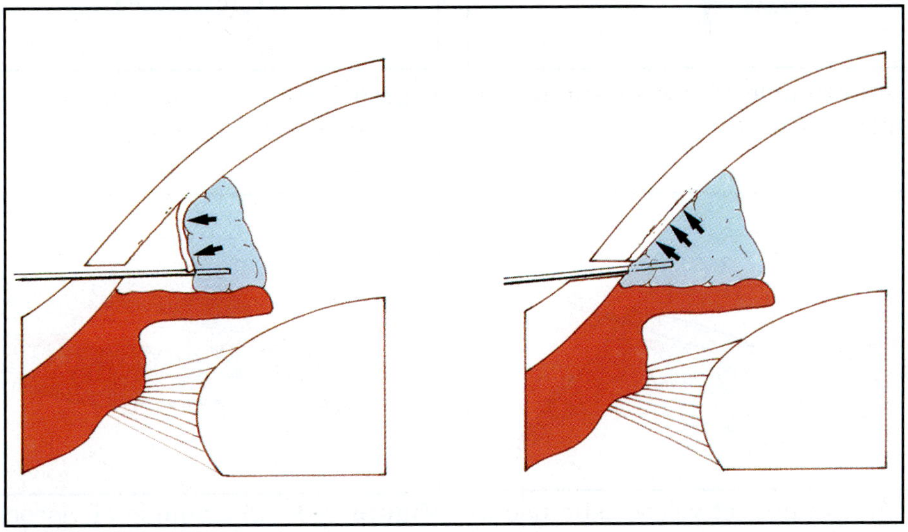

Figure 7-2. Viscoelastics can freeze tissue flaps, capsular flaps, and small foreign bodies, allowing the surgeon to retrieve them in the most comfortable and safe way possible.

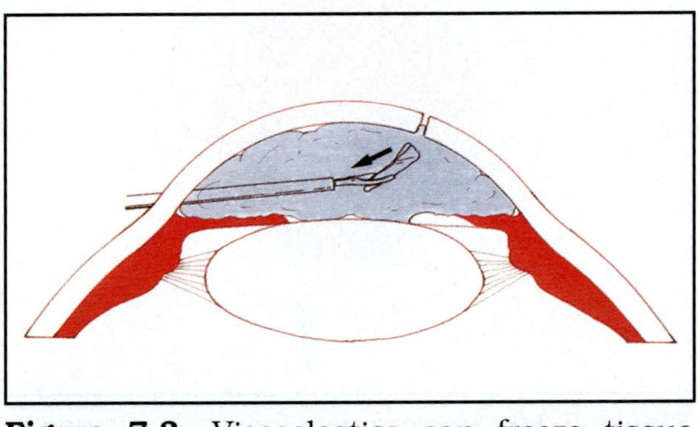

Figure 7-3. Viscoelastics can freeze tissue flaps, capsular flaps, and small foreign bodies, allowing the surgeon to retrieve them in the most comfortable and safe way possible.

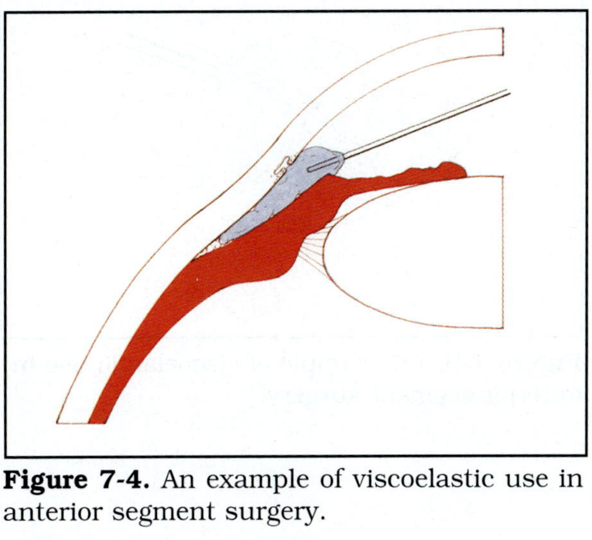

Figure 7-4. An example of viscoelastic use in anterior segment surgery.

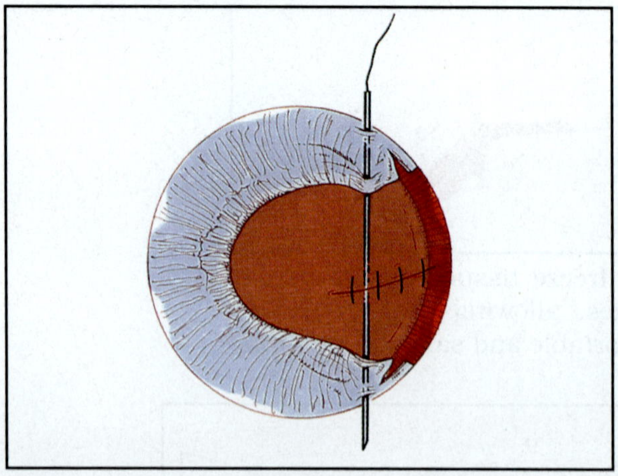

Figure 7-5. An example of viscoelastic use in anterior segment surgery.

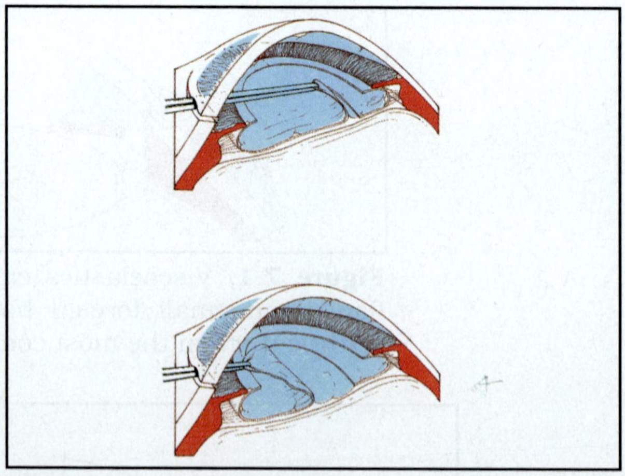

Figure 7-6. An example of viscoelastic use in anterior segment surgery.

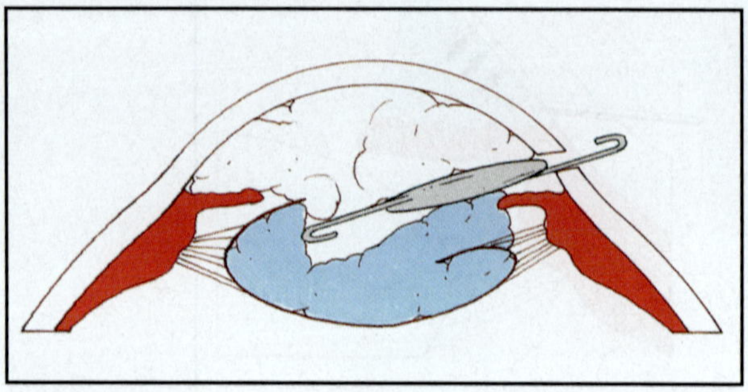

Figure 7-7. An example of viscoelastic use in anterior segment surgery.

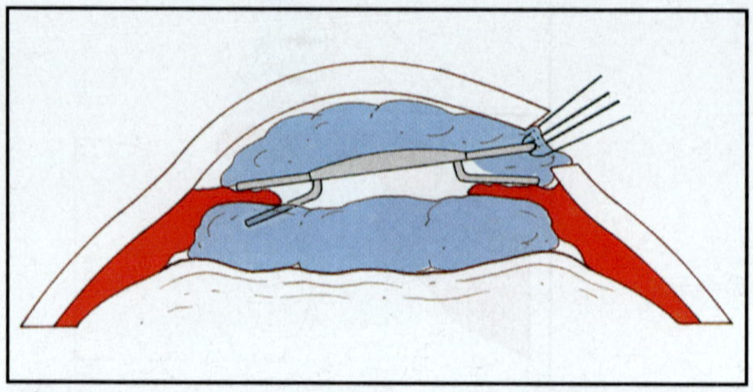

Figure 7-8. An example of viscoelastic use in anterior segment surgery.

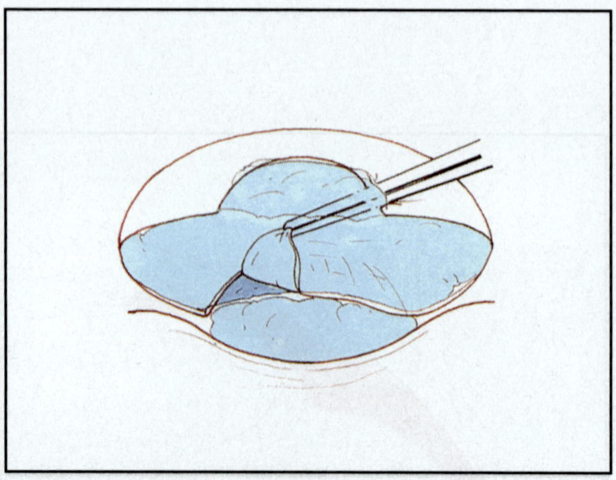

Figure 7-9. An example of viscoelastic use in anterior segment surgery.

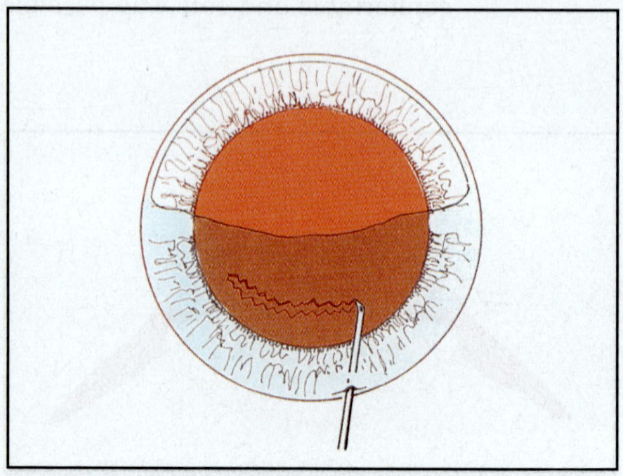

Figure 7-10. An example of viscoelastic use in anterior segment surgery.

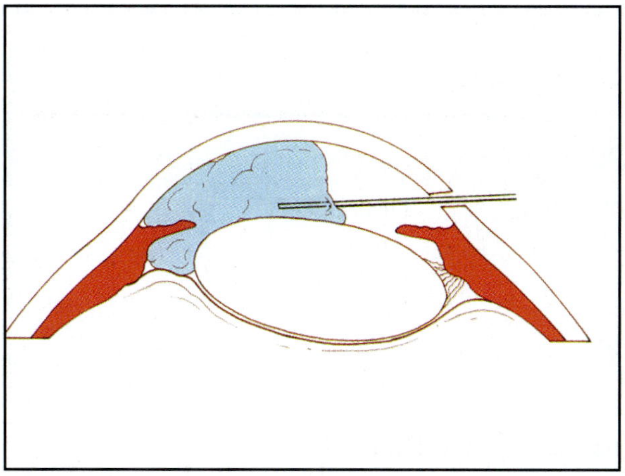

Figure 7-11. An example of viscoelastic use in anterior segment surgery.

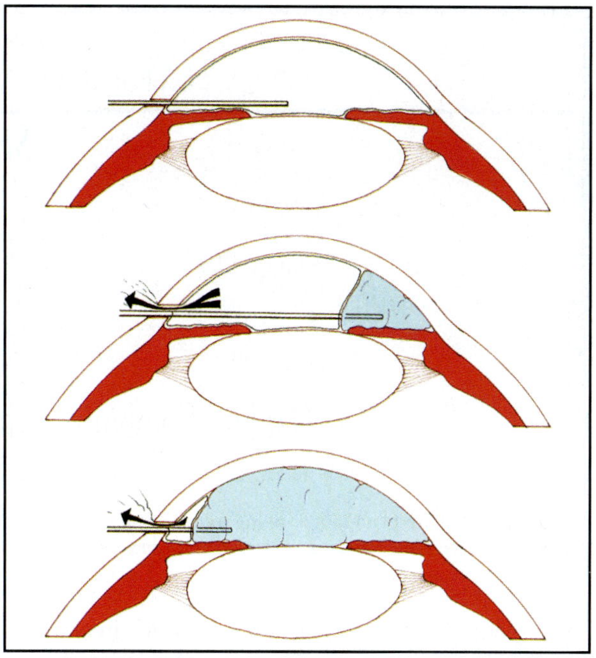

Figure 7-12. An example of viscoelastic use in anterior segment surgery. (The liquids present in the eye are pushed out and gradually replaced by the viscoelastic.)

When using a viscoelastic that is more cohesive, it can also be injected in the middle of the AC or localized in various spots—it will always tend to get compacted. When the injection of adhesive viscoelastic is not accomplished inside itself, the consequence will be a typical "stranding" effect, forming a tube-shaped amount of product, like toothpaste squeezed out of its tube.

A useful trick can be the injection of an air bubble that is then replaced by the viscoelastic, as the air/viscoelastic interface is more visible for the surgeon than the aqueous/viscoelastic interface (Figure 7-12). An air bubble is injected into the AC and filling is completed with air. The viscoelastic is injected inside the air and AC filling is visible. The air/viscoelastic exchange is completed while progressively retracting the cannula toward the paracentesis wound while the viscoelastic is being injected.

Should the surgeon believe that the filling is excessive, it is possible to allow a desired amount of viscoelastic to leak out of the paracentesis wound by pushing on the posterior portion of the wound with the cannula or some other tool.

In the Space Behind the Iris

In the early phase, it will be easier to direct the viscoelastic toward the lens so that it is depressed. The surgeon can then inject more viscoelastic in the space that has been created. However, if the surgeon starts injecting the viscoelastic near the pupillary border, some material may be placed on top of, instead of under, the iris, negating the viscoelastic's effect.

In the Capsular Bag

This is a very important maneuver because it aims to fill the bag completely before IOL implantation. The injection should be started in the middle of the bag and in the most distal position with respect to the entrance of the cannula. In some cases, a small amount of viscoelastic can be placed in the AC to create a sort of natural slope for the IOL toward the open bag (visco-glide). This technique is used particularly with rigid IOLs, whereas for soft lenses it is better to accomplish uniform and complete opening of the bag, starting by injecting the product in the middle. For a more detailed description of the application techniques in this phase of surgery, see the chapter devoted to IOL implantation.

In the Hyaloid–Capsular Space

To perform posterior capsulotomy without damaging the anterior hyaloid, the surgeon can puncture

Table 7-2.
CHOICE OF VISCOELASTICS

Single

Healon®	Healon® Yellow*	Healon® GV
Provisc	Viscoat	Amvisc
Amvisc Plus	Biolon	Hymecel
IAL	IAL Stron	Vitrax
Biogel	Occucoat	Collagel
Adatocel	Cellugel	

Double: Combining advantages of two materials

Duovisc

**Healon® Yellow is no longer being manufactured.*

the capsule with a very thin needle after injecting a small amount of viscoelastic over it. The cannula can then be used to lift the posterior capsule orifice gently at the site of incision and a small amount of viscoelastic can be injected under the capsule.

The next step is to inject a larger amount of viscoelastic to separate the posterior capsule and hyaloid. For a more detailed description of this maneuver, see the chapter on surgical techniques.

In rare situations, some viscoelastic material may open a valve (corneal or sclerocorneal), thus inhibiting contact between both planes of the incision. Fluid may leak between viscoelastic and wound. The exceeding material is to be removed.

REMOVAL OF THE VISCOELASTIC

Removal of very cohesive products (Healon®) tends to be simple. In fact, the material leaves its place inside the eye and comes out as a whole. Less cohesive and pseudoplastic materials (Viscoat) are more difficult to remove and require a longer time to complete the operation, while the irrigation cannula presses on the posterior portion of the surgical wound. The use of aspiration combined with irrigation quickens the procedure.

When removing more difficult materials—that is, poorly cohesive materials with short molecular chains—it is important to search thoroughly for any small portion of residual viscoelastic.

Irrigation will help create natural cleavage planes that the surgeon can follow and exploit to ease removal of the product. The reader is referred to the chapter focusing on surgical techniques, in which a more analytical description is made of the problems concerning viscoelastic removal.

AMOUNT OF VISCOELASTIC TO BE INJECTED

The viscoelastics available on the market are usually supplied in a syringe filled with 0.4 mL up to 2.0 mL of material. It has been calculated that the amount of viscoelastic required to perform routine cataract surgery with phacoemulsification ranges from 0.55 mL to 0.85 mL. Depending on the molecular weight of the substance, the surgeon uses significantly different amounts of material. The use of products with a higher molecular weight requires less material.

For instance, it takes 0.21 mL for Healon® but only 0.20 mL for Healon® GV to fill the AC before capsulotomy. As far as viscoexpression is concerned, the amount is 0.25 mL for Healon® and 0.22 mL for Healon® GV. The amount required to fill the capsular bag is 0.18 mL for both materials.

Table 7-2 provides a list of the main viscoelastic products available on the market and a comparison of the amounts supplied in the syringes. Multiple listings occur and it is possible to find packages with different amounts. When performing an extracapsular technique it is undoubtedly better to choose packages with smaller contents, whereas for phacoemulsification the surgeon requires a larger amount.

WHICH VISCOELASTIC?

In recent years, much has been published about the ability of viscoelastics to support cataract surgery. Each surgeon knows well how these products are helpful in the various surgical phases. Physical characteristics of viscoelastics are responsible for surgical effectiveness, whereas chemical features provide for safe application. Choosing a material from the wide range of products available on the market (Table 7-2) can be difficult.

There are 12 features that should be present in the ideal viscoelastic. A single material meeting all 12 requirements is not available. Most products perform excellently in some aspects but are weak in other respects due to physico–chemical characteristics. However, all viscoelastics must have one basic requisite—high viscosity at 0 shear rate—to stabilize and manage tissues and structures inside the eye while ensuring the presence of suitable space. Terms such as viscospatula, viscoblockade, viscotamponade, and viscospacing can all be summarized by this one characteristic—high viscosity at a low shear rate.

Of course, other physical features (ie, cohesiveness, adhesiveness, pseudoplasticity) also greatly influence the performance of the product's injectability, removability, and persistence in the eye during surgical maneuvers and must be taken into account by the surgeon.

Chemical features, which are mainly responsible for immunogenicity, toxicity, teratogenicity of the product, and its ability to induce inflammation, are often underestimated. It is often difficult to have obtain information about sterilization of the product and its assembly.

In many countries, viscoelastic materials are considered medications; however, they should be judged as atypical and independent products, separate from medications.

Particularly in recent years, due to the advent of several new products, the safety of viscoelastic materials has become as important as rheologic performance. In fact, in the last 15 years, almost all of these products have caused new complications in ophthalmic surgery. Some of these include the hypertension induced by Healon® (1980), the corneal precipitates of calcium phosphate caused by Viscoat (1985), the impurities detected in methylcellulose (1988), the severe glaucoma induced by Orcolon (1991), the problems of sterilization for Occucoat (1991), and the bacterial contamination of Microvisc Plus (1993).

Until recently, no one has asked the manufacturers to perform routine standardized controls on their products to test their biosafety. For instance, the owl monkey test (performed by Pharmacia & Upjohn), if considered the most reliable method, should be compulsory for all products currently marketed.

There are also problems concerning the application techniques of viscoelastic materials (ie, the capsular blockade following viscoelastic application). After correctly performing both capsulorhexis and implantation in the bag, capsular blockade can occur postoperatively due to the viscoelastic. If a large amount of material is left behind and around the IOL, the viscoelastic may absorb water, thus pushing the lens forward. Capsulorhexis may be occluded by the IOL and angle closure glaucoma may occur consequent to the expansion of the capsular bag.

Furthermore, regular controls regarding the standards of a certain product are still lacking. There have been reports that some materials were "adjusted" for molecular weight and some others showed very different physical and chemical characteristics according to the lots produced.

The ideal viscoelastic for cataract surgery should meet the following requirements:

- High viscosity at low shear rate—for space maintenance
- Moderate viscosity at a mean shear rate—to enable easy manipulation of instruments, IOL, and inside the viscoelastic solution
- Low viscosity at high shear rate—for easier injection–aspiration of the solution
- High elasticity rate—to protect tissues from accidental contact with surgical instruments
- Good cohesiveness—to aid in compacting the product and to enable easier aspiration from the eye (conversely, high cohesiveness hinders outflow through the trabecular meshwork, causing higher ocular hypertension in case of incomplete removal)

- Good adhesiveness—to be able to remain in the AC while surgical procedures are being performed, if possible

The following data were taken from the components of products that are most frequently used.

HYALURONIC ACID

- Natural component of connective tissue
- The main component in the vitreous and one of the components of the layer that coats anterior segment tissues
- It is not metabolized inside the eye—it passes with no change through the trabeculum and is then led by vessels to the liver
- When the concentration of hyaluronic acid is increased, its molecules, which form flexible spirals, are likely to compact and get superimposed, quickly increasing viscosity as well as elasticity

CHONDROITIN SULFATE

- Extracted from shark cartilage, it was first used in 1980 (to coat IOLs)
- It is a natural component of connective tissue
- Its molecular structure is similar to that of hyaluronic acid, the main difference being the presence of a sulfur and two negative charges in molecular subunit (according to supporters of the material this should be an advantage because it opposes the electrostatic fields of surgical instruments and IOLs)
- Its molecules are smaller than those of hyaluronic acid and therefore higher concentrations are required to obtain the same viscosity
- The material is less elastic than hyaluronic acid: to pass through a 30-G cannula, a 20% chondroitin sulfate solution needs to be compressed very strongly, and 50% solutions cannot pass at all; the material is more suitable for surface interventions rather than in spaces
- In Viscoat, sodium hyaluronate has been added to chondroitin sulfate to combine high viscosity of the former with wettability of the latter
- Sodium hyaluronate present in Healon® is derived from cockscomb, but in Viscoat the sodium hyaluronate is produced from bacterial fermentation of streptococcus cultivations; the chondroitin sulfate in Viscoat is obtained through enzymatic extraction of cartilage in shark fins

CHONDROITIN SODIUM SULFATE

- Preserves endothelial cells (product to preserve corneas: Optisol Chiron)
- Owing to high wettability, it protects the corneal endothelium
- As it is a Newtonian fluid, chondroitin sulfate is poorly pseudoplastic; therefore, viscosity decreases slightly with movement, and consequently it can maintain spaces longer

VISCOSITY

- Ability to resist shifting

PSEUDOPLASTICITY

- Variation of viscosity with increasing friction speed (ie, easy passage through a syringe)
- A material is very pseudoplastic when poorly deformable at rest (high viscosity at 0 shear rate) and very deformable when subjected to quick movement (low viscosity at 1000 shear rate)
- Healon® is far more pseudoplastic than Viscoat

NEWTONIAN PROPERTIES

- Hyaluronic acid is a non–Newtonian fluid (its viscosity changes according to friction speed)
- Chondroitin sulfate is a non-pseudoplastic Newtonian fluid (its viscosity remains unchanged independently of friction speed)
- While at rest, Healon® is very viscous, but with movement it becomes less viscous
- Viscoat (hyaluronic acid and chondroitin sulfate) is less viscous and less pseudoplastic (due to the presence of chondroitin sulfate) at rest; viscosity decreases less dramatically with movement and the material maintains position and space for a longer period

ELASTICITY

- Aptitude of a material to recover its original shape
- Elasticity allows the viscoelastic to restore it to its original form after being injected
- Elasticity depends on the viscosity and length of molecular chains; during surgery, it provides protection from mechanical vibrations

- When remaining in spaces, Healon® is very elastic; Viscoat is less elastic, but remains longer in the site of injection

COHESIVENESS

- Ability of molecules to adhere to one another
- Solutions with long molecular chains (Healon®) and high molecular weight are very cohesive and tend to come out of the eye as a whole mass when aspirated
- Materials with short molecular chains and low molecular weight are less cohesive and tend to leave the AC in lots (Viscoat)
- The more cohesive a material, the more difficult its outflow, which causes hypertension when not removed

BIOCOMPATIBILITY

- Both cohesive and adhesive products (Healon®, Viscoat) are physiologic

WETTABILITY

- Ability of a material to coat/wet a solid
- Compared with Healon®, Viscoat has a greater ability to coat

SUMMARY

The viscosity of cohesive products (Healon®) decreases when forces are applied; the viscosity of dispersive solutions (Viscoat) is less likely to decrease and, as a result, these tend not to leave the site where they have been placed.

Long molecular chains result in high viscosity, but also cause a remarkable increase in IOP in the postoperative period.

High cohesiveness favors aspiration maneuvers, but the poorer wettability of cohesive products results in greater ability to coat.

The viscoelastic solution must preserve spaces, protect endothelium, and enable maneuvers. It must not cause IOP increase.

Viscosity/elasticity preserves spaces, keeps the AC formed, eases injection, and causes postoperative pressure increase.

Low molecular weight results in low postoperative IOP; high allows easy aspiration.

Pseudoplasticity eases injection and IOL implantation.

Cohesiveness results in postoperative pressure increase when the material is not removed.

Wettability gives cell protection and helps coat surgical instruments and tissues (with low contact angle).

COHESIVE PRODUCTS, DISPERSIVE PRODUCTS

According to Arshinoff, viscoelastics can be categorized by two parameters: molecular characteristics, concentration, and length of polymer chain; and cohesiveness of the material.

Most viscoelastic materials consist of hyaluronic acid. As a result, more viscous products show pseudoplasticity, rigidity, and high elasticity at low shear rate. Then, if we consider viscosity at 0 shear rate and cohesiveness, we can immediately have a useful indication for our future surgical goals.

Very cohesive viscoelastics showing high viscosity, such as Healon® GV, Healon®, Amvisc, Amvisc Plus, Provisc, and Biolon, can be usefully employed to create spaces and stabilize tissues, enhance mydriasis, stabilize the lens during capsulorhexis, deepen the AC, dissect synechiae, widen and keep the capsular bag open during IOL implantation, and create counterpressure on the vitreous in case of capsular break.

Materials with lower viscosity and poor cohesiveness (dispersive), such as Viscoat, Vitrax, and methylcellulose, may easily get broken and consequently "scatter" in small fragments once injected in the eye. Their main use aims at protecting the endothelium during phacoemulsification, mobilizing and isolating selectively, and retrieving nuclear fragments.

In choosing a viscoelastic one considers its cost as related to the quality of the solution, syringe, and cannula, and the presentation of the whole package.

Some viscoelastics are better suited than others for different surgical needs. In case of complications occurring during surgery (presence of adhesions, positive vitreous pressure, small pupils, difficult capsulorhexis, or flattening AC), it is better to choose a highly viscous and cohesive viscoelastic. Conversely, in the presence of iris damage (for

Table 7-3.
VISCOELASTICS

Goal	Shear Rate	Characteristics
In ECCE		
Anterior chamber filling	1000	Pseudoplasticity
Capsulotomy	0	High viscosity, plasticity
Nucleus expression	2.5	Pseudoplasticity
Irrigation/aspiration of the cortex	Wettability	
Anterior chamber filling	1000	Pseudoplasticity
Keeping the bag open	0	High viscosity, elasticity
IOL implantation	2.5	Pseudoplasticity
Removal		Cohesiveness
In Phacoemulsification		
Anterior chamber filling	1000	Pseudoplasticity
Capsulotomy	0	High viscosity, elasticity
Emulsification of the nucleus	?	Low cohesion
I/A of the cortex		Wettability
Capsular bag filling	1000	Pseudoplasticity
Keeping the bag open	0	High viscosity, elasticity
IOL implantation	2.5	Pseudoplasticity
Removal		Cohesion

instance, when the phaco tip accidentally catches the iris), zonule disinsertion, posterior capsule break, nuclear fragment removal, or corneal endothelial damage, a less cohesive viscoelastic—ie, a dispersive and less viscous solution—is more useful. The ultimate cohesive viscoelastic is undoubtedly Healon® GV, but the ideal dispersive viscoelastic is Viscoat.

Each surgeon should be able to choose, based on the case and the surgical technique, which viscoelastic is best to use. Ideally, the surgeon should have more than one viscoelastic at his or her service during the same procedure. This would allow him or her to reap the benefits of each product without enduring its drawbacks.

Endothelial protection is a problem lacking a solution. On one hand, it is asserted that dispersive materials ensure greater protection; on the other hand, it is put forth that cohesive materials such as Healon® and Healon® GV have a protective effect on the endothelium while binding chemically with the cornea and protecting it from free radical release during phacoemulsification. This kind of bond should be far more protective for the endothelium than the bonds provided by more adhesive (dispersive) materials that stratify on the corneal posterior surface, providing only mechanical protection.

Nichols states that the drag forces acting on the cells of corneal endothelium when trying to remove dispersive viscoelastic would cause much greater damage. It must also be remembered that cataract surgery with phacoemulsification is very different from extracapsular techniques, especially regarding the shear rate involving the viscoelastic during the procedure (Table 7-3).

Our approach mostly concerns analysis of the following surgical steps: AC filling, capsulorhexis, cleavage of lens structures, phacoemulsification, irrigation and aspiration, capsular bag filling, maintenance of a fairly wide capsular opening during IOL implantation, and viscoelastic removal. We studied the expected needs of the surgeon and how these requirements can be met by the characteristics of viscoelastics.

CHAPTER EIGHT

Anterior Chamber Filling

In performing phacoemulsification, correctly filling the AC with a viscoelastic is a fundamental phase for the progression of surgery. When faced with a small pupil or a shallow chamber, or if the surgeon wishes to perform capsulorhexis with forceps, the surgeon must use a transparent material that is able to keep constant space in the AC and facilitates accomplishment of various surgical maneuvers.

There are three basic features required of the viscoelastic material: 1) excellent visualization of AC structures; 2) ease of injection; and 3) preservation of spaces. Consequently, the product requires three mechanical properties: 1) good transparency; 2) high pseudoplasticity; and 3) high viscosity at 0 shear rate.

VISIBILITY EQUALS TRANSPARENCY

The product should be very transparent to provide the surgeon with optimal visibility. It is possible that a dystrophic cornea or epithelial or tear film abnormalities (due to patient age or repeated instillation of topical anesthesia) may hinder visibility of both the iris and the AC. In the same way, imperfect coaxial arrangement of the microscope light and absent red reflex of the fundus, which often occur when very hard or intumescent cataracts are being extracted or when the pupil is particularly small, may render surgery even more difficult if a poorly transparent viscoelastic is used. For instance, in complicated cases where excellent visibility and high magnification of the surgical microscope are of fundamental importance, a poorly transparent product like Viscoat may not be indicated.

However, transparency also depends on the preparation of the viscoelastic solution and cannula and syringe use. In fact, some materials (ie, Viscoat) must be stored in a vertical position to allow air bubbles present in the syringe to gather in the upper portion and not toward the piston. Thus, it will be possible for the surgeon to allow small amounts of air to exit the syringe prior to assembly of the cannula on the syringe and injection in the eye. This is essential for the correct preparation of Viscoat (Figure 8-1). It will then be necessary to inject a small amount of viscoelastic outside the eye to ensure that the viscoelastic is completely present in the cannula when it enters the AC. Air may still be present, as some syringes are provided with a piston sliding very easily in the outer part and a rubber plug on the piston end that can be too soft. When the plug is pressed by the viscoelastic, it permits depression in the cannula with consequent air inflow (Figure 8-2).

Transparency will also be ensured by preventing cleavage lines of water and viscoelastic and by the formation of a single aqueous/viscoelastic interface while the product is being injected in the AC. If the product divides in lots and is poorly cohesive, it may render visualization more difficult. Therefore, it will be necessary, especially when using more dispersive products, to inject the material inside itself starting distal to the incision (Figures 8-3 and 8-4).

Another useful indication can be provided by the sequence following the injection of the viscoelastic as it relates to the formation of a tunnel in a clear cornea. In fact, many surgeons inject the viscoelastic after completing the tunnel and entering the AC. In our opinion, this is incorrect because while performing surgery under topical anesthesia,

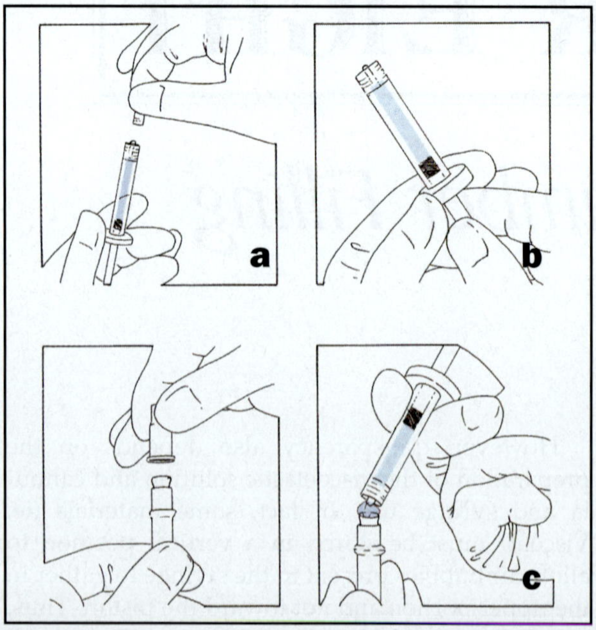

Figure 8-1. Correct preparation of Viscoat. (a) Remove the gray rubber cap from the syringe tip. (b) Keeping the syringe in the position shown, let air bubbles inside the syringe come out. (c) Inject Viscoat in the cone of the cannula and immediately screw the syringe on the cannula.

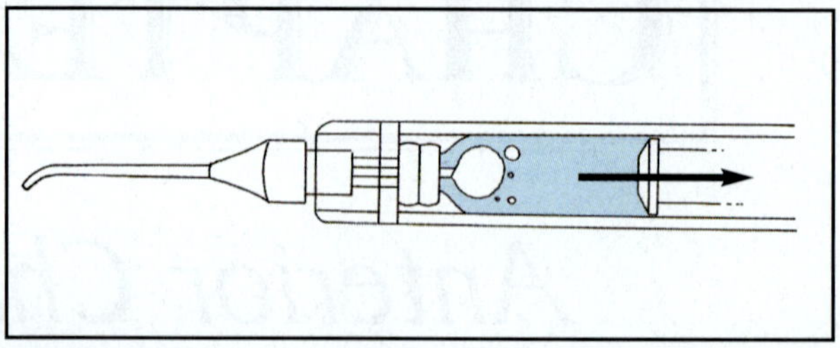

Figure 8-2. A cap that is too soft can be compressed by the viscoelastic material and consequently let the piston feed back, sucking air inside the cannula.

it is possible that positive pressure form the eye itself or blinking may empty the AC that has not yet been filled with the viscoelastic. It is better to accomplish a paracentesis incision first, then to inject the viscoelastic solution, and then to enter the AC through the main incision, while being protected by the viscoelastic injected.

Great care must be taken in the performance of the paracentesis incision: this should be neither too small nor too wide. If the paracentesis incision is too small, it could be difficult to introduce the cannula in the AC to inject the viscoelastic material, particularly when large cannulas are being used, for instance, to inject a poorly pseudoplastic and consequently barely injectable solution (HPMC). Furthermore, a small opening may be obstructed by the cannula, thus stopping the aqueous solution from leaking out of the chamber when pushed by the introduced viscoelastic. If the paracentesis incision is too wide, the AC might shallow during phacoemulsification as a result of fluid leakage. In addition, infectious material may be allowed to enter the chamber in the postoperative period. Therefore, in the performance of a paracentesis incision with correct dimensions, it is very important to fill the chamber correctly with the viscoelastic.

For surgeons not yet familiar with viscoelastic materials, a useful trick can be injecting air in the chamber before injecting viscoelastic. This way, the volume taken by the viscoelastic inside the air bubble is better demonstrated and the novice viscooperator can better appreciate complete viscoelastic filling (Figure 8-5).

Easy Injectability = High Pseudoplasticity

It has already been said that products with high pseudoplasticity (such as Healon® GV) are more easily injected (Figure 8-6), even through narrow cannulas, as they have a low viscosity at high shear rate. Therefore, the physical and rheologic features of a product favor optimal injectability. Consequently, more pseudoplastic products such as Healon® GV and Healon® are preferable to adhesive and less pseudoplastic preparations such as Viscoat and Vitrax, and others such as HPMC (Figure 8-7). Pseudoplasticity lets the material "stretch" inside the cannula and become compact in the AC, thus ensuring a good preservation of space.

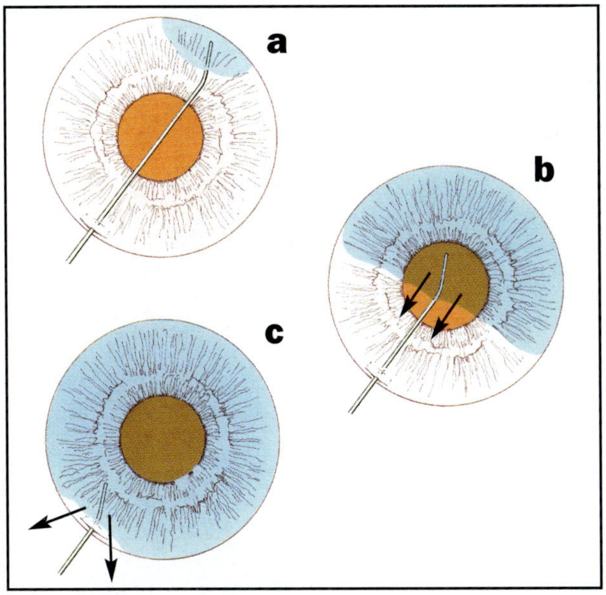

Figure 8-3. Correct filling with adhesive viscoelastic. (a) The viscoelastic product must be injected starting from the position distal to the paracentesis. In case of adhesive viscoelastics, the material is to be injected "inside itself." (b, c) The insertion of viscoelastic is completed by gradually retracting the cannula toward the entrance made in the AC.

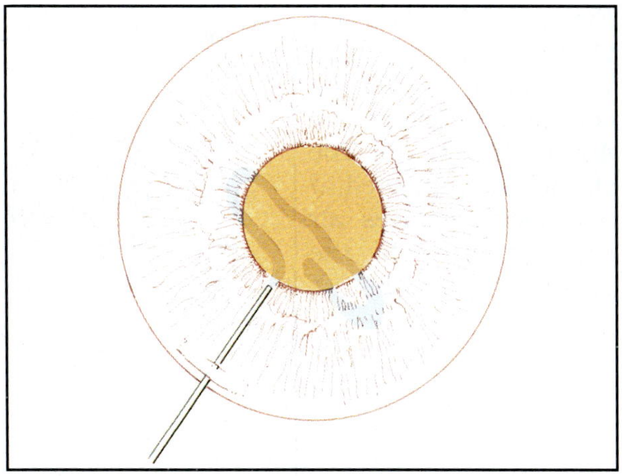

Figure 8-4. Incorrect filling with poorly cohesive material. Omitting injection of the viscoelastic "inside itself" causes a "stranding" effect.

Space Maintenance = High Viscosity at Zero Shear Rate

Space preservation is essential to the continuation of surgery. This allows the surgeon to introduce the knife through the main entrance with no damage to either the iris or the capsule, particularly when the AC is shallow. The viscoelastic solution should also provide and maintain optimal mydriasis, thus tamponading possible bleeding and enabling the operator to perform further maneuvers.

With the development of phacoemulsification techniques, it is now possible to treat even the smallest pupils and the most difficult nuclei. The management of small pupils is eased by the ability of the viscoelastic to keep space, as well as the effect of soft spatula to manipulate tissues and "fix" them into the desired position.

In recent years, the following maneuvers have been developed that permit the surgeon to dilate a small pupil. All these maneuvers depend on the use of viscoelastic materials.

- Mydriasis—This is accomplished through the use of a "heavy" viscoelastic, particularly when the pupil is poorly responsive to preoperative mydriatics. These pupils are atonic and, therefore, can be dilated and shaped by a viscoelastic material. High molecular weight, high viscosity at 0 shear rate, and excellent soft and permanent spatula effect are the basic requirements of the material. Among the viscoelastics currently available, Healon® GV is the ideal material under these circumstances. All other products follow in order, with the "dispersive" materials with lower viscosity at low shear rate (ie, Amvisc, Vitrax) being less suitable and HPMC being the least suitable. In Figure 8-7, the "soft spatula effect" provided by the various viscoelastics is compared.
- Removal of iris/lens synechiae—These are formed consequently to prolonged miotic treatment or uveal irritation. In this case, the viscoelastic is essential to tamponade possible bleeding following iris tissue traction or small vessel breaks as well as to mobilize the iris pigment released during synechiolysis or floating iris fragments. Also, an excellent soft and permanent spatula effect as well as good space

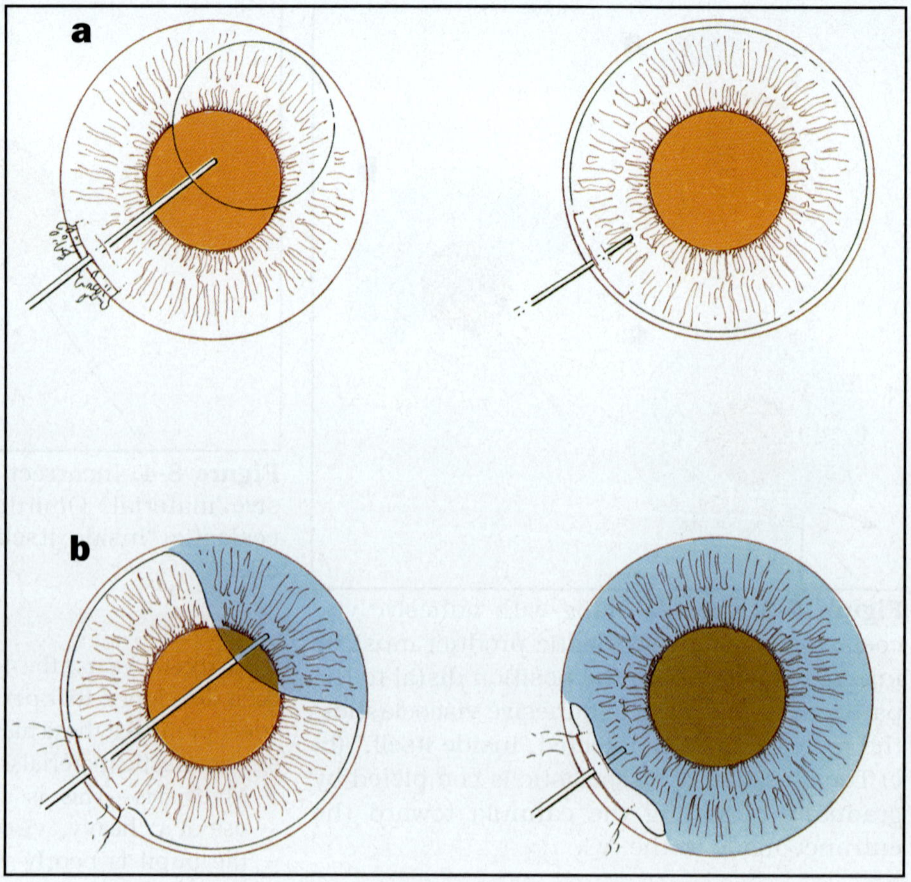

Figure 8-5. Anterior chamber filling with viscoelastic: air/viscoelastic exchange. (a) Air in the AC. (b) The viscoelastic, injected at 6 o'clock, replaces air leaving through the opening in the AC.

maintenance is necessary, provided that the viscoelastic does not leave the chamber while the surgical tools are being moved into the AC.

- Pupillary stretch—Completed by means of hooks and bimanual maneuver through the main incision and the paracentesis. This is accomplished by forcing the pupillary borders in opposite directions to achieve its enlargement (Figure 8-8). Stretching can also be performed with recently introduced devices, such as the one suggested by Zanini. This consists of a coaxial and monomanual system that is introduced through the main incision and, once opened, stretches the pupillary border along the axis of the device itself. Because the tool is more cumbersome than two single hooks, it will require a heavy viscoelastic to keep space and avoid contact between the device and the cornea on one side and the anterior capsule on the other (Figure 8-9).
- Removal of fibrotic pupillary membrane—When the membrane is present, its removal by forceps (for example, McPherson or Corydon forceps) can smooth the way for subsequent mydriasis with a heavy viscoelastic such as Healon® GV. When the fibrotic membrane is incised bleeding and the release of the iris pigment almost always occurs. It is paramount that the surgeon use a viscoelastic that is able to control these phenomena while providing good visualization. High viscosity at low shear rate and excellent soft and permanent spatula effect are basic requirements to perform the maneuver. In this respect Healon® GV is unrivaled.
- Multiple sphincterotomies—This procedure is more traumatic than the others. The surgeon is compelled to use microscissors, which, when introduced in the chamber under viscoelastic control, allow the surgeon to cut multiple, small, radial incisions in the pupillary border. He or she can then achieve partial dilation after the intro-

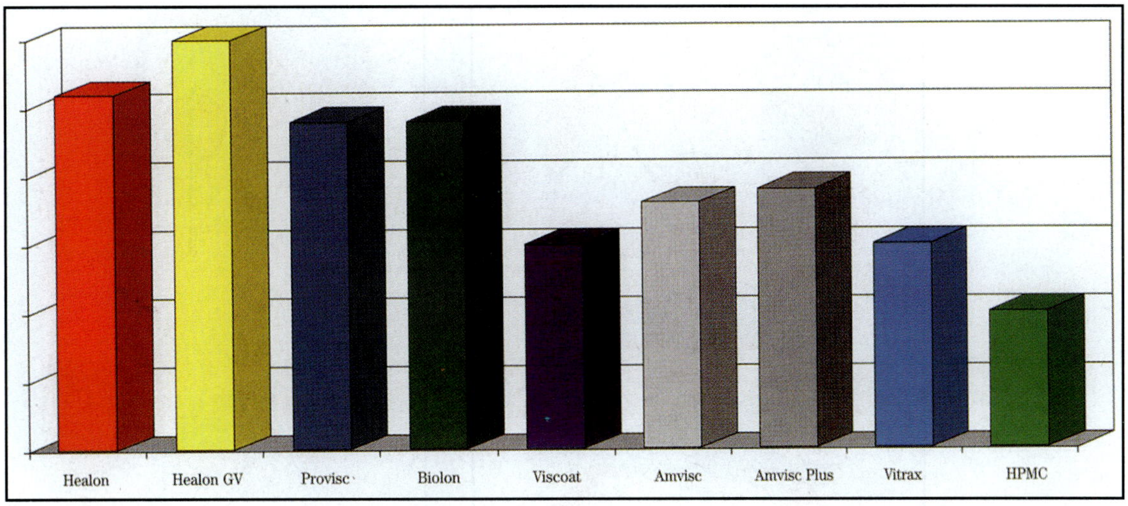

Figure 8-6. Injectability. Healon® = red; Healon® GV = yellow; Viscoat = blue; Provisc = octane; Amvisc = light gray; Amvisc Plus = dark gray; Vitrax = azure; Biolon = green; HPMC = pale green.

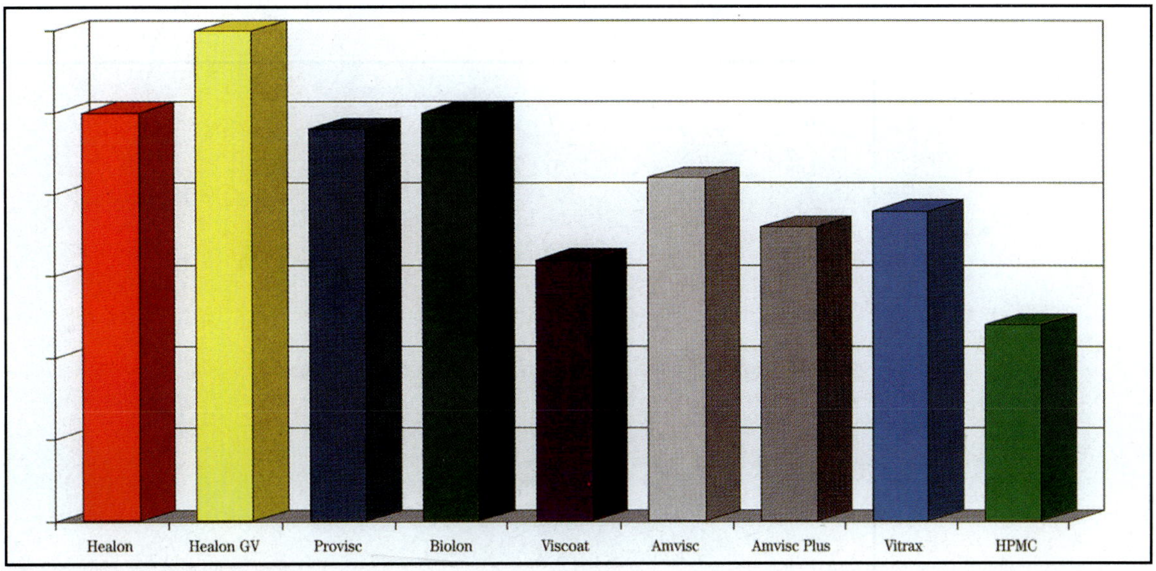

Figure 8-7. Mobilization of tissues (soft spatula).

duction of the viscoelastic. These sphincterotomies must be very short, small, and radially oriented in order to minimize bleeding or iris tissue damage that, besides causing postoperative inflammation, also impair the recovery of pupillary function (Figure 8-10). It is difficult for the surgeon to create a sphincterotomy in the subincisional iris. Although small and bent surgery scissors have been invented, the surgeon still may deform the tunnel to enter the AC and is then forced to adopt uncomfortable and unnatural positions which may cause a partial leakage of viscoelastic from the chamber. Therefore, it is necessary to use a heavy, transparent viscoelastic with high viscosity at a low shear rate that has the ability to "freeze" the situation for as long as possible with a deep chamber and strict tissue control. Again, Healon® GV is preferred.

- Mechanical mydriasis—This is accomplished by means of soft or rigid hooks, placed at the

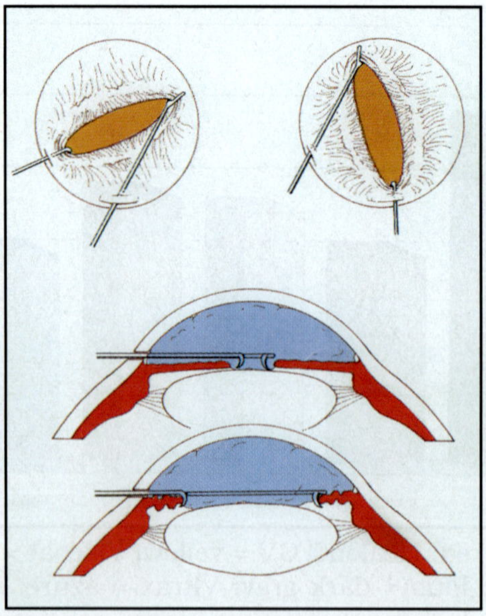

Figure 8-8. Pupillary stretching (bimanual maneuver with two hooks).

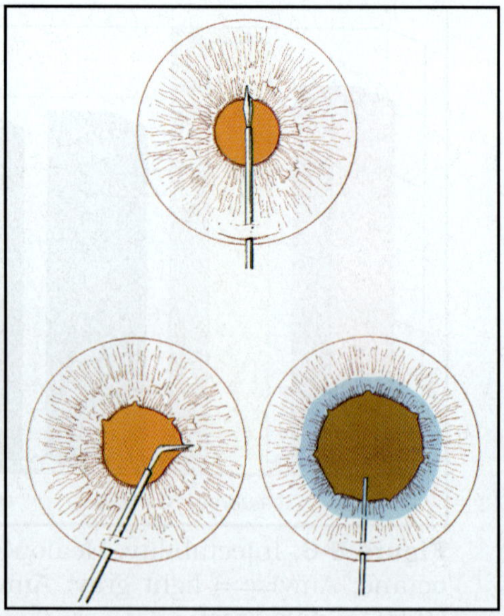

Figure 8-9. Pupillary stretching (one-handed maneuver).

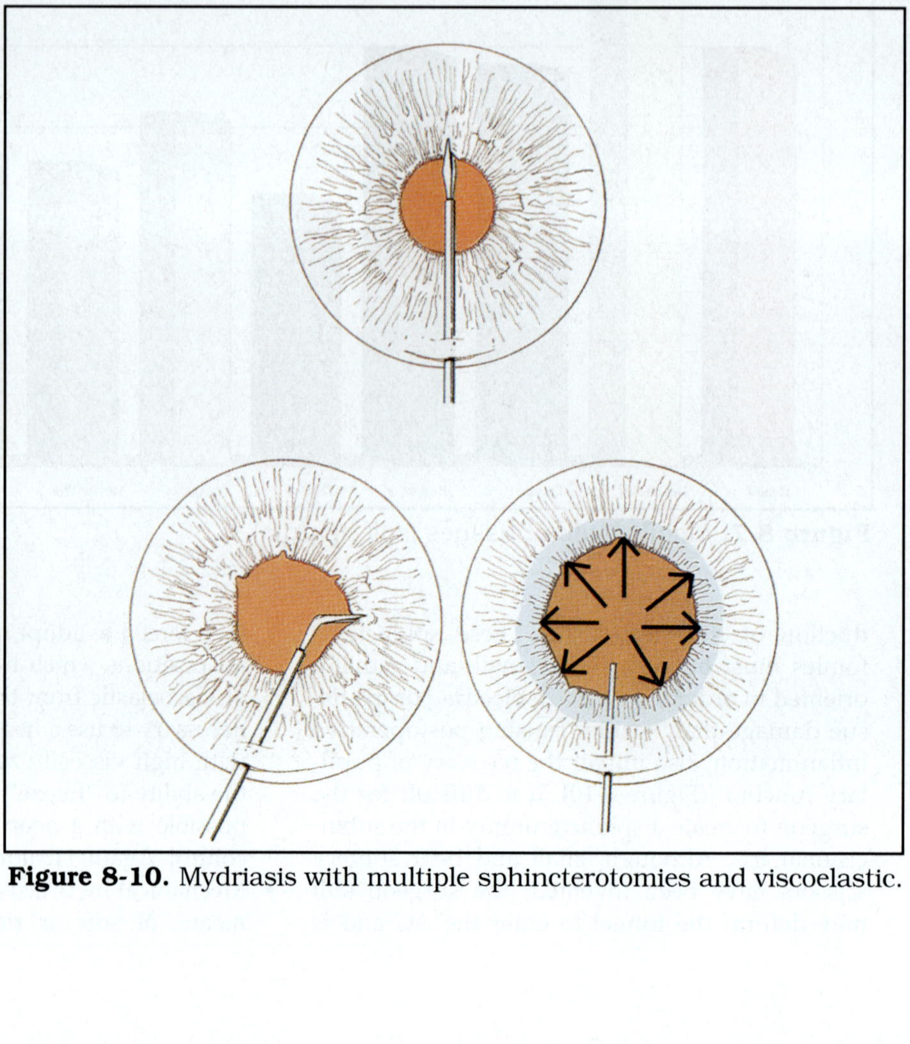

Figure 8-10. Mydriasis with multiple sphincterotomies and viscoelastic.

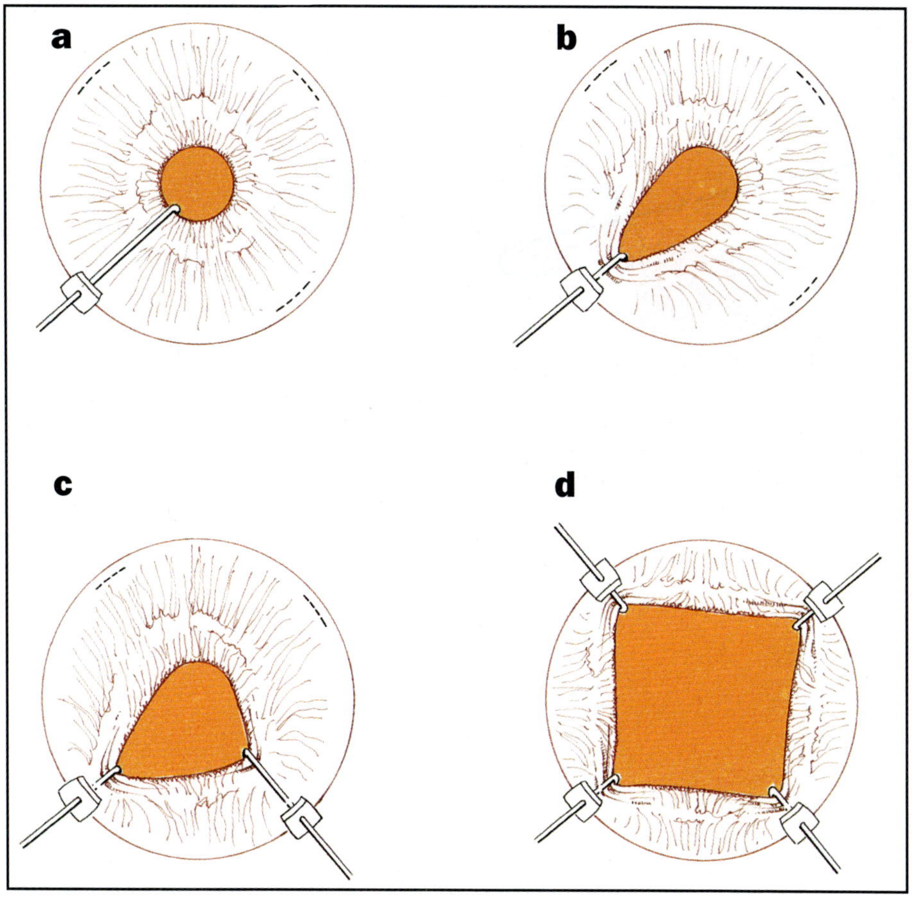

Figure 8-11. Mechanical mydriasis by means of hooks. (a) After creating a paracentesis incision and injecting a viscoelastic material to create an optimal working space in the AC, the first hook is introduced under the pupillary border. (b) The hook is retracted centrifugally, and once the desired mydriasis has been achieved, it is blocked with a small silicone clip. (c) The procedure is repeated in the four quadrants. (d) The four hooks in place.

beginning of surgery and left in place until IOL implantation has been completed. Various types of materials, flexible or stiff (made of nylon, prolene, or metal), have been suggested. These are placed (generally on four hooks) at the beginning of surgery, making four paracentesis incisions in the limbus at 2, 10, 4, and 8 o'clock with respect to the surgeon. Through these openings, the hooks are introduced in the AC after injecting a heavy viscoelastic. After hooking the iris, they are pulled toward the limbus and fixed by small clips inserted on their portion outside the eye (Figure 8-11). Healon® GV is particularly useful in this maneuver, where the risk of accidental contact between the hook and the corneal endothelium is high (Figure 8-12). The whole procedure can be easily controlled with no losses of chamber depth or trauma between the hook and iris anterior capsular corneal endothelium. It is important that the chamber is deep and bleeding is controlled. It is advisable to replace the viscoelastic (Healon® GV) with another one more likely to remain in the AC during phaco maneuvers. A more adhesive and less cohesive material, such as Viscoat or Vitrax, should be used. In case of hypotony during phacoemulsification, this will allow one to avoid accidental contact with the hook and the corneal endothelium.

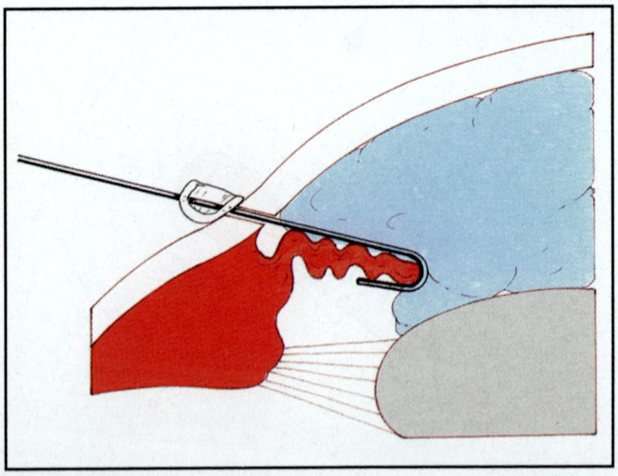

Figure 8-12. The viscoelastic material keeps a safe distance among hook, cornea, and lens.

CHAPTER NINE

Capsulorhexis

The ophthalmic surgeon must understand that the advent of capsulorhexis represents a milestone in contemporary cataract surgery. During the mid 1980s, Gimbel and Neuhann simultaneously developed the concept of continuous curvilinear capsulorhexis (CCC). The idea is one of the most significant innovations of the last 15 years. The advantages of capsulorhexis are widely known and include better IOL centering, more correct positioning in the capsular bag, and reduced incidence of secondary posterior capsule opacification. Owing to the stability of capsulorhexis, it has been possible for surgeons to develop endocapsular phacoemulsification, nucleofracture inside the bag, and modern chop techniques. Furthermore, it has enabled the improvement of delineation and dissection techniques with fluids inside the bag or the nucleus, to allow the surgeon to approach the nucleus and cortex together or separately. Capsulorhexis has facilitated the development of advanced extracapsular techniques using hydro- or viscoexpression and provided IOLs with valuable support in case of a posterior capsule break.

Moreover, the absence of free and irregular capsular flaps, which result from performance of the can-opener technique, reduces postoperative inflammation, thereby preventing the formation of posterior synechiae, pupillary deformations, and IOL capture by the pupil. In addition, capsulorhexis prevents and minimizes any contact between the iris and other structures in the posterior chamber, which limits the dispersion of pigment and glaucoma.

Implantation in the bag is a basic necessity for the surgical treatment of patients with uveitis or glaucoma. The stability of capsulorhexis enables the performance of all maneuvers for soft foldable IOL implantation—introduction inside the bag and then unfolding and centering using various systems for implantation, such as forceps and injectors. Therefore, capsule and bag, which were often a cause of anxiety in the past owing to the possibility of uncontrolled breaks, are now intrinsic elements of modern ophthalmic surgery.

The basic principle in the performance of capsulorhexis is that a tear in the AC can be accomplished at the surgeon's will, which produces the desired shape (which is that of CCC). There are two methods that may be employed to create the capsulorhexis execution: cystotome or forceps.

Arshinoff described the progression of capsulorhexis through tearing by shearing when the capsulorhexis is performed with a cystotome (Figure 9-1). Otherwise, capsulorhexis can be achieved through tearing by stretching that occurs when the rhexis is performed with a forceps (Figure 9-2). The forceps technique is considered much easier, as the surgeon can direct the capsular flap while exerting tractions that are tangential to the capsular surface but also perpendicular to it and therefore easier to control. This holds true particularly for difficult capsulorhexis performed in eyes with small pupils, because when the capsular flap is being torn upward it is automatically guided by the pupillary border itself. It is often possible to accomplish capsulorhexis that are larger than the pupil without losing control, as the flap is constantly guided and drawn by the pupillary edge. This technique is feasible provided that traction is exerted upward by means of a forceps. The forceps technique greatly eases the performance of capsulorhexis when a red reflex is poor or absent. The forceps used can have either convergent or coaxial jaws.

It preferable to use forceps as they provide a safer hold of the capsular flap. The performance of capsulorhexis by forceps requires an incision length of at least 2.5 to 3 mm that allows easy opening of

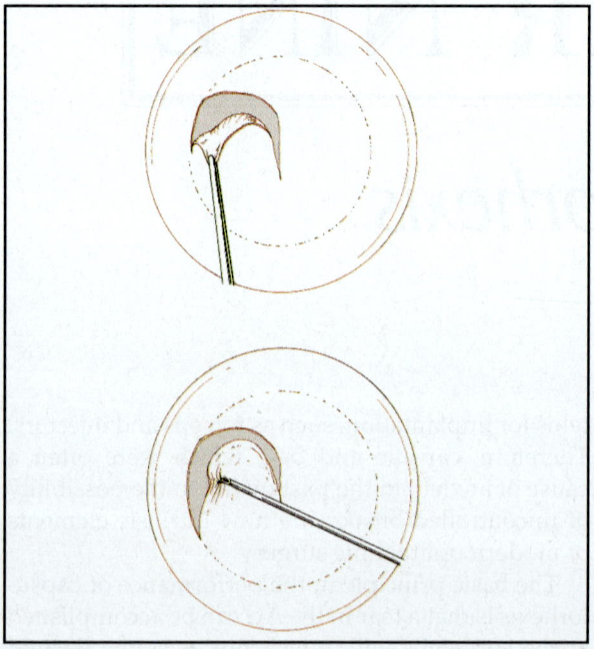

Figure 9-1. Capsulorhexis performed with tearing by stretching technique.

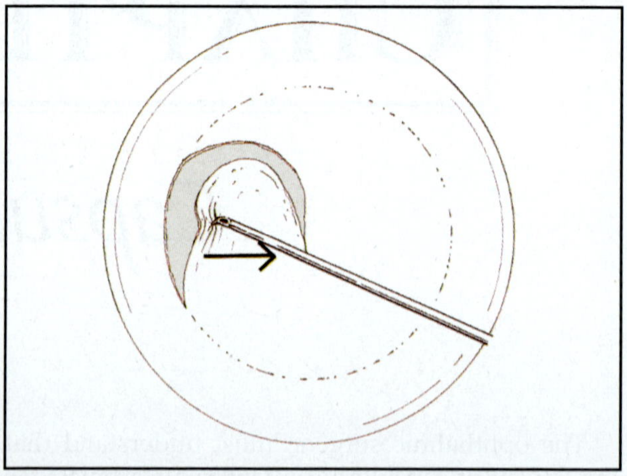

Figure 9-2. Capsulorhexis performed with tearing by shearing technique. Force generated by forceps.

the jaws and their rotating motion inside the AC while creating the CCC.

In this respect, the cystotome is more suitable, as it requires a very small opening and allows the surgeon to work in a closed chamber. Nevertheless, the cystotome does not provide a stable grasp of the capsular flap, results in poor control when the surgeon wishes to make a large rhexis, and does not permit modification of shape or diameter during performance of the rhexis. In addition, it can only be performed when the AC is homogeneous. Moreover, when an irrigating cystotome is used, it causes bothersome fluctuations of the flap. With respect to the cystotome, capsulorhexis by forceps does not posses these drawbacks. When beginners perform rhexis, forceps provide optimal and safe control during the procedure.

The contents of the AC are another basic element for the performance of a correct rhexis. BSS, air, or viscoelastic material can be used. BSS is generally used with the cystotome technique, and consequently presents the same limitations mentioned. Furthermore, in complicated cases (ie, remarkable vitreous pressure, juvenile cataract, or small pupil), BSS is not recommended. Air is likely to leave the AC, particularly when forceps are used to perform capsulorhexis. It may occasionally be advantageous when performing a difficult rhexis with poor red reflex, but requires an experienced surgeon and is not recommended for beginners.

It can therefore be concluded that capsulorhexis performed by forceps under viscoelastic is considered the easiest, safest, and most reproducible method in both routine surgery and difficult cases.

In the following, we examine which viscoelastic is ideal for the performance of safe CCC and the reasons the viscoelastic is fundamental in the performance of this phase of surgery.

The optimal width of capsulorhexis is controversial. Surgeons debate whether it should be equal to, slightly larger than, or smaller than the IOL diameter. The opening must be central and not too small. The surgeon must constantly control the development of the rhexis, avoiding potential loss of control extension toward the equator or convergence toward the center.

It is essential to understand that two forces act on the detached edge contributing to the direction and course of the rhexis. One force is the tension exerted by zonular fibers that generates a radial force. Once the first tearing on the anterior capsule has started, this force is applied on the most equatorial edge of the flap. The second force is generated at the spot of detachment caused by the traction exerted by the surgeon (Figure 9-3).

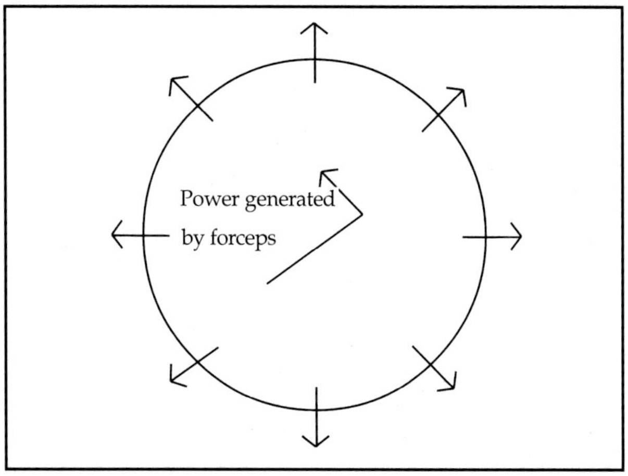

Figure 9-3. Centrifugal radial force generated by zonular fibers.

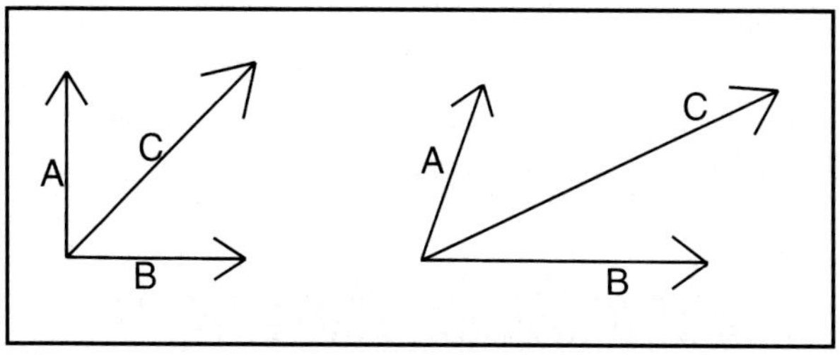

Figure 9-4. The higher the force of B (zonular fiber force), the more the rhexis will extend outward, thus driving it away from the direction impressed by A (forceps force).

When two forces act on one location it is possible to calculate direction, sense, and strength of the resulting vector. Therefore, an increase in the general force of zonular fibers is likely to shift the resulting vector toward that force (ie, outward) (Figure 9-4). When the zonular force is high, there is an increased tendency for the rhexis to escape control. The lower the force indicated with B (zonular force), the closer C is to the direction and force exerted by the forceps.

Thus, it is evident that the key to optimal control of the rhexis is control of zonular tension. If the lens moves anteriorly, zonular fibers are submitted to tension. On the contrary, when it shifts posteriorly, the zonular fibers are relaxed. Consequently, if remarkable vitreous pressure is present, the lens moves forward and zonular tension is increased. In this circumstance, any tearing on the anterior capsule moves toward the periphery in an uncontrolled fashion. Therefore, the performance of capsulorhexis intimately depends on the constant preservation of a deep AC (Figure 9-5).

The optimal viscoelastic must possess four basic features for the surgeon to perform a correct CCC. They are: 1) maintenance of a deep AC; 2) excellent visibility; 3) preservation of a stable capsular flap that does not fluctuate or push downward; and 4) ease of surgical maneuvers.

Maintenance of a Deep Anterior Chamber = High Molecular Weight and High Viscosity at Zero Shear Rate

The considerations previously made with respect to AC filling and preservation are also true in the case of capsulorhexis. High molecular weight and high viscosity at low shear rate are elements of basic importance. Healon® GV best demonstrates these characteristics. High viscosity also allows the surgeon to treat intumescent white cataracts successfully. When the anterior capsule is punctured, some milky cortical fluid leaks out. This is easily moved to the periphery by Healon® GV, thus allowing the surgeon to continue CCC with good visibility and to grasp the capsular flap created by early opening.

Optimal Visibility = High Transparency

The products containing hyaluronic acid are preferable and Healon® GV achieves optimal performance.

Capsular Flap Control = Soft and Permanent Spatula Effect

As the rhexis proceeds, it is important to be able to move the capsule without fluctuation, while keeping it pressed downward. When the surgeon pauses, the situation should be frozen in that position to allow a change in grasp (holding the flap with the forceps closer to its base) or a change of direction (in the traction exerted by the forceps). The viscoelastic material must provide the best soft and permanent spatula effect; once again, hyaluronic acid with high molecular weight is preferred.

EASE OF SURGICAL MANEUVERS = HIGH PSEUDOPLASTICITY, HIGH ELASTICITY

The viscoelastic material must, above all, protect the ocular structures from contact with the instruments introduced in the chamber, preserve optimal space, and allow the performance of precise movements. The high pseudoplasticity of Healon® GV, Healon®, and hyaluronic acid with high molecular weight generally meet these requirements.

PROPER CCC MANEUVER

The appropriate maneuver to perform a good CCC begins with puncture of the center of the anterior capsule. This can be accomplished with an insulin needle or by the closed jaws of the capsulorhexis forceps. The tip of the jaws is introduced at the puncture site, while lifting the capsule upward to create the edge of the capsular flap to grasp. The procedure continues by pulling the flap at its base in a circular motion, keeping in mind that some of the viscoelastic may leak out through the chamber opening as a result of the push of the forceps.

Partial viscoelastic leakage may reduce AC depth, thus increasing the traction force exerted by zonular fibers and favoring possible rhexis extension. If this occurs, the surgeon should refill the chamber with viscoelastic, grasp the flap at its base again, and exert traction in a centripetal direction. The surgeon should not hesitate to accomplish this maneuver as soon as the rhexis tends toward the periphery. This should also be performed in high-risk cases, such as congenital or juvenile cataracts, intumescent lens opacities, and highly myopic eyes in obese patients with difficult respiration, or in the presence of increased orbital volumes resulting from retrobulbar injection. If the surgeon observes these rules he or she will almost always complete a correct CCC (Figure 9-6).

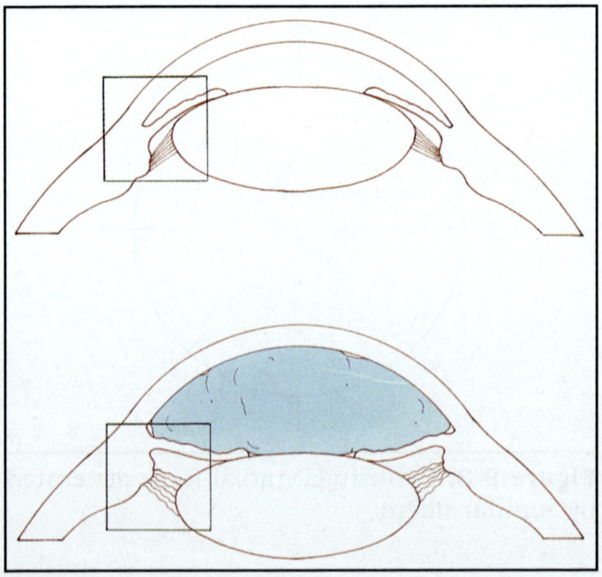

Figure 9-5. The viscoelastic material deepens the AC while relaxing zonular fibers.

In difficult cases with small pupils, white or brown cataracts, or poor red reflex of the fundus, the performance of diathermal capsulotomy may also be useful. Because small bubbles are created by the passage of diathermy on the anterior capsule, it is essential that the viscoelastic material does not trap air bubbles and preserves optimal space, permitting a precise and controlled movement of diathermy.

Based on our observations, Healon® GV is the ideal material to perform capsulorhexis in routine surgery as well as in complicated cases. The use of Viscoat is also acceptable, as it is less likely to leave the AC while the incision is being manipulated; however, this material has less pseudoplasticity, poorer soft and permanent spatula effect, and reduced transparency. The products containing hyaluronic acid with high molecular weight, such as Healon® and Provisc, are less desirable. Viscoelastic solutions containing HPMC are to be used as a last resort. In Figure 9-7, we list the various viscoelastics according to their ability to keep space, a basic feature for the performance of an optimal rhexis.

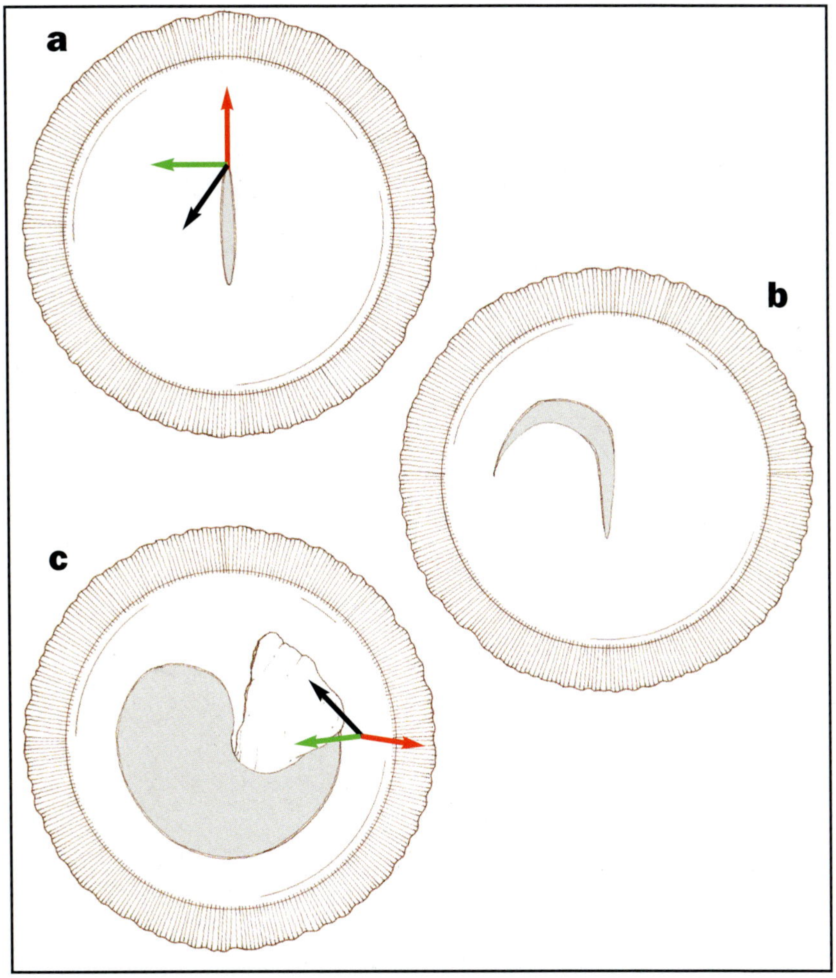

Figure 9-6. (a) Beginning of capsulorhexis. (b) Progression of capsulorhexis. (c) Completion of the rhexis. (The red arrows show zonular force, the green arrows show the direction of the traction exerted by the forceps, and the black arrows show the progression of the rhexis.)

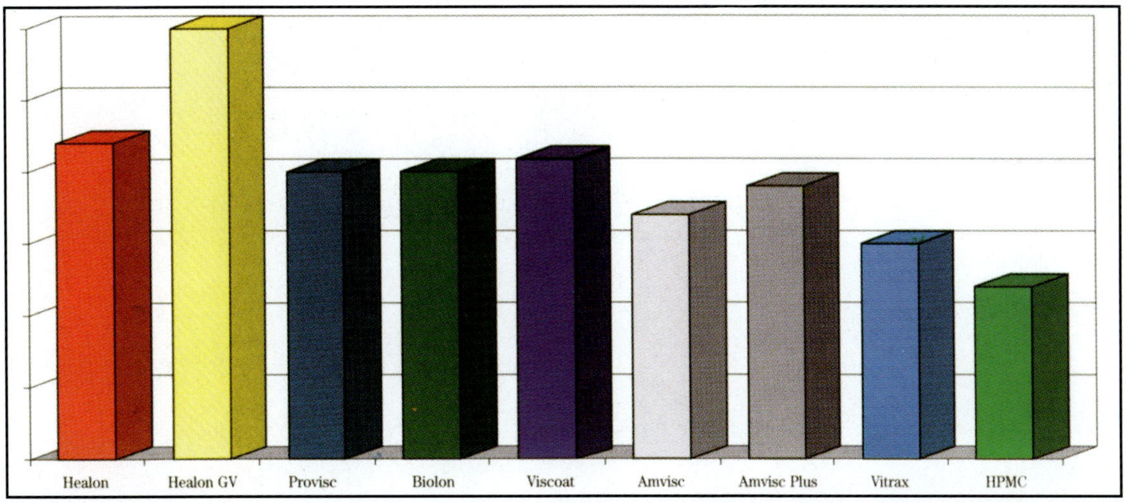

Figure 9-7. Space maintenance/tissue stabilization (permanent spatula effect).

Chapter Ten

Cleavage of Lens Structures

Modern surgical techniques allow the surgeon to detect and separate various parts of the lens. Such techniques were first studied by surgeons using the extracapsular technique, but then were rapidly expanded and applied to phacoemulsification, including nucleofracture and chop techniques. These cleavage techniques can be performed with viscoelastic materials or BSS.

Hydrodelineation

Hydrodelineation is the separation, by means of fluid injection, of the internal nucleus consisting of very compact and therefore inseparable lamellae and the external nucleus, or epinucleus, which consists of less compact lamellae.

Hydrodissection

Hydrodissection is performed by injecting BSS or viscoelastic under the anterior capsule; the fluid finds space between the cortex and the epinucleus. Contrary to popular belief, cleavage does not occur between the capsule and cortex. Fine recently asserted that it is possible to make a cortex/capsule cleavage by creating a very small capsulorhexis and injecting the fluid immediately under the lifted anterior capsule. This way, the amount of cortex aspirated with irrigation and aspiration cannula (no-cortex technique) is reduced. In fact, this can be accomplished in very old and hard cataracts where the nucleus is nearly the whole lens and in very soft juvenile or presenile cataracts, where decreased lamellar thickness allows the surgeon to delineate many lens components.

Hydrodelamination

Hydrodelamination is performed by splitting the superficial portion from the compact internal portion of the nucleus with a thin cannula that is advanced forward into the nucleus, inside the capsulorhexis, until it is opposed by resistance. The fluid is injected in an attempt to achieve cleavage, evidenced by a typical golden ring, between the nucleus and the epinucleus.

Hydrodelamination allows the surgeon to tackle the inner and harder nucleus (for instance, with a chop technique) independently of the outer and softer nucleus (with aspiration alone or with low power ultrasounds). Hydrodelamination is used to mobilize the nucleus so it can rotate inside the capsular bag and dissect most of the capsular/cortical adhesions, which eases the removal of residual cortical material. This procedure is also useful in creating a space between the capsule and nucleus in order to move the whole nucleus in front of the pupil when surgical complications force the surgeon to convert from phaco to ECCE procedures.

Surgeon's Needs With Relation to the Viscoelastic Material

The basic requisites for successful outcome of the procedures mentioned are that the wave of fluid injected is free to circulate, can divide the tissues to be separated, and is then able to leave toward the AC. Therefore, the ideal viscoelastic material must keep the AC shape unchanged during BSS injection and avoid remarkable pressure increase in the event that an excessive amount of BSS is injected (capsular blockade). The viscoelastic material must be able to preserve the AC (high viscosity at low shear rate) and leave the eye when too much BSS has been introduced (high cohesiveness and high pseudoplasticity).

Consequently, it is important to choose a product that is cohesive, is pseudoplastic, and shows high viscosity at 0 shear rate. Healon® and Provisc seem to fulfill these requirements fairly well. On some occasions, Healon® GV may turn out to be too heavy and cause the BSS "wave" to discharge with more difficulty from the bag.

A potential drawback to adhesive materials such as Viscoat and Vitrax is that they are less likely to leave the AC when an excessive amount of BSS is injected. This results in a severe pressure rise. Also with Viscoat, the wave of fluid injected may create cleavage lines, which make good visibility behind structures more difficult to achieve.

In addition to the use of a suitable viscoelastic (a fairly pseudoplastic and cohesive material), application of slight pressure on the posterior border of a surgical wound prior to hydrocleavage is useful because it allows a small amount of viscoelastic to leak out. This results in better circulation of the fluid wave injected, which will be easily discharged from the bag (Figure 10-1).

It has been suggested that hydrodissection could be performed with viscoelastic material. This would allow the surgeon to create a "safety space" in front of the posterior capsule that would make contact between the phaco tip and the posterior capsule less likely. We deem this procedure unnecessary and in some cases even dangerous. Corydon demonstrated that there is an inversely proportional relationship between the size of capsulorhexis

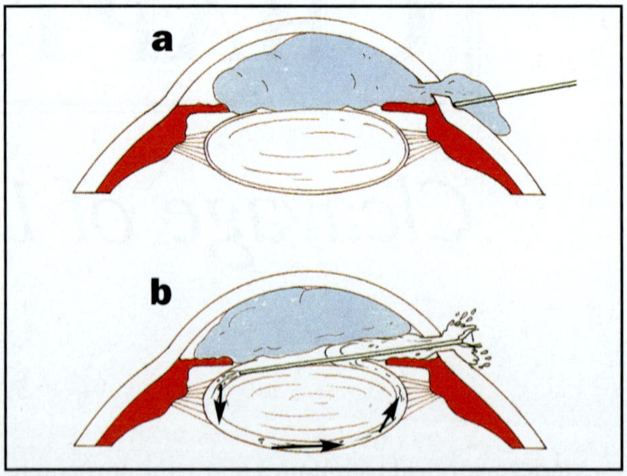

Figure 10-1. (a) Before performing hydrodissection, press the cannula on the posterior edge of the tunnel and let a small amount of viscoelastic leak out. (b) Inject BSS under the anterior capsule. The wave will go out of the capsular bag more easily, as an area free from viscoelastic has been created.

and the possibility that the viscoelastic injected into the bag may break the posterior capsule. In other words, the smaller the rhexis, the higher the possibility that the viscoelastic injected will break the posterior capsule and enter the vitreous space.

Viscoelastic injection in the capsular bag is a legitimate procedure only when a conversion from phaco to ECCE is required. In this event, the surgeon can luxate the nucleus outside the bag in the AC in order to perform viscoexpression later, when the incision is open wider. One can also try to accomplish a manual phacoemulsification in the AC (for example, by Kansas' trisector) (Figure 10-2).

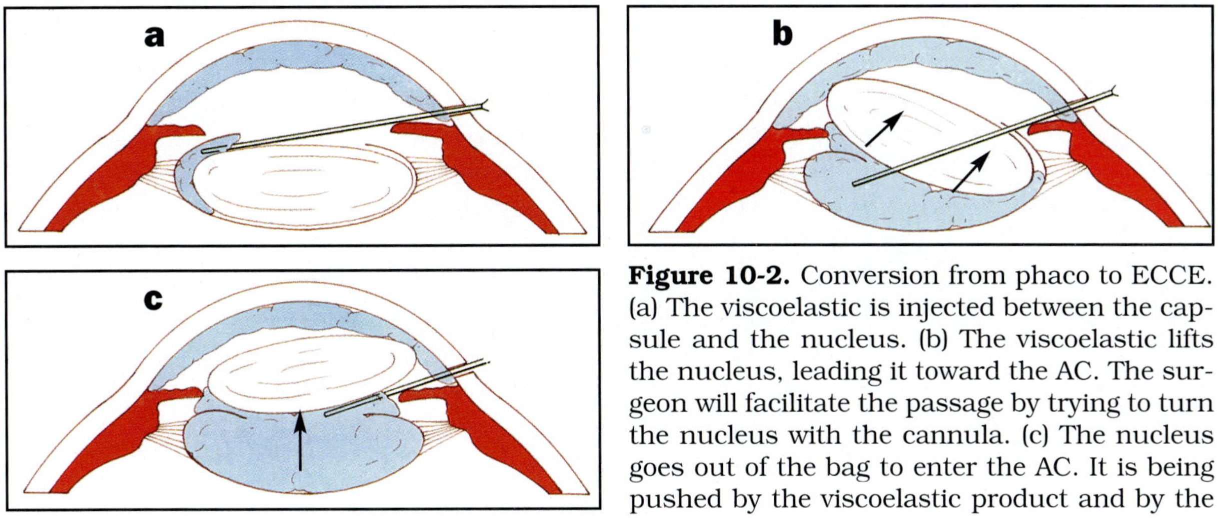

Figure 10-2. Conversion from phaco to ECCE. (a) The viscoelastic is injected between the capsule and the nucleus. (b) The viscoelastic lifts the nucleus, leading it toward the AC. The surgeon will facilitate the passage by trying to turn the nucleus with the cannula. (c) The nucleus goes out of the bag to enter the AC. It is being pushed by the viscoelastic product and by the rotation maneuver accomplished with one or both hands of the surgeon with cannula and spatula.

Chapter Eleven

Phacoemulsification

While the phase of real phacoemulsification is being performed (Figure 11-1), the basic requirements for the surgeon are the following:

- Preservation of space despite the movements of the phaco tip, the spatula, and the nucleus.
- Because phaco is a turbulent process with continuous high fluid irrigation and aspiration flows, it tends to remove the viscoelastic. To compensate for this, the surgeon needs a product that is able to resist these forces and remain in the eye for endothelial protection.
- The possibility of leakage, slow and controlled, during the whole phaco procedure, and complete removal on conclusion.
- Protection of surfaces, especially the corneal endothelium, because emulsification of the nucleus produces: collision of nuclear particles in the AC; air bubbles consequent to cavitation processes that may damage the endothelium; high fluid turbulence; and high hydric exchange, which also removes some of the viscoelastic material.
- Protection of the eye from the mechanical vibrations of the phaco tip produced by the ultrasounds that are transmitted to ocular structures.

In the following, we examine these five points in detail and determine which viscoelastic products are able to fulfill these requirements.

Preservation of Space: Phaco Parameters

Viscoelastic is not essential in the preservation of space. Once the phaco tip has been introduced in the AC, the elements responsible for constant AC depth are the machine settings (height of the bottle, flow rate, vacuum values, kind of pump, presence or absence of continued irrigation). These elements, rather than the presence of viscoelastic, actually permit the surgeon to work in a deep chamber. However, a product with poor pseudoplasticity is more likely to remain in the AC instead of leaking out of the eye. Therefore, products such as Viscoat, Vitrax, Amvisc Plus, and methylcellulose are preferred.

Low Cohesiveness: Product Remaining in the Chamber Despite High Irrigation Flow

As stated previously, the irrigation fluid of phaco tends to remove the viscoelastic from the AC. Materials with short molecular chains and low molecular weight are less cohesive and consequently remain in the chamber for a longer period of time. Therefore, Viscoat and Vitrax are particularly suited for this procedure as compared with other solutions with high cohesion and high molecular weight that come out as a whole mass (Figure 11-2).

Low Cohesiveness: Permanence in the Chamber While Instruments Are Being Introduced

Viscoat, which is poorly cohesive, is probably most effective in maintaining space without leaving the chamber during the introduction of the phaco

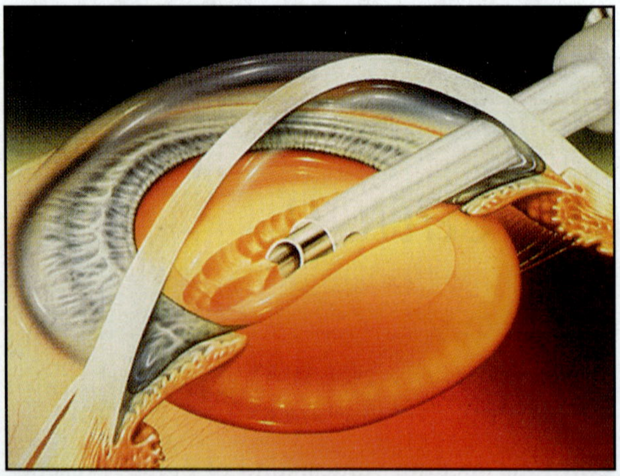

Figure 11-1. Phacoemulsification.

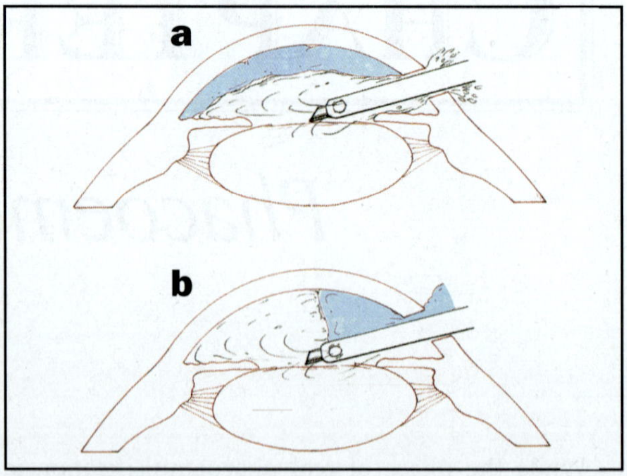

Figure 11-2. (a) Dispersive products leak out only partially due to the irrigation flow during phacoemulsification. (b) Cohesive products tend to come out of the chamber as a whole mass due to irrigation flow.

tip or the spatula. In the event that Viscoat does leak, it comes out little by little in a controllable way. On the contrary, cohesive products such as Healon® GV, Healon®, and Provisc are likely to leave the AC as a whole mass, owing to their long molecular chains and high molecular weight.

Adhesiveness: Protection of Corneal Endothelium

Adhesive materials such as Viscoat, Vitrax, and HPMC tend to protect corneal endothelial cells by adhering to them. High wettability is an essential feature in accomplishing this.

The subject of endothelial protection is controversial. Some researchers assert that the presence of Viscoat in the chamber until the end of the procedure ensures endothelial protection. In practice, they support a "mechanical protection" of endothelial cells, which is accomplished by stratifying the viscoelastic upon them. The low wettability of Healon®, Healon® GV, and Provisc results in their poor ability to coat surfaces. However, other researchers claim that, despite this, Healon® and Healon® GV provide excellent endothelial protection because of three main characteristics:

- Scavenger effect—Capture of free radicals released during phaco with consequent inactivation.
- Binding sites—Chemical receptors for viscoelastic materials on the corneal endothelium. A molecular bond seems to occur between the viscoelastic solution and the corneal endothelium that can persist up to several hours after phacoemulsification. This protection would be much greater than that provided by the mechanical stratification of adhesive materials such as Viscoat, Vitrax, or HPMC on the endothelium.
- High elasticity—found in Healon® and Healon® GV, this would also smooth possible impacts of lens material against the endothelium provided that they occur when the viscoelastic is still present in the chamber.

The question of endothelial protection still exists; however, it seems that the permanence of a viscoelastic on the corneal endothelium during the whole phaco procedure is a favorable element. From this point of view, adhesive materials such as Viscoat, Vitrax, and HPMC are preferable.

High Elasticity: Protection From Mechanical Vibrations of the Phaco Tip

The phaco tip vibrates when it is operated. Because it is inside a closed system, its vibrations

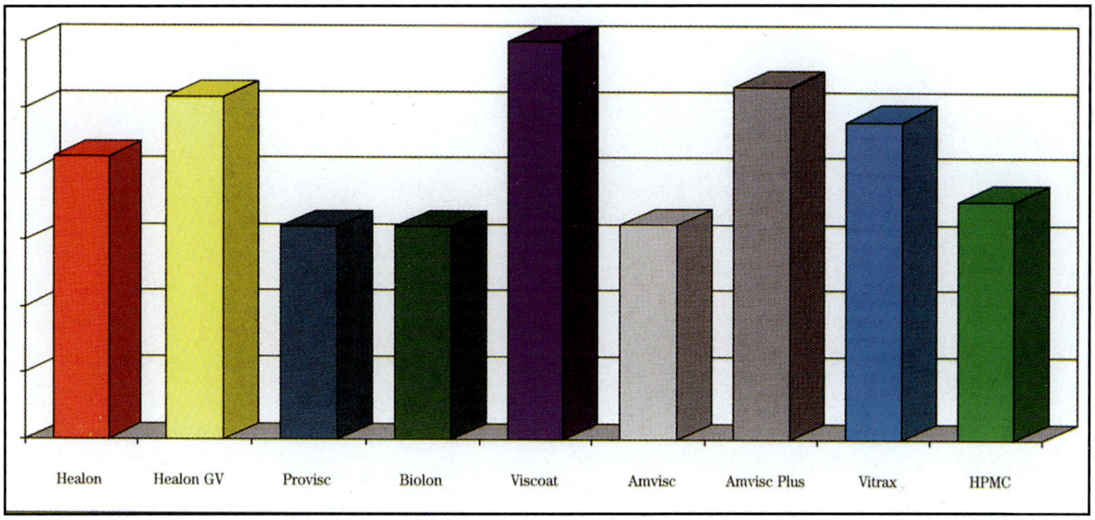

Figure 11-3. Phacoemulsification.

are transmitted to the internal structures of the eye. The viscoelastic must provide a smoothening shield against them. In this case, the question is whether highly elastic materials such as Healon® GV or Healon® are preferable to less elastic materials such as Viscoat. It must be considered that more elastic products are also more cohesive because they have longer molecular chains. They also leave the AC more quickly during phacoemulsification. Therefore, a less elastic product that remains in the AC is preferable to a highly elastic material that quickly leaves the chamber.

In Figure 11-3, viscoelastic materials for phacoemulsification are listed in order according to preference. Viscoat tops the list. However, this product has some negative aspects that should be pointed out:

- Although the material remains in the AC, air bubbles already present in the product that are not accurately discharged from the syringe or that are created by cavitation of the phaco tip may be trapped in Viscoat and could obscure visibility during surgery.
- Product transparency is limited owing to the intrinsic features of the material and because during surgery some irregular cleavage lines may occur and form irregular surfaces in the Viscoat/irrigation fluid interface. At times this results in poor visibility and obliges the surgeon to remove the layer of product in contact with the nuclear material at the beginning of the phaco.
- Usually considered an advantage, Viscoat's endurance to removability may also be a drawback in that the product requires a longer time for removal at the end of surgery. Several maneuvers to ease viscoelastic removal at the end of surgery have been described. However, all of them are characterized by high flow and a long irrigation and aspiration time that has been found to cause endothelial damage.
- Viscoat may be likely to occlude the phaco tip. This occurs particularly in "slow motion" techniques, in which low flow and low or zero vacuum values are used. Thus, at the beginning of the procedure, it is important to remove the layer of viscoelastic in contact with the nuclear material by using a suitable vacuum and flow setting for a few seconds.

Chapter Twelve

Irrigation and Aspiration

Most of the capsular breaks that occur during phacoemulsification take place during irrigation and aspiration of residual epinuclear or cortical material. Complete removal results in reduced postoperative inflammation and decreased incidence of posterior capsular opacification. The surgeon should take all the time needed to accomplish this phase thoroughly and accurately.

A single probe or a two-way system may be used. The two-way system uses a separate line for infusion and another for aspiration, which are inserted through two different paracentesis incisions. It is also possible to accomplish aspiration of residual cortex fragments adjacent to the surgical port by using a one-way cannula mounted on a syringe that is operated under viscoelastic protection.

Irrigation and aspiration is commonly performed both in ECCE and in phacoemulsification cataract surgery. There is generally less cortical material left over at the end of nuclear phacoemulsification than there is after removal of the nucleus by the extracapsular technique. This is because hydrodissection in phacoemulsification is often more complete and effective and because repeated rotation of the nucleus allows the surgeon to remove the cortical material adherent to the capsule by using the phaco tip (no cortex technique).

In addition, most surgeons perform ECCE with a can-opener or envelope capsulotomy and not with capsulorhexis. Consequently, the margins of capsulotomy are more indented and irregular, which makes mechanical irrigation and aspiration more difficult.

Additionally, unlike in phacoemulsification, the opening made in the AC for ECCE is wider and the system is not closed. As a result, some of the irrigation fluid leaks out, the capsular bag is less formed, and the capture of cortical masses is more difficult to accomplish.

The surgeon has a variety of interchangeable tips to fix on the handpiece (straight, curved, angled, and U-shaped). Tips without sleeves are thinner and enter through the surgical wound with more ease; however, they do not keep the chamber as well formed as do tips with sleeves, particularly under topical anesthesia. On the contrary, tips with sleeves always ensure the presence of a deep AC and a well-formed bag, even in the presence of posterior vitreous pressure. The aspiration port ranges from 0.2 mm to 0.7 mm. The most commonly used size is 0.3 mm. Vacuum values for tips with such holes are generally 300 to 400 mmHg.

Aspiration of the cortex is usually started at the area most distal to the surgical wound, whereas the subincisional cortex is left for last because it is the most difficult to remove and further imbibition facilitates its aspiration. Two kinds of material can be removed with irrigation and aspiration. At the end of phacoemulsification and after expression of the nucleus in ECCE, a "bowl" of epinucleus occasionally remains with or without cortical material, depending on surgical technique. In addition to the irrigation and aspiration systems mentioned, the support provided by a viscoelastic material can also help the surgeon in some situations. Preservation of a deep AC and a well-formed bag depend mostly on the height of the irrigation bottle, the selected values of flow and vacuum, and the tightness of the incision. As previously stated, in phacoemulsification the viscoelastic plays a less important role than in other phases of the procedure, such as capsulorhexis or IOL implantation.

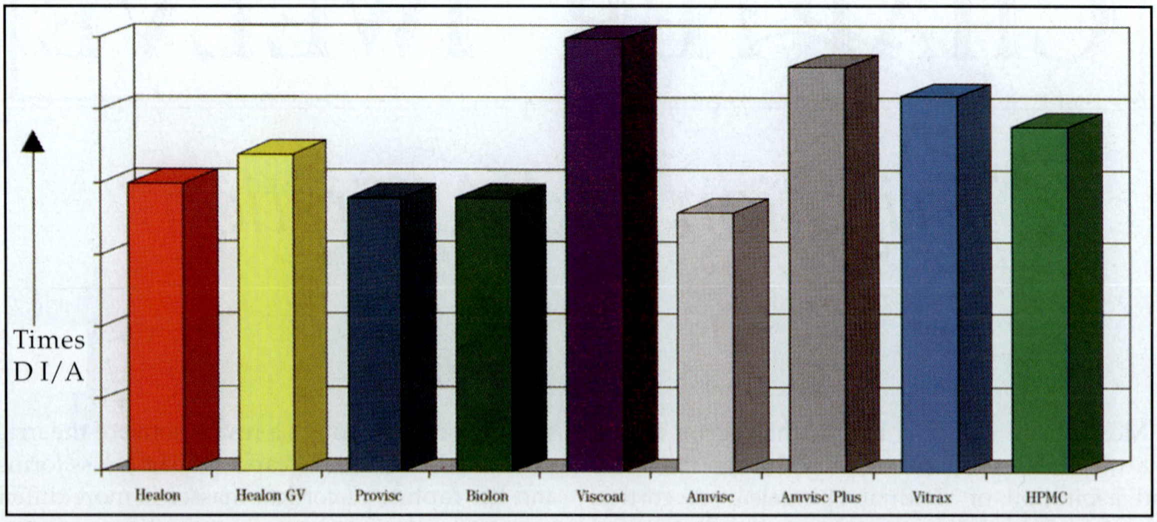

Figure 12-1. Relationship between adhesiveness and permanence in the chamber.

The ideal viscoelastic to use during irrigation and aspiration of the cortex possess the following features:

- Ability to resist high BSS flows inside the AC to provide constant endothelial protection
- Ability to remain where it has been placed (on the endothelial surface) without mixing with the cortex and interfering with cortical removal
- Ability to be cleared gradually, rather than coming out of the chamber as a whole mass when the probe is introduced

Endothelial Protection = High Adhesiveness

It is preferable to use a material that adheres to the endothelium and remains in the AC, despite high BSS flows (ie, Viscoat). The surgeon should also consider the endothelial protection provided by Healon® GV and Healon® (binding sites, scavenger effect, and elastic protection).

In any case, we prefer a material with high adhesiveness (Viscoat, Vitrax).

Ability to Remain Where Placed Without Mixing With the Cortex = Poor Cohesiveness

The viscoelastic material should enable easy removal of the cortical material, but avoid being aspirated with it. In this case, a material with poor cohesiveness is preferable.

Ability to Leave the Anterior Chamber Gradually = Poor Removability

A material showing dispersive features (ie, a poorly cohesive product with short molecular chains) is preferable. However, its complete removal at the end of surgery will be difficult, and the longer irrigation and aspiration time needed to remove the viscoelastic, the more danger to the corneal endothelium. Nevertheless, adhesive and poorly cohesive products are the most suitable. Our first choices are Viscoat, Vitrax, Amvisc Plus, and HPMC, as is evident in Figure 12-1.

This discussion may be academic, at least in part, as at this point of surgery if some residual viscoelastic is still present after phaco, as often happens with Viscoat, the surgeon is not likely to

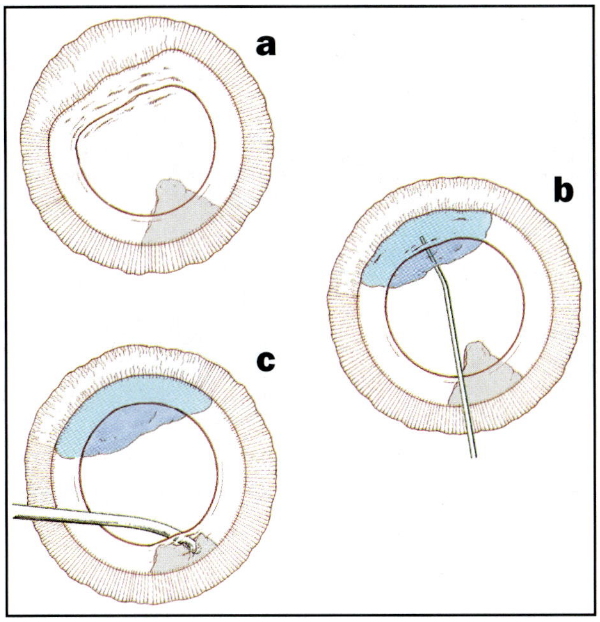

Figure 12-2. (a) Capsular disinsertion. (b) The viscoelastic stretches the partly disinserted bag. A cohesive viscoelastic is required to fill the whole bag, whereas a dispersive material is necessary only when the disinserted zone needs to be filled. (c) Aspiration of the cortical material is accomplished with the "dry" technique.

choose to remove it and replace it with a more suitable viscoelastic material. Therefore, the viscoelastic chosen to accomplish phacoemulsification remains the same also for the following phase of irrigation and aspiration.

In the presence of a well-stretched capsular bag, aspiration of residual cortical fragments will not cause surgical problems and does not require further support by the viscoelastic. If the bag appears atonic or partially disinserted, it may be essential to use a viscoelastic to keep the bag stretched. In this situation, it is necessary to work with low vacuum and very low flow. At the same time, the bag is constantly kept open and stretched toward the area of disinsertion by means of an adhesive viscoelastic that does not leave the site of injection (ie, Viscoat).

Aspiration of the cortex can be accomplished using the "dry" technique without an irrigation line or with a cannula mounted on a syringe. The viscoelastic should be constantly added when accidentally aspirated and is fundamental to keeping the bag open and stretched to prevent any further disinsertion (Figure 12-2). This allows complete aspiration of cortical material. In this situation, it is useful to implant a PMMA ring (Morcher Ophthec) in the bag, constantly controlled by the viscoelastic, which if positioned at the equator and stretched inside the bag will restore the partially disinserted bag and facilitate IOL implantation.

Viscoelastic material also enables the surgeon to perform special maneuvers—for instance, if at the end of a phaco technique with residual epinucleus he or she is unable to remove it from the bag, perhaps due to a too small rhexis or strong adhesion to the capsule.

Some of the techniques currently used (chip and flip, crack and flip) involve aspiration of the epinucleus with the phaco handpiece at the end of nucleus removal, occluding the phaco tip with low vacuum values and with minimal or no ultrasound. At this phase of surgery, occluding the phaco tip may causes dangerous traction on the zonules or the posterior capsule. An attempt to mobilize the epinucleus can be made by introducing a spatula through the paracentesis. However, at times, this maneuver may cause damage to the posterior capsule.

Another option recently suggested by Singer is to disconnect the aspiration tube of the phaco and aspirate the epinucleus with passive vacuum and low ultrasound. This maneuver appears to be effective, but the danger of causing accidental capsular break or zonular disinsertion is present, as high hydric charge would rapidly worsen the problem.

A good alternative is to use the viscoelastic to create a cleavage between the epinucleus and the posterior capsule so that the epinucleus is lifted to the same level as the rhexis, facilitating its safe aspiration (Figure 12-3). This procedure may be useful for the surgeon, especially when performing the chop technique, which often requires hydrodelineation to separate the nucleus to be chopped and often results in a large amount of residual epinucleus. Occasionally, the epinucleus is aspirated and the bag is cleared very easily. However, in the presence of small rhexis or epinuclei consisting of hard, "dry" material that is less likely to create occlusion, its viscomobilization far from the capsule allows the surgeon to remove it safely.

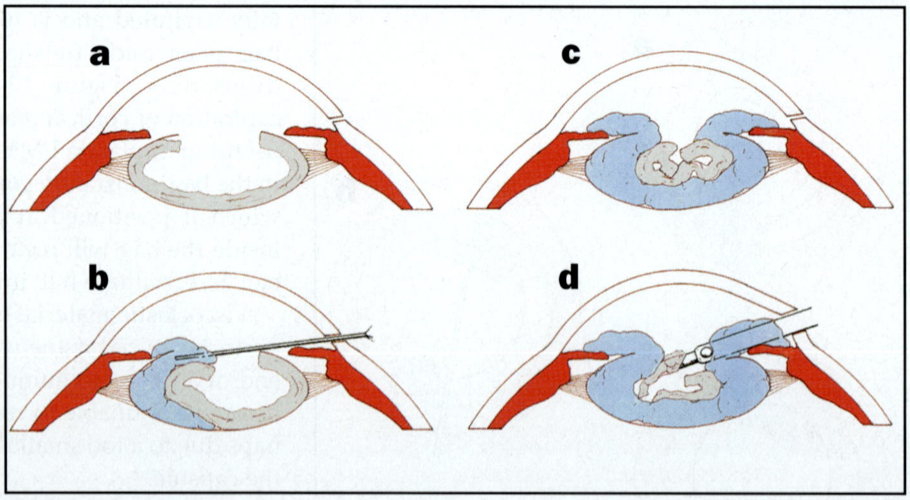

Figure 12-3. (a) The epinucleus strongly adheres to the capsular bag. (b) The viscoelastic is used to create cleavage between epinucleus and capsule. (c) The viscoelastic lifts the epinucleus that separates it from the bag. (d) Aspiration of the epinucleus is completed safely with little or no ultrasound, owing to the protection provided by the viscoelastic layer.

CHAPTER THIRTEEN

Capsular Bag Filling

After completing phacoemulsification and aspiration of the residual cortical material, it is necessary to expand the capsular bag with a viscoelastic to prepare it for IOL implantation. The viscoelastic product allows the surgeon to keep the bag well opened and formed, easing the introduction of the IOL inside the bag with respect to both the loops and the optic plane. The material enables correct IOL positioning and centering and allows for possible rotation maneuvers.

The basic requisites of the ideal viscoelastic for capsular bag filling are:

- Easy injectability of the material
- Filling the volume and remaining still
- Providing good visibility
- Ability to be easily removed from the bag after IOL implantation has been completed

EASY INJECTABILITY = HIGH PSEUDOPLASTICITY

The observations previously made about AC filling with viscoelastic material are also valid in this case. The products with high pseudoplasticity (Healon® GV, Healon®, and Provisc) are preferable to those with low or no pseudoplasticity (Vitrax, HPMC).

After filling the AC with viscoelastic to protect the cornea, the bag can be filled by using either the rigid or soft lens technique.

If a rigid lens is used, it is better to create a sort of "slope" with the injected viscoelastic material. This encourages placement of the lens inside the bag and minimizes friction between the IOL and the cornea, the iris, and the margin of the capsulorhexis. The surgeon begins by injecting viscoelastic in the middle of the bag (Figure 13-1) to deepen the posterior chamber. This protects the posterior capsule while the IOL is entering the bag, preventing capsular breaks or zonular disinsertion. As the surgeon continues to fill the bag, he or she must progressively open the bag inferiorly. At this point, an attempt is made to "close" the bag slightly superiorly or alternatively in the portion of the bag closest to the surgical incision. This allows the surgeon to create a sort of slope along which the IOL glides without getting entangled in any part of the bag. The amount of viscoelastic slightly closing the bag superiorly must not be excessive. Too much viscoelastic in this area can force the anterior and posterior portions of the capsule together with consequent difficulty in positioning the proximal loop.

The technique employed for bag filling when using a soft IOL (Figure 13-2) slightly differs from visco glide. Viscoelastic injection is started in the middle of the bag on the posterior capsule to stretch it. The procedure is then continued so that the bag is opened as much as possible by the viscoelastic both in the most distal and in the proximal position, closest to the surgeon. It is important to lift the anterior capsule with the viscoelastic to have the bag well opened when the soft IOL unfolds after being placed inside the bag. An incomplete bag opening may cause a collision of the IOL or its loops against the margin of the rhexis, thus causing dangerous tractions and consequent positioning of the unfolding lens inside the sulcus instead of the bag.

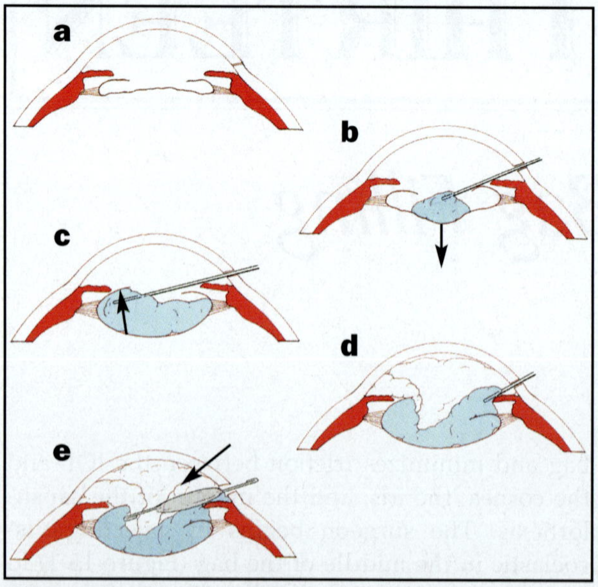

Figure 13-1. (a) Empty bag. (b) The surgeon injects viscoelastic onto the posterior capsule. (c) Bag filling is completed, opening carefully at 6 o'clock. (d) The bag is slightly closed at 12 o'clock, placing some viscoelastic on the anterior capsule. (e) The IOL glides gently on the viscous slope.

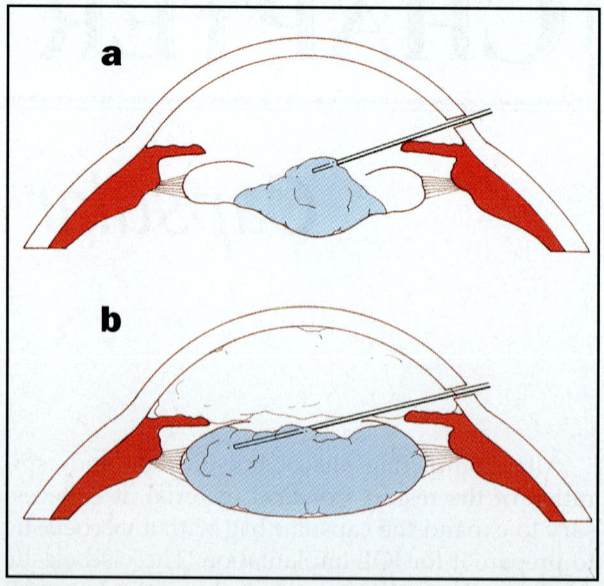

Figure 13-2. (a) The operation is started by injecting the viscoelastic on the posterior capsule and in the middle to stretch it. (b) The whole bag is carefully filled by lifting the AC with the viscoelastic material.

Permanent Spatula Effect: The Product Must Fill The Volume While Remaining Still

A material with the permanent spatula effect is one with high viscosity at 0 shear rate. In this respect, the best product is Healon® GV, followed in order by Healon®, Provisc, and the like, to Vitrax and HPMC, which demonstrate this feature less. High molecular weight, high elasticity, and high viscosity at low shear rate make Healon® GV the ideal material for this purpose. Incomplete removal of Healon® GV from the bag may cause remarkably high postoperative hypertension. Lighter materials that have a good permanent spatula effect, such as Healon® and Provisc, can have an excellent effect and cause less hypertension when not thoroughly removed.

Good Visibility = Transparency

The product must provide good transparency to allow precise control of the capsular bag during implantation, unfolding, and rotation of the IOL. Ideal materials, like Healon® GV, Healon®, and Provisc, are very transparent. Viscoat and HPMC are not as suitable.

Easy Removal From the Bag = High Cohesiveness

Once implantation of the IOL has been completed, the surgeon has to remove the viscoelastic solution from the AC and the bag. This is easily performed in the AC, but is more difficult in the bag due to the presence of the lens. The surgeon must clear the capsular bag with the utmost care, even reaching under the optic plane of the IOL, to

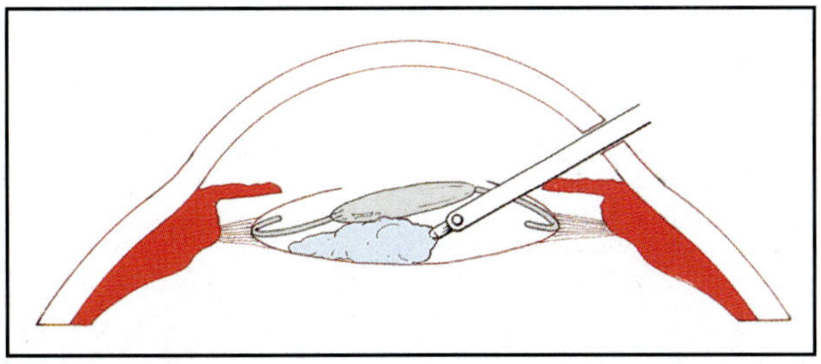

Figure 13-3. The viscoelastic must be completely removed (even from under the IOL).

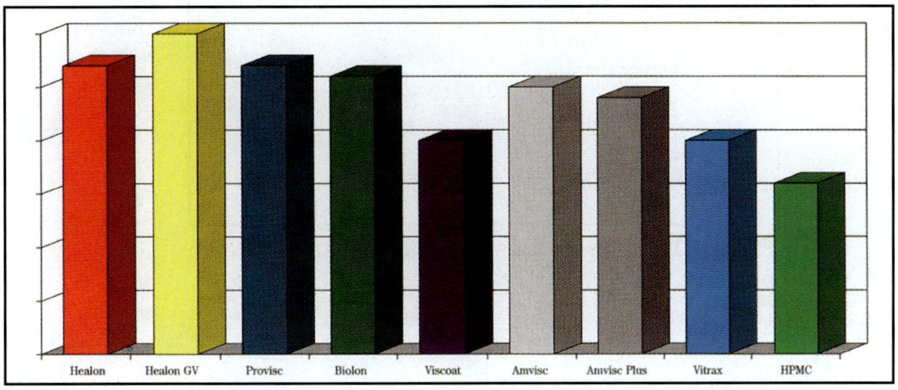

Figure 13-4. Bag filling.

remove any viscoelastic trapped between the posterior capsule and the implant (Figure 13-3).

The materials that best meet this requirement are the most cohesive ones, such as Healon® GV, Healon®, and Provisc. The worst materials for this use are poorly cohesive products, such as Viscoat, Vitrax, and HPMC.

We have listed our choices of the optimal viscoelastics for bag filling in Figure 13-4. Healon® GV and Healon® top the list because of their easy injectability (pseudoplasticity) and excellent permanent and soft spatula effect (high molecular weight, high viscosity at low shear rate). Additionally, these materials are very transparent and cohesive; as a result, their aspiration from the bag is completely free from complications.

DOUBLE FILLING

A poorly adhesive material is less likely to stratify and adhere to the corneal endothelium than is a material with high ability of mechanical adhesion to the endothelium. Therefore, some surgeons deem it useful to fill the capsular bag with a cohesive viscoelastic, a heavy and pseudoplastic material such as Healon® GV, Healon®, or Provisc, placing over it in the AC another, more adhesive product, such as Viscoat, Vitrax, or HPMC (Figure 13-5). This solution is more expensive as it implies the use of two products, but it offers several advantages.

Double filling allows the surgeon to use a heavy, cohesive viscoelastic with high viscosity at low shear rate in the bag. These features mostly facilitate stretching of the bag to receive the IOL, dampening its entrance into the bag. The material is also more easily aspirated outside the bag, owing to its high cohesiveness. In the AC, the adhesive viscoelastic, especially when provided with good ability to form space (Viscoat or Vitrax), creates mechanical protection of the corneal endothelium and the iris, protecting them from passage of the IOL. In addition, these materials are less likely to leak out of the chamber when pressure is exerted at the entrance of the wound. When the surgeon

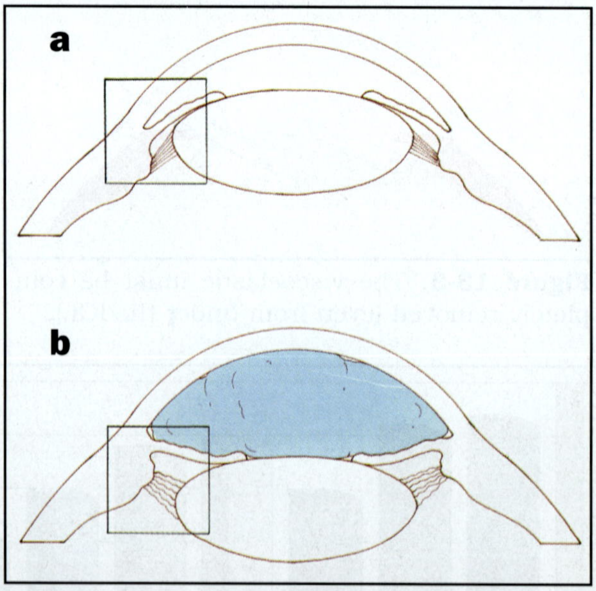

Figure 13-5. (a) Adhesive product. (b) Cohesive product.

inserts a soft IOL through a very small incision, these materials allow maintenance of the AC even when IOL unfolding is taking place.

Chapter Fourteen

Maintenance of Good Capsular Opening During IOL Implantation

In recent years, soft, foldable IOLs have become very popular. Initially, these IOLs supplemented the use of rigid PMMA lenses, but with time their position in the market has become increasingly prominent.

Implanting a rigid lens in the capsular bag presents complex problems. The viscoelastic is particularly important for space maintenance when implanting rigid lenses; however, this is not the case for soft lenses. In fact, these are introduced folded and when they open inside the eye, more significant dynamic problems may present (Figure 14-1).

The requirements of a viscoelastic concerning IOL implantation are as follows:

- Space maintenance, to preserve both the AC (to avoid traumatic contacts of the IOL with cornea and iris) and optimal opening of the capsular bag during all implantation procedures
- Good visibility
- Must permit easy introduction of the IOL without obscuring its passage
- Must oppose quick unfolding of the lens (when foldable) and sudden "lashes" by the distal loop of the IOL when it is released in the bag (soft lenses implanted with longitudinal technique)
- Must not oppose IOL shifting inside the bag, which permits optimal centering

Space Maintenance = High Viscosity at Low Shear Rate, High Molecular Weight

A viscoelastic material with very high molecular weight (ie, Healon® GV, Healon®) and high viscosity at 0 shear rate provides optimal space maintenance. This is beneficial because it constantly maintains a safe distance between the implant and the corneal endothelium and the underlying iris surface when the IOL is introduced into the AC. This prevents any accidental contact of the loops or the optic plate and the cornea or the iris.

It also allows the surgeon to perform bimanual techniques to support IOL implantation by introducing a spatula into the paracentesis incision. For instance, when the corneoscleral tunnel is "long," the IOL is likely to go up toward the cornea, after being introduced into the AC. If the viscoelastic maintains a proper space, it will be easier to move it down toward the capsular bag. Therefore, materials such as Healon® GV and Healon® are preferable, whereas materials with poor ability to create space, such as HPMC, should be used as a last resort.

Good Visibility = Transparency of the Viscoelastic Material

Each maneuver must be visible in order to be optimally controlled. Hence, less transparent materials such as HPMC or Viscoat are not preferable in this respect, particularly when compared with other more transparent products such as Healon® GV, Healon®, or Provisc. Furthermore, some materials may trap small air bubbles (ie, Viscoat), which may further limit visibility.

Easy Introduction of the IOL = High Pseudoplasticity

Some products, such as Healon® GV and Healon®, have high pseudoplasticity and low viscosity at zero shear rate. These features, which enable the viscoelastic to pass through easily, facilitate the introduction of the IOL. More adhesive and less pseudoplastic products, like Vitrax or Viscoat, or materials with no pseudoplasticity, like HPMC, should be considered the second choice.

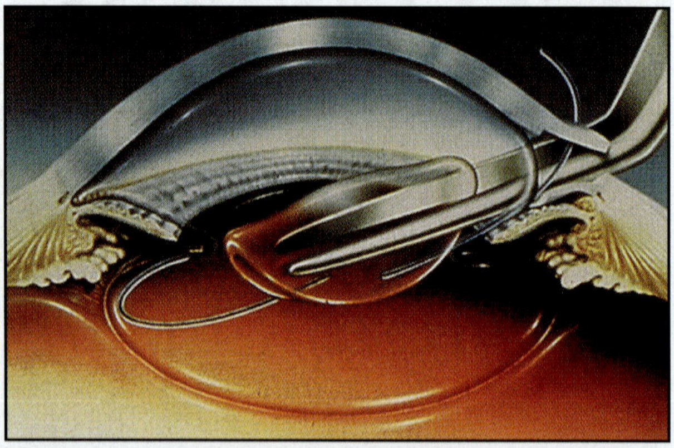

Figure 14-1. Soft, foldable IOLs.

Dampening of IOL Unfolding = High Elasticity, Low Pseudoplasticity

The desirable features of a viscoelastic that will serve to dampen IOL unfolding are opposite to those features that facilitate IOL introduction. If the surgeon wants a viscoelastic that does not oppose introduction of the IOL into the chamber and that can act as a cushion that dampens the potentially sudden and explosive IOL unfolding, particularly with silicone lenses, a product with low pseudoplasticity is preferable. However, the elastic features of the product are of greater importance because they better absorb the shock of the rapid unfolding of the lens. Therefore, we prefer the high elasticity of Healon® GV, and place products such as Amvisc Plus, Vitrax, and HPMC at the end of the list because of their poor or nonexistent elasticity.

Need to Shift the Lens Easily = High Pseudoplasticity, High Viscosity

Once the lens has been completely introduced in the capsular bag, it may be necessary to perform some maneuvers to center it. High pseudoplasticity allows the surgeon to accomplish this maneuver easily. However, high viscosity at low shear rate, which contributes to the creation of high pseudoplasticity, is also important. For instance, if a loop has gone in the sulcus and the surgeon needs to reposition it, a highly viscous viscoelastic will ease these maneuvers. Therefore, Healon® GV, Healon®, and Provisc are our first choices, leaving materials with poor or nonexistent pseudoplasticity and low viscosity as a last resort.

When the surgeon wants to wrap and cover the IOL with a viscoelastic to ease its introduction into the AC and cause less trauma to the access tunnel, products with high wettability and greater adhesiveness, such as Viscoat, are preferable. In IOL implantation, products showing high molecular weight, high viscosity, high elasticity, and high pseudoplasticity are undoubtedly our first choice.

Healon® GV, Healon®, and Provisc are ranked highly, whereas products made of HPMC are ranked the lowest.

In the following section we focus briefly on how IOL implantation can be correctly supported by the viscoelastic substance.

Rigid Lenses

After filling the capsular bag correctly, as described in the previous chapter (visco-glide technique), the distal loop of the IOL is inserted inside the surgical wound. Occasionally, viscoelastic may be useful for slightly opening the incision and permitting softer introduction of the loop.

If properly positioned, the viscoelastic should allow the IOL to enter the capsular bag easily. We almost always prefer performing a bimanual technique (Figure 14-2), constantly controlled by a

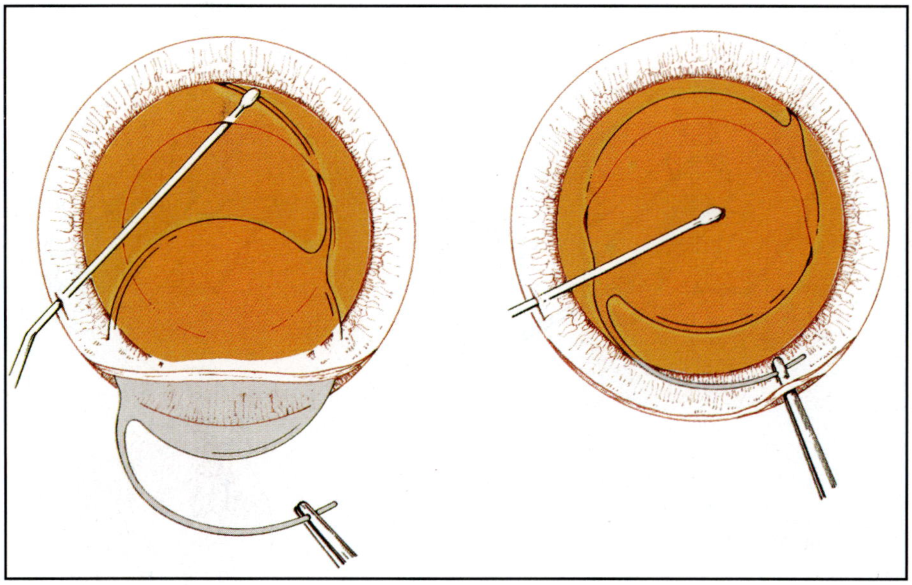

Figure 14-2. Bimanual technique.

Buratto's spatula introduced through the paracentesis. This maneuver permits correct positioning of the distal loop under the margin of the rhexis and proper entrance of the optic plate inside the bag. With light pressure on the tip, the IOL is rotated slightly and then the proximal loop is released in the capsular bag by McPherson forceps. Lens centration can then be performed with a spatula or a hook.

SOFT LENSES

Implantation of soft foldable lenses can be accomplished in two ways: by means of an injector or a forceps.

INJECTOR

The most widely used and well-known injector is the device marketed by Staar, which consists of a cartridge of plastic material. One section is opened to receive the lens, which is a one-piece silicone IOL. In two small longitudinal grooves, the surgeon must inject many small streaks of viscoelastic to ease injection and dampen IOL shifting. The part of the cartridge entering through the incision and then appearing in the AC has a slightly conical shape, cut in the terminal portion like a flute to enter the tunnel. Inside it passes the IOL, partly rolled along its longitudinal axis. A metal piston pushes the lens until it comes out of the cartridge. The piston is contained in an injector where the cartridge itself is placed. The piston is moved forward by a worm-screw that is operated bimanually (Figure 14-3).

The presence of viscoelastic in the cartridge is important because it permits a smoother passage of the IOL, dampens possible contacts of the piston and the terminal surface of the IOL, and makes lens unfolding softer when the implant has come out of the cartridge and entered the capsular bag. The ideal viscoelastic for this purpose must be very pseudoplastic and elastic; therefore, Healon® GV, Healon®, and Provisc are preferable. It is also possible to accomplish this maneuver by placing BSS in the cartridge, but we do not advise this procedure because it involves a greater potential of damage to the IOL.

Chiron Vision Corporation (Claremont, Calif) recently presented its injector (Pass-port) designed for one-piece silicone IOL implantation. The advantage of such a system is that, unlike with the Staar injector, it consists of a disposable sterile syringe, which allows the surgeon to implant with one hand instead of two. In this case, it is important to inject the viscoelastic inside the terminal portion of the system (about 0.2 mL) (Figure 14-4). The function of the viscoelastic is to enable the lens to pass smoothly from the proximal portion of the Pass-port, which contains the open IOL, to the distal portion, pushed by the piston of the syringe. IOL folding occurs smoothly and progressively,

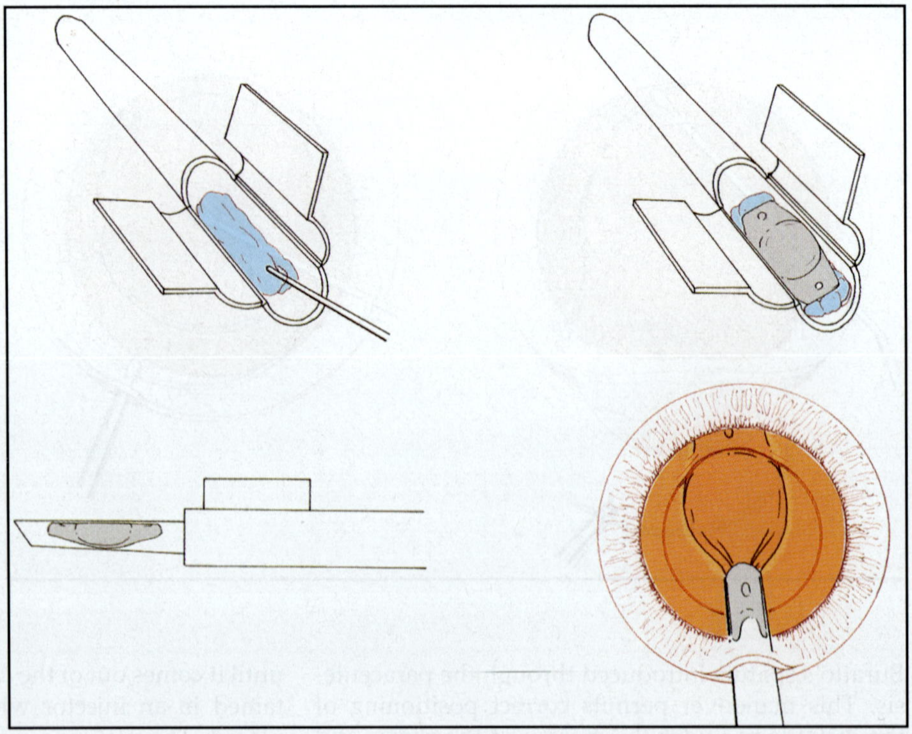

Figure 14-3. The piston is moved forward by a wormscrew that is operated bimanually.

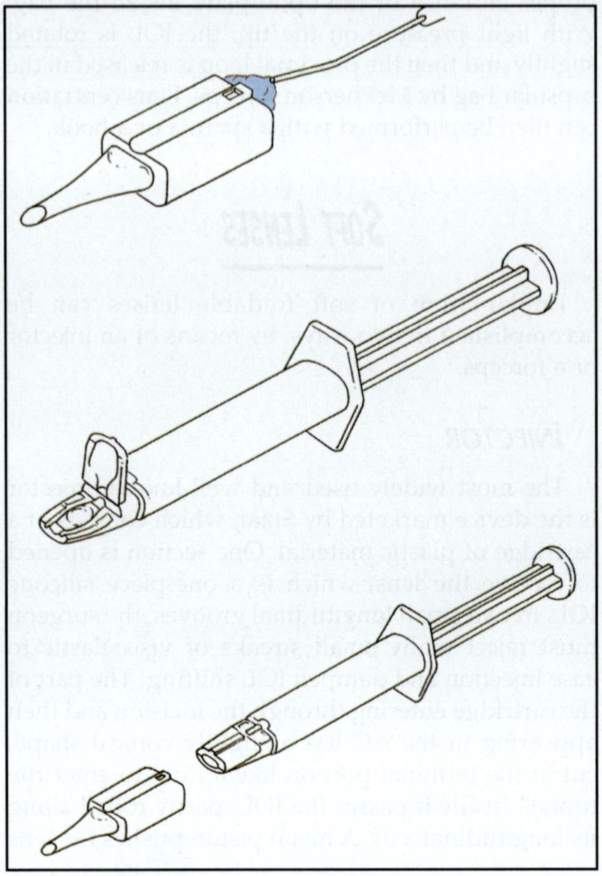

Figure 14-4. It is important to inject the viscoelastic inside the terminal portion of the system.

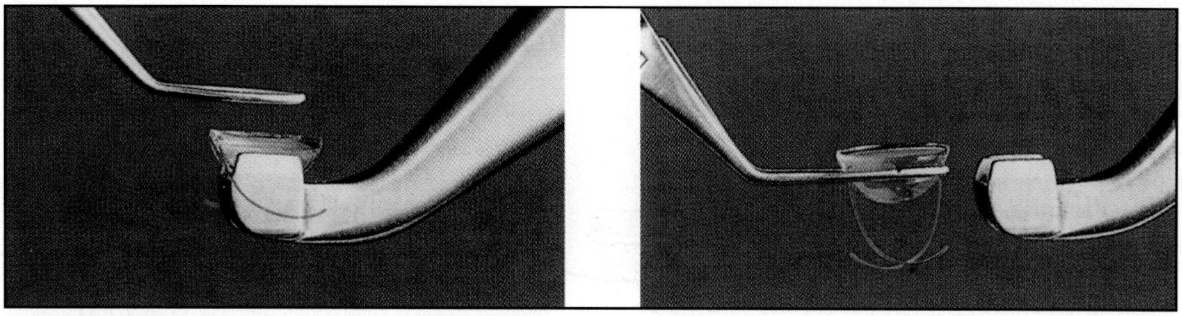

Figure 14-5. Buratto's folder and holder.

also because it is dampened by the viscoelastic. Once it has reached the final cylinder, the IOL is ready for injection, with the same modalities described for Staar's injector. As previously stated, the viscoelastic permits soft progression of the piston and eases the course of the IOL inside the system until it reaches the opening. It protects the IOL and makes its unfolding softer in the eye, inside the capsular bag. The ideal viscoelastic should be pseudoplastic and transparent, like Healon® GV, Healon®, and Provisc.

FORCEPS

This system is mostly used to implant soft IOLs provided with loops. The optic part of the IOL can consist of silicone, PoliHema, or acrylic. The loops may be made of prolene or PMMA. Soft IOLs range from 6.0 to 5.5 mm in diameter and are introduced folded through incisions that are generally no smaller than 3.2 mm. They are folded by special forceps (folders), which are available in various models (Figure 14-5), but all have the ability to fold the lens in two, leaving one portion exposed so that it can be grasped with another forceps with thin jaws (holder), which inserts the lens into the capsular bag. This procedure is heavily viscoelastic-dependent when performed with a longitudinal technique but even more so when a transverse technique is employed (Figure 14-6).

The lens is grasped with the folder and kept in a longitudinal position; the folder holds the IOL at 3 and 9 o'clock. At this point, a small amount of viscoelastic can be placed on the folded portion of the IOL in order to ease the entrance of the IOL in the incision and to protect against accidental contact between lens and iris or lens and corneal endothelium. This procedure should definitely be considered when implanting IOLs made of acrylic material or PoliHema, but must be assessed carefully when implants are made of silicone. Silicone IOLs require a dry environment for implantation and, therefore, wetting forceps and lenses with BSS or viscoelastic may jeopardize optimal hold of the IOL.

At this point, the capsular bag should be completely filled with a cohesive viscoelastic with high molecular weight and pseudoplasticity (ie, Healon® GV, Healon®, Provisc) in order to keep the bag open and stretched during implantation. This ensures that both the cornea and its endothelium are kept separate and far away from the rotation of forceps and IOL. The first difficulty the surgeon has to face is the entrance of the holder forceps, which contains the folded IOL, through a small incision. It is important to start making the distal loop of the IOL enter the AC without "stressing" it. Then a stronger pressure can be applied to let the optic plate enter the chamber as well. In this phase, light and poorly viscous viscoelastics are likely to leak out of the chamber or the eye when even the slightest pressure is applied. On the contrary, when a high molecular weight product such as Healon® GV is used, the surgeon can achieve the best performance. This material hardly leaves the AC and, when forceps and folded IOL are introduced in the chamber, the space is well maintained.

In addition to being soft enough to dampen possible contacts, the viscoelastic should be heavy and highly viscous at low shear rate to keep the space formed and poorly viscous at high shear rate to allow the lens to pass through it. When being introduced, the IOL must be positioned like a "D" with the folded part toward the left. The distal loop should be led into the bag with a Buratto's blunt

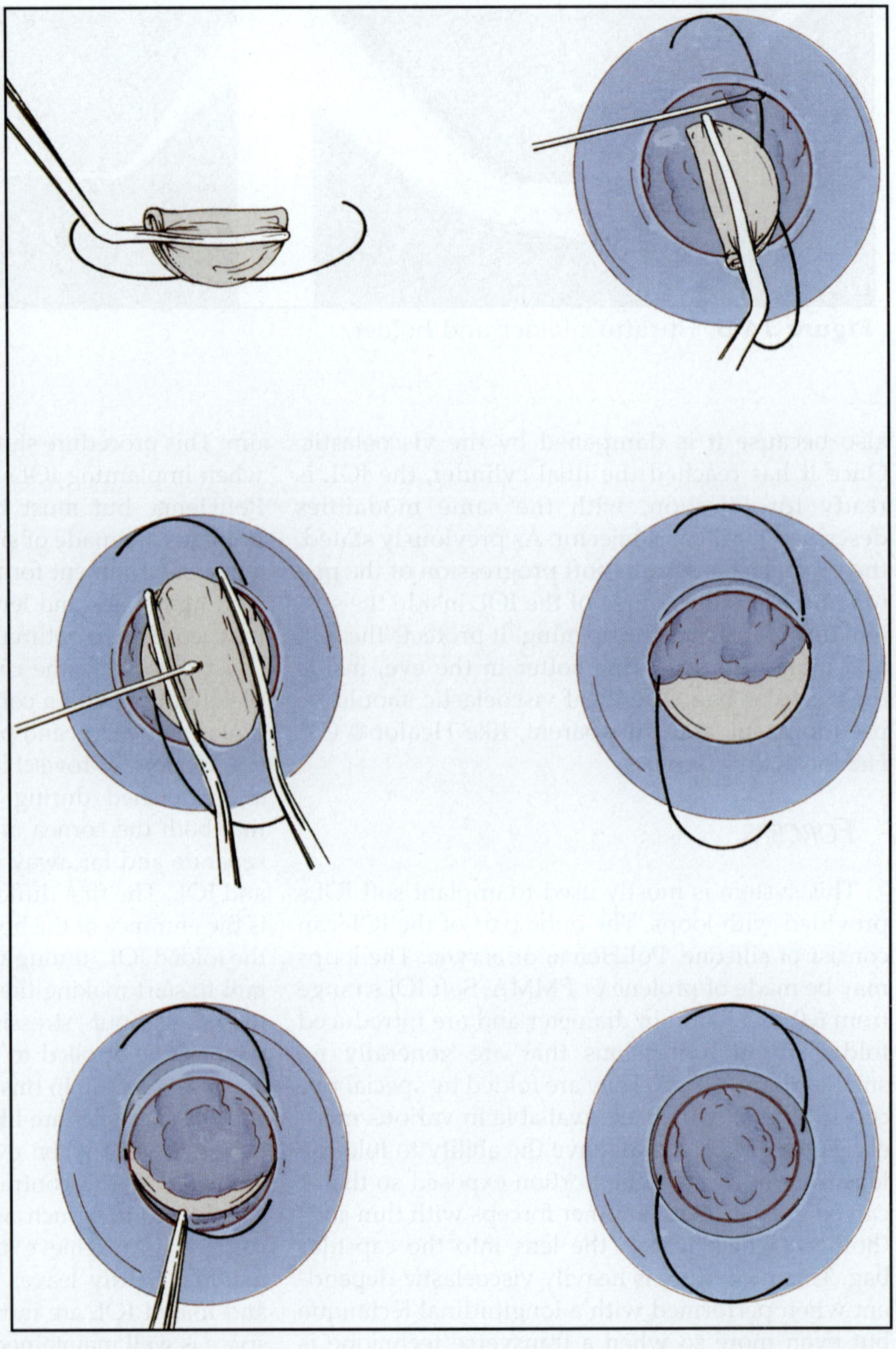

Figure 14-6. This procedure is heavily viscoelastic-dependent when performed with a longitudinal technique but even more so when a transverse technique is employed.

spatula inserted in the paracentesis. Then rotation toward the left should be accomplished so that the folded IOL is placed in a vertical position inside the bag. In this phase, the ability of the viscoelastic to maintain the space formed is important, as it is when the forceps starts opening, releasing the IOL that unfolds inside the capsular bag controlled by the spatula.

The dynamics of this phase differ greatly depending on the material that makes up the artificial lens. Acrylic material unfolds in the slowest, most controlled fashion, whereas silicone shows the highest "explosivity." PoliHema falls somewhere in between the other two materials. When working with silicone implants, the viscoelastic used must be highly elastic so it is able to dampen and smooth

IOL unfolding and consequent positioning of the distal loop in the bag equator. The ideal product for this application is Healon® GV, whereas the least convenient materials for this application are those made of HPMC. IOL insertion is completed with the insertion of the proximal loop in the bag by a forceps or a furcula.

Occasionally, the performance of these maneuvers causes greater stress to the tunnel than implantation of rigid IOLs because larger instruments (forceps with IOL) fill up the AC and the capsular bag. The use of a proper viscoelastic is crucial to prevent AC shallowing, which could result in contact among forceps, IOL, and the corneal endothelium. In this situation, the viscoelastic should not leak out of the chamber, but must maintain space and protect intraocular structures. As previously mentioned, the most suitable viscoelastic materials are Healon® GV, Healon®, and Provisc. The least suitable, in this case, are Amvisc Plus, Vitrax, and HPMC.

TRANSVERSE MANEUVER

The IOL is placed on the folder transversally (Figure 14-7); the folder holds the optic plate at 6 and 12 o'clock. The IOL is grasped with the forceps and both loops cross with a slight touch. After placing a moderate amount of viscoelastic material on the apex of the IOL (except for silicone lenses), the implant is introduced into the incision, while the loops are brought close to the incision in an attempt to introduce them into the wound together. The IOL contained in the forceps is folded like a "D" and the portion introduced into the incision is the curved, folded part. Next, the IOL is rotated to make the tip of the forceps and the IOL enter the tunnel, while the surgeon starts increasing pressure on the incision. At this time, the surgeon must make sure that the viscoelastic filling the capsular bag and AC does not leak out. After entering the bag, the surgeon rotates the IOL by leading the curved portion of the IOL toward the posterior capsule and letting the IOL unfold, while the jaws of the holder forceps are opened. The IOL must be unfolded with forceps and IOL inside the bag, possibly controlled by a Buratto's spatula inserted in the paracentesis.

After this procedure, the whole IOL should be immediately positioned in the bag along with its loops. It is essential that in this phase the bag is always well open, stretched and formed by the viscoelastic to allow the loops to make a transverse movement in the bag. In fact, the loop may trickle in folds of the capsule, causing damage or breaking of the capsule itself. Moreover, the opening of the optic plate inside the bag may be explosive, particularly when silicone IOLs are being implanted, and the impact inside the bag or against the margins of the rhexis may be traumatic. In this situation, the viscoelastic must be elastic, heavy, and able to preserve space. Healon® GV possesses ideal characteristics, whereas Healon®, Provisc, and HPMC are less suitable because of their poor or nonexistent elasticity and low pseudoplasticity. In particular, the transverse maneuver must be protected and supported by viscoelastic products, perhaps even more so than in the longitudinal procedure. The dynamic action inside the bag is greater in the transverse maneuver, owing to the longer excursion of the loop that leads to complete positioning of the IOL in the capsular bag.

The viscoelastic must be highly elastic and have the ability to create space. Our ranking of the products is depicted in Figure 14-8. Healon® GV, Healon®, and Provisc rank the highest, owing to their ability to preserve space, transparency, high viscosity, and high pseudoplasticity. Vitrax, Viscoat, and HPMC are less desirable because they are adhesive solutions, which are less or not pseudoplastic or elastic.

The choice of which viscoelastic to use in IOL implantation is largely determined by ability to be removed as completely as possible after implantation has been accomplished.

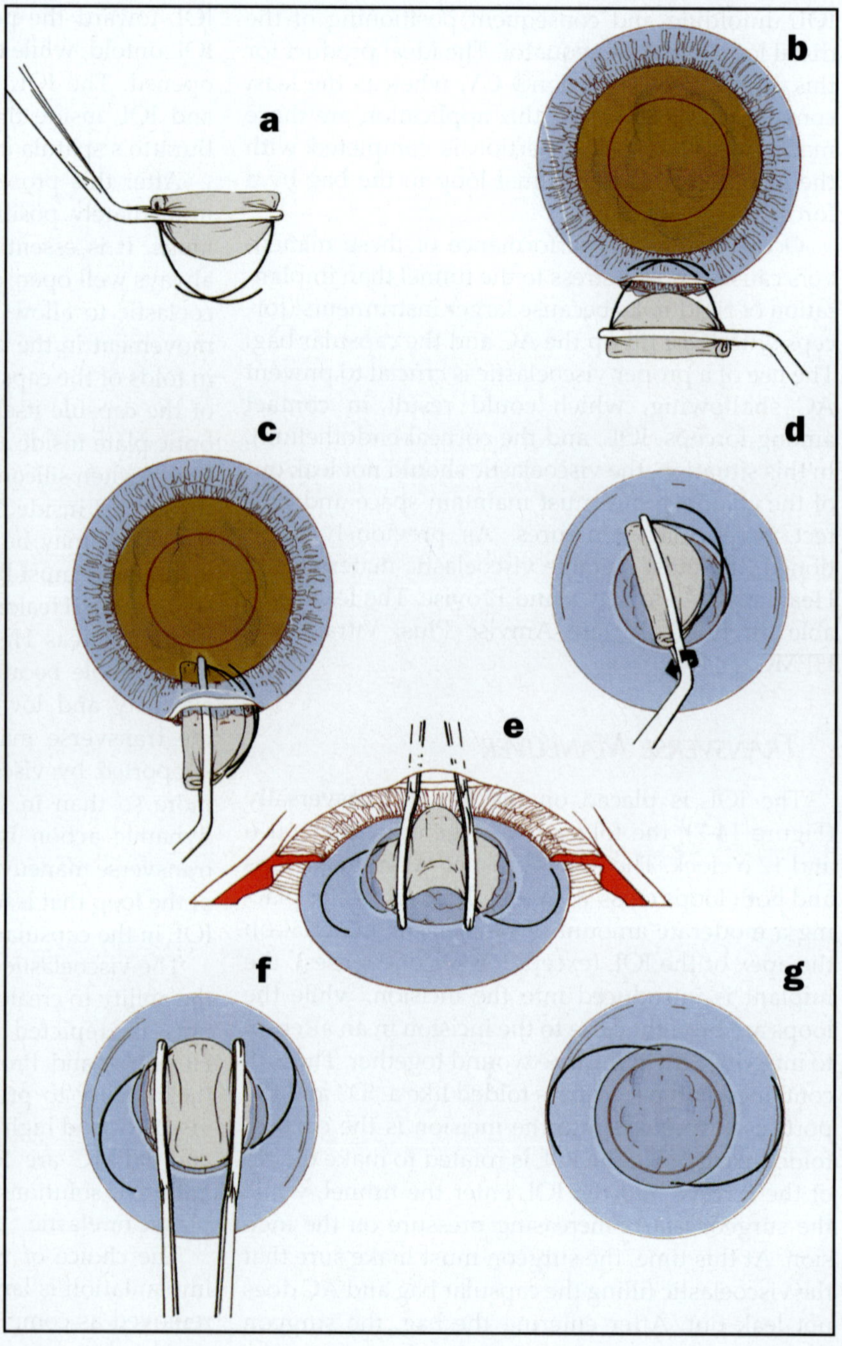

Figure 14-7. a) The IOL is placed on the folder transversally. The IOL is grasped with the forceps and both loops cross with a slight touch. b) After placing a moderate amount of viscoelastic material on the apex of the IOL (except for silicone lenses), the implant is introduced into the incision, while the loops are brought close to the incision in an attempt to introduce them into the wound together. c) The IOL contained in the forceps is folded like a "D" and the portion introduced into the incision is the curved, folded part. d, e) Next, the IOL is rotated to make the tip of the forceps and the IOL enter the tunnel, while the surgeon starts increasing pressure on the incision. At this time, the surgeon must make sure that the viscoelastic filling the capsular bag and AC does not leak out. f) After entering the bag, the surgeon rotates the IOL by leading the curved portion of the IOL toward the posterior capsule and letting the IOL unfold, while the jaws of the holder forceps are opened. The IOL must be unfolded with forceps and IOL inside the bag, possibly controlled by a Buratto's spatula inserted in the paracentesis. g) After this procedure, the whole IOL should be immediately positioned in the bag along with its loops.

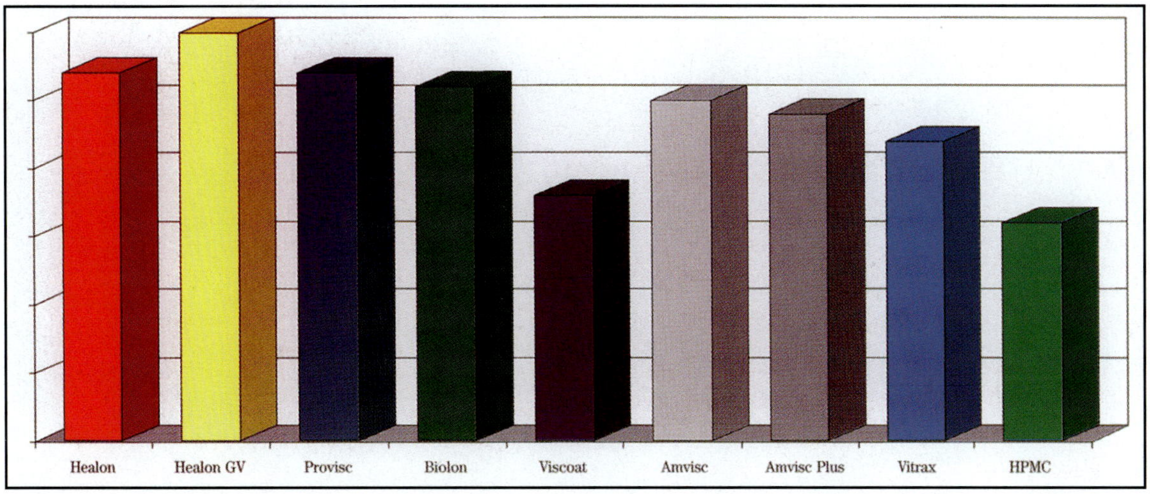

Figure 14-8. Rankings of viscoelastic elasticity and ability to create space.

Chapter Fifteen

Importance of Viscoelastic Removal

Viscoelastic materials are useful for easing surgical maneuvers as well as protecting and manipulating tissues. However, leaving these materials inside the eye can cause complications, such as intraocular hypertension in the postoperative period.

As formerly demonstrated by Fry, Roberts, and Alpar, the occurrence of postoperative hypertension is caused by poor outflow of the solution through the trabecular meshwork. The degree of intraocular hypertension is related to the amount of viscoelastic left inside the eye and the chemico–physical characteristics of the material. More adhesive products with high molecular weight, such as Healon® GV, Healon®, and Provisc, cause a remarkable pressure rise when not completely removed. Less cohesive materials, such as Viscoat, Vitrax, and HPMC, cause less hypertension because they tend to leave the eye through the trabecular meshwork.

In most cases, hypertension is easily controlled with beta blockers and carbon anhydrase inhibitors. Hypertension is generally a transient phenomenon that disappears within 24 to 72 hours. However, such pressure peaks may be very dangerous for patients with glaucoma because they might worsen visual field defects and visual function in addition to causing acute postoperative pain.

To minimize the possibility of postoperative hypertension, the surgeon should always completely remove the viscoelastic material. A basic requirement of the viscoelastic is easy removal from inside the eye, considering both the time needed and difficulty level for the surgeon to perform this maneuver. The viscoelastic should possess features that ease its removal, including low viscosity at high shear rate and low cohesiveness. All maneuvers for irrigation and mechanical aspiration of the viscoelastic are performed with viscoelastics that have high shear rates and low viscosity, which allows the product to be easily cleared through the aspiration line. Cohesiveness of the product and the length of its molecular chains are equally as important. A highly cohesive product with long molecular chains will be likely to come out of the eye en bloc. On the contrary, adhesive and poorly cohesive materials are divided in lots during irrigation and aspiration. This can make removal particularly difficult when devices with peristaltic pumps are used. These machines require good occlusion to let the vacuum rise, and the surgeon must look for the viscoelastic, directing the tip in the fornix of the bag, under and behind the IOL, and toward the chamber angle.

In a study by Assia et al, the time required to remove different viscoelastics from the capsular bag after IOL implantation was compared using Miyake's video technique. Five different materials were considered: Healon® GV, Healon®, Viscoat, Occucoat, and Orcolon. Healon® GV and Healon® consist of sodium hyaluronate, Viscoat is made of sodium hyaluronate and chondroitin sulfate, Occucoat consists of HPMC, and Orcolon is made of polyacrylamide. All of the viscoelastics were dyed with fluorescein. A PMMA one-piece IOL was implanted in the capsular bag and each product was used to fill the capsular bag. The time needed to completely and partially remove the viscoelastic using a vacuum level of 250 mmHg was then studied. The results are shown in Table 15-1.

Materials with high cohesiveness and low viscosity at high shear rate, such as Healon® GV and Healon®, are aspirated quickly. Partial and complete removal occur almost simultaneously. The clearing time of less cohesive viscoelastics (Viscoat, Occucoat, and Orcolon) is three times longer for partial aspiration, six to eight times longer for complete removal.

Table 15-1.
TIME FOR VES REMOVAL

Product	Partial	Complete
Healon®	20 seconds	20 seconds
Healon® GV	24 seconds	24 seconds
Viscoat	1 minutes	3 minutes
Occucoat	1 minutes	3 minutes
Orcolon	35 seconds	3 minutes

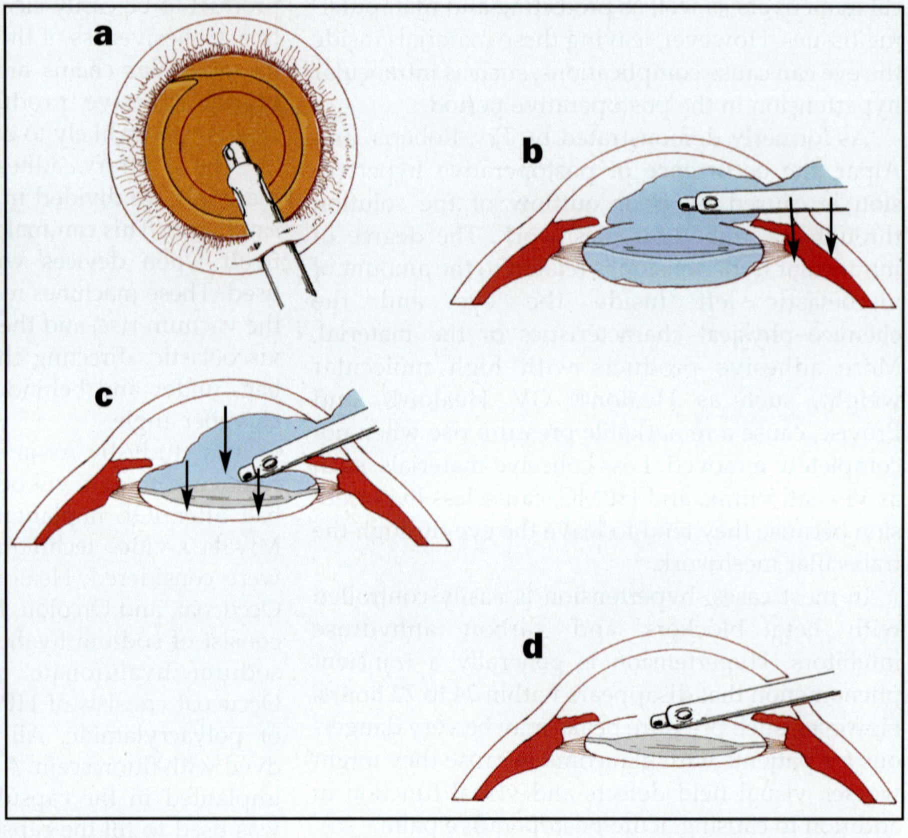

Figure 15-1. Viscoelastic removal with a cohesive product. (a) With the irrigation and aspiration handpiece in the middle of the pupillary field, above the IOL, the surgeon operates with the pedal in position 2, aspirating viscoelastic. (b) The viscoelastic comes through the aspiration line, but also as a whole mass through the surgical wound, led by the irrigation flow, while the surgeon depresses the posterior margin of the incision. (c) To clear the viscoelastic from the bag, some pressure is exerted on the IOL and then released. Optimal clearing is achieved by repeating this maneuver. (d) Viscoelastic removal has been completed.

High irrigation and aspiration times result in long flow times inside the eye and greater damage to endothelial cells. The protection provided by adhesive products may result from the longer times required to remove the viscoelastic completely.

COHESIVE PRODUCTS

In the presence of cohesive products like Healon® GV and Healon®, it is often sufficient for the surgeon to place the irrigation and aspiration handpiece over the IOL on the pupillary plane and operate the pedal in position 2 to see the viscoelastic product partially aspirated and partially come out "like a bolus" through the surgical wound. This can be accomplished by depressing the proximal margin of the incision (Figure 15-1). The viscoelastic that occupies the AC and the upper part of the bag will come out first. Slight and repeated pressure exerted on the IOL causes the viscoelastic located between posterior capsule and IOL to be removed as well.

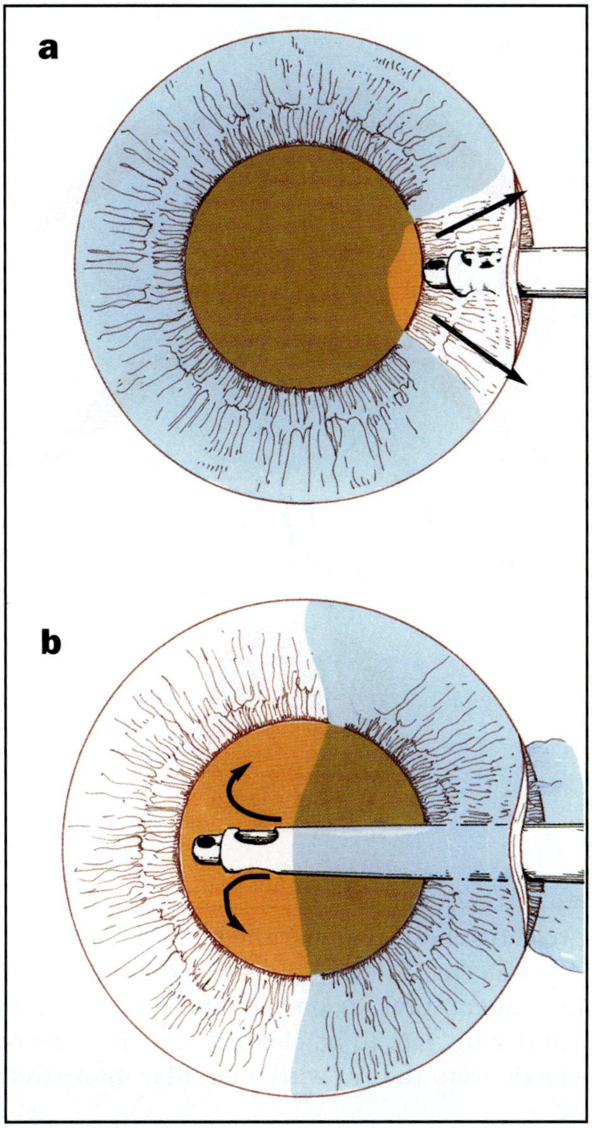

Figure 15-2. Viscoelastic removal with a cohesive product. (a) Correct position: The irrigation and aspiration handpiece is deep inside the AC. The viscoelastic comes out as a whole mass. (b) Incorrect position: The irrigation and aspiration handpiece is just on the threshold of the AC. A small amount of viscoelastic is cleared.

The pressure applied on the lens moves the viscoelastic from the posterior portion of the bag forward along the IOL borders and by pushing and releasing the IOL the bag is quickly free of viscoelastic. The irrigation flow then takes the viscoelastic outside, along with the aspiration handpiece. It is important not to leave the irrigation and aspiration handpiece on the threshold of the AC. In this situation the irrigation flow is partially obstructed by the viscoelastic and consequently clearing is reduced.

If the handpiece is introduced deeper into the AC, the irrigation flow will push the product outside the eye more effectively (Figure 15-2).

A modified version of this maneuver is the "rock and roll" technique (Figure 15-3). After pressing the irrigation and aspiration handpiece downward on the IOL in the bag to make the viscoelastic come out of the space between the IOL and the posterior capsule, pressure is exerted toward the margin of the IOL, first on the left then on the right, tilting the lens.

This procedure releases more viscoelastic from the fornix of the bag. Next, rotation should be performed above the iris to complete removal from the AC and the angle recess.

POORLY COHESIVE PRODUCTS

Referring again to the results of Assia's study concerning the times required for viscoelastic removal, products that are poorly cohesive (Viscoat, Occucoat) require long removal times owing to their adhesive properties. Furthermore, Assia emphasizes that poorly cohesive viscoelastics do not spontaneously come out from the space between the posterior surface of the IOL and the posterior capsule, but remain adherent to the lens and the capsule.

It is therefore up to the surgeon to push the handpiece to reach that area and inside the fornix of the bag. As the irrigation flow creates cleavage lines in the product, it may be necessary to aspirate the material in lots, searching for it in the AC and in the bag. When the phaco machine has a peristaltic pump, the surgeon must try to achieve good occlusion of the irrigation and aspiration tip with the viscoelastic, exactly as if the viscoelastic was cortical material.

The viscoelastic solution should be diluted with irrigation to make aspiration easier (Figure 15-4). Regardless, the surgeon must try to achieve complete removal to prevent side effects. Because adhesive products remain stratified in the bag recess and under the IOL, the surgeon should accomplish gen-

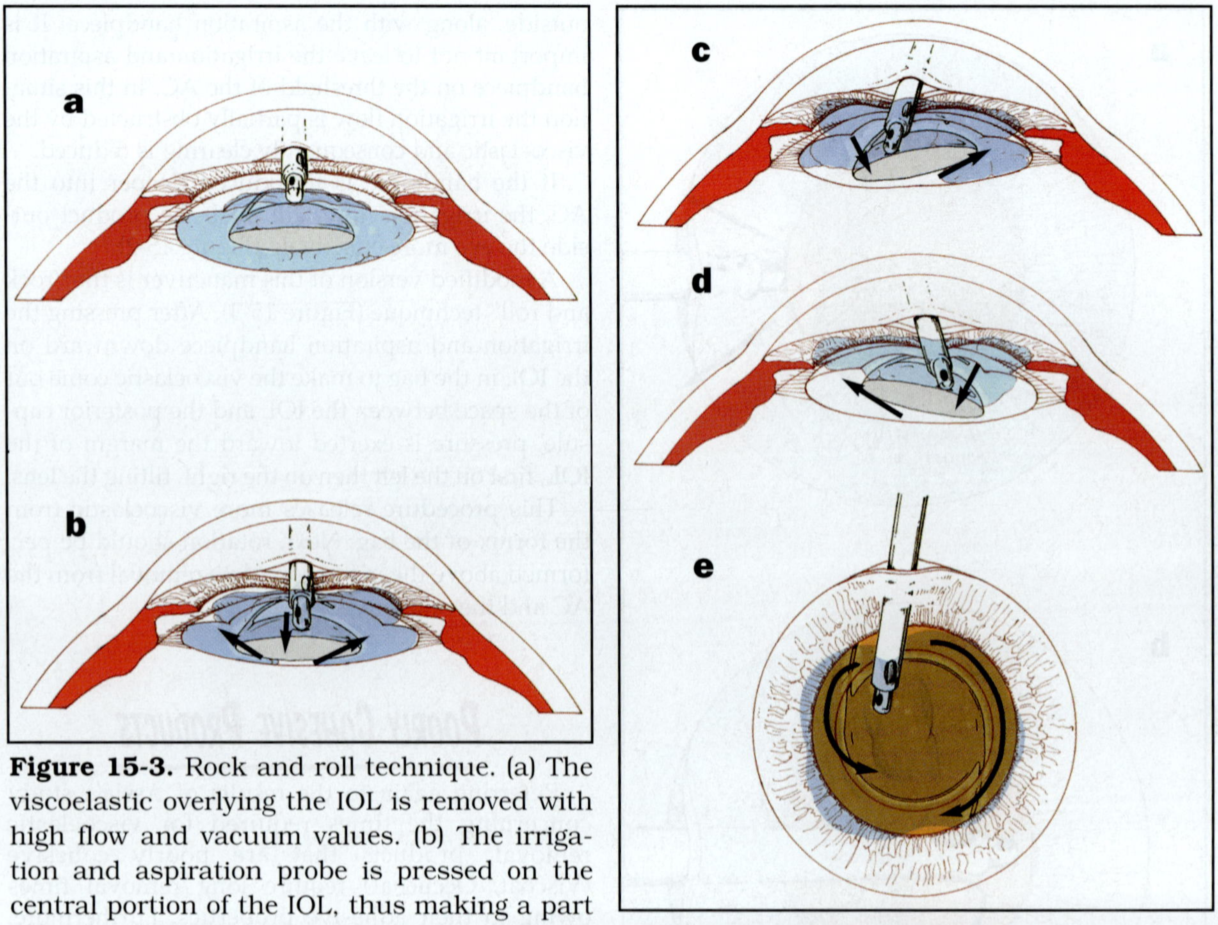

Figure 15-3. Rock and roll technique. (a) The viscoelastic overlying the IOL is removed with high flow and vacuum values. (b) The irrigation and aspiration probe is pressed on the central portion of the IOL, thus making a part of the viscoelastic in the bag come out. (c) Gentle pressure is exerted near the margin of the IOL, inclining it and making the trapped viscoelastic come out on the opposite side of the IOL between the posterior capsule and the IOL. (d) The surgeon presses on the opposite portion of the IOL, thus allowing the viscoelastic in the bag under the IOL to be cleared. (e) It is possible to achieve complete removal of the residual viscoelastic from the AC with a circular maneuver.

tle and careful lifting of the optical plate with the handpiece itself, controlled with a spatula introduced through the paracentesis. This will facilitate complete removal of the product (Figure 15-5).

This maneuver is dangerous, however, with risk of posterior capsule rupture, accidental luxation of the IOL outside the bag, and dangerous zonular traction. Removability is an important criterion to consider when selecting which viscoelastic to use (shown in Figure 15-6).

Provisc, Healon®, and Healon® GV can be removed rapidly and completely, whereas more adhesive products such as Vitrax, those made of HPMC, and Viscoat are more difficult to remove.

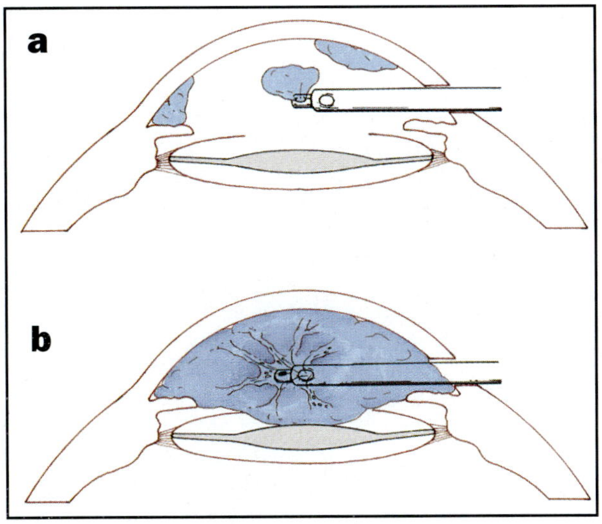

Figure 15-4. Removal of poorly cohesive viscoelastic. (a) Dilution of the viscoelastic with the irrigation flow to create cleavage lines, which facilitate its aspiration. (b) The surgeon systematically searches for occlusion caused by a single block of viscoelastic inside the AC divided into lots by the aspiration line.

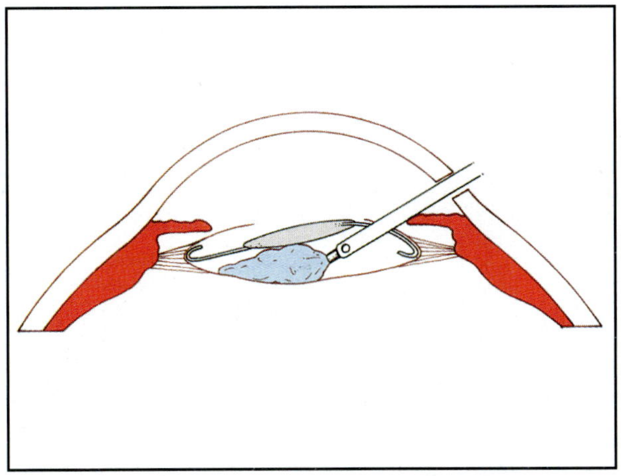

Figure 15-5. While gently lifting the optic plate of the IOL, the viscoelastic lying between posterior capsule and the lens is removed.

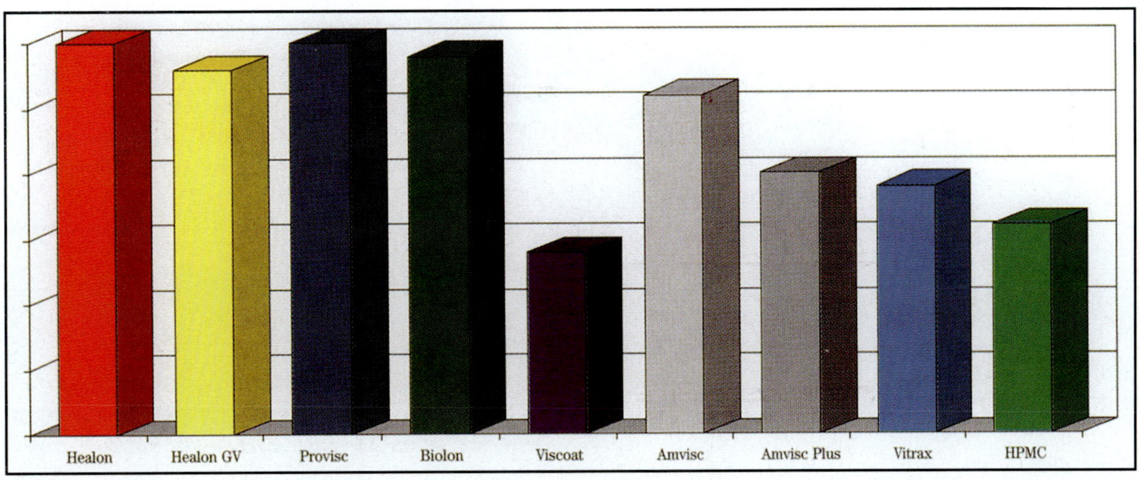

Figure 15-6. Easy removal of the viscoelastic material.

CHAPTER SIXTEEN

Double Viscoelastic

In each phase of surgery, certain aspects bring out some chemicophysical characteristics of a viscoelastic and reject others (Table 16-1). In particular, we have observed that:

- High viscosity and elasticity result in increased ability to form space, soft and permanent spatula effect, fair dampening effect, and postoperative IOP increase
- High molecular weight results in easy injection, easy removal, and good space maintenance
- High pseudoplasticity results in easy injectability and easy penetration by instruments and IOL
- High cohesion results in easy removal and high IOP increase when left inside the eye
- High wettability results in remarkable cell protection, good ability to coat surgical tools and IOL, and difficult removal

It is evident that once a viscoelastic has been chosen there will be phases in surgery when its particular characteristics are not favored. However, it is possible to combine the use of viscoelastic materials to enhance advantages and reduce drawbacks (Figures 16-1 and 16-2).

Simultaneous Application of Two Products During the Same Surgical Phase

It can be helpful to combine the use of an adhesive and a cohesive product in capsulorhexis, hydrodissection, and phacoemulsification. The overlying product must be more adhesive and have a lower molecular weight to remain in the site during the entire intervention.

For instance, the upper layer may be made of a product such as Viscoat that has greater adhesion, less pseudoplasticity, and lower molecular weight. This will help form the bag, coat the IOL, and ease penetration of the implant inside the capsular bag and make its rotation–manipulation easier. The underlying product must improve visibility during the rhexis, enhance instrument manageability, and be easily removed during the early phase of phaco. The lower layer may be made of products such as Healon® GV, Healon®, or Provisc, which have better transparency, greater pseudoplasticity, higher molecular weight, lowered cohesiveness, and greater adhesion to tissues.

The use of double viscoelastic facilitates removal of the material. Underneath, in the bag, there is a cohesive material such as Healon®, Healon® GV, or Provisc that is easily removed from under the IOL. However, above the bag, there is a material such as Viscoat that is more difficult to remove but is clearly visible (it is in the higher portion of the AC) and can be found and removed. Therefore, it is beneficial to have two different viscoelastics available to meet the various requirements of surgery.

Capsulorhexis and Phacoemulsification

In this case, it is possible to place materials such as Healon® GV, Healon®, or Provisc in contact with the lower AC (Figure 16-2, a and b). These materials have excellent transparency, high pseudoplasticity, and high molecular weight. These features allow the surgeon to see the capsular flap (even in conditions of poor visibility), easily accomplish the maneuvers of capsulorhexis, block or move the cap-

Table 16-1.
VISCOELASTIC APPLICATIONS

Features	Results
Viscosity	Keeps spaces and a deep chamber Eases insertion Implies postoperative IOP rise
Molecular weight	Eases injection Eases aspiration Implies high postoperative IOP
Pseudoplasticity	Eases injection Eases IOL implantation
Cohesiveness	Eases removal Implies high postoperative IOP
Wettability	Provides cell protection Coats instruments and tissues (when the contact angle is small)
Elasticity	Protects from mechanical vibrations

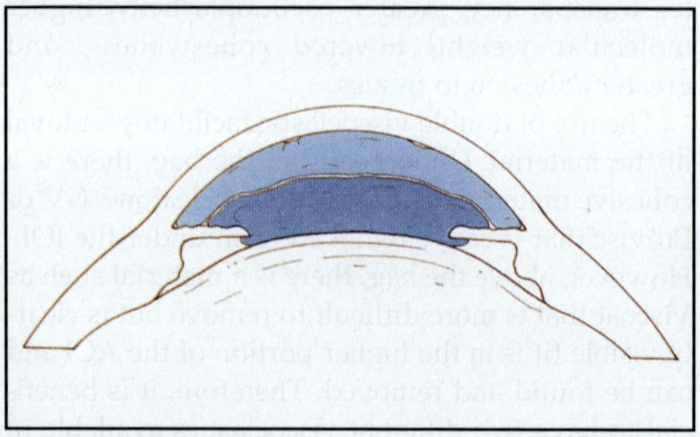

Figure 16-1. Double viscoelastic. Bottom: Product with high molecular weight, high viscosity at 0 shear rate, and high pseudoplasticity. Top: Adhesive product that remains in place even during surgical maneuvers.

sular flap, and control the leakage of milky endolenticular fluid in intumescent cataracts.

In the overlying position could be placed an adhesive product such as Viscoat or Vitrax, which ensures high adhesiveness, low pseudoplasticity, and lower molecular weight.

Hence, it will be possible to make the best use of the features provided by the different types of materials designed for corneal endothelial protection. The underlying product can leave its place during hydrodissection and phaco, thus allowing the BSS wave to leave the capsular bag while hydrodissection is being accomplished. The performance of phacofragmentation is favored because maneuvers are not hindered by the presence of the viscoelastic. The overlying product remains in contact with the endothelium and protects it during the whole phaco procedure.

IOL IMPLANTATION

Underlying, Healon® GV, Healon®, or Provisc may be used because they have high pseudoplasticity, high molecular weight, and high elasticity. This will ease implantation by providing optimal dampening of forces while soft IOLs unfold, providing excellent IOL centering and ensuring preservation of the space formed (Figure 16-2c).

Overlying, Viscoat or Vitrax may be used because they have poor cohesiveness and high

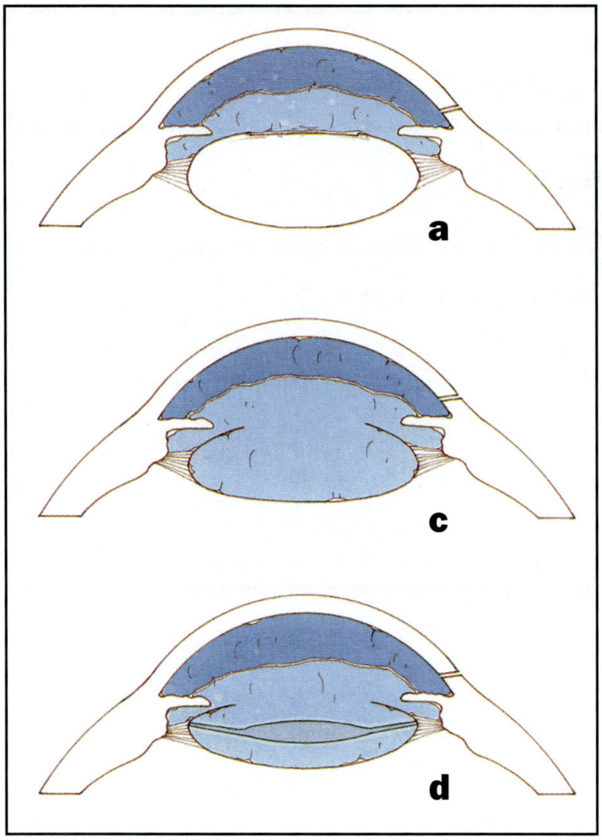

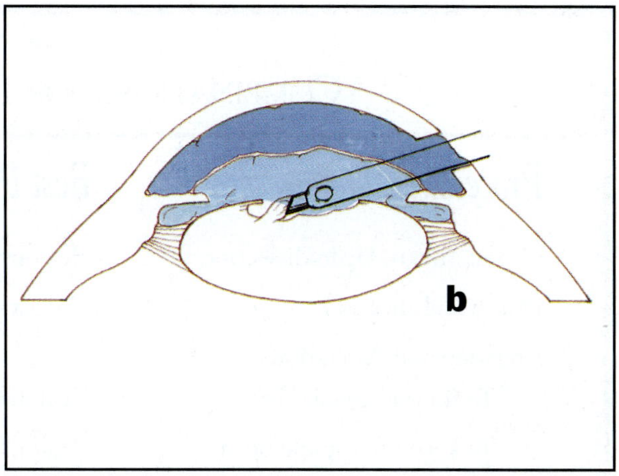

Figure 16-2. Double viscoelastic. (a) Capsulorhexis and phaco: Viscoat above, Healon® GV below. (b) Phacoemulsification: Viscoat above, Healon® GV below (it is discharged as soon as the irrigation flow starts). (c) Capsular bag filling and IOL implantation: Viscoat above, Healon® GV below. (d) Viscoelastic removal: Viscoat above, Healon® GV below.

adhesion to tissues. In this case, the protection that is provided by an adhesive product is optimal.

REMOVAL

This procedure also improves removability (Figure 16-2d) because underlying, in the bag, there is a cohesive material such as Healon®, Healon® GV, or Provisc that is easily cleared from the bag and even from under the IOL. Overlying, there is a product such as Viscoat, which is more difficult to remove, but is well visible because it has been placed in the top portion of the AC and therefore can be found and removed.

It is beneficial to have two different viscoelastics available at all times to best meet the different requirements of surgery (Table 16-2).

Table 16-2.
COMBINATIONS FOR DIFFERENT PROCEDURES

Procedure	Best Products
Capsulorhexis, Hydrodissection	Healon® GV, Healon®, Provisc, or other cohesive products
Phacoemulsification	Viscoat or other dispersive products
Irrigation and Aspiration	
To fill the capsular bag	Healon® GV, Healon®, Provisc, or other cohesive products
To keep the capsule open	Healon® GV, Healon®, Provisc, or other cohesive products
For IOL insertion, unfolding, and centering	Healon® GV, Healon®, Provisc, or other cohesive products
To remove the viscoelastic	Healon® GV, Healon®, Provisc, or other cohesive products

Chapter Seventeen

Intracapsular Cataract Extraction

Even though in contemporary surgery intracapsular cataract extraction has been almost completely abandoned, it is useful to remember that in some cases of severe lens luxation, it remains the technique of choice.

Viscoelastic material can be used after lens cryoextraction to push the vitreous back in case of positive vitreous pressure or to reposition a prolapsed iris. The material should have high molecular weight and high viscosity at 0 shear rate (Healon® GV) and must be able to keep the space formed for when the surgeon intends to perform implantation in the AC.

Implantation with scleral fixation can also benefit greatly from this material. In this setting, the pseudoplasticity, elasticity, and cohesiveness of Healon® GV are unrivaled. This material maintains a large space and is easily removed.

Should the vitreous prolapse from the pupil in the AC or leak out of the surgical wound, it is possible to distinguish vitreous from Healon® using a Merocel stick. Healon® separates from Merocel easily. Vitreous forms a thread and remains stuck to the Merocel sponge.

At the end of surgery, the viscoelastic needs to be removed from the AC. The high cohesiveness and pseudoplasticity of Healon® GV make it easy to remove at the conclusion of this type of procedure.

Healon®, Provisc, Biolon, and Amvisc provide less effective space maintenance. However, they are easily removed. Viscoat is very good for vitreous control, preservation of space, and protection from surgical maneuvers, but its removal takes much longer and is more difficult. Amvisc Plus and Vitrax are ranked next on the list because their medium and low cohesiveness also present difficulties in of removal. Products made of HPMC such as Occucoat, Hymecel, and Adatocel are ranked last because they provide poor space maintenance, cannot oppose vitreous pressure, and cause problems for removal due to their adhesiveness.

CHAPTER EIGHTEEN

Extracapsular Cataract Extraction

In recent years, ECCE surgery has been overshadowed by phacoemulsification procedures. These procedures allow the surgeon to create smaller wounds and, therefore, better control astigmatism. They also enable one to work in a closed chamber, thereby alleviating problems of positive vitreous pressure. Modern phacofracture techniques and refined machinery offer safe phaco procedures even in white and black nuclei and in small pupils. At the same time, ECCE surgery has evolved and improved owing to the advent of viscoelastic materials. These materials allow the surgeon to perform extracapsular techniques with capsulorhexis, nuclear viscoexpression, small and sutureless wounds, and manual phacodissection with functional results that are comparable to those achieved with phacoemulsification.

With respect to the techniques of AC filling with viscoelastic and irrigation and aspiration procedures, we refer the reader to our former statements concerning phacoemulsification (Chapter 11). Here we make some observations concerning capsulotomy in extracapsular cataract surgery and the use of the most suitable viscoelastic.

ANTERIOR CAPSULOTOMY

The most commonly known techniques for anterior capsulotomy (Figure 18-1) are the can-opener technique, envelope technique, pocket technique, and capsulorhexis.

CAN-OPENER TECHNIQUE

The can-opener is the most widely known technique and is easily performed in a well-formed chamber with a sharp cystotome. The drawback is that it often creates an irregular margin that often makes irrigation and aspiration of cortical material difficult to perform. Moreover, it cannot ensure implantation in the capsular bag and sometimes results in iris/capsular synechiae, IOL decentration, and greater postoperative inflammation. It can be performed in a closed chamber with an irrigating cystotome or in an open chamber under air or viscoelastic. In the latter case, it would be useful to choose a product with high molecular weight, high pseudoplasticity, high elasticity, and high viscosity at 0 shear rate, as previously mentioned regarding capsulorhexis in phaco. The significant observation in this respect is that the use of a product with high weight or high viscosity can provide optimal space and excellent protection, but it makes it difficult to perform the subsequent maneuvers of nuclear expression owing to the pressure exerted by the viscoelastic. Therefore, we prefer using products with good ability to form space, like Healon® and Provisc, which are easily removed from the AC and do not inhibit nuclear expression to a large extent. Hence, products with very high molecular weight, such as Healon® GV, or high adhesiveness, such as Viscoat, should not be considered.

ENVELOPE TECHNIQUE

The envelope technique allows the surgeon to work in the bag under the protection of the anterior capsule and, at the same time, have support of the anterior capsule in case of accidental break of the posterior capsule.

POCKET TECHNIQUE

The lower capsular pocket technique is a seldom used technique that need not be discussed here.

CAPSULORHEXIS

The use of capsulorhexis in ECCE allows the surgeon to achieve a more precise removal of the cortex and achieve accurate IOL centration, but it may be difficult to lead the nucleus outside the bag. However, it is the basis of modern extracapsular extraction and must be expanded upon. In this type of capsulotomy, it can be useful to let viscoelastic injection follow the insertion of a large air bubble in the AC, particularly when the surgeon is inexperienced. This will allow the surgeon to replace the air with the viscoelastic and inject it distal to the surgical wound (Figure 18-2). The procedure enables the surgeon to assess how the AC is filling with viscoelastic. The air–viscoelastic exchange gives a sense of how the viscoelastic is filling the chamber and empty spaces. For instance, starting to inject the product at 6 o'clock and withdrawing the cannula toward 12 o'clock at the wound will make the air escape as a result of the viscoelastic injection.

Once filling with the viscoelastic has been completed, anterior capsulotomy is begun. In this case, the surgeon performs an envelope capsulotomy and avoids complete filling with viscoelastic material, as the technique is applied from about 10 o'clock to 2 o'clock. It is possible to exploit the ability of the material to form space by injecting a large air bubble in the AC and using the viscoelastic only in the upper third portion of the chamber. This permits the introduction of an insulin needle with which linear capsulotomy shall be performed (Figure 18-3). The insulin needle or the cystotome used to perform capsulotomy can be mounted directly on the syringe of the viscoelastic, rendering it possible to inject the desired amount of viscoelastic in case of reduction or loss of space in the AC.

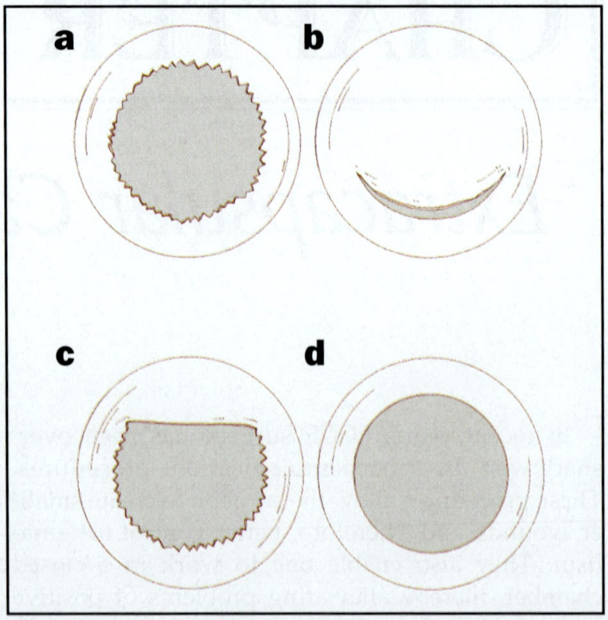

Figure 18-1. a) Can opener capsulotomy, b) envelope capsulotomy, c) capsular pocket technique, and d) capsulorhexis.

NUCLEOREMOVAL

Once the capsulotomy has been completed, removal of the nucleus can be started. The removal must be accomplished with no trauma to anterior segment structures, such as the zonules, capsule, iris or corneal endothelium.

The forces possibly acting to remove the nucleus are:

- Forces transmitted onto rigid structures—applied on cornea and sclera, they are transmitted to the lens nucleus (Pascal's law)
- Forces using the kinetic energy of a fluid in motion (BSS)
- Forces transmitted by the pressure exerted by a viscoelastic material (ie, Healon®)

The nucleus is expressed as a result of one or a combination of such forces. In the typical case, pressure and counterpressure are applied at 6 o'clock and 12 o'clock and the nucleus is expressed. Due to Pascal's law, the pressure exerted in the chamber at 6 o'clock and the counterpressure in the sclera at 12 o'clock are passed on the vitreous inside the eye. This enables the surgeon to remove the nucleus.

When the hydrodynamic technique is used, the active effect is a result of forces transmitted by fluids in motion: BSS is injected under the nucleus or distal to it and streams are provoked that flow toward the surgical wound, carrying the nucleus with them.

In the case of nucleus viscoexpression, the viscoelastic materials act through a mechanism similar to that of fluids with low viscosity like BSS. They also act as mediators that transmit forces applied on rigid structures, and they reduce friction between the nucleus and cornea, iris, and pos-

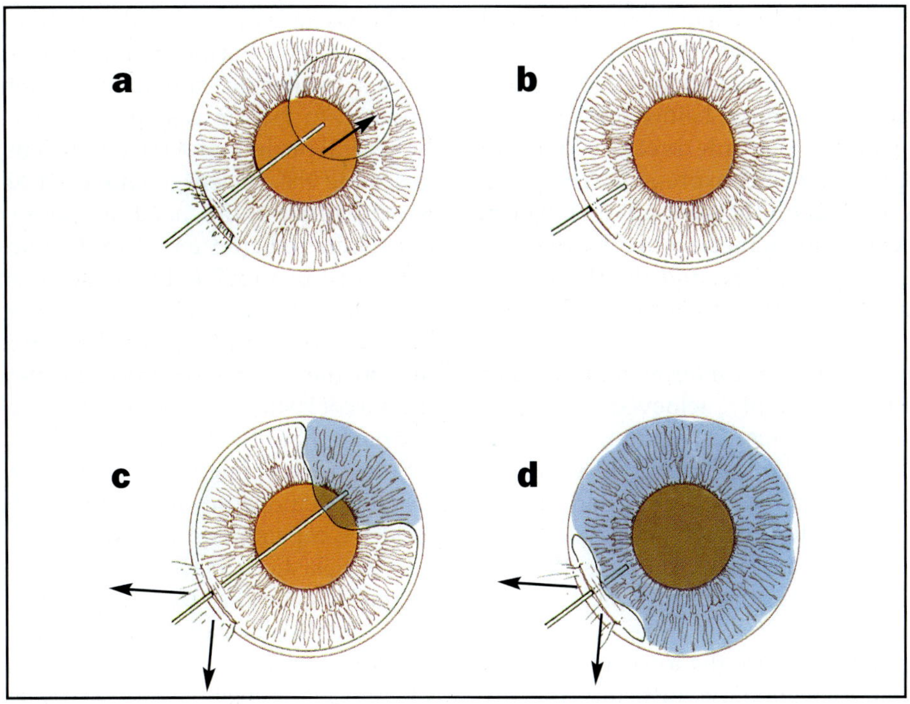

Figure 18-2. AC filling with viscoelastic: air–viscoelastic exchange. (a, b) Air in the AC. (c, d) The viscoelastic, injected at 6 o'clock, replaces the air going out through the AC opening.

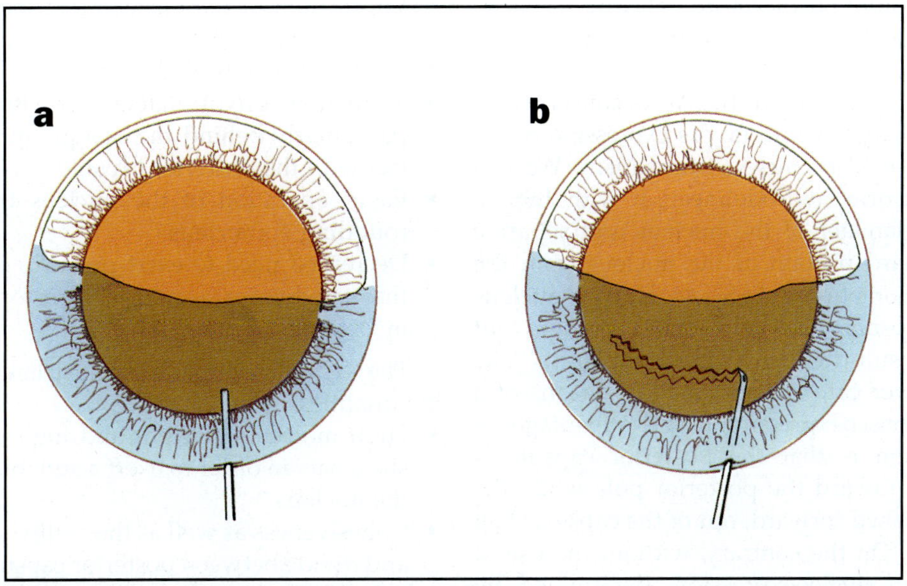

Figure 18-3. Envelope technique capsulotomy. (a) The chamber is filled only in part with viscoelastic. The rest of the volume is filled with air. (b) Envelope technique capsulotomy accomplished with an insulin needle under viscoelastic protection.

terior capsule while the nucleus is being moved. The forces necessary to express the nucleus must exceed those opposing its removal. Nevertheless, such force must also remain below the level that might cause posterior capsule breaks. There are three forces opposing nucleoexpression. The first is the resistance applied on the surgical opening; the second is the elastic resistance exerted by the margins of anterior capsulotomy; and the third is the resistance caused by adhesions of the nucleus and the cortex.

It is known that optimal centering and positioning of the IOL are mainly achieved by capsulorhexis. Besides phacoemulsification, the technique can be used in planned ECCE. Viscoelastics provide the surgeon with decisive support. In fact, removal of the nucleus through a capsulorhexis, particularly when small sized, requires that the force the rhexis opposes to nucleoremoval is overcome.

In the attempt to increase the force applied outside the globe to overcome this difficulty, the surgeon might cause zonular disinsertion, vitreous loss, or unexpected intracapsular extraction and in turn possibly cause nuclear dislocation into the vitreous. Thus, some surgeons cut relaxing incisions in the capsulorhexis, but these incisions, besides being rather dangerous, may also extend to the posterior capsule. Furthermore, relaxing incisions jeopardize the geometry of capsulorhexis, limiting its advantages.

As far as the opening in the AC is concerned, it is true that a larger width favors expression of the nucleus, but it also causes astigmatism. We can therefore perform hydrodelineation with BSS to reduce the diameter of the nucleus and separate the central hard portion of the nucleus from the epinucleus. Sometimes, BSS can lift the nucleus from the capsular bag and make it come out through capsulorhexis (hydroexpression). The same maneuver can be performed by means of a viscoelastic (viscoexpression). The advantage of viscoexpression is that the posterior capsule is pushed back toward the posterior pole while the nucleus is pushed forward, out of the capsular bag (Figure 18-4). On the contrary, without the use of viscoelastic in nucleoexpression, determined by pressure and external counterpressure, both capsule and nucleus are pushed forward by the vitreous, thereby causing stress to the zonules.

The viscoelastic material greatly limits stress on zonular fibers. Furthermore, viscoexpression provides a further advantage in relation to hydroexpression. In fact, in case of persistent adhesion of the central nucleus and the epinucleus, BSS tends to go around the nucleus, coming out of the bag. This usually implies the need to perform additional maneuvers to better mobilize the nucleus. The surgeon must manipulate the nucleus with the cannula, pushing the cannula between the nucleus and the posterior capsule. Often the cannula is not visible and there is risk of posterior capsule rupture. The viscoelastic, on the contrary, creates cleavage and push that lifts the nucleus.

Some experimental works conducted by Corydon demonstrate a direct relationship between posterior capsular rupture due to the pressure of the viscoelastic injected between the capsule and the nucleus and the size of capsulorhexis.

The smaller the capsulorhexis, the higher the viscous force applied for viscoexpression. Therefore, it is beneficial to create a wide rhexis when performing such a technique.

Thus, we can summarize the advantages of viscoexpression in extracapsular surgery as follows:

- Decreased zonular stress during removal of the nucleus; therefore, reduced risk of zonular disinsertion
- Lubrication of the nucleus and increased likelihood of expression
- Gentle and controlled expression
- Reduction of hydromaneuvers with the cannula, particularly behind the opaque nucleus in contact with the posterior capsule
- Easy separation of the nucleus from the surrounding epinucleus
- Decreased need to exert pressure on the cornea that can deform it and cause postoperative folds in Descemet's membrane

The viscoelastic material must have the following qualities:

- High molecular weight and high viscosity at 0 shear rate in order to exert a suitable pressure on the nucleus
- Cohesiveness as well as the ability to be compact and divide between posterior capsule and nucleus, in order to facilitate expression
- High pseudoplasticity so it can create a cleavage between hard nucleus and epinucleus and achieve their viscoseparation

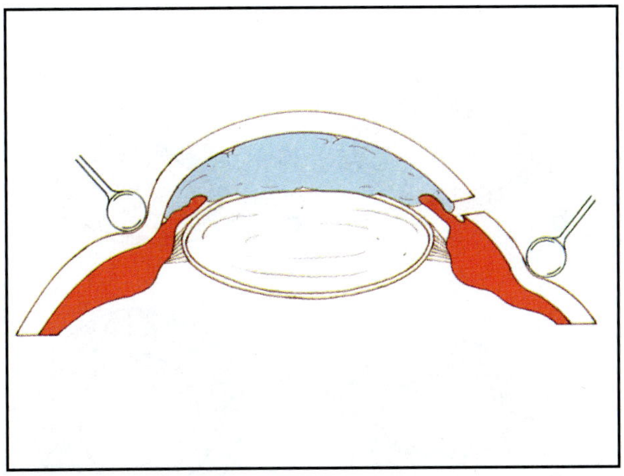

Figure 18-4a. Nucleoremoval accomplished by means of an external pressure and counterpressure (pressure is transmitted onto the whole lens).

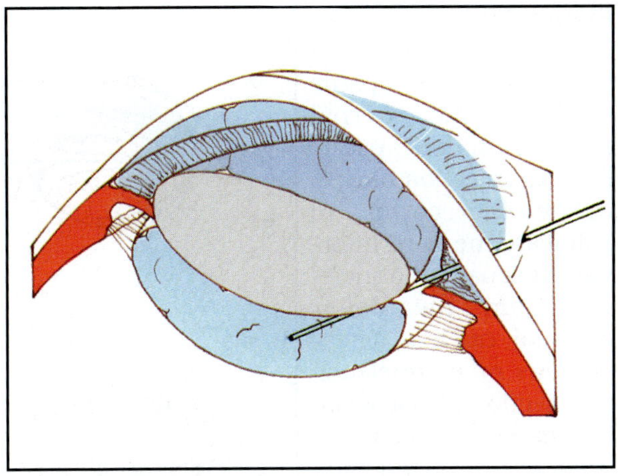

Figure 18-4b. Viscoexpression. The viscoelastic pushes the capsule down and the nucleus up, outside the capsular bag.

- High elasticity to allow a dampening action of possible maneuvers performed with the cannula or the loops
- Excellent soft and permanent spatula effect in order to mobilize the nucleus and block it in the desired position

The products that best meet these requirements are Healon® and Provisc. Nonpseudoplastic products, such as HPMC, or adhesive products, such as Viscoat or Vitrax, are unsuitable for this procedure.

Some basic rules must also be followed:

- The opening in the anterior capsule must be in proportion with the nucleus to be viscoexpressed. A soft nucleus surrounded by abundant cortex requires a small opening. A hard nucleus with little cortex needs a larger opening. Once the nucleus has been mobilized in the AC, the surgeon should assess its dimensions and consider enlarging the incision if necessary.
- The wider the mydriasis, the easier the luxation and removal of the nucleus. It is important to achieve optimal preoperative mydriasis, as well as to avoid maneuvers causing trauma to the iris which, when stimulated, may cause miosis. Should the pupil shrink during surgery, the surgeon should not hesitate to make some sphincterotomies or a radial iridotomy with eventual pupilloplasty when necessary.
- It is also important to mobilize the nucleus inside the bag. In this way, one can reduce adhesions between nucleus and cortex, thereby easing viscoexpression.

It is useful to lift the portion of nucleus closest to the surgical wound, using a curved cannula, like the Corydon type. Once the nucleus has been lifted in that area, the surgeon should try to achieve the same result on the lateral portions. When the nucleus is fairly free, it will be easy to increase the amount of viscoelastic in the interspace between nucleus and posterior capsule in order to complete passage of the nucleus in the AC through the rhexis (Figure 18-5).

As the nucleus is expressed into the AC, the application of slight pressure on the margin of the surgical wound proximal to the surgeon should have the double effect of opening the incision favoring nuclear engagement and transmitting an additional pressure to the viscoelastic, making it exit the eye with the nucleus (Figure 18-6).

In this phase, the function of the viscoelastic is to exert a positive push, to lubricate the nucleus so that it can slip outside the eye, and to protect the corneal endothelium from accidental contact with the nucleus. This might be very harmful, particularly in the presence of hard nuclei.

If the nucleus is not expressed out of the chamber, the cause may be an insufficient amount of viscoelastic or too small of an opening. The surgeon should try to increase pressure on the posterior lip of the incision at 2 to 3 mm and apply gentle pressure

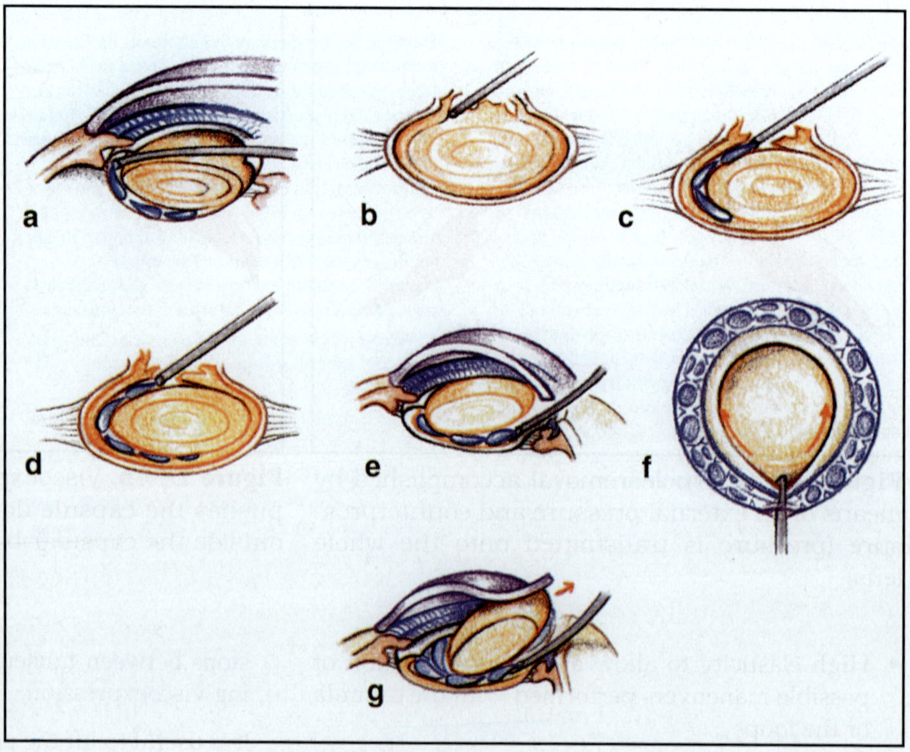

Figure 18-5. Hydrodissection. (a) Injection of BSS under the capsule to detach the external cortex from the capsule. (b, c, d) Injection of BSS inside the cortex to delineate the hard internal nucleus (endonucleus) from the softer external nucleus (ectonucleus or epinucleus). (e) Injection of viscoelastic material under the nucleus, passing through the capsulorhexis, eases the expulsion of the nucleus from the capsular bag. (f, g) Mobilization of the nucleus with the cystotome eases further injection and the expulsion of the nucleus first from the rhexis and then from the AC.

at 6 o'clock if necessary. This pressure also causes the margin of the nucleus to pull up toward the incision, thus favoring its expression (Figure 18-7).

When the nucleus is not particularly large, such a procedure can be coupled with techniques of sclero–corneal tunnel, which may not require sutures. If the nucleus is particularly large, is not well mobilized, or its expression is slowed down by dense cortical material, the surgeon can ease its outlet with knurled loops, irrigating loops, or a bimanual maneuver (loop under the nucleus, spatula on it). This is supported by a viscoelastic with excellent ability to preserve spaces and high pseudoplasticity (ie, Healon® or Provisc).

This technique of viscoexpression, along with capsulorhexis, had an important role in the revolution of extracapsular surgery in the 1980s. In that period, the intervention consisted of extracapsular extraction with manual techniques and IOL implantation in the bag. In 1988, there was a transition to an intervention performed with instrument technique and IOL insertion in the bag. Currently, it is performed with a small incision, capsulorhexis, viscoexpression, and often with sutureless wound closure.

Capsulotomy has become continual circular capsulotomy. Expression is accomplished atraumatically by means of a viscoelastic. Irrigation and aspiration is performed with automatic devices operating in a closed chamber. The IOL is implanted in the bag and centering is ensured by the presence of the rhexis.

Owing to the advent of viscoelastic materials, surgery is no longer performed without space, under air, or with risk of contact between corneal endothelium and IOL, instruments, or nuclear material. These materials allow the surgeon to perform every step safely.

Traditional extracapsular techniques and the phase of irrigation and aspiration of cortex do not appear to be particularly viscodependent.

Implantation of the IOL in the bag does not differ from the process described in phacoemulsification (Chapter 11) regarding the support provided by viscoelastics.

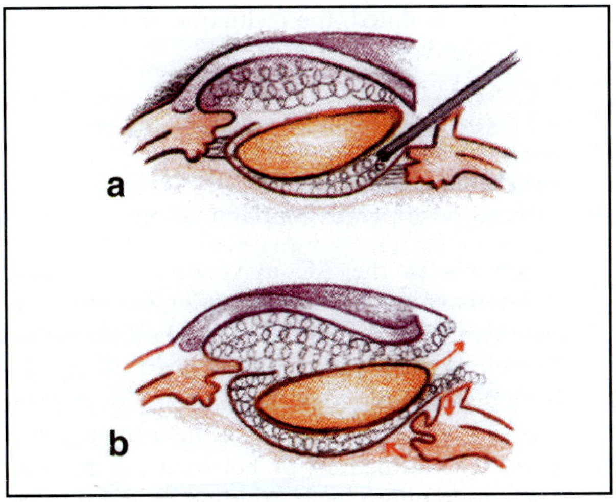

Figure 18-6. Viscoluxation. (a) The viscoelastic material is first injected into the AC, keeping its volume below physiologic level, and then under the nucleus. The latter is effected with a push upward. (b) Little by little, luxates, especially when a scleral pressure is applied, are transmitted to the vitreous and consequently to the posterior capsule and the viscoelastic material present between capsule and nucleus.

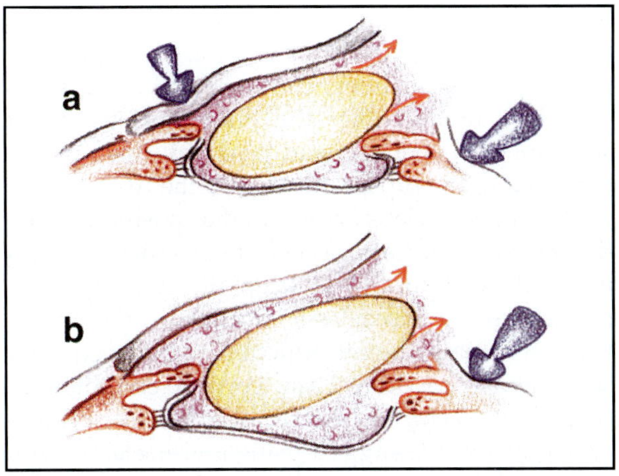

Figure 18-7. (a, b) Expression of the nucleus can also be achieved by means of double pressure. The application of double pressure placed inferiorly on the cornea (the endothelium is protected by the viscoelastic) and posteriorly on the sclera helps in leading the nucleus out of the bag. Usually, pressing on the sclera is all that is needed to draw out the nucleus.

MANUAL NUCLEOSECTION TECHNIQUE

Small-incision surgery with phacoemulsification is undergoing a period of enormous development. However, the technique requires the use of very expensive equipment and demands a learning curve that cannot be accomplished by all surgeons. Furthermore, in several cases the nucleus is too hard to permit safe phacoemulsification. Financial limitations may prevent many hospitals from adopting new technologies, especially in countries with slow industrial development.

Manual nucleosection is a feasible technique in nearly all cataract cases, excluding dark cataracts and cases with extremely shallow ACs and subluxated nuclei.

The procedure requires several more maneuvers than in the classic extracapsular technique, but it allows the surgeon to operate through a very small, sometimes even sutureless, incision.

There are various methods to dissect the nucleus. One was suggested in 1992 by Peter Kansas. It consists of a scleral tunnel incision with length ranging from 3.2 to 7 mm, followed by capsulorhexis under viscoelastic. Capsulorhexis is wide (approximately 6 to 7 mm in diameter). Then hydrodelineation is performed to separate the harder nuclear layers from the outer and softer portions as well as the cortical layers.

Correct performance of hydrodelineation is fundamental to the continuation of the procedure. We usually employ a 3-cc syringe with 27-G cannula. The tip of the cannula is inserted where the central hard nucleus is expected to end and held in that position. The injection of BSS is performed until a golden ring is visible, indicating cleavage between the internal hard nucleus and the surrounding soft nucleus.

The procedure continues with further BSS infusion under the capsule to delaminate the outer cortical layers. This next point marks the beginning of the most delicate phase of surgery. With Kuglen hooks and the support of viscoelastic, the nucleus is prolapsed from the capsular bag.

This maneuver is achieved by rotations made with hooks and injection of a very pseudoplastic viscoelastic (Healon®, Provisc) with a Corydon's bent cannula under the margin of the rhexis closest to the surgical wound. This will raise its equatorial portion, thus enabling the surgeon to insert a straight cannula under the lifted nucleus, inject some more viscoelastic, and then make the nucleus come out of the capsulorhexis into the AC.

When the nucleus arrives in that position, using the most appropriate viscoelastic is crucial. In this phase it is important to keep the nucleus "suspended" in the viscoelastic, injecting some underneath to permit the introduction of the vectis and some above to protect the corneal endothelium from the trisector or bisector, which may accidentally touch it. We suggest using a viscoelastic with a great ability to create space, a high permanent spatula effect, and elasticity. Healon® GV possesses these qualities.

It is also possible to use two viscoelastics, placing a more adhesive product (ie, Viscoat) immediately in contact with the corneal endothelium. Then the bisector is introduced in the space marked by the viscoelastic between the cornea and nucleus, and the rigid vectis in the space formed by the viscoelastic between the capsular bag and nucleus. Then the trisector is pressed toward the vectis and reversed. The nucleus is pressed between them and the trisector is thrust into the nucleus, thereby cutting it into three pieces.

The central piece remains trapped in the trisector and is extracted from the AC. The other two pieces are removed with special forceps with 9 mm toothed jaws to provide an optimal grasp of the remaining nuclear portions. In this phase, the surgeon must not hesitate to use the viscoelastic as a real surgical tool, moving the pieces to be removed with the viscoelastic material so they are oriented along the 6 to 12 axis and their orientation is parallel to that of the forceps' jaws. The viscoelastic must often be replaced, as some leaks out of the opening each time the surgeon extracts the forceps holding the piece of nucleus. The keystone of the procedure is to work in a very deep chamber and float fragments in the viscoelastic.

At this point, mechanical irrigation and aspiration of the residual cortex is accomplished, new viscoelastic is added to fill the capsular bag and the AC, the IOL is implanted, the viscoelastic is accurately removed, and tunnel tightening is checked. If the walls of the tunnel show no damage and the valve has been correctly made, the surgeon can leave the incision sutureless (Figure 18-8).

As has been stated, the technique allows one to achieve a number of results:

- Decreased induced astigmatism
- Fast visual rehabilitation
- Fast recovery of the patient
- Quick local healing
- Reduced postoperative inflammation

Maneuvers in the AC may sometimes cause corneal damage in the days following surgery, particularly when not supported by the best viscoelastic. Therefore, such interventions must always be performed with optimal space control. The surgeon must avoid contact between the instruments and the corneal endothelium or between the nucleus and the endothelium itself. Abiding by these rules, the functional outcome should be comparable to that achieved with phacoemulsification.

Irrigation, Aspiration, IOL Implantation, Viscoelastic Removal

With respect to the ideal viscoelastics for these phases of surgery, we refer the readers to the chapter concerning phacoemulsification (Chapter 11).

Complications of Extracapsular Technique

There are many complications of extracapsular cataract surgery. These vary in severity, but the most threatening is undoubtedly posterior capsular rupture. The techniques through which one can obviate, with viscoelastic support, the complications occurring during ECCE are in most cases similar to those already discussed for phacoemulsification. Therefore, questions concerning problems during capsulotomy, management of the nucleus, irrigation and aspiration maneuvers, capsular break, and IOL implantation are referred to the chapter on phacoemulsification (Chapter 11).

Conclusions

In extracapsular surgery, there are phases in which the presence of a viscoelastic plays a primary

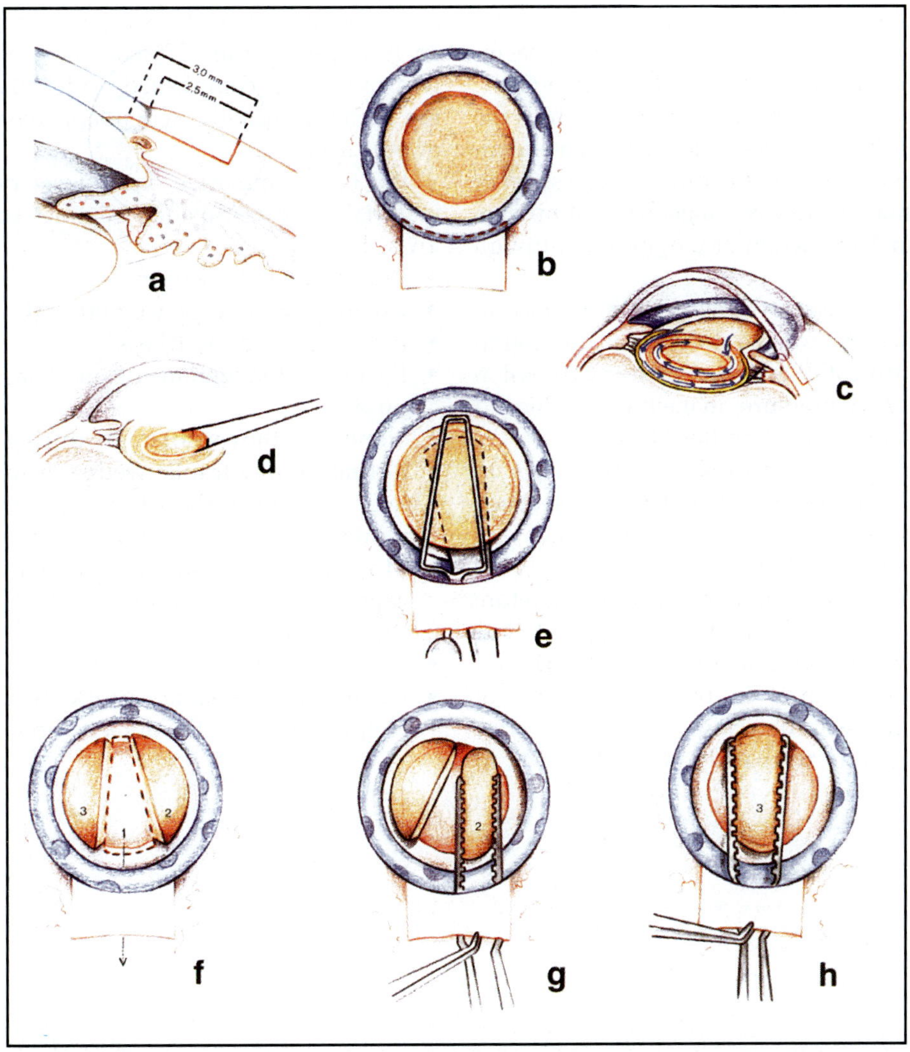

Figure 18-8. (a) Straight tunnel incision in half scleral thickness, self-closing internal incision in the cornea. (b) Continuous tearing capsulotomy performed by a forceps. The width of a capsulorhexis performed by forceps is usually greater than the width created by a cystotome. (c) Hydrodissection and hydrodelamination. (d) Luxation of the nucleus in the AC helped by two Kuglen hooks, under the protection of Healon®. (e) Kansas' trisector nucleotome (over the nucleus) and Kansas' solid vectis spatula (under the nucleus). (f) Trisection: the first fragment has been extracted by the trisector. (g) The special forceps for fragments removes the second portion. The chamber is maintained formed by Healon®. (h) The forceps removes the third fragment.

role (ie, capsulotomy, IOL implantation, or viscoexpression of the nucleus). All these phases are facilitated by the employment of viscoelastic material.

On the other hand, there are phases in which the presence of an improper viscoelastic from a chemical–physical point of view (ie, during expression of the nucleus) may be disadvantageous, as it hinders engagement and extraction of the nucleus through the surgical wound.

A study by Rappazzo showed no difference in terms of corneal thickness, endothelial cell count, and postoperative IOP between nuclear expression (by pressure and pressure maneuvers) achieved with Healon® or with BSS in the AC.

We find employing adhesive viscoelastics in extracapsular surgery inconvenient, as has been demonstrated by Alpar. Cohesive materials are unquestionably preferable in this case because they are likely to leave the AC as a whole mass, therefore keeping the space formed and showing good elasticity. In the above mentioned work, Healon® and Viscoat were compared in the performance of ECCE. Healon® was determined to be superior except for its ability to coat the IOL. However, in advanced extracapsular surgery, many maneuvers such as capsulotomy, viscoexpression, and trisection must be accomplished under viscoelastic and are therefore heavily dependent upon these kinds of products.

We can summarize the effects of viscoelastic materials in extracapsular cataract surgery as follows:

- Protecting endothelium
- Creating working space in the AC
- Inducing good mydriasis
- Easing achievement of mydriasis in miotic pupils
- Stabilizing the capsular flap during capsulotomy
- Acting as a hydraulic wedge in some phases of lens luxation in the AC or favoring and determining its expression outside the eye
- Moving the nucleus away from the posterior capsule, enabling the surgeon to perform phacosection maneuvers
- Slowing motion of fragments floating in the AC
- Acting as a mechanical shock absorber
- Helping separate the nucleus from the cortex

CHAPTER NINETEEN

Anterior Chamber Intraocular Lens Implantation

In recent years, AC IOL implantation has become less popular. IOL implantation in the AC is largely reserved for selected secondary cases.

INDICATIONS

The occasions in which AC implantation can be considered useful are as follows:

- After intracapsular cataract extraction—This technique is currently performed only in cases of extremely subluxated lenses. In this setting, the surgeon cannot implant a posterior chamber lens because of absence of capsular support. In such cases, IOL implantation in the AC can be considered. Cystoid macular edema is one of the major complications of intracapsular surgery. Intracapsular extraction, especially in highly myopic eyes, exposes the patient to a much higher risk of retinal detachment than does other cataract procedures. It is also known that the presence of an IOL in the AC may result in progressive corneal endothelium cell loss, leading to complications such as corneal decompensations and bullous keratopathy months or even years after the surgery. Based on the above reasons, intracapsular extraction is used only in carefully selected cases. In our opinion, IOL implantation after intracapsular cryoextraction can be accomplished in the AC provided that a good corneal endothelium is present and the patient is aged. In the treatment of younger patients or older patients with various problems of corneal endothelium, we prefer IOL fixation in the sclera.
- In aphakic patients, for secondary implantation—The guidelines for secondary implantation in the AC are patient age, relative integrity of the anterior segment, presence of a pupil without surgical mydriasis, absence of angle synechiae that may jeopardize proper IOL placement in the AC, sufficient endothelial cell amount, and absence of glaucoma. If these criteria are not met, it may be convenient to perform secondary implantation with scleral fixation.
- After capsular breaks during extracapsular extraction or phacoemulsification—In case of capsular break during extracapsular extraction or phacoemulsification, an AC lens can be considered if there is inadequate support for a posterior chamber lens. AC lenses have evolved tremendously from the early designs of Strampelli, Choyce, and, later, Kelman. With time, angle support has become increasingly gentle and less invasive for angle structures. As far as AC lenses with iris fixation are concerned, the number and severity of their negative consequences have been such that they have been almost completely abandoned. The advent of viscoelastic materials has resulted in a turning point for AC IOL implantation. In the past, implantation was performed under the protection of air or BSS in the AC. Currently, the viscoelastic ensures atraumatic maneuvers, space, tamponading of blood, and protection of the corneal endothelium. In a work by Lazembly, it was observed that corneal endothelium cell loss due to secondary IOL implantation in the AC under BSS is 13.5%, whereas the rate under Healon® is 9.7%.

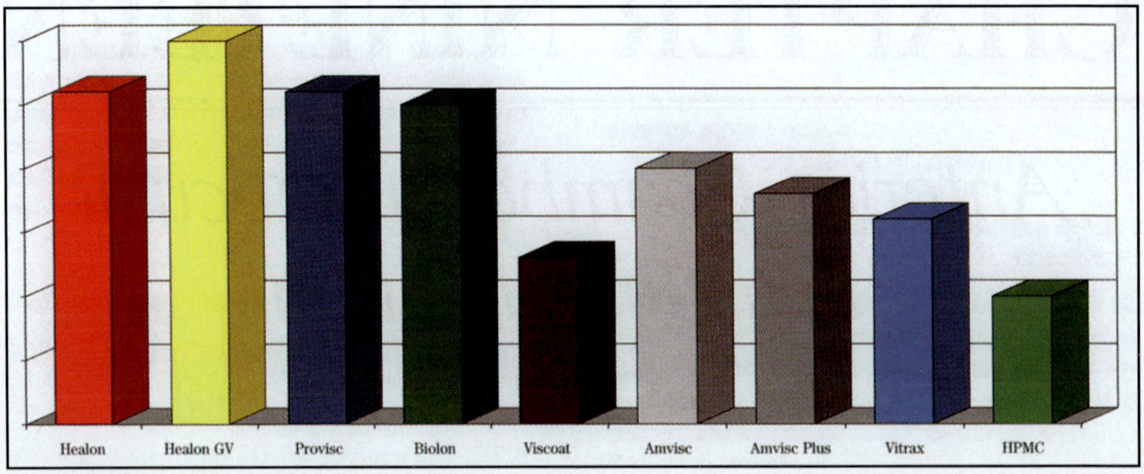

Figure 19-1. AC implant.

Viscoelastic Features Required

Surgeon requirements concerning the use of viscoelastic in these types of surgery are:

- Space maintenance—A material with high molecular weight and high viscosity at low shear rate is mandatory to create and maintain a large volume in the AC between the corneal cupule and the iris. Moreover, the chamber angle must be kept wide and possible synechiae must be detached.
- High elasticity—The product must be able to dampen potential collisions and friction of the IOL loops against angle structures and cushion the introduction of guides and instruments.
- Good transparency—The product must allow the surgeon to visualize the pupil, iris, and IOL correctly in order to lead it into its site in the best and most atraumatic way possible.
- High pseudoplasticity—The product must be easily injected even in difficult conditions and must favor passage of the IOL when one is being inserted.
- Removability—High cohesiveness enhances removability at the end of surgery.
- Avoidance of hypertension—Easy and complete removal is the best insurance that the incidence of postoperative hypertension is reduced.

Healon® GV is the product that best meets all the above requirements. Products made of HPMC are ranked the worst because they fail to meet these requirements (Figure 19-1).

The viscoelastic material is used to reduce herniated vitreous to a position behind the iris plane before the introduction of the AC IOL. This is true whether AC implantation is being performed after intracapsular cryoextraction, after completing extracapsular extraction, after phaco with capsular break, or to accomplish secondary implantation in the chamber.

Before viscoelastic injection, the surgeon can check for the presence of vitreous strands by inserting a Buratto's spatula through the paracentesis incision. Using the spatula, the pupil can be swept to ensure that the vitreous body is posterior to the iris plane. One can also check for vitreous by injecting an air bubble in the AC. Healon® Yellow* may be useful in this type of surgery because it can be distinguished easily from vitreous material.

When reforming the AC with viscoelastic (Figure 19-2), care must be taken to reduce the vitreous behind the pupillary plane. A temporal incision with a tunnel into clear cornea is preferable as it provides optimal astigmatism control. A two-plane limbal opening or a short corneoscleral tunnel may be used.

AC filling with the viscoelastic must be carefully accomplished, according to the techniques we previously described. Special care must be taken to fill the chamber so that there is a flat iris plane. This favors optimal IOL positioning. Furthermore, par-

**Healon® Yellow is no longer being manufactured.*

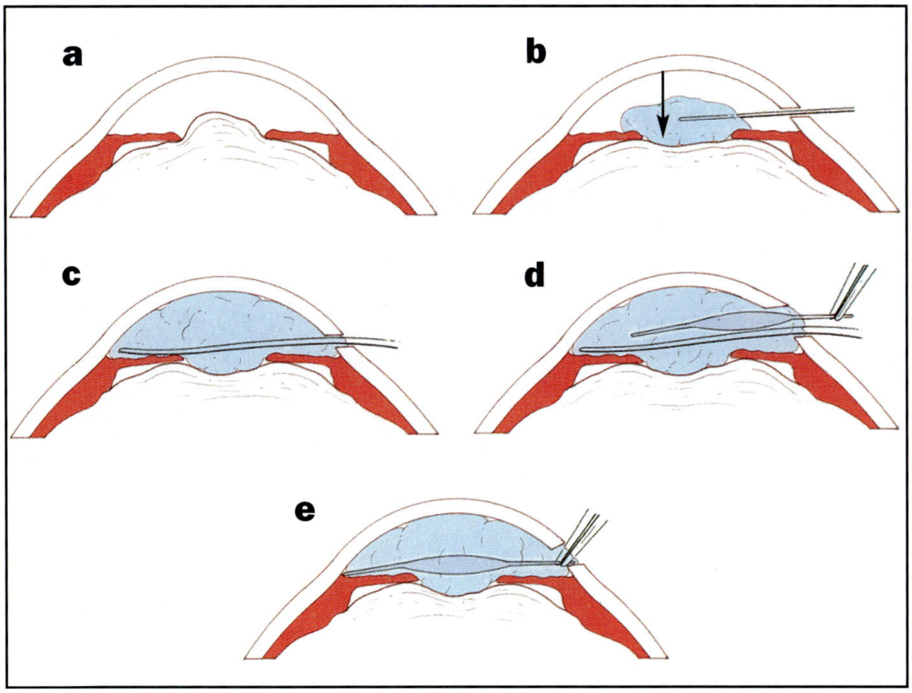

Figure 19-2. IOL implantation in the AC under viscoelastic protection. (a) Intra-capsular aphakia: the vitreous tends to prolapse through the pupillary foramen. (b)Viscoelastic is injected, controlling the vitreous and creating space in the pupillary chamber. (c) A Sheet's glide is inserted. (d) The IOL is implanted, making it slip on the glide, which is then removed. (e) Positioning of the proximal loop of the IOL and removal of the viscoelastic are performed.

tial AC deepening might compress the vitreous, thus favoring its prolapse through the pupil foramen. When the viscoelastic is present in the chamber, a Sheet's glide is inserted in the AC, allowing it to slide gently on the iris until it reaches the angle recess opposite to the entrance area. At this point, a thin layer of viscoelastic should be placed on the anterior surface of the IOL to prevent contact with the endothelial surface. The IOL is then inserted. Gently lifting the flap, the IOL is advanced on the slide until the ends of the distal loop are placed in the opposite angle. While holding the IOL, the surgeon removes the Sheet's slide. During the maneuvers for IOL insertion and slide removal, a part of viscoelastic may leak out. In this event, it must be replaced, particularly to lower the iris under the entrance in the AC.

With a toothed forceps, the posterior flap of the incision may be grasped to introduce the proximal loop of the IOL into the proximal chamber angle. It is always necessary to make an iridectomy. The iridectomy must be placed far from the supporting area of the loop feet to avoid incarceration of the loop in the iridectomy. This helps prevent lens malpositioning and pupillary block. Then the viscoelastic is removed and the opening sutured.

CHAPTER TWENTY

Phacoemulsification Complications

Phacoemulsification enables the surgeon to achieve quick and excellent functional results provided that each passage, from incision to suturing, is performed flawlessly. A problem in a single step may jeopardize the positive outcome of the following phases, whereas in the extracapsular technique there are more "ways out" for the surgeon if one of the various passages of the procedure is not performed with exact precision.

The following is an overview of the complications of phacoemulsification that may be solved with the use of a suitable viscoelastic.

GENERAL CONCEPTS

Possible requirements of the surgeon include: the possibility for conversion (in this event, the surgeon must perform rotation, manipulation, and movement of the nucleus in the capsular bag or in the AC as well as viscoexpression); shallow AC (to reform the chamber); vitreous push (to push the capsular diaphragm back); removal of the nucleus in the presence of posterior capsule break (to remove the nucleus and close the hole); and removal of cortical material in the presence of capsular breaks (to perform dry aspiration of cortex).

CONVERSION

The best viscoelastic to employ in this case should have the following features:

- High elasticity
- High pseudoplasticity
- High molecular weight
- Good soft spatula effect
- Good permanent spatula effect
- Good removability
- Good ability to protect the corneal endothelium

The products that best meet these requirements are those made of hyaluronic acid (particularly with high molecular weight, such as Healon® GV and Healon®).

In case of conversion, the surgeon must be able to move portions of or the whole nucleus in the desired direction, in addition to performing, if necessary, mechanical dissection or viscoexpression of the nucleus. Therefore, the ability to mobilize, protect, and cushion possible contacts between nuclear portions or surgical tools and ocular structures is extremely important. Healon® GV, Healon®, and Provisc are the products that best meet these requirements. Nonpseudoplastic products, such as HPMC, or poorly elastic materials, such as Viscoat, lack these necessary features. Furthermore, the poor removability of these latter products may result in problems if the surgeon, during conversion, must manage complications (which differ from case to case) that may require a change of strategy and partial removal of the viscoelastic from one position to another. Table 20-1 lists the viscoelastics in order of preference.

Although the chemical and physical characteristics of Healon® GV are preferable to those of Healon®, Healon® GV was placed second after Healon® because its incomplete removal (which is more likely in the presence of complications) generally causes much higher postoperative hypertension than Healon®. The corneal endothelial protection provided by Viscoat is rather good despite its low ranking in Table 20-1, and in our list the product may be underrated. However, we believe that its

Table 20-1. Conversion: Viscoelastics in Order of Preference
Healon®
Healon® GV
Provisc
Amvisc
Amvisc Plus
Vitrax
Viscoat
HPMC

Table 20-2. Flat AC: Viscoelastics in Order of Preference
Healon® GV
Healon®
Provisc
Amvisc
Amvisc Plus
Viscoat
Vitrax
HPMC

poor soft and permanent spatula effect along with high adhesiveness could cause difficulty in the maneuvers required to move the nucleus and its viscoexpression.

Flat Anterior Chamber

A good viscoelastic in this application will have the following features:

- High pseudoplasticity
- High viscosity at low shear rate
- High permanent spatula effect
- Good endothelial protection
- Ability to remain in the place where it was injected

In Table 20-2, the viscoelastic materials are ranked, according to our opinion, from best to worst.

It should be noted that some features counteract each other. In fact, easy injectability, good transparency, and high pseudoplasticity are not compatible with the need for a product to remain in site, which is adhesive and protective. We therefore consider Healon® GV and adhesive products such as Viscoat to be excellent provided that the surgeon chooses the product based on the specific procedure. If the surgeon must perform invasive and protracted phaco maneuvers, products with adhesiveness, such as Viscoat, are recommended. On the contrary, if the surgeon must perform a viscoexpression during conversion, Healon® GV would be a good product to use.

Posterior Capsule Holes with Intact Hyaloid

In case of capsular break, a product with the following features is required:

- High molecular weight
- Excellent ability to create space

Table 20-3.
CAPSULAR RUPTURE

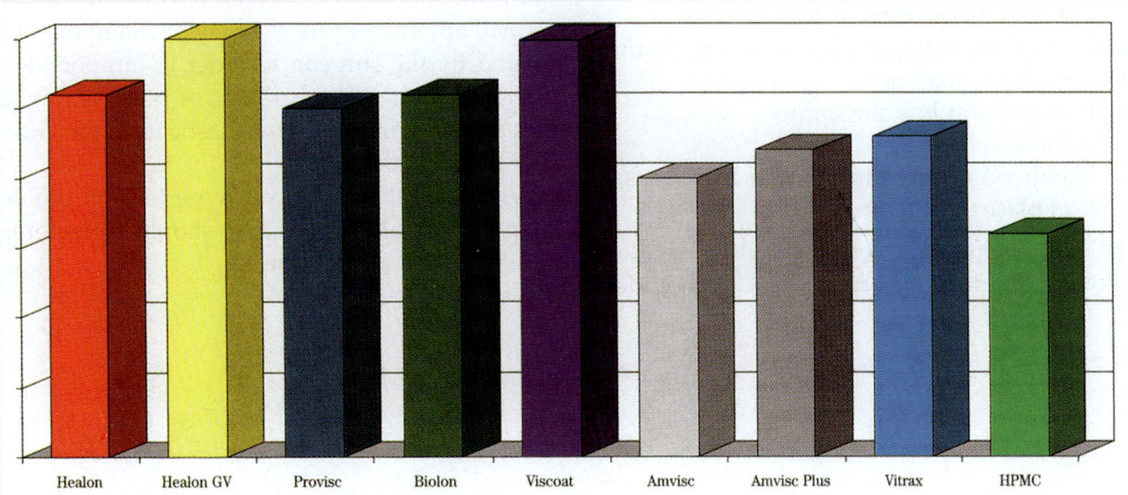

- Good ability to act as permanent spatula
- No likelihood of causing hypertension when left in place and mixed with vitreous
- No tendency to leave the site where it has been placed

A product with these features must keep the vitreous controlled in its place and exert a remarkable counterpressure; however, it must also be able to counterbalance vitreous push, be easily drained through the trabecular meshwork, and allow the surgeon to continue maneuvers to remove residual nucleus and cortex. Viscoat, despite its inferiority to Healon® GV with respect to transparency, molecular weight, and ability to push back the vitreous, is considered to be an excellent product because it has greater adhesiveness that enables it to remain in the injection site for a longer period of time. This seems to be an important feature because, unlike more cohesive products, it allows the surgeon using dry techniques to continue with residual work (removal of nucleus fragments, aspiration of cortical material) without removing an excessive amount of product. Because the counterpush that Healon® GV is able to exert may be advantageous in many circumstances, it may be necessary to combine both products. Table 20-3 suggests a ranking order of various viscoelastic products that may be used in case of capsular breaks. Products with low molecular weight and poor ability to create space are ignored or ranked last.

IRIS PUSH, VITREOUS PUSH

Choosing between Healon® GV and Viscoat may depend on the specific surgical circumstance. If a remarkable counterpressure is required to allow implantation of an IOL, it is best to use a product with high pseudoplasticity, such as Healon® GV. On the contrary, if the surgeon needs to perform maneuvers with irrigation and aspiration to complete clearance of difficult subincisional cortex, it is better to use Viscoat because its adhesiveness allows it to remain in place despite irrigation and aspiration flows. The irrigation and aspiration flows could potentially remove a more cohesive product like Healon® GV. Choice of viscoelastic may be made according to Table 20-3. The surgeon may prefer Healon® GV or Viscoat depending on the circumstance.

REMOVAL OF CORTICAL MATERIAL IN THE PRESENCE OF CAPSULAR BREAKS

In this case, the following are necessary features of the viscoelastic material:

- High viscosity at low shear rate
- High cohesiveness
- No likelihood to cause intraocular hypertension if left in place

The permanent spatula effect should be marked; therefore, a product like Healon® GV should be considered, although its high cohesiveness may render it easily removable. The surgeon may prefer a product that has a poorer ability to create space but is more adhesive, such as Viscoat. Furthermore, a small amount of product may be intentionally left behind by the surgeon in order to tamponade, for instance, a small hemorrhage, or because it is difficult to distinguish the viscoelastic from the vitreous due to poor visibility.

Viscoat will cause fewer hypertension problems than will Healon® GV and should, therefore, be considered as a first choice.

Chapter Twenty-One

Possible Applications of Viscoelastic Materials to Treat the Main Complications of Phacoemulsification

Mistakes in Incision

Even though a common limbal approach cannot be performed, one of the advantages of phacoemulsification is the formation of small openings in the AC that heal rapidly and are stable, thereby causing no astigmatism. These characteristics allow the surgeon to reduce surgical trauma and increase postoperative control, and favor a quick, functional recovery for the patient. Moreover, the creation of a tunnel incision provides constant and complete control of AC depth and consequently of all surgical maneuvers.

It is known that the tunnel incision also allows the surgeon to avoid suturing the wound margins, as the eye pressure itself will press the inside flap against the outside flap of the valve and achieve a fully tightened incision. Of course, construction of a tightened tunnel is based on precise concepts; namely, tunnel dimensions, depth of preincision, and tunnel procedure.

Tunnel Dimensions

When the tunnel starts from the sclera (sclerocorneal tunnel) or in the cornea (clear cornea), what matters most is the formation of a valve inside the AC that creates a flap that remains closed under the push of IOP, thus allowing the wound to heal without sutures. Some time ago it was thought that sclerocorneal tunnels should be made posterior to the limbus for the sake of tightening. It was later demonstrated that the scleral path could be remarkably reduced, provided proper entrance in the AC. However, the distance from the limbus is directly proportional to the width of the incision (Koch's funnel). Also, in clear cornea, the tunnel should resemble a square in order to be tightened. Therefore, the smaller the incision length, the shorter the pathway in the cornea to ensure tightening of the valve.

Depth of Preincision and Tunnel Procedure

Early tunnels were constructed with only one cutting plane, but after surgeons recognized the importance of the valve there was an evolution to two and later three cutting planes. When applied to clear cornea, the first cut is made parallel to the limbus, 250 to 300 µm deep. Recently (hinge technique), a deeper precut has been suggested, with the second part of the incision starting about midthickness of the precut. The second part continues in the corneal stroma, running parallel to the corneal surface itself, angling downward and entering the AC, achieving the third portion of the cut. If an incision is in a single plane, the contact surface between the two flaps is small and pressure from inside or outside will open the wound (Figure 21-1). On the contrary, when the incision is performed

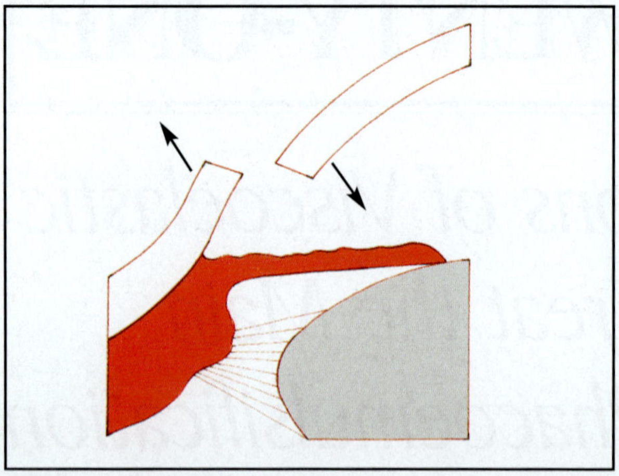

Figure 21-1. Single plane incision. There is little contact between both flaps. The AC opens.

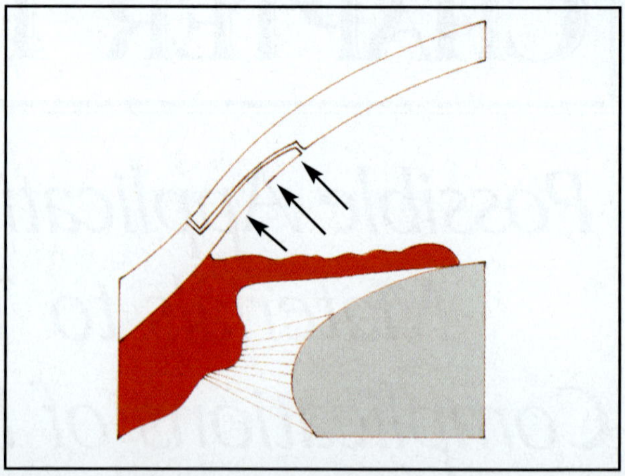

Figure 21-2. Corneal tunnel incision. The area of contact of both flaps is large and IOP itself keeps the opening closed.

correctly, the internal flap will lean on a wide external support area and IOP itself will keep the wound closed (Figure 21-2).

Any mistake in the formation of the tunnel can cause problems. When the incision is too short the tunnel might not tighten properly. When the incision is too superficial it may lacerate due to friction with the phaco handpiece, heat generated, or trauma caused by toothed forceps. When the entrance to the AC is placed too posteriorly, iris engagement is also possible; the iris, stressed by contact with the sleeve of the phaco tip, will undergo progressive friction, thereby rendering it atonic. While the procedure continues, the iris will be more likely to become incarcerated in the surgical wound. The iris can be repositioned with a spatula and kept in place using a heavy, space-creating viscoelastic such as Healon® or Healon® GV (Figure 21-3). In addition, iris atony and its tendency to be incarcerated in the wound makes it likely that the phaco tip will engage iris tissue while the handpiece is entering the eye. This can cause iridodialysis and severe bleeding (Figure 21-4). Putting viscoelastic on the iris, once the iris has been repositioned, will facilitate introduction of the phaco tip. The surgeon can start the infusion with the tip already in the chamber, as irrigation flow and the push of the iris might cause the viscoelastic (particularly when cohesive) to come out of the AC. This may cause iris prolapse.

Therefore, great care must be taken to introduce the phaco tip so that the sharper apex is distant from the iris and then to rotate it 90°, repositioning it correctly once the prolapsed iris has been overcome and the instrument has entered the AC. Only then should infusion be started. AC depth is maintained by the presence of the viscoelastic material.

Detachment of Descemet's membrane is another complication related to incorrect tunnel incision. This may occur because the phaco tip was not positioned correctly while entering the incision. This may also occur when irrigation is not done while entering or if the tunnel is too long. In this situation, the tip tends to "go up" toward the corneal endothelium, with higher risk of endothelial damage on entry.

Following are the possible methods for repositioning Descemet's membrane:

- Injection of an air bubble—This method can be harmful to corneal endothelial cells.
- Suturing the detached Descemet's membrane with 10-0 nylon sutures.
- Reattaching the detached membrane with viscoelastic (Figure 21-5)—The ideal material should have a good soft spatula effect as it must gently "unroll" the detached membrane and reposition it. The viscoelastic must also have good permanent spatula effect, as it must keep Descemet's membrane in that position for as long as possible. The hypertension the viscoelastic causes must not be significant, as it is purposefully left in the AC. A suitable product, in this case, is Provisc, because it possesses the fea-

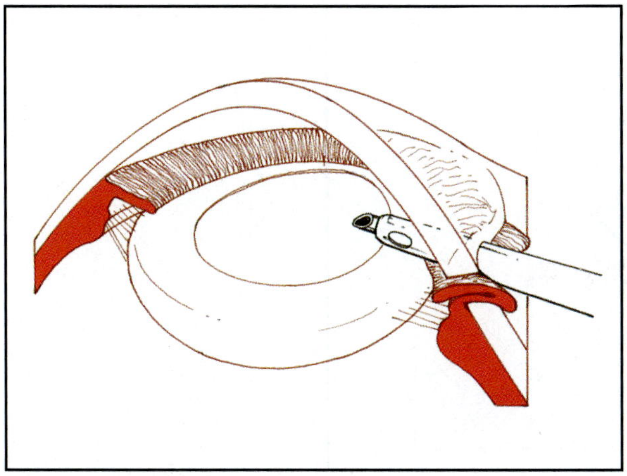

Figure 21-3a. Short tunnel: the iris prolapses through the opening.

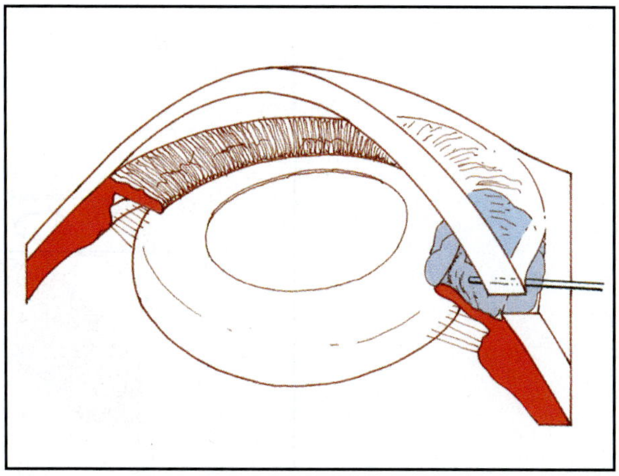

Figure 21-3b. The iris is repositioned and kept in place by the viscoelastic.

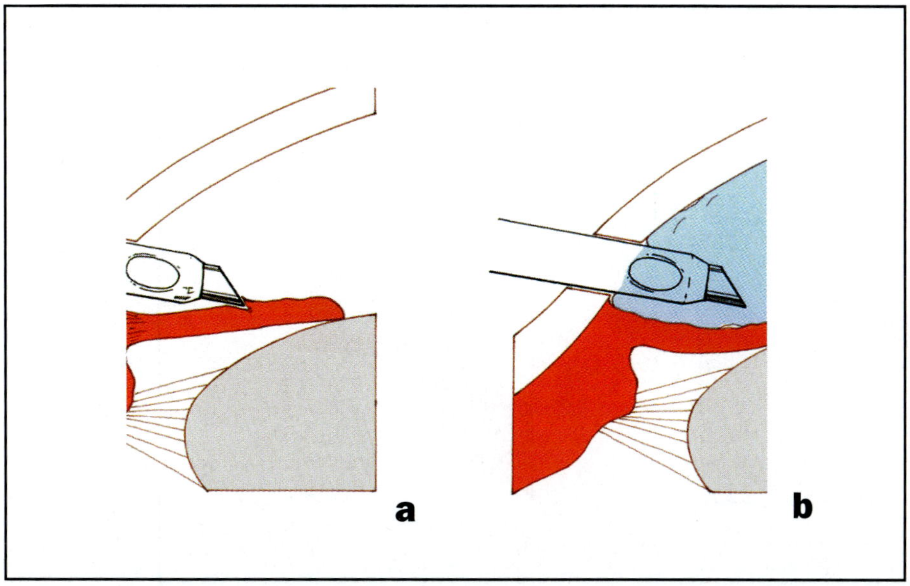

Figure 21-4. (a) The phaco tip makes contact with the iris, damaging it or causing iridodialysis. (b) The viscoelastic is injected in order to form a large space between cornea and iris, thus allowing atraumatic introduction of the phaco tip.

tures required for reattachment of Descemet's membrane and weighs less than Healon®, causing a lower IOP increase when left in the chamber. Even if the surgeon intends to suture the membrane in place, Descemet's membrane reattachment with viscoelastic is still necessary. In fact, more precise and atraumatic suturing is ensured when the membrane is stretched in the anatomic position and there is sufficient space between cornea and iris.

Wound burns have been reported with both corneal and sclerocorneal tunnels. According to some authors, this is due to overheating caused by the viscoelastic material. This thesis suggests that the burn is a consequence of an obstacle in the irrigating flow caused by the viscoelastic or an occlusion in the aspiration line by the viscoelastic and resulting turbulence in the water flow necessary to cool the tip in contact with the tunnel flaps. In our opinion, burns can be mainly attributed to low irrigation bottle height, lack of use of cold BSS, very low flow rate setting, or zero vacuum combined with a wound opening that is too small related to the size of the phaco tip. In addition, a sleeve that is

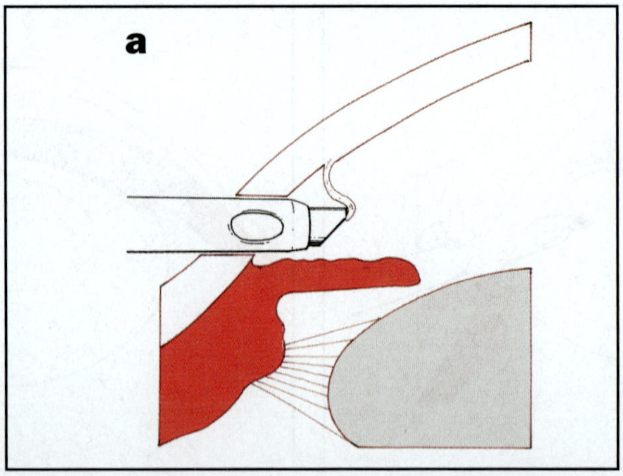

Figure 21-5a. Descemet's membrane is detached by the phaco tip.

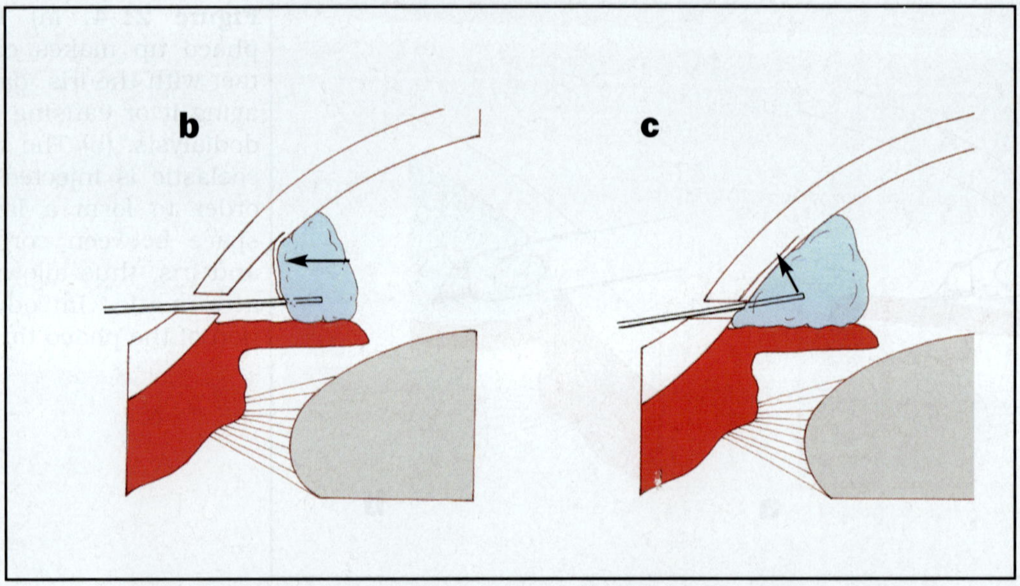

Figure 21-5b and c. (b) Descemet's membrane is detached by the phaco tip. (c) Reattachment of Descemet's membrane.

repeatedly sterilized becomes too soft, atonic, and likely to collapse. These important elements may be the reason for scleral and corneal burns rather than the use of a viscoelastic material.

MISTAKES IN CAPSULORHEXIS

An intact capsulorhexis is crucial to the completion of safe and successful phacoemulsification. Other types of capsulotomy, such as can-opener, envelope, etc, do not allow the margins of the anterior capsule to retain the same geometric shape and soundness that allow endocapsular maneuvers, such as hydro- and viscocleavage of the nucleus, nucleofracture, and correct IOL centration.

Dimensions of the capsulorhexis usually range between 5 mm and 6 mm in diameter. The zonular fibers extend only about 2 mm beyond the lens equator. Therefore, the 6-mm central area is always

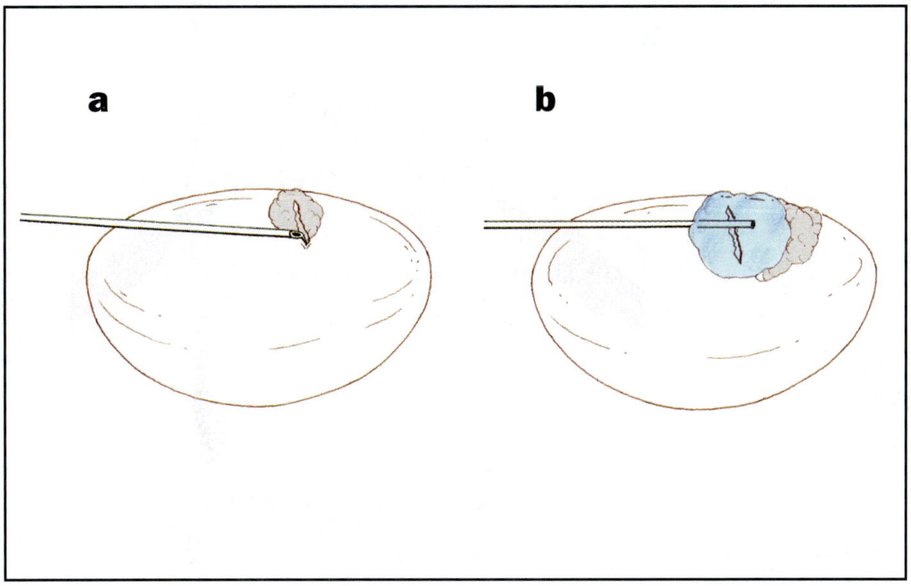

Figure 21-6. (a) Leakage of the cortical material obscures visualization of the capsulorhexis. (b) Injection of viscoelastic shifts the cortex and restores good visibility to continue the rhexis.

free from zonular fibers and the surgeon can be sure that there is no fiber interference. In such a safe environment, the surgeon should be able to accomplish a regular, centered, round capsulorhexis with regular margins.

Therefore the surgeon must perform this maneuver with great concentration and care. As previously noted, AC depth is a determining element for good control of capsulorhexis. In fact, when the depth of the AC is maximized, the strain on the zonular fibers is released and the vectorial force that makes the rhexis likely to escape toward the periphery becomes negligible in comparison to the force the surgeon exerts while performing the rhexis itself.

The ideal viscoelastic for performance of the rhexis is Healon® owing to its high molecular weight, high viscosity at 0 shear rate, excellent transparency, high pseudoplasticity, and excellent soft and permanent spatula effect. When the surgeon has difficulty performing the rhexis, he or she should not hesitate to inject Healon® GV or another product showing similar chemicophysical characteristics. Using the cystotome and forceps under viscoelastic is the most popular technique for performing capsulorhexis.

We focus here on how viscoelastics may help alleviate potential problems that occur with such a technique. Capsulorhexis is started after the AC has been completely filled with viscoelastic. With the cystotome or the capsulorhexis forceps with closed jaws, the surgeon incises the capsule in its central portion, and a small lateral incision, 1.5 to 2 mm in length, is cut. The surgeon then lifts the anterior capsule and creates a small triangular flap, which he or she can then lead in a circular fashion to create the capsulorhexis.

Occasionally, the incision performed with the cystotome is too superficial. More commonly, a deep incision may release cortical material, thus impairing visualization of the capsular flap. It is necessary to inject viscoelastic again in that area, to move the leaked cortex and visualize the portion of capsule to be grasped with the forceps (Figure 21-6). The maneuver should also be performed in cases of intumescent cataract from which milky, white fluid is released and mixed with the viscoelastic in the AC. The injection of a further amount of viscoelastic in the AC restores optimal visualization and deepens the AC, allowing the surgeon to continue the rhexis. In the presence of intumescent cataracts, particularly in young patients, the nucleus is not perfectly formed and a large amount of white fluid will be released from the bag.

This maneuver may also be preferred by surgeons who aspirate the milky material in the bag with a cannula introduced through the first opening in the central anterior capsule. This improves visibility, decompresses the capsular bag, and allows the surgeon to detect dimensions and consistency of the nucleus itself.

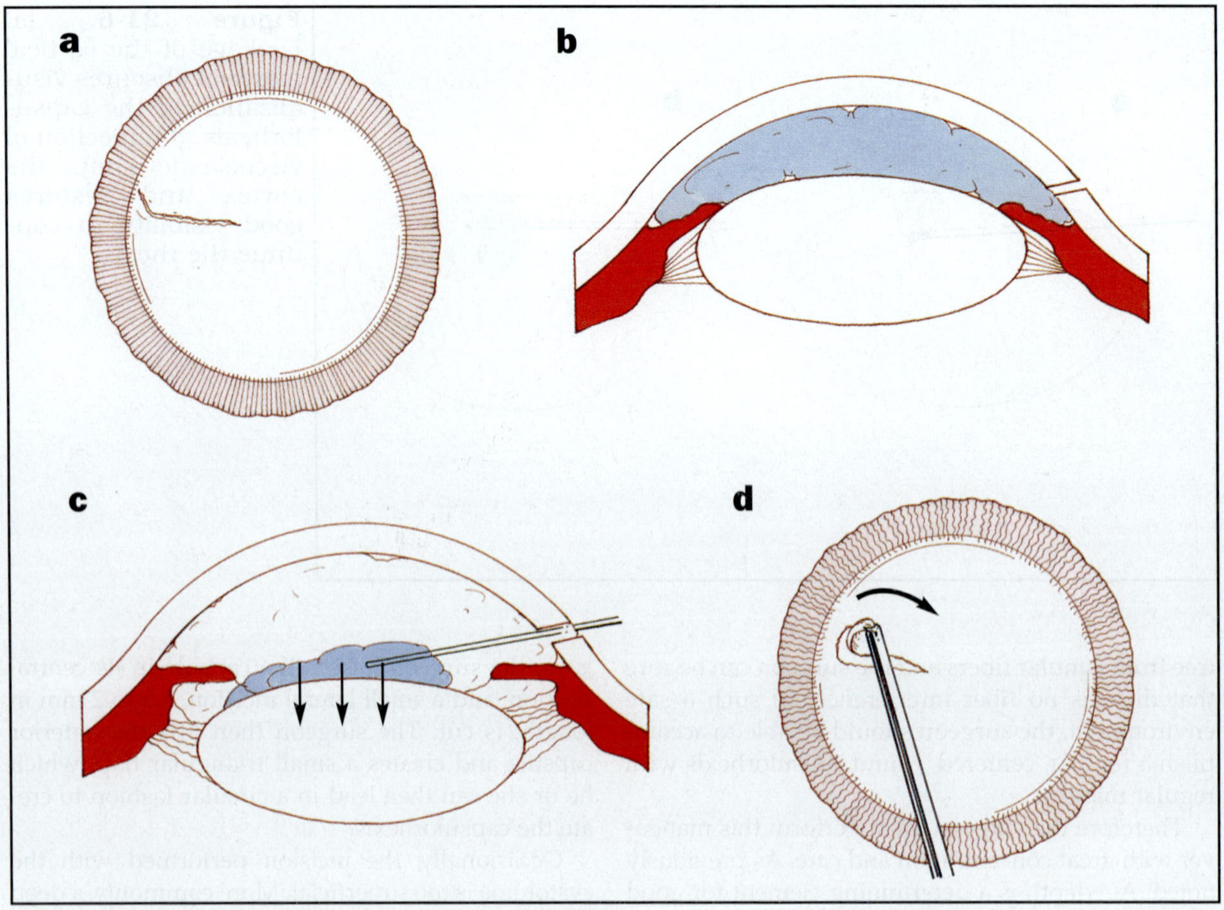

Figure 21-7. (a) The rhexis tends to extend toward the zonular fibers. (b) The AC is not deep enough and zonular fibers are on stretch. (c) Viscoelastic is further injected to relax the zonules and deepen the AC. (d) The margin of the rhexis is held again by exerting centripetal traction with forceps.

In some cases, enough endocapsular material is removed from the bag that subsequently the bag contracts at least in some areas. In such an event, it may be appropriate to inject a small amount of viscoelastic into the bag to reform it. In fact, a partially collapsed bag does not allow the surgeon to complete the capsulorhexis correctly.

If the early pathway of the rhexis turns out to be too small, it should be continued and enlarged. On the contrary, if the early pathway of the rhexis is too large, it is necessary to inject viscoelastic in the AC to relax the zonules and to exert centripetal traction with the forceps to prevent the rhexis from becoming uncontrolled (Figure 21-7).

Once completed, the rhexis may turn out to be too small. This will make it difficult to work in the capsular bag. In particular, once phacofracture has been accomplished, the aspirating maneuvers outside the bag will be challenging. The easiest maneuver is to widen the rhexis after IOL implantation. However, in special cases, the surgeon may decide to enlarge it immediately.

After further injection of viscoelastic, widening is performed with microscissors by cutting a small incision in the margin of the rhexis and tearing it concentrically to the previous small rhexis with the forceps (Figure 21-8).

In the event that the capsulorhexis is too large, the nucleus may prolapse out of the capsular bag. If the nucleus is soft or of medium density, it is possible to perform phacoemulsification outside the bag. However, when the nucleus is hard, it is always bet-

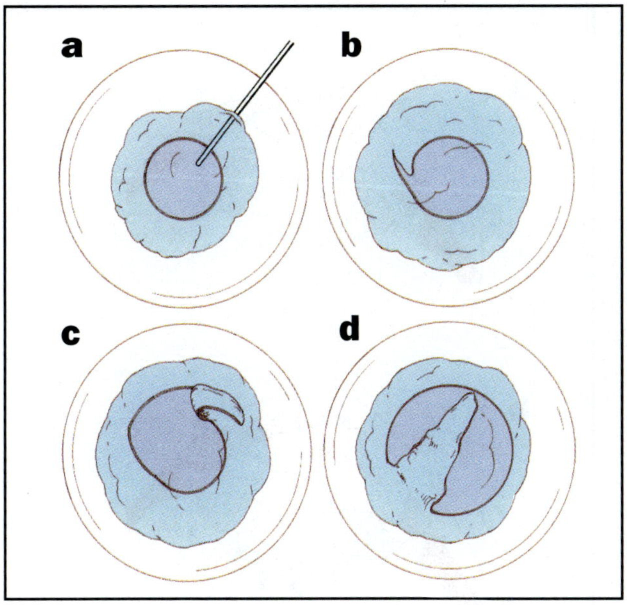

Figure 21-8. (a) A small rhexis. (b) After injecting further viscoelastic, the margin of the rhexis is incised with microscissors. (c) A second capsulorhexis is started with forceps, concentric to the first. (d) Capsulorhexis is completed.

ter to attempt to reposition it with a spatula and viscoelastic injected over the nucleus. It may be necessary to repeat this maneuver a number of times to reduce the nucleus inside the capsular bag.

Occasionally when the rhexis is performed with a diathermic capsulotome, the margins of the rhexis may be irregular. This may result in extension of the rhexis during maneuvers in the bag, as these microincisions may occur at places where the mechanical resistance of the rhexis margins is weaker. While advancing, the capsulotome produces microbubbles along its course of capsulotomy that impair visualization of the rhexis. Therefore, it is useful to inject some more viscoelastic above the capsule, to visualize the development and completeness of the rhexis.

If the capsulorhexis extends peripherally, there are three possible strategies that may be employed. In all cases, it is essential to deepen the chamber as much as possible to counteract zonular tension. The surgeon may continue the rhexis on the side opposite to the initial incision or cut the anterior capsule with microscissors immediately distal to the extension and continue with a new one. Alternatively, in the presence of optimal mydriasis and excellent visibility of zonular fibers, some of the fibers can be cut immediately beyond the area where the rhexis has extended and the surgeon can continue with forceps, grasping the capsule corresponding to the last zonular fiber dissected.

In eyes at risk of rhexis extension (ie, with congenital or juvenile cataract, or white or hypermature cataracts with poor visibility), it is a good rule to perform a small rhexis and then widen it, when necessary, after IOL implantation.

MISTAKES IN HYDRODISSECTION

The hydric cleavage of lens portions, performed with suitable cannulas while injecting BSS, is a very important phase of phacoemulsification. Mobilization of the nucleus inside the bag allows the surgeon to perform phacofracture maneuvers and distinguish the hard nucleus from the surrounding epinucleus and cortex. This maneuver can be performed by flat or round irrigating cannula, depending on the kind of flow the surgeon desires.

Hydrodissection can be accomplished with a flat cannula by lifting the margin of capsulorhexis and injecting the fluid so as to visualize a wave that passes posteriorly along the capsule. Gentle downward pressure applied by the cannula on the nucleus itself causes the fluid to leak out of the rhexis, which enhances the effectiveness of the hydric cleavage. Alternatively, the surgeon can use a round cannula placed at the outer one-third of the lens to inject fluid inside the lens and to reach a certain depth in order to obtain the formation of a "golden ring," which indicates completed cleavage between the nucleus and epinucleus. The use of viscoelastic materials instead of BSS to achieve "viscocleavage" of ocular structures has also been suggested.

Listed in the following are the possible problems that may result from mistaken hydrodissection and how viscoelastic products can help solve them.

POSTERIOR CAPSULE BREAK

If the capsulorhexis is small, particularly when the surgeon has elected to inject a viscoelastic material to achieve separation of the soft epinucleus and the capsule, and the amount of viscoelastic is too large, the pressure generated in the bag may cause the capsule to break. This is especially true when a poorly pseudoplastic product is being used that inadequately separates the surfaces (Figure 21-9).

If the break in the posterior capsule is large, the nucleus may dislocate into the vitreous. Management of this complication will be described in the following sections.

INCOMPLETE HYDRODISSECTION

If fluid is incorrectly or insufficiently injected and cleavage is not achieved, maneuvers that rotate the nucleus may not be possible. Therefore, the surgeon should not hesitate to repeat hydro- or viscodissection until successful completion occurs. Incomplete cleavage may result in additional cortex adhering to the capsule, making it difficult to remove subincisional cortex. Moreover, forced rotation may cause zonular disinsertion. Should this occur, the surgeon should repeat hydrodissection and inject viscoelastic into the AC to relax the zonular fibers. The surgeon can then proceed cautiously with phacoemulsification while minimizing pressure on the bag and rotation maneuvers. To accomplish complete cleavage, the surgeon can use a curved Corydon cannula, which eases subincisional fluid passage.

ZONULAR DISINSERTION

If zonular disinsertion occurs, the surgeon should gently remove the nucleus and the residual lens material from the bag, using suitable parameters (low bottle height, low flow and vacuum). During this maneuver, the bag must remain stretched to prevent the vitreous from passing through the zonular disinsertion into the AC.

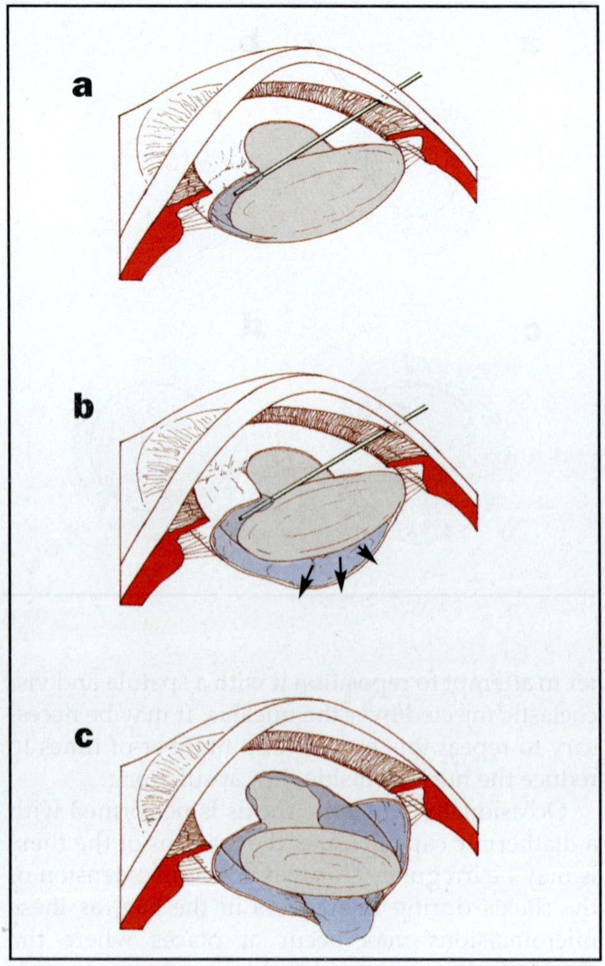

Figure 21-9. (a) In the presence of a small rhexis, a viscoelastic product is injected to obtain viscocleavage. (b) An excessive amount of viscoelastic exerts strong pressure on the posterior capsule. (c) The posterior capsule breaks. The viscoelastic contacts the vitreous and the nucleus may dislocate into the vitreous cavity.

In cases of large disinsertion, the surgeon must consider converting to a no irrigation "dry technique" to prevent vitreous hydration. It is critically important to maintain capsular bag formation. This

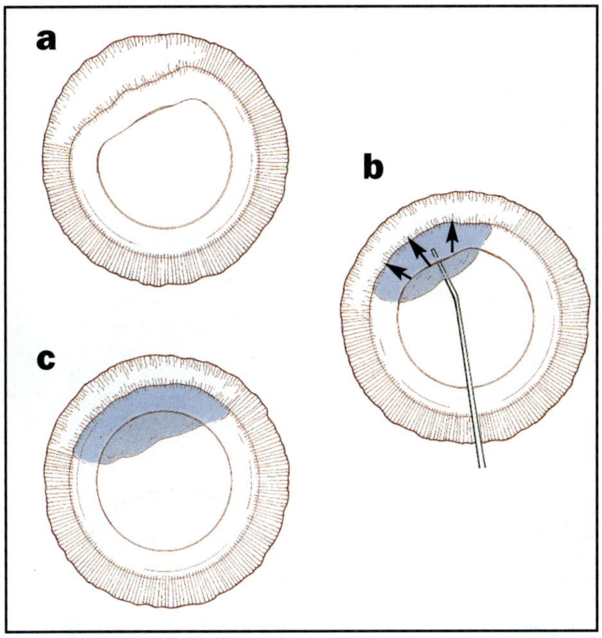

Figure 21-10. Stretching a disinserted capsular bag using viscoelastic. (a) Partly disinserted capsular bag. (b) An adhesive viscoelastic is injected inside the bag to stretch it. (c) Capsular morphology is restored and the viscoelastic keeps the bag stretched.

can be achieved by continuous injection of a very adhesive viscoelastic material that is also pseudoplastic and will remain inside the bag during maneuvers, regardless of whether low or no irrigation is used. Viscoat is ideal for this maneuver.

The viscoelastic should be continuously injected inside the bag into the site where the bag tends to curl up due to the disinsertion (Figure 21-10). It is essential to continue creating a pressure that counterbalances the vitreous pressure that would otherwise widen the disinsertion. The viscoelastic tamponades the bag fornix, allowing the surgeon to complete the maneuvers to remove lens fragments.

Before IOL implantation, the surgeon should consider insertion of a PMMA ring (manufactured by Ophthec and supplied with its special injector) designed to keep the disinserted bag well stretched to receive the implant. Available in two sizes (for "big" bags, typical of myopic eyes, and for "normal" bags), the ring is inserted by a special injector or by McPherson forceps and an IOL hook, following accurate filling of the bag with viscoelastic material (Figure 21-11). The material should be pseudoplastic, with good soft and permanent spatula characteristics, high viscosity at low shear rate, and cohesiveness that eases removal. Healon® and Provisc are the preferred materials in this situation. The bag should be filled completely in order to keep it well stretched and permit insertion of the ring, while avoiding any contact with the corneal endothelium or further damage to the zonules.

NUCLEUS LUXATION IN THE AC

This occurs mainly as a result of an abnormally large capsulorhexis or overly vigorous hydro- or viscodissection when BSS or the viscoelastic pushes the nucleus outside the capsular bag. The surgeon must then reposition the nucleus, which is usually accomplished by pressing a spatula downward onto the nucleus. If too much viscoelastic has been injected behind the nucleus and the surgeon wishes to continue with phacoemulsification, the excessive viscoelastic can be aspirated with a cannula. This maneuver can be dangerous and the surgeon might therefore consider keeping the luxated nucleus in the AC and converting to viscoexpression or a manual nucleofracture technique.

If the nucleus is not particularly dense and the corneal endothelial cell count is high, phaco can be performed in the AC, protecting the endothelium with an adhesive viscoelastic such as Viscoat. Occasionally, it may be possible to "lighten" the nucleus in its equatorial portion by means of ultrasound until it is repositioned in the bag and the techniques of endocapsular phacoemulsification can be started again.

RHEXIS EXTENSION

In the rare case of a potentially "weak" rhexis—for instance, one made by diathermic capsulotome (characterized by slightly irregular and weak margins)—rhexis extension may occur. The surgeon should manage this complication in the same manner as he or she would an uncontrolled rhexis.

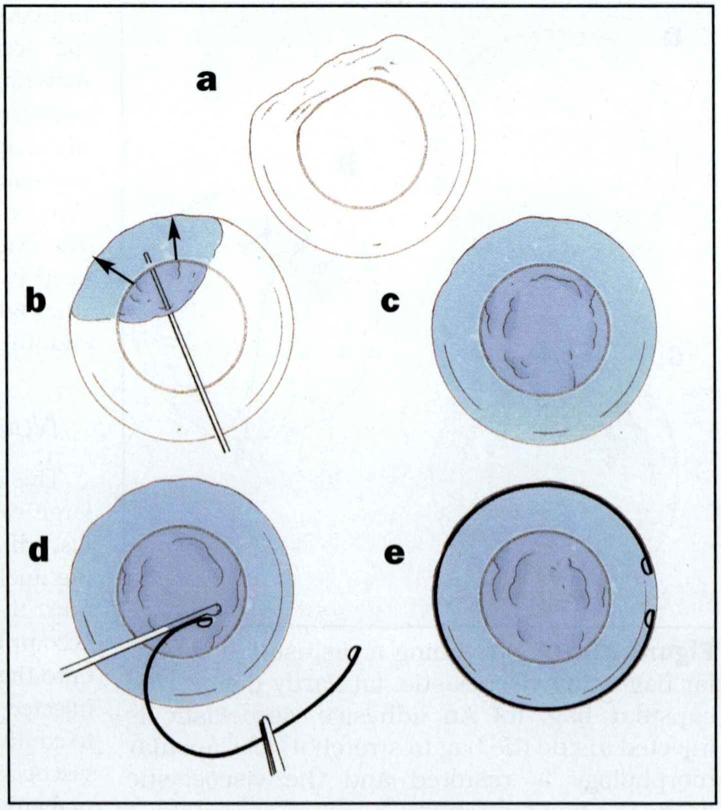

Figure 21-11. A ring for capsular bag dilation is positioned by viscoelastic in case of partial disinsertion. (a) Partly disinserted bag. (b) The bag is stretched by a viscoelastic. (c) The bag is completely filled with viscoelastic. (d) The ring is introduced in the capsular bag. (e) Ring in place.

MISTAKES IN PHACOEMULSIFICATION AND IRRIGATION AND ASPIRATION

During phacoemulsification of the nucleus and irrigation and aspiration of residual cortex, a number of complications may occur. These can be divided into three main groups:

- Nucleus shift and luxation—The management of a subluxated lens with the help of a viscoelastic was previously described. The next step is to complete phacoemulsification of the nucleus by using a few gentle maneuvers and correct machine parameters (low bottle height, low flow, low aspiration, and low ultrasonic power). Chop techniques are preferable because they do not require rotation of the nucleus in the presence of damaged zonules.
- Rhexis extension and capsular disinsertion—The use of the most suitable viscoelastic facilitates surgical maneuvers, as previously described.
- Capsular break due to phaco or irrigation and aspiration—In such severe complications, the viscoelastic material plays a decisive role. It must be able to counterbalance positive vitreous pressure, and therefore it should possess high molecular weight and high viscosity at 0 shear rate. This ensures that suitable counterpressure will be applied to the remnants of the broken capsule, the vitreous that tends to pass through the break, and the iris. The material must remain in place without being easily removed by irrigation or aspiration. These characteristics are fulfilled by an adhesive material. In the event that material is left behind, it must not cause postoperative hypertension. Viscoat is preferable. However, in selected cases where pseudoplastic features and soft or permanent spatula effect are required, Healon® GV can be used.

The reported incidence of capsular break in ECCE and phacoemulsification ranges from 0.05 to 10%. The main complications related to capsular break include cystoid macular edema (sometimes chronic), retinal detachment, uveitis, secondary glaucoma, and progressive corneal decompensa-

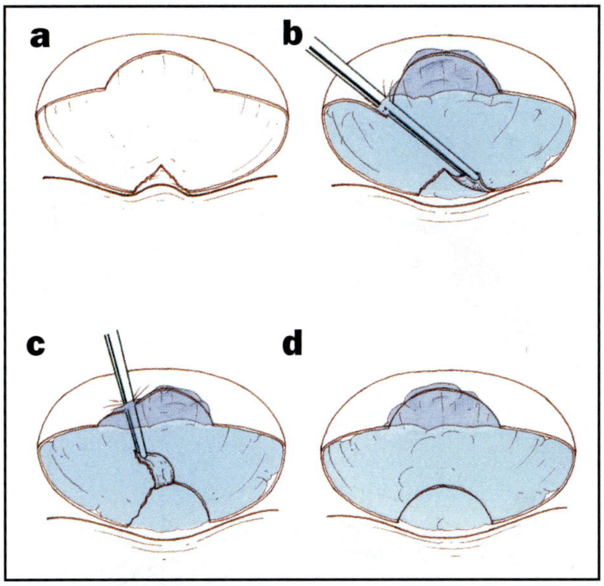

Figure 21-12. Posterior capsulorhexis. (a) Posterior capsule break (intact anterior hyaloid face). (b) Posterior capsulorhexis is started with a forceps, under viscoelastic protection. (c) The posterior rhexis is gradually accomplished. (d) Finished posterior capsulorhexis.

tion. In all cases, correct management of the capsular break is fundamental to ensuring a good functional result.

The surgeon should always try to accomplish IOL implantation in the AC, with scleral fixation or in the ciliary sulcus (over the rhexis). The main advantage of preserving the posterior capsule, even when broken, is the ability to implant the IOL in the posterior chamber.

The surgeon must recognize the capsular break immediately, during phacoemulsification of the nucleus or during capsular cleaning. Capsular breaks occur most frequently during irrigation and aspiration of cortex, particularly when removing subincisional material. The subincisional cortex can be difficult to manage owing to poor visibility caused by the wound, a small rhexis, or incomplete hydrodissection. However, a capsular break is not always followed by vitreous loss. In a study by Osher, 62% of capsular breaks occurred without vitreous loss. Gimbel reports a 0.5% incidence of capsular break. In 38% of these cases, no vitrectomy was required.

When the capsular break occurs during irrigation and aspiration or capsular cleaning, the surgeon can easily recognize the location and extension of the break. Initially, most breaks are small. They are often significantly enlarged by mistaken maneuvers made by the surgeon. In case of a small posterior capsule break, Gimbel suggests that a posterior capsulorhexis be made.

POSTERIOR CAPSULORHEXIS

A viscoelastic with optimal characteristics should be used to perform this technique. The material should have high molecular weight, be highly viscous, and be very transparent, in addition to being easily removed. In the presence of an intact hyaloid, this technique is performed in the following manner. A viscoelastic with high molecular weight (ie, Healon® GV) is injected into the AC and onto the posterior capsule to stretch the capsule and relax the zonular fibers that are stretched by vitreous pressure. A small amount of viscoelastic is also injected through the hole in the posterior capsule and onto the hyaloid to displace the hyaloid as far away as possible.

After grasping one of the flaps where the capsule has been broken, the surgeon performs a posterior capsulorhexis with the forceps under the protection of a heavy viscoelastic. This should be small (from 1.5 to 3 mm in diameter) and central, if possible. Posterior capsulorhexis can also be eccentric, provided that the visual axis is clear.

It is also important to keep the AC formed with heavy viscoelastic while pushing the vitreous toward the posterior pole (Figure 21-12).

It is essential to keep the capsular bag stretched to create a posterior capsulorhexis that is as round and centered as possible.

When possible, the viscoelastic material should be injected through the capsular break to keep the vitreous located as far posteriorly as possible. This ensures that the vitreous will not be inadvertently grasped or dragged by the forceps while the rhexis is being created.

Posterior capsulorhexis under viscoelastic can be performed with capsular breaks, both with and without vitreous prolapse through the capsular hole. In fact, the viscoelastic provides counterpressure that opposes the vitreous pressure and keeps the capsular bag stretched. Posterior rhexis has the same advantages as the anterior rhexis (eg, better durability). This results in a capsular opening that remains unchanged without extending toward the zonular fibers from vitreous pressure.

In addition, it is possible to perform a vitrectomy safely through the posterior rhexis because capsular damage is less likely to occur during maneuvers. This also ensures correct IOL positioning and avoids posterior rhexis extension during IOL implantation.

Posterior capsulorhexis should also be performed when removing fibrotic opacities of the posterior capsule, in congenital cataract surgery, or in very young patients to prevent the occurrence of secondary fibrotic opacities, as an alternative to later YAG laser capsulotomy.

Posterior capsulorhexis can be performed even when the break is not centrally positioned.

BIMANUAL LIMBAL ANTERIOR VITRECTOMY

To protect the integrity of a posterior capsular break it is useful to convert it into a posterior capsulorhexis. The surgeon should take great care to avoid widening the break. Above all, this can be achieved by tamponading the vitreous with a viscoelastic material with high molecular weight, as described previously.

The surgeon should not perform a vitrectomy with coaxial infusion. The fluid infusion through the vitrector tip will further hydrate the vitreous, which will subsequently prolapse through the capsular break and enlarge the hole. It is preferable to place an irrigation line through the paracentesis or as far away as possible from the capsular break. This is performed with a 23-G cannula and the infusion bottle is kept very low. The vitrector is then inserted through the main incision (Figure 21-13). It is preferable to use the guillotine type rather than the rotative model. The vitrectomy should be performed by pulling the vitreous posteriorly, starting anteriorly and proceeding posteriorly. The general tendency is to do the opposite; most sur-

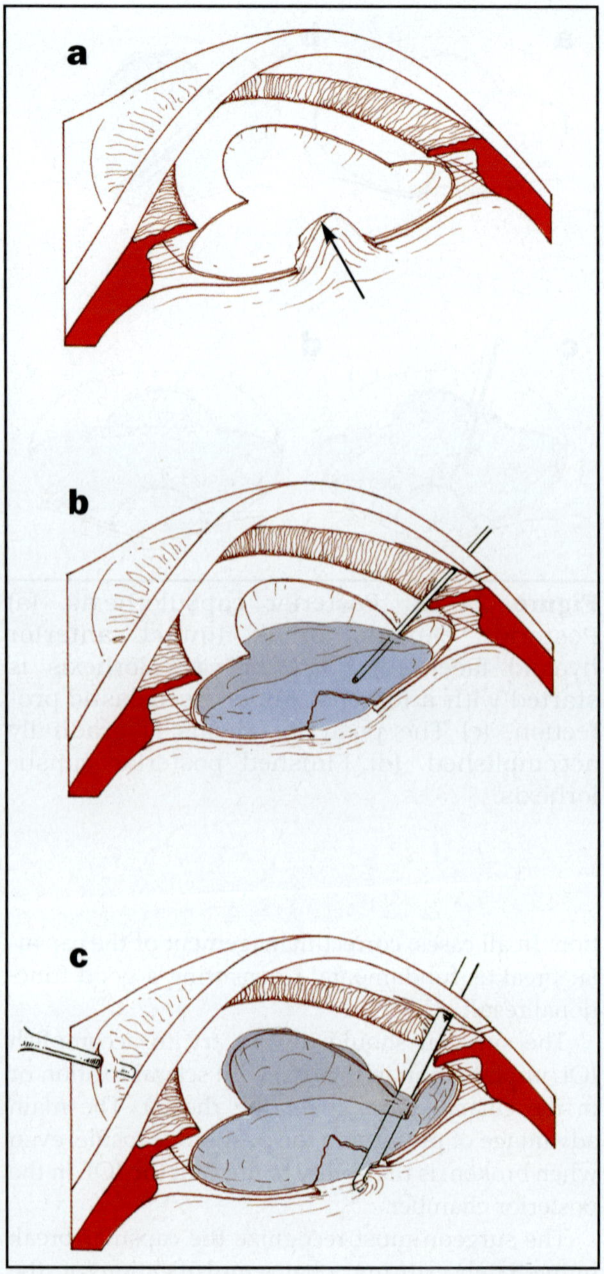

Figure 21-13. Bimanual anterior vitrectomy via the limbus. (a) The vitreous passes through the posterior capsule break. (b) The viscoelastic repositions the vitreous and counterbalances the positive pressure. (c) The viscoelastic allows the surgeon to start the vitrectomy as posteriorly as possible after placing a separate infusion line. Bimanual anterior vitrectomy via the limbus: under viscoelastic control, an infusion system is placed and the vitrectomy is performed through the main incision.

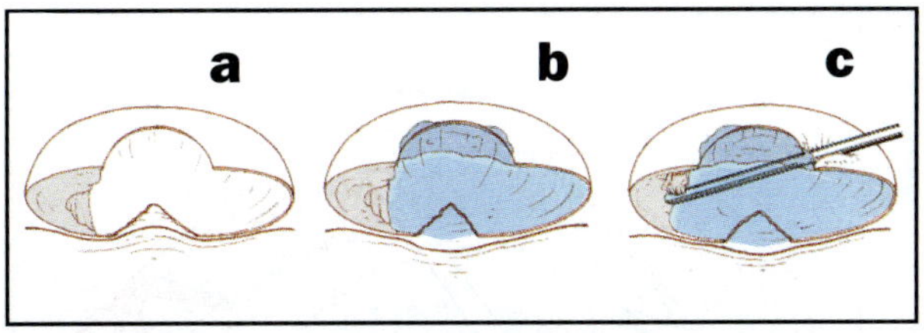

Figure 21-14. Removal of cortical material. (a) Capsular bag with posterior break and residual cortex with no presence of vitreous. (b) The bag is reformed with viscoelastic and the vitreous is tamponaded. (c) Cortex is aspirated under viscoelastic protection.

geons leave the vitrector in the AC in an attempt to clear the vitreous from the AC. However, this results in more vitreous prolapse. The pars plana approach may, in some cases, result in a more effective vitrectomy, but the anterior segment surgeon's lack of technical expertise often prevents him or her from performing this technique. In addition, the level of anesthesia may be insufficient for a pars plana vitrectomy, which may take a longer time.

Bimanual vitrectomy can also be performed in dry conditions. Viscoelastic with high molecular weight is injected, pushing the vitreous posteriorly, while the vitreous is removed with a vitrector that is directed posteriorly. This technique may permit IOL implantation in the capsular bag or the ciliary sulcus.

Scleral fixation of the IOL is also made easier by accurate vitrectomy.

Removal of Cortical Material

After completing the vitrectomy and adequately removing the vitreous that prolapsed through the posterior capsule break, the surgeon turns his or her attention to the cortical material. The viscoelastic plays a fundamental role in permitting removal of the cortical material without also aspirating the vitreous. In fact, when viscoelastic is injected to fill the capsular bag, it serves to keep the bag open and well-formed and to tamponade the vitreous behind the plane of the capsular break (Figure 21-14).

Such maneuvers can be performed after injecting the viscoelastic material, which should have good molecular weight and adhesive characteristics so that it will not be easily aspirated in the event that the aspiration cannula is plunged into it. Aspiration can be accomplished with the same irrigation and aspiration handpiece after disconnecting the infusion line, repeatedly filling the bag whenever the viscoelastic is accidentally aspirated with the cortical material.

Otherwise, the surgeon can perform a technique with two separate Buratto's cannulas: one infusing with low bottle height and very reduced flow rate through the paracentesis and the other aspirating through the main incision. It is possible to invert the position of both cannulas, according to the location of residual cortex, creating additional paracenteses when needed to facilitate cortical removal.

Occasionally, it may be convenient to perform a "mixed" technique, which involves alternating the vitrector with the aspiration cannula. If the cortical material is mixed with the vitreous in the presence of viscoelastic, it may be difficult for the surgeon to distinguish the three elements. Therefore, to prevent dangerous vitreous traction, it may be useful to remove some of the residual cortex with the vitrector.

The surgeon should always abide by four basic rules:

- Always exert traction toward the break, not away from it
- Give up removing innocuous cortical fragments that are located peripherally or difficult to remove
- Add viscoelastic frequently to maintain vitreous tamponade and bag formation
- When necessary, alternate use of the irrigation and aspiration system and the vitrector if the cortex is mixed with vitreous

Posterior Capsule Breaks During Phacoemulsification of the Nucleus

If the posterior capsule break occurs when the whole nucleus or fragments of it are still in the capsular bag, the conditions are different from those that have been considered previously as the surgeon cannot be aware of the extent of capsular damage.

Following are some clues that may suggest a break has occurred in the posterior capsule:

- Ineffectiveness of phacoemulsification
- Unexplained shifting of the nucleus and AC deepening
- Sudden and unaccountable increase of pupillary diameter

In this case, viscoelastic material must be injected immediately without extracting the phaco tip from the eye (Figure 21-16). If the vitreous is already trapped by aspiration, it might be pulled out of the eye, causing dangerous traction on the retina. Even when the vitreous is not engaged in the aspiration hole of the phaco tip, sudden extraction of the tip from the eye may leave a void inside the eye that the vitreous fills, widening the capsular break and causing the nucleus to fall into the vitreous cavity.

The situation is slightly different when a phaco system with continual irrigation is present in the eye. In this event, it is mandatory to extract the phaco tip from the eye immediately to avoid widening the capsular break with irrigation.

Most importantly, the surgeon must prevent the nucleus from falling into the vitreous cavity.

Removal of the Nucleus

In the presence of capsular break, there are two possible approaches to removing the nucleus:

- Widening the incision and extracting the nucleus in one piece
- Preserving the same incision size and extracting the nucleus in fragments or continuing phacoemulsification (in selected cases)

Widening the Incision

In the event that the capsular break is very large, the surgeon should widen the small incision to be equal to or slightly larger than the nuclear diameter. The viscoelastic material should be injected in an effort to achieve cleavage between the broken posterior capsule and the overlying nucleus (Figure 21-17). In this situation, it is preferable to use a very pseudoplastic viscoelastic with high molecular weight, transparency, and a soft and permanent spatula effect (ie, Healon® GV). The viscoelastic should be injected in an attempt to lift the nucleus and separate it from the broken posterior capsule. This serves the dual purpose of preparing extraction of the nucleus and counterbalancing vitreous pressure. The surgeon should be careful not to inject excessive amounts of viscoelastic, to avoid widening the capsular break.

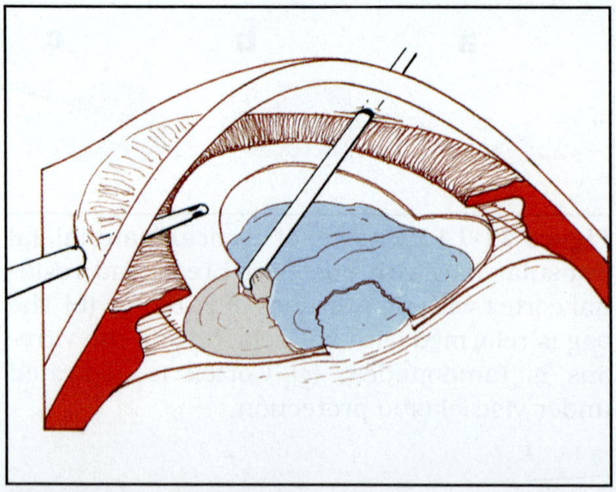

Figure 21-15. Removal of cortical material by Buratto's two-way system. Under viscoelastic protection, the residual cortical material is removed even from the most inaccessible positions.

It may be useful to insert a Sheet's glide between the posterior capsule and the nucleus to keep the vitreous behind the posterior capsule, create a "supporting plane" for surgical maneuvers, and facilitate nucleus extraction.

Extraction of the nucleus is then accomplished, with the protection of Healon® GV, by placing a loop below the nucleus and a Sinskey hook above. This maneuver results in a relatively atraumatic nucleus extraction.

Healon® GV should also be injected adjacent to the corneal endothelium to prevent friction of the nucleus against the endothelium and create a "viscoelastic passage" of the nucleus outside the eye. Healon® GV, when placed over and under the

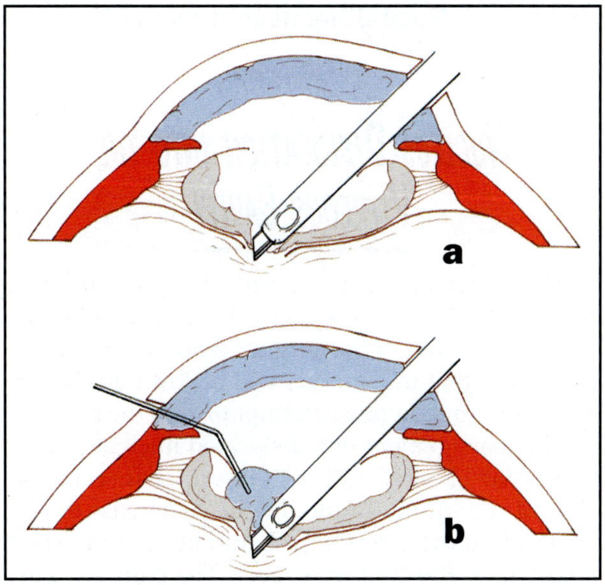

Figure 21-16. (a) Capsule rupture during phacoemulsification: the phaco tip must not be extracted suddenly, as it may drag some vitreous out of the eye. (b) The surgeon should stop and introduce viscoelastic before extracting the phaco tip. This does not apply when using continuous infusion.

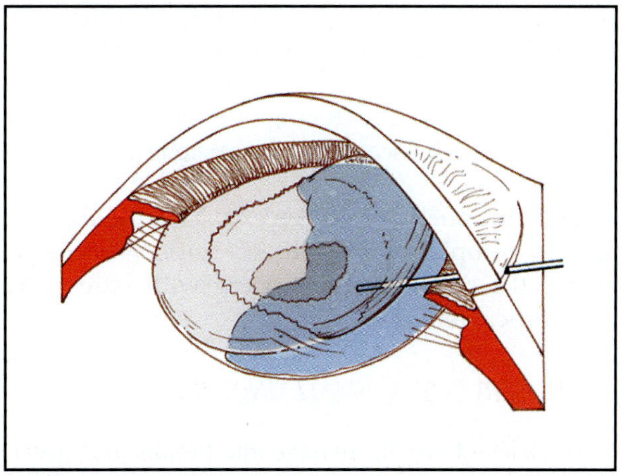

Figure 21-17a. Capsular break and extraction of the nucleus by a loop. The viscoelastic is placed between the nucleus and posterior capsule.

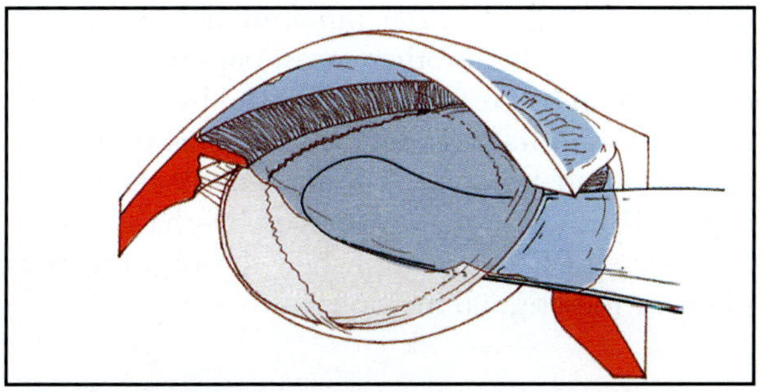

Figure 21-17b. Capsular break and extraction of the nucleus by a loop. After injecting viscoelastic, a Sheet's glide is inserted between the broken posterior capsule and the nucleus.

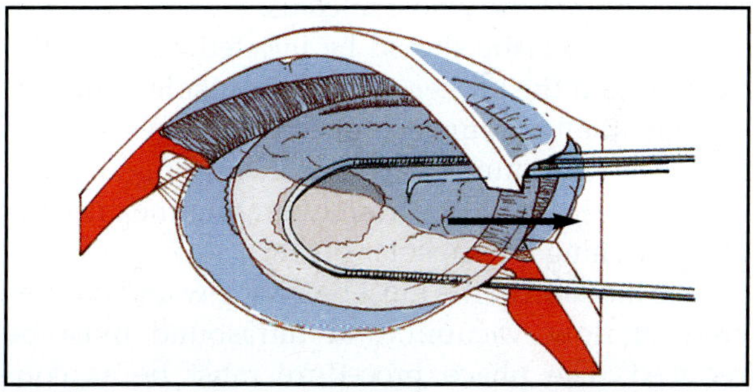

Figure 21-17c. Capsular break and extraction of the nucleus by a loop. The nucleus is extracted using a Sinskey hook and loop.

nucleus, permits the nucleus to slide out of the eye easily. The surgeon should avoid any maneuvers involving pressure and counterpressure, which increase the risk of widening of the capsular break and potential dislocation of the nucleus into the vitreous cavity.

Once the nucleus has been extracted, the surgeon should completely fill the AC with viscoelastic, suture the opening, and proceed with vitrectomy and cortical removal.

PRESERVING A SMALL INCISION

In cases of small, manageable breaks and given the protection of a Sheet's glide, another procedure is possible. Manual nucleosection with the technique suggested by Kansas allows the surgeon to extract the nucleus while keeping the incision and providing greater control of astigmatism. Trisection or bisection is feasible only after "suspending" the nucleus between an overlying and underlying layer of Healon® GV. Nucleus suspension creates space and avoids trauma to the cornea or the underlying capsular bag, which is protected by the Sheet's glide. Occasionally, phacoemulsification may be continued in cases where the capsular break is small, the nucleus not difficult to fragment, or when the break occurs in the presence of nuclear fragments and not the whole nucleus.

The viscoelastic should be injected between the nucleus and the broken posterior capsule to dampen potentially traumatic phaco maneuvers. This also serves to counterbalance vitreous pressure and prevent irrigation flow from hydrating the vitreous and widening the capsular break.

The infusion bottle must be very low and parameters of flow, vacuum, and ultrasound must be reduced. The phaco procedure must be as controlled as possible.

The ideal viscoelastic under these circumstances should be adhesive so that it remains in place even during irrigation flow. Viscoat is the material of choice. Occasionally, it will be necessary to replace the viscoelastic, because the material may be partially removed despite its high adhesiveness.

Michelson suggests continuing phacoemulsification after introducing a Sheet's glide under the nucleus. He asserts that the glide provides capsular support on which the phaco is accomplished, which ensures greater safety by limiting vitreous and preventing accidental dislocation of the nucleus into the vitreous cavity.

NUCLEUS DISLOCATION INTO THE VITREOUS CAVITY

The surgeon must prevent the nucleus from falling into the vitreous cavity. Even when vitreous is prolapsing out of the surgical wound, if there is a possibility that the nucleus will be lost into the vitreous the surgeon must attempt to grab the nucleus.

The management of a dislocated nucleus is controversial. Some authors assert that removal should be done immediately, whereas others believe that the procedure should be accomplished a few days after initial surgery. The patients must be carefully monitored for signs of phacoanaphylactic inflammation such as iritis, vitritis, and secondary glaucoma.

Fastenberg describes 13 cases in which the posterior capsule broke during phacoemulsification with fragments of nucleus (from 20 to 80% of the whole nuclear volume) falling into the vitreous. Two patients with fragments smaller than 25% responded to medical therapy and no vitrectomy was required. When the nuclear fragment is small and results in minimal ocular inflammation, it may be left in the site. In all other cases, pars plana vitrectomy should be performed, followed by retrieval of the nucleus or its fragments by means of perfluorocarbon liquid injection. The nucleus floats on this material and can then be removed by phacoemulsification, which is accomplished through the pars plana or the original incision.

CONVERSION

Conversion refers to transition from phacoemulsification to manual removal of the nucleus due to complications brought about by phacoemulsification. These complications include a very dense nucleus, anesthesia problems, lengthy ultrasound time, poor visibility, and inability to mobilize the nucleus. When these complications occur, the surgeon may elect to convert phacoemulsification into extracapsular technique.

In some cases, when the capsulorhexis extends with consequent subluxation of the nucleus into the AC, it may be possible to complete phacoemulsification in the AC. The corneal endothelium and the underlying structures should be protected by a suitable viscoelastic (ie, Viscoat). The viscoelastic used, in this case, must be able to remain where it has been injected to protect the ocular structures without being aspirated or washed away by the irrigating flow of the phaco. Other viscoelastic materials with high or medium adhesiveness, such as Vitrax and Amvisc Plus, can also be considered.

If endocapsular maneuvers are too difficult, the surgeon may deliberately luxate the nucleus into the AC. The surgeon can depress the nucleus with a spatula opposite the incision while lifting the subincisional pole by impaling it at the equator with the phaco tip. Alternatively, he or she can dissect a cleavage plane (hydric or viscoelastic) by irrigating with BSS or viscoelastic, lifting the nucleus in place and creating a protective cushion between nucleus and the underlying posterior capsule.

Once the nucleus has been lifted, injection of viscoelastic is continued in order to lift it completely, and then, with gentle rotation maneuvers, luxate it outside the capsular bag. In this case, the ideal viscoelastic should have high molecular weight, have high pseudoplasticity, and show soft and permanent spatula effect. In this respect, Healon® and Provisc are preferred.

After the nucleus is in the AC, experienced surgeons can perform a manual nucleofracture technique with suitable viscoelastic protection. Alternatively, the procedure can be converted into extracapsular extraction with a large incision. To convert the incision, the AC must be appropriately reformed with a viscoelastic that shows fair ability to create space and can be partially removed in the event that its presence interferes with luxation of the nucleus in the AC. A sclerocorneal tunnel is easily converted to a wide limbal opening by making two radial cuts on the margin of the tunnel and then continuing with curved corneal scissors along the limbus. A biplanar limbal opening is easiest to widen, whereas the corneal tunnel may create problems on the posterior aspect.

The surgeon could also close the original surgical site with sutures and create a new incision to perform extracapsular extraction. All these procedures should be performed in the presence of a chamber that is well formed by viscoelastic.

After displacing the nucleus into the AC, the surgeon can take advantage of the pressure exerted by the viscoelastic present under and behind the nucleus itself. This facilitates nuclear expression simply by pressing on the posterior lip of the wound. If the surgeon is not familiar with this technique, he or she can extract the nucleus with a loop, protected by the viscoelastic present adjacent to the posterior capsule and the corneal endothelium. Healon® and Provisc, the most pseudoplastic products, are the ideal viscoelastics for this procedure.

Alternatively, the nucleus can be expressed by using pressure and counterpressure applied at 6 and 12 o'clock. Once the nucleus has been expressed, irrigation and aspiration of the cortex can be performed.

CHAPTER TWENTY-TWO

Demanding Cases

The ideal viscoelastic for use in difficult cases has the following features:

- Easy injection
- Optimal preservation of spaces
- Endothelial protection
- Coatability
- Resistance to shifting
- Effective manipulation of tissue
- Chemical and physical stability during use
- Easy removal at the end of surgery

These features are important in difficult cases in which the viscoelastic functions as a surgical instrument. In cases where positive vitreous pressure must be effectively opposed; bleeding must be tamponaded; a damaged tissue must be protected, shifted, or manipulated; or difficult implantation must be accomplished, the surgeon should use the most effective viscoelastic. Demanding cases are situations in which routine maneuvers are difficult to perform owing to the complexity of the case or in which special procedures must be introduced to finish the intervention.

The following is a list of demanding cases:

- Congenital cataract
- Cataract in diabetic patient
- Cataract in eye with glaucoma or previously operated on for glaucoma
- Cataract in uveitis
- Cataract and keratoplasty
- Cataract with retinal detachment
- Cataract with vitrectomy
- Implantation of IOL with scleral fixation
- IOL extraction
- IOL replacement

In all these cases, the surgical complications differ; however, the viscoelastic must always have the ability to preserve space, move tissues, and provide excellent visibility. These features are particular to products with high viscosity at 0 shear rate, strong "soft spatula" effect, and excellent transparency. Therefore, materials with high molecular weight (ie, Healon® GV) and high viscosity at low shear rate are preferable. Adhesive materials (ie, Viscoat), which are less likely to be removed en bloc, are effectively used for protection and maintenance. The ease with which the viscoelastic is removed at the end of surgery is a function of its cohesiveness. In this respect, highly cohesive products, such as Healon®, are preferable. We suggest that the surgeon choose a viscoelastic according to the order of our list, starting with the most suitable viscoelastic and ending with the least suitable material (Table 22-1).

In this section, we analyze how various viscoelastics can be successfully employed in different cases. We refer our readers to Chapters 24 to 35 for information on problems concerning cataracts associated with glaucoma surgery, keratoplasty, retinal detachment, or vitrectomy.

CONGENITAL CATARACT

In recent years, pediatric cataract surgery has undergone major changes owing to the evolution of modern techniques including small incisions and the development of modern IOLs. One main problem is the control of very plastic ocular tissues. The performance of capsulorhexis in the presence of high capsular elasticity is very difficult. In eyes with congenital cataracts, many factors contribute

Table 22-1.
DEMANDING CASES

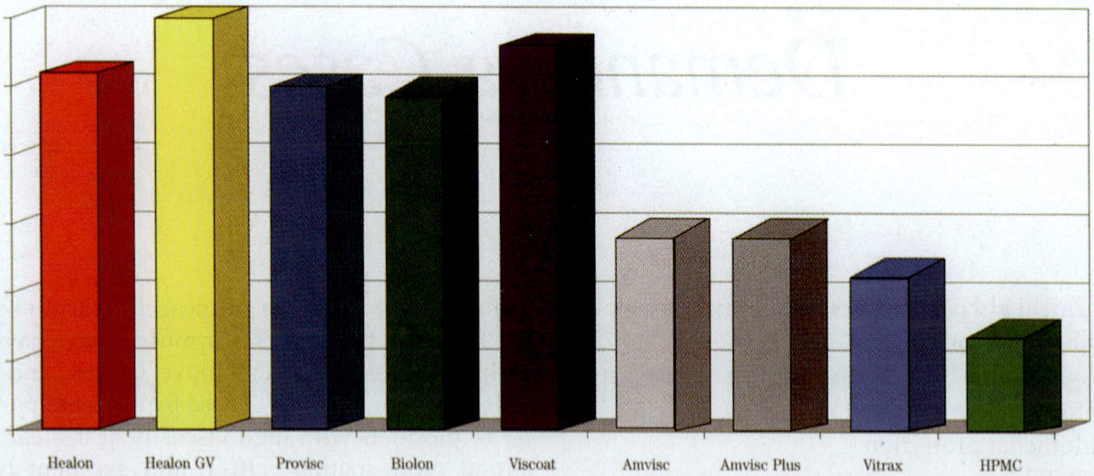

to the difficulty involved in performance of optimal capsulorhexis. A softer sclera and greater vitreous pressure tend to curve the anterior capsule, which enhances the vectorial forces pushing the rhexis outward.

The effective push in the opposite direction provided by the viscoelastic is fundamental to correct completion of the rhexis. The AC should be carefully and completely filled with viscoelastic with high molecular weight (Healon® GV). The rhexis must be started in the central portion and not toward the equator in order to prevent it from escaping control and extending radially. In pediatric implantology, an optimal rhexis ensures correct positioning and centering of the implant inside the bag. Moreover, owing to its high cohesiveness, Healon® GV can be easily removed at the end of surgery, including material behind the IOL. This prevents the occurrence of capsular blockade, particularly in eyes where a small rhexis may often extend significantly over the IOL optic. Maintenance of a deep AC and the absence of contact with iris tissue also guarantee that optimal mydriasis is maintained, as these eyes tend to get miotic during surgery. Healon® GV helps maintain a good intraoperative mydriasis.

When removing a soft cataract, the surgeon can use low vacuum values and the phaco tip set only on aspiration, very low-powered ultrasound pulses, or the irrigation and aspiration tip alone. In cases with polar cataracts placed posteriorly or with membranes, the performance of posterior capsulorhexis followed by partial vitrectomy may be mandatory.

Posterior capsulorhexis can best be performed if the forceps do not grasp the vitreous along with the posterior capsule. Vitreous will not be grasped when Berger's space is visualized and partly filled with viscoelastic. To accomplish this, the capsular bag is stretched with viscoelastic and the surgeon incises the posterior capsule with a thin needle. A small cannula is introduced into this incision in the posterior capsule and viscoelastic (ie, hyaluronic acid) is gently injected between the posterior capsule and hyaloid. The posterior capsule is pushed upward by the viscoelastic, which forms a cushion underneath and thus prevents the vitreous from being grasped along with the posterior capsule when the posterior rhexis is being performed (Figure 22-1).

A viscoelastic with great ability to form space and high transparency, such as Healon® GV, allows the surgeon to complete posterior capsulorhexis with control. Membranous cataracts occasionally oblige the surgeon, after aspiration of all possible lens material, to remove the membranous portion completely (Figure 22-2). It is also possible to isolate

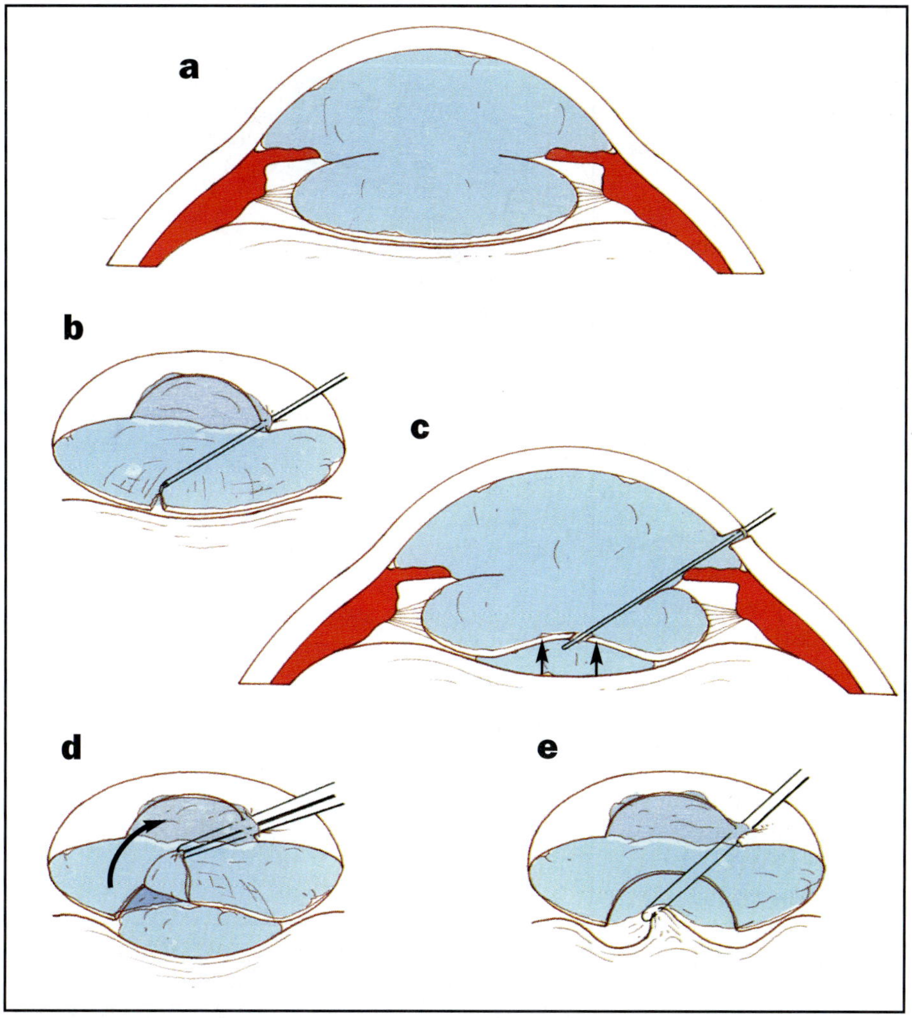

Figure 22-1. Posterior pole or membranous cataract: Posterior capsulorhexis and posterior vitrectomy under viscoelastic control. (a) The viscoelastic keeps the bag stretched and the AC formed. (b) The posterior capsule is incised by a thin needle. (c) In the hole made in the posterior capsule, some viscoelastic material is injected to display Berger's space. (d) Posterior capsulorhexis is completed with forceps, while Berger's space is formed by the viscoelastic, which keeps the vitreous far away as the posterior rhexis is being accomplished. (e) Partial posterior vitrectomy.

the portion to be removed by injecting some viscoelastic around and under it, thus controlling the vitreous.

When cataract extraction is followed by IOL implantation, particularly in the presence of posterior capsulorhexis and partial vitrectomy behind the posterior capsule, it is necessary to keep the bag open and well formed and prevent the vitreous from prolapsing into the bag itself. This ensures a successful and safe implantation in the bag.

The use of a viscoelastic like Healon® GV is fundamental because its high molecular weight and high viscosity at 0 shear rate provides good space maintenance and excellent vitreous control during implantation. Furthermore, it can be easily removed, owing to its high cohesiveness.

CATARACT IN THE DIABETIC PATIENT

In diabetic patients, cataract surgery is influenced by iris alterations (nonproliferative iridopathy, proliferative iridopathy) as well as by diabetic microangiopathy and the fundus (simple diabetic retinopathy, proliferative diabetic retinopathy).

Diabetic iridopathy may lead to the formation of subatrophic areas, bleeding from neovessels, and the formation of iris/lenticular synechiae. This will sometimes make the pupil difficult to dilate and cause bleeding when the surgeon performs maneuvers in an attempt to dilate the pupil (ie, pupillary stretching, sphincterotomies). A product with high molecular weight and high viscosity at low shear rate is preferable when performing maneuvers in the AC to achieve good hemostasis in case of bleeding. The viscoelastic also must be highly cohesive to prevent it from getting mixed with blood, which could form cleavage lines and consequently hinder visibility.

Healon® GV best meets these requirements. The presence of Healon® GV also facilitates preservation of the widest mydriasis possible. A larger pupil can result in a larger capsulorhexis and yield better postoperative visualization of the diabetic retina. Additionally, it ensures that the IOL can be implanted in the position preferred by the surgeon either in the bag or the sulcus. Only good mydriasis and well-formed bag and good visibility of both the anterior and posterior capsule allow the surgeon to position the IOL where he or she deems it appropriate. Implantation in the sulcus facilitates better vision of the retina during postoperative photocoagulation, whereas implantation in the bag prevents contact between the iris and IOL and consequent increased incidence of cystoid macular edema. Preoperative fluorescein iridography allows the surgeon to plan appropriately. However, Healon® GV or products consisting of hyaluronic acid with high molecular weight are preferable.

It may be beneficial to remove the viscoelastic to perform a surgical iridectomy, which we recommend in the presence of extensive diabetic iris vessel pathology. The presence of a heavy viscoelastic in the AC may keep the iris away from the surgical opening, making it difficult for the surgeon to grasp, particularly when a tunnel procedure is being performed. Should abundant bleeding occur after iridectomy, one can inject more viscoelastic into the AC, leaving it there for some minutes for hemostatic action. The presence of a heavy viscoelastic will also be useful in case of cataract extraction followed by vitrectomy for diabetic retinopathy. In this case, the surgeon can perform an anterior phaco, leaving Healon® GV in site to keep the chamber deep, even during scleral indentation and application of lenses used during posterior vitrectomy. The heavy viscoelastic also ensures good mydriasis, which will provide better visibility during pars plana vitrectomy. The employ of lighter viscoelastics may be useless, as they are more likely to come out through the surgical wound in the AC during maneuvers that exert pressure during vitrectomy. After completing the vitrectomy and implanting the IOL, the surgeon will have to remove the viscoelastic material.

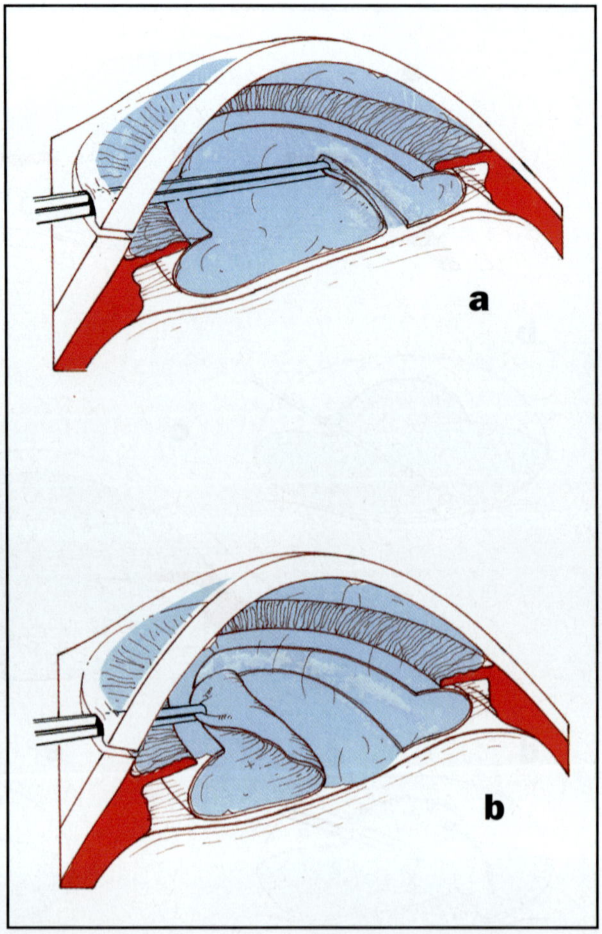

Figure 22-2. Removal of membranous cataract with viscoelastic. (a) Removal is started gently with a forceps. The viscoelastic keeps the AC and the bag formed. (b) The viscoelastic allows complete removal, keeping the vitreous controlled.

The viscoelastic will be useful in case of a silicone oil tamponade because it will prevent the oil from passing into the AC. Once oil filling has been completed, iridectomy performed, and the sclerotomies closed, the viscoelastic in the AC is replaced with BSS. In this situation, the exchange will be easier if a cohesive product, such as Healon® GV, is present.

CATARACT AND UVEITIS

Cataract extraction in eyes with uveitis may cause surgical problems, particularly associated with iris damage possibly caused by uveitis. Cataracts frequently occur in intermediate uveitis (40 to 50%), whereas the incidence is lower in anterior uveitis (25%) and even less in posterior uveitis (5%). The intervention is often considered high risk.

The most frequent morphologic alterations that affect the iris tissue are iris atrophy with consequent atony, sclerosis of the pupil, posterior synechiae, pupillary cyclitic membranes, glaucoma, iris neovascularization, and hypotony. Even when correctly performed, intervention may lead to severe complications involving the globe, which may evolve into phthisis with total loss of visual function.

In such cases, viscoelastic products can help the surgeon accomplish maneuvers as cleanly and atraumatically as possible, with the greatest respect for ocular structures.

Viscoelastics can act as a valuable surgical tool that can control hemostasis during sudden bleedings, enhance poor mydriasis, achieve viscodissection of possible synechiae, ease invasive maneuvers in the AC such as cutting or suturing the iris, and preserve correct anatomic relationships in eyes in which inflammation often causes morphologic alterations.

The main surgical problems can be summarized as follows:

- Difficulty in achieving optimal mydriasis
- Shallow AC
- Presence of posterior synechiae
- Difficulty in the performance of correct capsulotomy
- Difficult extraction of the nucleus
- Difficult removal of lens masses due to poor visibility
- Difficult reconstruction of a correct iris plane before the IOL
- Difficulty in assessing correct IOL positioning in the posterior chamber

OPTIMAL MYDRIASIS

Please refer to the chapter on working techniques in narrow pupils with viscoelastic support.

SHALLOW AC

The application of a viscoelastic with great ability to form space, high viscosity at low shear rate, high molecular weight, and high soft and permanent spatula effect is helpful in the management of a shallow chamber and in enlarging a small pupil. Our first choice in this situation is Healon® GV, followed by Healon®, Viscoat, and Provisc. Products made of HPMC are the last resort because they possess only half of the features needed in these situations.

POSTERIOR SYNECHIAE

The viscoelastic must have the same characteristics that will facilitate removal of synechiae with a spatula and tamponade possible bleeding originating from the synechiae or neovascularization.

CAPSULOTOMY

Our first choice is again Healon® GV because it meets capsulotomy requirements in difficult conditions.

DIFFICULT EXTRACTION OF THE NUCLEUS

In this case, the choice of the most suitable viscoelastic depends on the technique that is employed. The surgeon may prefer not to use a viscoelastic to perform cryoextraction of a severely subluxated brown cataract. Otherwise, when extracapsular technique with expression is performed, it is beneficial to use a viscoelastic product made of hyaluronic acid that is pseudoplastic with molecular weight that is not too high. Our first choices, in this situation, are Provisc or Healon®, whereas products with greater adhesiveness such as Viscoat, Vitrax, and Amvisc Plus should not be considered because they could hinder surgical maneuvers.

Should the surgeon decide to use phaco that is expected to be difficult and invasive, a product that remains longer in the AC and on the corneal endothelium, such as Viscoat, is preferable.

DIFFICULTIES IN THE REMOVAL OF CORTICAL MASSES

A viscoelastic may help keep the pupil round and mydriatic. This makes it easier for the surgeon to perform bimanual maneuvers with a spatula, iris hook, or push/pull, which, depending on the case, the surgeon may use to visualize residual cortex hidden behind the iris. Our recommendation is to use Healon® GV when a soft spatula effect is desired to mobilize tissues and Viscoat when longer permanence of the product in the AC is required.

DIFFICULT RECONSTRUCTION OF A CORRECT IRIS PLANE BEFORE IOL INSERTION

At the end of surgery, the iris tissue may appear damaged and atonic as a result of surgical manipulation. Procedures such as pupillary stretching, removal of pupillary hyalinosis, mechanical mydriasis, and posterior synechiolysis may cause damage to the iris.

When the iris is damaged or atonic, inadvertent capture of iris tissue by the irrigation and aspiration tip or the phaco tip may be rather frequent. At the conclusion of the surgery, the surgeon must reposition the iris plane before the IOL. In the presence of severe damage or remarkable atony, the surgeon may decide to perform pupilloplasty with 10-0 nylon or 10-0 prolene.

Flat iris tissue will be maintained with very pseudoplastic viscoelastics employed after a miotic is used. These materials provide an excellent soft and permanent spatula effect and can be easily removed at the end of surgery. Healon® is the ideal viscoelastic for this procedure.

If an iris suture is difficult to accomplish due to the presence of a shallow chamber, products with higher molecular weight, such as Healon® GV, are best. Iris suturing should be a last resort owing to the frequent presence of fibrin in the pupillary field in the days following the intervention.

The additional trauma caused to the iris while suturing it increases the amount of fibrin produced. The viscoelastic should be removed on completion of the procedure, regardless of which intervention and viscoelastics are used. However, in some cases of atonic iris, the surgeon can leave a small amount of viscoelastic on the iris to keep it in that precise position. In this case, the most suitable products are those that can be easily discharged through the trabecular meshwork and cause less pressure rise when not removed, such as Viscoat or the HPMC products.

DIFFICULTY IN THE ASSESSMENT OF CORRECT IOL POSITIONING

The ideal viscoelastic is one that facilitates better bag filling and easier IOL positioning, even in difficult conditions such as in complicated cataracts in uveitis.

High molecular weight, high viscosity at low shear rate, and high pseudoplasticity favor correct implantation and provide good mydriasis. High cohesiveness enables easy aspiration of the viscoelastic from the posterior chamber even with poor visibility, because the material tends to be removed en bloc. The product that best meets the requirements for performing implantation in difficult conditions is Healon® GV.

EXPLANTATION AND REPLACEMENT OF AN IOL

Explantation and replacement of an IOL have become much safer than in the past. The systematic use of viscoelastic materials is mainly responsible for this advance. Other fundamental factors are improved surgical techniques and better understanding of the conditions that require IOL removal and exchange.

In 1983, Freeman defined the basic elements that the surgeon considers when determining whether to explant or replace an IOL:

- Postoperative recurrent and persistent iritis
- Persistent or recurrent cystoid macular edema
- Dislocated IOL (ie, IOL with iris fixation)
- Subluxation of the IOL
- Drews' intermittent contact syndrome
- Erosion of supporting tissues
- Damage to the IOL
- Chronic pain
- Uncontrolled pain
- Toxic syndrome
- Incorrect IOL power

Even when protected by a suitable viscoelastic, IOL explantation is always far more traumatic and invasive than implantation.

The IOL is often tenaciously attached to the angle chamber structures, iris, ciliary bodies, or vitreous, which may make its removal very invasive.

After releasing the IOL from possible tissue adherence, under the protection of a viscoelastic, explantation is accomplished by slipping off the IOL or performing some rotation maneuvers, following the curve of the haptics and never in the opposite direction.

The requirements of a viscoelastic material for IOL removal are:

- Good transparency
- High molecular weight
- High viscosity at low shear rate
- High pseudoplasticity
- Strong soft and permanent spatula effect
- Easy removability

The ideal viscoelastic follows the same order that was indicated for demanding cases described previously; Healon® GV and Healon® on the top on the one hand, and Viscoat on the other, with products such as those made of HPMC considered last.

The surgeon should always have wide spaces available where explant or filling maneuvers can be performed safely (high ability to form space), consistent good visibility of the IOL and the position of tissues (good transparency, absence of air or bubbles), and control of tissue pushes and bleeding with the ability to shift and guide the IOL owing to the viscoelastic material (good soft and permanent spatula effect). In addition, the viscoelastic should protect the corneal endothelium and other ocular structures from friction against the IOL (adhesiveness and endothelial protection) and be easy to remove at the end of surgery (high cohesiveness).

Healon® GV seems to be the viscoelastic that best meets such requirements. Because Healon® is slightly less adhesive than Viscoat, it is better able to remain in place during maneuvers, slip the IOL out of the eye, and implant the new lens. Healon® has better transparency, pseudoplasticity, ability to form space, soft and permanent spatula effect, and removability at the end of surgery.

When discussing the various viscoelastics and their role in IOL exchange, a distinction should be made among the various locations of the IOL to be removed:

- IOL in the AC with angle support
- IOL in the AC with iris fixation
- IOL positioned in the sulcus
- IOL positioned in the capsular bag
- IOL luxated in the vitreous

IOL in the AC With Angle Support or Iris Fixation

The severity of surgical difficulties is related to the tenacity of adhesions the IOL may have created with ocular structures, which mostly depends on the duration that the implant has been in the eye. The incision should be oriented in the direction of the longer axis of the IOL to avoid rotation maneuvers, which produce damage to iris structures and dangerous bleeding. If the surgery is performed a few days after the intervention of implantation, the surgeon may consider using the same surgical wound.

First, the surgeon should inject a viscoelastic with the necessary features between the IOL and cornea to create a safety space and between the IOL and iris to lift the IOL from the iris. This also ensures that the loops or the optic plate of the IOL do not get entangled in the pupillary border, iris folds, or previous surgical iridectomies.

The IOL can be lifted by injecting the viscoelastic through a paracentesis 90° from the opening through which the surgeon intends to remove the IOL. In the space created by the viscoelastic, it is possible to insert a small spatula, which is used in bimanual technique to shift and lead the IOL in order to grasp it with the forceps through the main incision. Therefore, the surgeon should try to grasp the proximal loop of the IOL support and make it come out through the main hole.

During this procedure some viscoelastic may leak out and the surgeon may need to add more material. At this point, the surgeon should assess whether it is possible to extract the IOL gently or whether it would be better to insert a Sheet's glide under viscoelastic protection on which the IOL may slide during explantation. This maneuver may be helpful in the presence of posterior vitreous pressure or irregular iris surface.

In the beginning, traction must be gentle, in order to check for the presence of tissue adhesions to the distal loop of the IOL and to avoid breakage of one of the loops, which would cause trauma to ocular structures (Figure 22-3). Once the IOL has been extracted, the surgeon must judge whether new implantation is feasible in that moment or must be delayed. Should vitreous be present in the AC, the surgeon should remove it according to the indications suggested in the chapter concerning capsular breaks and anterior vitrectomy.

If an iridectomy is not already present, it may be useful to perform one. If the surgeon deems new implantation to be possible, the procedure is performed following the schemes formerly described for various implant techniques.

IOLs with large supporting surfaces may require removal of the loops when adhesions are too tough to be removed with the viscoelastic or the spatula and repeated tractions. In this case, excision of the loop must be accomplished in the presence of a large amount of viscoelastic, as a space must be provided for contemporaneous management of scissors and IOL and to avoid dangerous contact between the cornea and iris.

It has been suggested that the YAG or Argon laser be used to cut pigmented loops, but it is often difficult for the surgeon, even after accurate gonioscopy, to define the actual toughness of adhesions preoperatively. Therefore, complete removal of the IOL must always be attempted.

A wide space containing a highly pseudoplastic and space forming viscoelastic, such as Healon® GV, must be created to remove lenses with iris fixation such as Medallion or Iris–Claw lenses, as these rarely can be removed by simple traction or one-handed maneuvers. Moreover, the steel structures that sometimes fix these lenses to the iris require the use of stronger scissors and the introduction of bulkier instruments in the AC. In this situation the viscoelastic must maintain a large space in the AC.

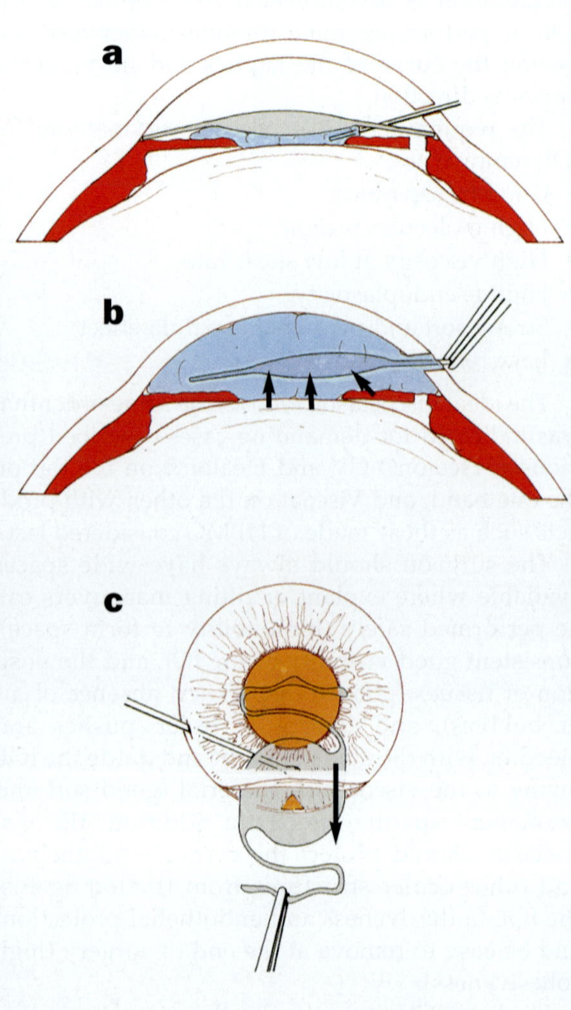

Figure 22-3. Explantation of an AC IOL with angle support. (a) The viscoelastic is injected under the IOL to control the vitreous and separate the IOL from the iris. (b) Lifting the IOL with viscoelastic or a spatula, the proximal loop of the IOL is extracted through the main incision. The viscoelastic injected over the IOL keeps the AC formed and protects the corneal endothelium. (c) The IOL is gently extracted with gentle bimanual technique. It is also possible to insert a Sheet's glide under the IOL to prevent the distal loop from hooking up the iris.

IOLs Placed in the Iridociliary Sulcus

The loops of IOLs positioned in the sulcus usually should be cut to permit IOL explantation. Adhesions are almost always very tough and after some time the loops penetrate in the uveal tissue and cannot be removed without severe bleeding.

After forming a stable space in the AC with the viscoelastic, the surgeon should try to inject the material under the IOL to separate it from the posterior capsule. After locating the loop closer to the surgical wound, the surgeon can try to rotate the IOL, but if resistance is great, it is better to dissect the loops and cut them as far as possible from the optical plate so that the loop portion left inside the eye is as small as possible. When the optic plate of the IOL is free from loops, the surgeon gently slips it off under viscoelastic protection in front of and behind the IOL (Figure 22-4).

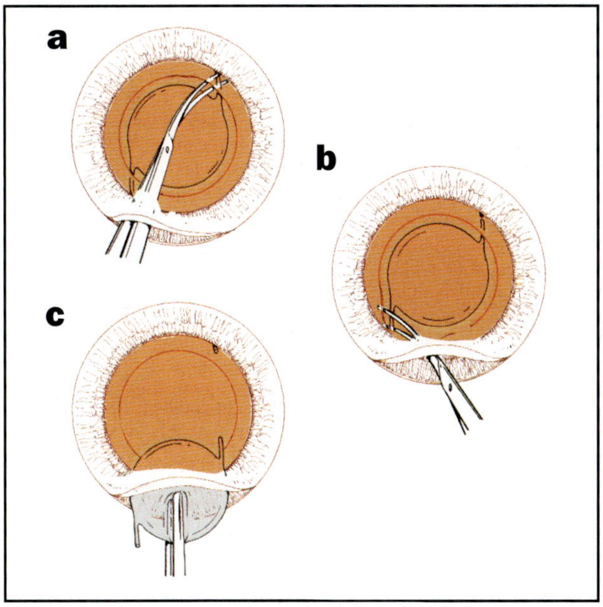

Figure 22-4. An IOL placed in the ciliary sulcus after dissection of support loops. (a) After injecting enough viscoelastic in front of the IOL to keep the AC formed and behind the IOL to separate it from the posterior capsule, the distal loop is cut with scissors. (b) Always under viscoelastic protection, the proximal loop is also excised. (c) The surgeon grasps the optical plate of the IOL with forceps and slips it out gently.

IOLs Positioned in the Capsular Bag

The same maneuver described for sulcus IOLs can be employed to explant IOLs positioned in the capsular bag. In this case, it is mandatory that the surgeon check the adhesion between IOL and bag. If these adhere completely and long-standing saccular fibrosis is present, it is not possible to separate the IOL from the bag.

For instance, when faced with an Anis' or a Galand disk lens, the surgeon should consider the IOL–bag complex as a whole and the IOL should be removed with the capsular bag. This can be accomplished using forceps and cryoextractor. When the IOL and capsular bag are removed together, the use of a viscoelastic is controversial as there might be confusion between the viscoelastic and vitreous, and the surgeon might accidentally create traction on the vitreous while removing the IOL–bag complex. Sometimes it is possible to detach the capsule little by little, thus saving some posterior capsular support for the new IOL.

When one-piece IOLs with smaller dimensions (ie, 5-mm optics), soft lenses that adhere less to the bag (ie, PoliHema implants), or recently implanted IOLs are removed, their extraction from the capsular bag will be eased by the protection of a viscoelastic.

The best material is Healon® GV, which, owing to its physical and chemical features, creates space, holds and lifts the IOL, keeps the bag formed, protects the corneal endothelium, and is easily removed from the bag at the end of surgery. In cases of recent corneal incisions, the surgeon can use the same opening for explantation. When one-piece IOLs are being removed, the surgeon can inject viscoelastic in the AC to form it and keep it formed during the following maneuvers. A cannula is then passed between the margin of capsulorhexis and IOL, and viscoelastic is injected behind the IOL to stretch the bag and lift and separate the IOL from the bag. With a spatula or the same cannula, the proximal loop of the IOL is found and brought above the iris, extracting it from the bag. Forceps are then used to grasp the loop, and with a clockwise rotation the IOL is extracted into the AC (Figure 22-5).

The capsulorhexis will always be strong enough to permit outward passage of the IOL. If the IOL is small (ie, a 6.0-mm optic or smaller), it has usually been through a small incision. In these situations it is possible to section the IOL in the AC with scissors, thus avoiding the need to enlarge the incision. The fragments obtained can then be extracted one by one through the small incision. To accomplish this maneuver, the requirements of the viscoelastic are similar to those discussed previously for manual nucleosection (ie, the Kansas' technique).

Viscoelastics make procedures such as cutting an IOL in the AC feasible, in contrast to air or BSS. After taking the soft IOL outside the capsular bag with the maneuvers described for one-piece IOLs, the lens is suspended by the viscoelastic between the underlying iris plane and the overlying cornea. Healon® GV's properties make it the recommended material for this procedure.

The fundamental properties are the ability to keep space, high pseudoplasticity that permits cutting of the IOL, corneal endothelial protection, and soft and permanent spatula effect that facilitates placement of the IOL fragments in the most convenient position to be grasped and extracted from the AC.

As previously described, the IOL is dissected after being extracted from the bag and positioned in the iris plane. If the AC is deep enough, the whole optic plane of the IOL can be dissected in just one maneuver, proceeding gradually with scissors. Otherwise, the surgeon can cut the lens from the optic margin to its center, then rotate it gently 180° under viscoelastic protection, taking care to avoid contact between the IOL and the cornea, iris, and angle structures. The opposite portion of the IOL is then cut from the optic margin to the center, thus joining the other half cut.

After the AC is refilled to replace viscoelastic that may have leaked out during the cutting of the IOL, the surgeon grasps both halves of the IOL with forceps and gently slips them out of the incision. The highest viscoelastic protection is always needed in order to avoid contact between the irregular cut surfaces of the IOL and the corneal endothelium or iris, and to prevent the ends of the haptic loops from entangling with ocular tissues (Figure 22-6).

After the bag and the AC are reformed with viscoelastic, it is usually possible to implant a new soft foldable IOL through the same small incision, which has not been enlarged. The surgery is concluded by complete removal of the viscoelastic material.

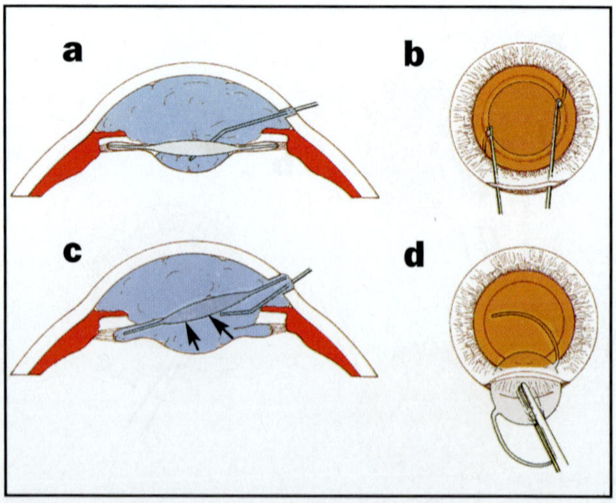

Figure 22-5. Explantation of PMMA IOL from the capsular bag. (a) Viscoelastic is injected under the IOL to separate it from the bag and lift it over the lens to keep the AC formed and protect the corneal endothelium. (b) The surgeon then lifts the proximal portion of the IOL and brings the first loop out of the capsular bag. (c, d) While protecting the cornea from friction and contact with the viscoelastic on the IOL, the surgeon removes the implant.

IOLs Dislocated into the Vitreous Cavity

The surgeon should not attempt to retrieve an IOL that has dislocated, completely or partially, into the vitreous cavity. Although some surgeons advocate a transpupillary approach, we believe that dangerous vitreal traction is exerted while attempting to retrieve the IOL in this manner. A pars plana vitrectomy allows better control by using the vitrector to release adhesions of the IOL with the vitreous vitrector. Once the IOL has been freed of vitreal adhesions and the surgeon is certain that no vitreous traction may cause retinal detachment, he or she can then retrieve and explant the artificial lens.

In some cases, a partial vitrectomy is enough, provided that a portion of the IOL still appears in the capsular bag and taking into account that excessive posterior vitrectomy may cause the IOL to dislocate further toward the posterior pole. Should the IOL be completely dislocated into the vitreous, posterior vitrectomy must be complete to retrieve the lens with perfluorocarbon liquids, using the technique previously described to retrieve the nucleus or its fragments dislocated into the vitreous.

Once the IOL has been removed, regardless whether an AC lens or a lens with fixation in the sulcus or in the bag, the surgeon should consider the placement of another IOL. This can be implanted in the AC, in the sulcus or in the bag, within the capsulorhexis or with scleral fixation, depending on the circumstances.

When an IOL is replaced, the surgeon can also plan to upgrade the IOL, and replace an older concept IOL with a modern lens. For instance, when an

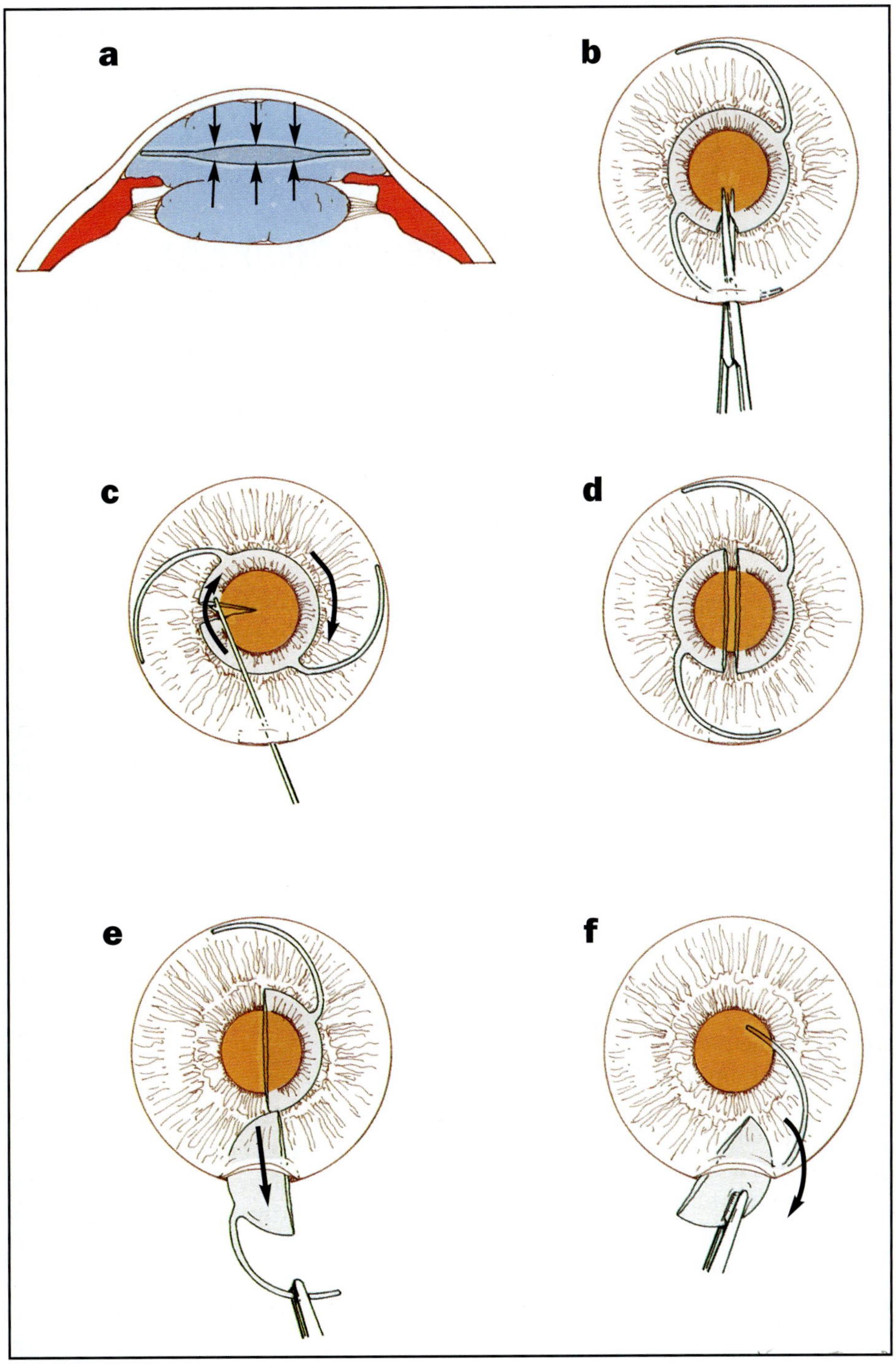

Figure 22-6. Explantation of soft IOL through a small opening by dissecting it in two. (a) Under the protection of a viscoelastic, the soft IOL is led out of the capsular bag and positioned in the AC. The IOL appears "suspended" in the viscoelastic, which pushes it upward, far from the iris plane, and downward, far from the cornea. (b) The proximal portion of the IOL is dissected with scissors, up to the center of the optic plate. (c) Under constant protection of a viscoelastic, the IOL is turned 180°. (d) The part opposite to that already cut is dissected, thus joining it. (e) Under viscoelastic protection the first dissected half of the IOL is slipped out through the tunnel. (f) The other half of the IOL is removed with a forceps.

iris fixated IOL is removed the surgeon should try to implant a posterior chamber IOL. Whenever it is possible, the surgeon must try to implant the IOL behind the iris. In the presence of early signs of corneal decompensation, the surgeon should not hesitate to explant an AC IOL. Also, when intermittent contact syndrome is present with cystoid macular edema, despite a quiet anterior segment and a transparent cornea, explantation must be considered to prevent any permanent macular damage.

TRAUMATIC CATARACT

The treatment of a traumatic cataract often requires particular effort on the part of the surgeon, as he or she must use his or her knowledge of corneal, lens, and vitreal surgery. It often occurs that in the same intervention the "double personality" of anterior and posterior segment surgery must coexist. Problems are varied and often due to difficult visualization of tissues blocked by tissue opacities, scars, blood, foreign bodies, lenticular masses, or vitreous. Furthermore, anatomic relationships are often unclear or upset.

In their report on 419 eyes with severe trauma, Stegman and Miller report that 17% of all interventions failed. The failure rate would have been much higher had viscoelastic solutions not been available.

The basic needs of a surgeon who approaches a traumatic cataract are the following:

- Good visibility of any surgical maneuver
- Protection of the corneal endothelium and the other ocular structures
- Ability to shift membranes, damaged tissues, intraocular foreign bodies, and blood clots
- Application of a force that permits formation and maintenance of space, as well as to block tissue in the desired position and counterbalance positive vitreous pressure
- Ability to perform all the intraocular maneuvers required without being hindered by the viscoelastic material
- Use of a product that is not toxic to the eye and can be completely or partially left inside the eye at the end of surgery
- Easy removability of the product in case the surgeon decides to clear it at the end of surgery
- Ability to distinguish the viscoelastic from the vitreous

Viscoelastic materials meet these requirements in the following ways.

GOOD VISIBILITY EQUALS TRANSPARENCY OF THE VISCOELASTIC

During the performance of traumatic cataract surgery, corneal damage may render it difficult to visualize lenticular structures. In fact, blood, fibrin, and vitreous may be present in the AC, and the viscoelastic must act to shift, control, and immobilize them in the most convenient way for the surgeon. Therefore, it is evident that a poorly transparent product (ie, Viscoat) may hinder visibility. Moreover, adhesive products such as Vitrax and Viscoat are likely to trap air bubbles, further worsening visibility. Some cleavage lines between BSS and these adhesive viscoelastics may form, which also limits visibility.

The viscoelastic material must support and not present a further obstacle to surgery. Owing to their decreased transparency, the products mentioned (Viscoat, Vitrax) are not preferred in cases where surgical visualization is already impaired for other reasons.

ENDOTHELIAL PROTECTION EQUALS ADHESIVENESS

As has been discussed, it is questionable whether the best endothelial protection is provided by mechanical stratification of viscoelastic on the tissue (which is ensured by adhesive products such as Viscoat) or the chemical protection of Healon® GV and Healon® (binding sites, free radicals). Depending on specific surgical needs and the maneuvers to be accomplished, a product with poorer ability to form space but greater adhesiveness, such as Viscoat, is preferred. Under other circumstances, a heavier and more pseudoplastic product such as Healon® GV may be desired.

ABILITY TO SHIFT TISSUES THROUGH THE USE OF A SOFT SPATULA

A fair soft spatula effect is needed to tamponade AC hemorrhage, to mobilize damaged iris tissue, to shift and visualize intraocular foreign bodies, and to lyse anterior and posterior synechiae. Products with high molecular weight, high viscosity at 0 shear rate, and high pseudoplasticity are preferred. Healon® GV, Healon®, and Provisc are ideal in these situations, whereas poorly pseudoplastic, adhesive products with low molecular weight are to be considered a second choice. Consequently, HPMC, Viscoat, and Vitrax are not preferred.

ABILITY TO FORM SPACE, BLOCK TISSUES, AND COUNTERBALANCE PUSHES EQUALS A PERMANENT SPATULA

Very high molecular weight and high viscosity at zero shear rate materials are of fundamental importance for this purpose. The ability to form space is enhanced by these features. The best product for this function is undoubtedly Healon® GV. In fact, it is the product that can best block tissues, "freezing" them in the position desired by the surgeon and exerting maximal control on vitreous pressure.

Healon® GV's high cohesiveness, which in some circumstances makes it come out of the eye like a bolus, may sometimes be disadvantageous. To avoid this inconvenience, it is preferable to use a less cohesive product such as Viscoat, even though it has a much lower molecular weight and less viscosity at 0 shear rate.

POSSIBILITY TO PERFORM ALL SURGICAL MANEUVERS EASILY EQUALS HIGH PSEUDOPLASTICITY

Healon® GV provides the best pseudoplasticity among all the viscoelastics currently available. It is undoubtedly the material that best allows the surgeon to perform all maneuvers without obstacles and in guaranteed wide spaces. As has been stated, it sometimes leaves the eye en bloc, and therefore must be replaced by a material that has less or no pseudoplasticity and remains in the place where it has been positioned.

NO TOXIC EFFECT IF THE PRODUCT IS LEFT INSIDE THE EYE EQUALS HIGH BIOCOMPATIBILITY

Products with high biocompatibility are preferred because they are in direct contact with damaged ocular tissues and may be left inside the eye. Surgeons have had experience using sodium hyaluronate in ocular trauma surgery. Among sodium hyaluronate materials there are differences with respect to production. For example, products derived from bacterial fermentation may be more allergenic. In addition, there are significant differences between manufacturers regarding quality control.

EASY REMOVABILITY EQUALS HIGH COHESIVENESS

Highly cohesive products such as Healon®, Healon® GV, and Provisc are more easily removed at the end of surgery. Nevertheless, it may be useful occasionally for the surgeon to leave a small amount of product inside the eye to tamponade tissues or bleeding in the hours following surgery. In that case, it is better to choose more adhesive materials such as Viscoat, which can be easily filtered by the trabecular meshwork and cause lower postoperative hypertension.

EASY DETECTION OF THE VISCOELASTIC EQUALS A DYED PRODUCT

After years of viscosurgery techniques, surgeons are now able to see and distinguish the viscoelastic after injecting the material inside the eye. Nevertheless, there may be circumstances where the viscoelastic cannot be easily distinguished from the vitreous, as in situations when corneal transparency is diminished or when blood and iris pigments are present inside the eye. The only product available that obviates the problem is Healon® Yellow*. Owing to its yellow color, it can be easily distinguished from the vitreous. Its usefulness, effectiveness, and tolerability are the same as those of Healon®.

**Healon® Yellow is no longer being mannufactured.*

In cases of traumatic cataracts, viscoelastic products are ranked according to their suitability in the following order:

- Healon® GV
- Viscoat
- Healon®
- Provisc
- Amvisc
- Amvisc Plus
- Vitrax
- HPMC

Healon® GV is most preferable owing to its high molecular weight, high pseudoplasticity, and viscosity at 0 shear rate. This enables it to form space, have permanent and soft spatula effect, and provide excellent transparency and high biocompatibility. In some cases, high internal cohesion may be a handicap; Viscoat is preferred in these situations. Viscoat is less desirable than Healon® GV for the features described, but provides a much higher adhesive capacity, which allows it to remain longer where it has been placed without coming out of the eye like a bolus.

All the products with less ideal features than those of the two leaders of cohesive and adhesive solutions (ie, Healon® GV and Viscoat) are to be considered a second choice, although in many circumstances they can be effective.

PATHOGENESIS OF MECHANICAL TRAUMAS

These can be a consequence of contusions or perforating wounds with or without intraocular foreign body.

CONTUSIONS

Contusions may be produced directly on the globe or caused indirectly by the adjacent bony structures of the orbit. Furthermore, the trauma may cause a concussion mechanism, following the acceleration and deceleration of the foreign body during the traumatic event.

The result may be trauma to the cornea, especially involving Descemet's membrane, the iris (with dialysis, breaks, bleeding, synechiae), the chamber angle (with its consequent recession and hyphema), the ciliary body (with ciliary shock and hypotony), the lens (with damage to the zonular system and consequent luxation or subluxation of the lens), the vitreous (with vitreous hemorrhage, avulsion of the base, prolapse between iris and lens), or the retina (with breaks, dialysis, detachment). In all these cases the role played by viscoelastics is fundamental as they help the surgeon restore the correct anatomy of the eye, which is often altered by the lesion. The viscoelastic maintains spaces formed and enables the surgeon to continue the procedure.

PERFORATING WOUNDS

In this case, damage is caused directly by the object, and the severity depends on the dimensions of the foreign body along with its kinetic energy. Thus, a very small foreign body may have great kinetic energy and penetrate to the posterior portion of the globe after passing through cornea, iris, and lens. In contrast, a larger foreign body traveling more slowly may stop in the anterior segment. Sometimes, there is a combination of contusive and perforating damage.

The most frequent damage that occurs to the lens consists of damage to the zonules, which may be perforated by the foreign body, with consequent dissection of zonular fibers and subluxation of the lens.

The anterior capsule may be broken and the object may come to rest inside the lens itself or may pass through the lens completely, breaking the posterior capsule and resulting in leakage of lenticular material into the vitreous.

Contusive or perforating alterations of the lens capsule can cause damage to the "pump and leak" action that regulates the fluid balance inside the lens. Consequently, the lens retains water, proteins are agglutinated, and lens fibers are separated. All these things lead to decreased transparency and cataract development. The extent of cataract formation is mostly related to the severity of the damage caused to capsule and lens epithelium. Damage can be localized, resulting only in a small lenticular opacity, or there can be total opacification, often along with the release of lens material inside the eye, with inflammation and increased IOP.

Hypertension may be also caused by luxation of the lens in the AC or by the presence of blood.

A small capsular break usually can be easily controlled without widening it by using appropriate surgical techniques and tamponading the vitreous with an adhesive viscoelastic such as Viscoat, to prevent the vitreous from penetrating the break and widening it. Should the lens material dislocate into the vitreous, the surgery should be converted into a pars plana vitrectomy. If the vitreous enters the bag through the posterior opening, the surgeon should tamponade it with Viscoat and perform a dry vitrectomy, as described in the chapter on capsular breaks.

When traumatic cataract occurs in an older patient, a formed nucleus that cannot be removed with aspiration only will be present. Phacoemulsification with reduced parameters (low bottle, low flow rate, low aspiration) should be performed to make the procedure more controlled, even in the presence of posterior capsular damage that was not readily apparent at the beginning of surgery. Viscoelastic should be repeatedly injected whenever the integrity of the capsular bag is in question. A poorly cohesive product (Viscoat) is preferred so it can remain in place longer without being removed by the irrigation flow. A pseudoplastic product like Healon® or Provisc is employed if the surgeon intends to perform viscoexpression with a larger and extracapsular technique. During nuclear expression the pressure and counterpressure technique must be avoided so that no stress is applied to weak zonules and the nucleus is not dislocated into the vitreous cavity as a result. Viscoexpression offers the advantage that the viscoelastic exerts equal pressure upward on the nucleus and downward on the vitreous. This tamponades the vitreous well and does not permit vitreal prolapse into the capsular bag and widening of the posterior break.

A posterior capsular break should be circularized with more regular margins by means of posterior capsulorhexis. Viscoat is the ideal viscoelastic for this maneuver. A small amount must first be injected in the capsular hole, to better visualize Berger's space, and then posterior rhexis is accomplished using forceps. Once the lens material is cleared, the surgeon can attempt IOL implantation if possible. The ideal position is in the capsular bag. If the bag is damaged, the surgeon may place the IOL on the anterior capsule (in the ciliary sulcus), in the AC, or with scleral fixation. The location of IOL placement depends on a number of factors, including corneal endothelial cell count, the conditions of the iris, and the possible presence of retinal problems.

If the cataract appears subluxated and the surgeon decides to perform phacoemulsification, rotation of the nucleus in the capsular bag must not be performed, to avoid exerting dangerous traction on the zonules. Phacofragmentation chop techniques are preferred, as they exert less stress on the zonular apparatus.

If the cataract is dislocated into the AC, cryoextraction can be performed. Alternatively, viscoelastic can be injected under the nucleus, toward the iris, surrounding the nucleus to protect the corneal endothelium from contacts with the nucleus. Then the AC is opened proportionally to the size of the nucleus, and, applying gentle pressure on the posterior lip of the surgical wound, the viscoelastic is employed to accomplish viscoexpression of the nucleus from the AC. In this situation a pseudoplastic, high molecular weight viscoelastic should be used; Provisc and Healon® are most suitable. Once the nucleus has been expressed out of the AC, more viscoelastic is injected to reform the chamber and assess the conditions and position of iris, pupil, and vitreous. If vitreous prolapses into the AC, it must be tamponaded with Viscoat, and anterior vitrectomy is performed as previously described in the chapter on capsular breaks.

TRAUMATIC CATARACT ASSOCIATED WITH DAMAGE TO OTHER OCULAR STRUCTURES

Traumatic cataract may be associated with damage involving the anterior segment, the posterior segment, or a combination of both.

DAMAGE TO THE ANTERIOR SEGMENT

Cornea, sclera, iris, and chamber angle may be damaged. In particular, the iris, which is very vascular, may be damaged and often results in severe bleeding. When iris damage is not associated with perforating wounds that require surgery, the hyphema can be treated for some days with antifibrinolytic medication along with antihypertensive drugs to control IOP rise and mydriatics to prevent the formation of posterior synechiae. An enzymatic activator of thrombolysis may also be injected in the AC, although the efficacy of this procedure is controversial.

When blood has been reabsorbed, cataract surgery can be performed. If the blood persists, however, surgery should be performed earlier. Viscoelastic is injected through a limbal incision or through the traumatic corneal wound, if possible. The viscoelastic forms the AC homogeneously, shifts blood to aid in visualization of obscured structures, and restores tone to the globe. This filling procedure must be performed cautiously if a subluxated cataract is present, as excessive pressure may cause lens dislocation into the vitreous cavity. The ideal viscoelastic for this phase must create space, have pseudoplasticity, and have good soft spatula effect. Furthermore, high internal cohesiveness eases removal in case an excessive amount is injected. Healon® and Provisc are preferred in this situation. The viscoelastic, acting as a very soft spatula, allows the surgeon to explore the iris, previously obscured by blood. The advantage of using the viscoelastic in this early phase is twofold. Immediate removal of blood and clots with irrigation and vitrector or with irrigation and aspiration may cause rebleeding. This does not occur when a viscoelastic is employed to tamponade the bleeding. Furthermore, it is possible to mobilize tissues without touching them, which results in gentler handling of traumatized tissue. Restoring tone of a hypotonic globe also permits better realignment of the margins of the corneal or corneoscleral wounds to be sutured, thus ensuring better, more anatomic wound closure.

Once the wound is sutured, viscoelastic can be used as an alternative to BSS to assess wound closure, submitting the wound to the pressure of the viscoelastic. If iris tissue prolapses through the corneal wound, the surgeon may try to reposition the tissue using viscoelastic. If the tissue is not excessively atonic, it may remain in its anatomic position after repositioning. In recent years, viscosurgery has allowed repositioning of iris tissue which in the previscosurgery era would have been excised, as the surgeon would not have succeeded in repositioning the tissue using only air or BSS.

It is best to avoid repositioning the iris with viscoelastic through the same perforating wound through which iris protrudes; in fact, this may cause bleeding of the iris and further damage. Moreover, the repeated passage of instruments through wounded tissue may further damage the wound margins, and increase scarring. The viscoelastic therefore should be injected through a limbal incision.

To prepare for subsequent cataract extraction, mydriatics can be placed inside the AC to facilitate the release of iris tissue protruding through the central corneal wound. Miotics should not be used for this purpose as the miosis would most likely hinder the following phases of cataract extraction. Once the iris is repositioned and the viscoelastic is reinjected, the surgeon can proceed to cataract removal. If corneal damage is irreparably severe and visibility precludes performing cataract extraction, immediate keratoplasty should be considered.

If iris damage is significant and the surgeon fears that AC bleeding may begin again postoperatively, it is possible to leave some viscoelastic inside the eye, to create hemostasis by direct pressure of the viscoelastic on the bleeding area. Easily cleared viscoelastics (ie, Viscoat) are preferred in this situation.

On occasion the surgeon may complete surgery with viscoelastic in the AC, mixed with blood. This will be aspirated and replaced with clean viscoelastic. If after removing blood it is clear that vitreous, lenticular material, or foreign bodies remain in the AC, the surgeon should remove them.

Vitreous

Anterior vitrectomy has been discussed at length previously. This should be performed with the dry technique, with frequent injection of adhesive viscoelastic (ie, Viscoat) in the AC. Alternatively, it can be performed with gentle infusion, separate from the vitrector, so that there is no irrigation near the vitrector port. Irrigation near the vitrector port hydrates the vitreous and causes more vitreous leakage. Vitrectomy must be continued until the surface of the cataractous lens is free of vitreous, so that subsequent maneuvers on the lens do not cause vitreal traction.

It may be difficult to isolate these different maneuvers for different materials because blood, vitreous, and lens material often are mixed together and tissue damage is varied. Repeated injection of viscoelastic in the AC will help define the anatomic relationships of the tissues altered by trauma.

Lenticular Material

If the lens consists of soft cortical material, it can be removed by the vitrector, along with the vitreous. When nuclear fragments are present, they are first isolated from the surrounding the vitrector and then grasped by a toothed forceps under viscoelastic protection and removed from the eye. Nuclear fragments can also be removed using a suitable viscoelastic product with a fair soft spatula effect (ie, Healon®). It is also possible to apply a mixed technique, according to the situation. The surgeon can remove material separate from the vitreous with a dry technique with the vitrector only aspirating or through an aspiration cannula. Materials closer to or mixed with vitreous areas are removed with the vitrector (set on cut and aspiration) with the support of viscoelastic, constantly replaced or with a separate infusion system.

Healon® Yellow may be used, as it easily distinguishes the viscoelastic from the vitreous, owing to its yellow color.

During the vitrectomy, the viscoelastic also must keep the lens structure far from the vitrector tip to avoid capsular damage that could jeopardize cataract removal.

Complete vitrectomy should be performed, as persistent vitreous strands may cause cystoid macular edema in the postoperative period.

Foreign Bodies

Perforating trauma is often associated with the presence of intraocular foreign bodies. If these are in the AC, they should be removed immediately. If they are in the posterior segment of the eye, however, extraction is generally performed later, after the primary wound heals.

A foreign body is often visible on slit-lamp examination. Other times a foreign body is suspected based on breaks in the pupillary border, iris damage, or other clues suggesting its presence and location. Some foreign bodies (ie, glass fragments), may be extremely difficult to find.

Because viscoelastic smoothes and stretches tissues, it may help detect a hidden foreign body. It is important that the viscoelastic used in these situations provides a strong soft spatula action. For instance, Healon® is very helpful, as it shifts and mobilizes tissues easily. By compressing the iris, we can sometimes visualize a protrusion on the iris that suggests the presence of an underlying foreign body. The viscoelastic itself may be used to shift the foreign body and place it, whenever possible, in the most opportune position to be grasped by forceps and extracted.

After repairing the corneal or corneo–scleral wound and removing an anterior segment foreign body, the surgeon can proceed with cataract removal, as previously described.

A limbal incision is preferred but in the presence of severe posterior capsule break and lenticular material in the vitreous, a pars plana approach is indicated.

When the anterior segment is remarkably compromised, and the whole lens has been removed with anterior or total vitrectomy, immediate implantation of an IOL is not advisable. This can be accomplished later with scleral fixation, after assessing the possibility of functional visual recovery.

If the corneal damage is irreparable a double procedure (ie, keratoplasty and cataract extraction) should be performed. In some cases, a triple procedure (ie, keratoplasty, cataract extraction, and IOL implantation) is feasible.

After positioning a Flieringa ring when required, the surgeon performs corneal trephination, at least 7.5 mm in diameter. With such a large opening, the surgeon can be certain that he or she can successfully extract a senile, large-sized nucleus with open-sky technique. Synechiotomy performed with viscoelastic and spatula follows, if necessary. Then, open-eye capsulotomy and extraction of the nucleus by hydro- or viscoexpression or cryode is accomplished.

The surgeon then aspirates the cortical material and implants an IOL after injection of a viscoelastic. A peripheral iridectomy is then performed and the donor cornea is sutured, generally 0.5 mm larger than the explanted corneal button. The donor cornea is fixed in place with four cardinal stitches that will be removed later, followed by continuous 10-0 nylon suture.

The surgery is concluded with removal of the viscoelastic; it is advisable to use a cohesive product to facilitate viscoelastic removal and avoid long maneuvers needed to remove more adhesive materials.

Once IOL implantation is completed, the surgeon can then repair iris damage. Abundant viscoelastic that is able to form space and with high viscosity at low shear rate is very helpful for this phase of the procedure. The surgeon may prefer Healon® GV, although during some maneuvers it may partially come out of the AC owing to its high internal cohesion, therefore requiring frequent reinjection. A more adhesive product, such as Viscoat, can also be used but it is less able to form space than is Healon® GV.

Repair of iris damage should be performed after the cataract has been extracted and the new IOL implanted, to have adequate support for further maneuvers. Nevertheless, the iris is sometimes so damaged and the tissue so atonic that flaps of tissue float, pushed by the motion of the irrigation fluid or inescapably aspirated into the opening of the aspiration line. In such an event, the surgeon should try to stabilize the tissues by injecting viscoelastic to block them. An adhesive viscoelastic is preferred when the surgeon uses an infusion line. With a dry technique (without an infusion line), one can also use a cohesive product such as Healon® GV. In both cases, however, the viscoelastic will be added frequently.

When the iris is being sutured, no infusion is present. Therefore, a product with very high molecular weight, high pseudoplasticity, high ability to form space, and strong permanent spatula action is preferred. The ideal product for this purpose is Healon® GV. Owing to Healon® GV's protection and space formation, for instance, the surgeon can suture an iris coloboma with a long straight needle STC-6 and 10-0 prolene. The needle is introduced through a small corneal opening and emerges on the opposite side. The thread is retracted through the incision, and both ends are tied outside the globe. The knot is then tightened and replaced inside the eye.

In this technique space maintenance is mandatory, as is the preservation of a smooth and stretched iris, in order to approach the iris with the needle precisely to reappose tissue and restore correct tissue anatomy.

Permanent spatula action is equally important; Healon® GV is the product of choice.

The same viscoelastic characteristics must be possessed by the viscoelastic used for iridodialysis suturing. When they are small, iridodialyses may sometimes be left in place. They must be sutured when they may cause monocular diplopia, for cosmetic reasons, and to free the pupil when encumbered by vitreous tissue. It may be easier to perform cryopexy with viscoelastic control and scissors.

If the surgeon needs to suture the iris root of a large iridodialysis, accurate injection of viscoelastic on the iris is mandatory before suturing with 10-0 prolene. This stretches the iris and allows it to approach the original site of anatomic insertion.

If the surgeon is faced with traumatic cataract surgery in the presence of old scars in the anterior segment, the use of overwhelming viscoelastic may help clarify the anatomic relationships that have been subverted by trauma and the consequent cicatricial process.

The viscoelastic is used above all to remove anterior synechiae and to create the space required for this maneuver. In addition, the material stops the bleeding that originates from synechiolysis. If the synechiae cannot be removed with a spatula, they must be cut with scissors. The presence of a very heavy, pseudoplastic viscoelastic that forms space is fundamental for this procedure.

Some synechiae may be left in place, particularly when they are peripheral. Central synechiae, however, must be removed. Tissue bridges must be visualized and tented by injecting viscoelastic between cornea and iris, and then cut with microscissors.

After anterior synechiae are released, the surgeon can then concentrate on posterior synechiae. All iridolenticular synechiae should be detached to facilitate cataract surgery. The surgeon must therefore search for a cleavage plane to introduce the thin cannulas for viscoelastic, either through an iris coloboma or the pupillary border. The progressive injection of viscoelastic material opens the way for a spatula that will remove the synechiae.

The surgeon must try to remove the synechiae as completely as possible, leaving only the paracentral ones. This ensures enough support for the IOL in case of severe damage to the capsular bag.

Once synechialysis is completed, the cataractous material, often consisting of a hard white/yellow buffy coat, is removed. Its central portion is often cut with scissors and removed by forceps or a vitrector. The persistence of peripheral material may be useful support for the IOL.

CATARACT WITH POSTERIOR SEGMENT INVOLVEMENT

Cataract generally can be associated with vitreous hemorrhage, retinal detachment, intraocular foreign body, and lens dislocated into the vitreous cavity.

Cataract and Vitreous Hemorrhage

Phacoemulsification with limbal approach can be performed; then, after IOL implantation and sutured wound closure, a heavy viscoelastic is left in the AC. Its aims are to maintain mydriasis, provide a constantly well-formed chamber (even in the moments of hypotony that may occur during vitreous surgery), visualize the fundus, and facilitate scleral indentation maneuvers. Pars plana vitrectomy follows to clear the vitreous hemorrhage. At the end of surgery all the viscoelastic is removed.

The surgery is usually postponed until complete posterior vitreous detachment occurs, unless retinal problems coexist. A surgical approach through only the pars plana is also possible, which involves cataract removal by phacoaspiration (in young patients) or by pars plana phacoemulsification (in patients with harder nuclei).

Traumatic Cataract and Retinal Detachment

Similar to patients with vitreous hemorrhage, phacoemulsification through a limbal incision, followed by pars plana vitrectomy, is performed. Again, both procedures can be accomplished through a pars plana incision. The retinal detachment may be rhegmatogenous or tractional. Vitrectomy is followed by retinopexy of the retinal breaks by laser endophotocoagulation or ab externo cryocoagulation. Then an internal tamponade with limited action (gas) is used. If an epiretinal membrane is peeled or in the presence of giant retinal tears, the gas can be replaced with silicone oil.

Sometimes a scleral buckle is applied to tamponade the retinal breaks. Removal of the lens is necessary when the vitreoretinal periphery is compromised and complete cleaning of the vitreous base is required. In such cases IOL implantation is generally not performed, and it is better to defer IOL placement until the retinal conditions are stable and the tamponading means has been removed.

Cataract and Intraocular Foreign Body

After extracting the cataract as previously described, the intraocular foreign body is removed via pars plana vitrectomy. Performing cataract extraction first confers a number of advantages: the foreign body and possible retinal damage are better visualized and lenticular material dispersed in the vitreous can be removed. In addition, the foreign body, a possible source of infection and development of proliferative vitreoretinopathy, can be removed.

Cataract and Dislocation of the Lens Into the Vitreous Cavity

This topic has been discussed previously in the chapter concerning posterior capsular rupture.

It is important to note that gases or liquids used in vitreoretinal surgery can be found in the anterior segment postoperatively. Viscoelastic materials can be used to void the AC of gas or silicone bubbles. The gas or silicone oil is lighter than the viscoelastic and "floats" upon it. If the surgeon keeps the anterior incision open and elevated, silicone and gas are easily discharged through it. On the contrary, heavier tamponading means, such as perfluorocarbonates, may be blocked by the viscoelastic in a precise position and can then be aspirated by the cannula.

CHAPTER TWENTY-THREE

Secondary Implantation of Posterior Chamber IOL with Scleral Fixation

IOLs with both angle support and iris fixation implanted in the AC have marked an important phase in the evolution of implantology. However, over the years, their role has gradually diminished. Currently, they are mostly used for the treatment of rare cases of secondary IOL implantation in aged patients showing a fair corneal endothelial cell count or in the management of eyes with accidental posterior capsule rupture when it is not possible to position the IOL in the sulcus or on the anterior capsule. Their use has become limited 1) because they may cause corneal complications (bullous keratoplasty, friction intermittent syndrome), 2) because of difficulties affecting the iridocorneal angle (recession of the angle, formation of synechiae, glaucoma), and 3) because of complications, including those involving the iris (iris erosion and atrophy); uveitis; uveitis, glaucoma, and hyphema syndrome; or retinal problems (cystoid macular edema).

Since 1985, Wong, Hall, Drews, and several other authors have suggested that an IOL with loops sutured to the sclera be implanted to permit implantation and correct centration of the IOL in the posterior chamber, even in the absence of capsular support.

Suturing is generally accomplished using 10-0 prolene and variously shaped needles—straight, curved, or short—according to the technique used by the surgeon.

Preoperative examination is important to assess transparency of the cornea, corneal endothelial cell count, iris damage, anterior or posterior synechiae, free or incarcerated vitreous strands in the AC, intact hyaloid, presence of intraocular inflammation, and residual cortex and fragments or portions of AC that remain in site, which may be useful in supporting one or both IOL loops. The ocular fundus must be carefully inspected and checked for the possible presence of vitreoretinal traction, posterior detachment of the vitreous, cystoid macular edema, or rhegmatogenous problems in the periphery.

When choosing an IOL, the surgeon should not use lenses with prolene loops because they are too soft and flexible. It is better to use a PMMA one-piece lens with holes at half loop, through which the suture passes, to ensure that it is correctly positioned in the medial portion of the loop and not alongside it (which would cause IOL decentration). Furthermore, the hole also permits the surgeon to be sure that the suture cannot slip off the loop. The suggested size of the implant is at least 13 mm with an optic diameter not less than 6.5 mm.

There are a variety of implant techniques, all of which require viscoelastic support. The surgeon must consider, in each circumstance, the viscoelastic's ability to preserve space, control the vitreous, and protect ocular structures during maneuvers.

REQUIREMENTS OF THE IDEAL VISCOELASTIC MATERIAL

The following is a list of the of the surgeon's needs and the features that the viscoelastic must possess:

- Good visibility
- Creation of space in which various surgical maneuvers can be performed

- Vitreous control
- Protection of ocular structures from trauma caused by needles, forceps, sutures, and IOL
- Ability to mobilize tissues (shifting them)—This enables the surgeon to place tissues in the most convenient position to accomplish the various maneuvers and then to immobilize them in the ideal posture
- Biotolerability of the product—This is necessary in case some of the viscoelastic gets lost in the posterior chamber or is poorly distinguished from the vitreous and the surgeon decides to leave it inside the eye
- Easy removability of the product at the end of surgery—This limits the occurrence of postoperative hypertension in eyes that may have already been damaged

Good Visibility = Transparency

Transparent products that rarely trap bubbles, do not form cleavage lines with BSS, and homogeneously fill the AC are preferable. For this reason, Healon® GV and Healon® are the first choices. Viscoat is less desirable because it is less transparent, forms cleavage lines, may trap air bubbles, and has to be injected "inside itself." In the implantation of posterior chamber IOL with scleral fixation, these characteristics of the viscoelastic may be disadvantageous. The surgeon might desire early placement of the product in a particular portion of the anterior segment; for instance, to reveal synechiae, to further deepen an area of the AC, to lift the iris, and so on.

Placement of the viscoelastic in a specific intraocular location, which we call "parceling out," can be achieved with Healon® GV and Healon®, but not with Viscoat.

When using Viscoat the surgeon must achieve complete AC filling; otherwise, the product causes a "stranding" effect. Viscoat has some beneficial features that will be referred to later, but for purposes of this procedure, it is a second choice product.

Ability to Form Space and Accomplish Maneuvers = High Viscosity at Low Shear Rate, High Molecular Weight, and High Pseudoplasticity

In this type of surgery, the presence of a deep AC is essential. The surgeon must avoid contact with and trauma to iris and cornea while introducing needles, forceps, and IOL into the AC. Furthermore, the surgeon must be able to lift the iris to facilitate the passage of a needle or an IOL underneath it.

Products with high molecular weight and high viscosity at 0 shear rate are most suitable for this maneuver. Healon® GV is a leader among these products because its high pseudoplasticity facilitates the performance of almost all surgical maneuvers inside the eye as well as passage and positioning of the IOL. However, one disadvantage of Healon® GV is its high cohesiveness, which occasionally causes it to leak out of the eye. If viscoelastic leakage is a problem, double viscoelastic can be used. Healon® GV is placed in contact with iris and vitreous and Viscoat is placed over the Healon®, in contact with the corneal endothelium, filling the upper portion of the AC.

Vitreous Control = High Molecular Weight and High Viscosity at Low Shear Rate

Healon® GV best meets the requirements for vitreous control. However, owing to its high internal cohesion, Healon® GV can leave the place where it has been injected, particularly when submitted to irrigation flows. Healon® GV must be combined with a product showing greater adhesive ability, such as Viscoat. Viscoat is less able to create space and is less pseudoplastic, but has great adhesiveness that enables it to stay in place.

Healon® GV is helpful when the surgeon needs to create space while tamponading the vitreous. On the contrary, if the surgeon must complete a vitrectomy and aspirate residual masses, Viscoat is more suitable.

Protection of Ocular Structures From Contacts and Traumas = Ability to Form Space and Adhere Well

Alternating or combining Viscoat with Healon® GV best protects ocular structures from trauma. Healon® GV can be useful for forming wide spaces, which may be necessary to protect the eye during passage of a needle or introduction of forceps into the AC. Healon® GV is also highly elastic, which may prove to be a beneficial asset in some cases (ie, to achieve shifting of the kinetic energy of a compressed loop, which is then released by the surgeon). However, if the surgeon wants a protective layer with a mechanical action, a product with greater adhesiveness, such as Viscoat is preferable.

Ability to Mobilize Tissues and Fix Them in the Desired Position = High Ability to Act as Soft and Permanent Spatula

In the early phases of the intervention, the surgeon may want to lower the iris surface in order to form space in the AC. Alternatively, during the phases when the suture passes under the iris, the surgeon may want to create a space between vitreous and posterior surface of the iris. Mobilization of iris tissue and its optimal positioning are achieved most easily with a product like Healon® GV, owing to its very high soft and permanent spatula effect.

Fair Tolerability When Partially Left Inside the Eye

The material must result in minimal or no IOP rise and be nontoxic to intraocular structures. A serious drawback of products with very high molecular weight and high viscosity, such as Healon® GV, is that they may cause a very high IOP rise if not removed completely at the end of surgery.

The way a viscoelastic appears on the trabeculum (as a bolus if cohesive and with long molecular chains, or more fragmented if adhesive and with shorter molecular chains) influences its ability to be cleared and, therefore, determines the eventual severity of ocular hypertension. Less cohesive products, like Viscoat, are preferable in this respect. The surgeon must be certain that the product, when left in the eye, does not cause toxicity, allergy, or processes related to poor biocompatibility of the material employed.

Not all manufacturers of viscoelastic materials provide detailed information concerning tests on product sterility and the methods used to achieve sterility or individual lot-by-lot testing of biocompatibility. As previously discussed, all products, with the exception of Healon® GV, have been recalled at some point for problems of various natures. These problems have resulted in modifications of the product, vial, and package, and, in some instances, withdrawal of the product from the market. The surgeon must carefully consider the biologic safety of the product as well as its safety level in surgical performance before use.

Easy Removability = High Cohesion

High internal cohesion is synonymous with easy removal of the viscoelastic. Less cohesive products such as Viscoat and Vitrax may be more difficult to remove, but cause less hypertension. Thus, it can be concluded that a highly cohesive product such as Healon® GV must not be purposely left inside the eye. It is more beneficial to use a material that causes less hypertension—such as Viscoat—if the surgeon intends to leave the material behind. If the surgeon plans to remove the material completely, Healon® is preferred for its ease of removal. The following focuses on how the use of viscoelastics may facilitate the various surgical techniques for scleral fixation of the IOL.

The phases of the intervention are as follows:

- Opening and viscoelastic injection in the AC
- Dissection of possible synechiae
- Anterior vitrectomy and eventual removal of residual lenticular material
- Implantation and fixation of the IOL
- Suture and removal of the viscoelastic product

Opening and Viscoelastic Injection in the Anterior Chamber

After opening the conjunctiva at the limbus, the surgeon prepares a short scleral tunnel or cuts a limbal opening with a two-plane incision. The length of the opening must correspond to the diameter of the IOL to be implanted.

This intervention is generally performed at 12 o'clock, but can also be accomplished at the temporal or oblique position. The site is chosen based on anterior segment damage and the capsule remnants that the surgeon hopes to use as IOL support. The opening through which the IOL is inserted must be at 90° relative to the lamellar sclerotomies, where the loops of the IOL are sutured. The surgeon can decide to open the conjunctiva for 180°, exposing the portion of sclera at 12 o'clock where he or she desires to implant the IOL, and, at the same time, the portion where he or she intends to make the scleral flaps. Alternatively, the surgeon should

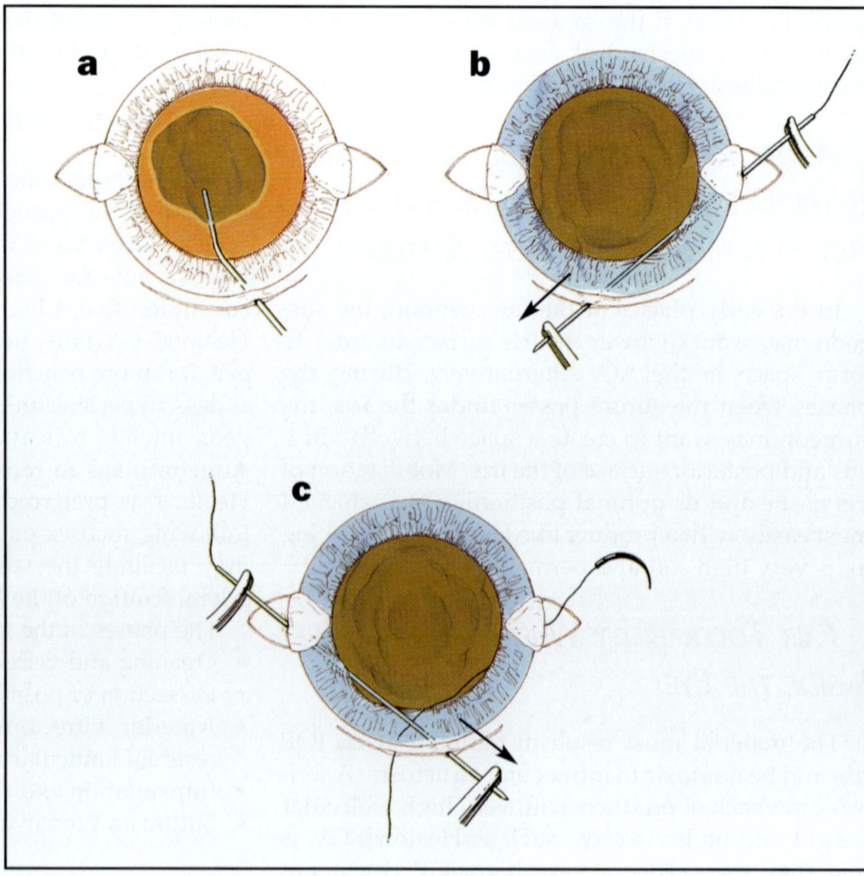

23-1a, b, and c. Implantation of an IOL with scleral fixation. (a) The conjunctiva is opened, two triangular lamellar sclerotomies, sclerocorneal tunnel, viscoelastic injection. (b) Passage of the first stitch applied with a straight needle, 10-0 prolene, under viscoelastic protection. The needle is extracted through the main opening. (c) Passage of the second needle with the same technique as the first, from the outside toward the inside.

make three separate openings in the conjunctiva. The two small triangular lamellar sclerotomies are generally performed at 9 and 3 o'clock, in order to immerse the knot suturing the loop of the IOL (Figure 23-1a). Next, the surgeon creates a paracentesis and enters the AC through the main opening with a 3.2-mm calibrated cutter.

The surgeon then injects an abundant amount of viscoelastic in an effort to deepen the AC and search for possible anterior synechiae and other scars that may not be readily apparent.

Excision of Possible Synechiae

In the presence of traumatic aphakia, the viscoelastic can help demonstrate any adhesions between iris and cornea and facilitate synechialysis. If the adhesions are particularly strong, lysis can be accomplished using a spatula or microscissors, or by using the viscoelastic alone. The viscoelastic must be particularly volumegenic and pseudoplastic with high soft and permanent spatula effect, like Healon® GV.

In the next step of the procedure, the surgeon dissects possible angle synechiae that may result in poor functional and cosmetic results if they distort the pupil. The viscoelastic is used to cut such synechiae or create volume, enabling the surgeon to perform gentle traction with the spatula or forceps to remove adhesions. These maneuvers must be performed gently to avoid bleeding. If bleeding occurs, the surgeon can tamponade it by introducing additional viscoelastic. The injection of additional viscoelastic will stop bleeding via mechanical action and via an increase in IOP. The surgeon can wait a few minutes, with the viscoelastic in site, until bleeding stops.

The surgeon should always refill the viscoelastic, particularly in the central portion of the AC over the pupil, to control possible vitreous push and pre-

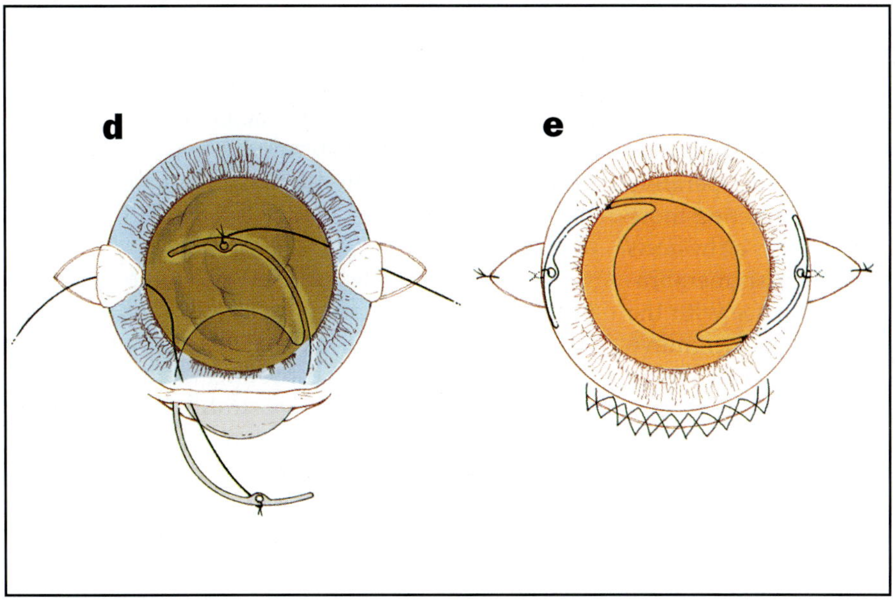

Figure 23-1d, and e. Implant of an IOL with scleral fixation. (d) Both prolene threads are tied with the rings positioned on the IOL loops. Under viscoelastic protection, the IOL is introduced by a forceps and traction is exerted on both prolene threads coming out of the scleral small flaps. (e) The IOL is rotated in position and correctly centered. The suture is fixed with the short curved needle. The main opening is sutured, removing the viscoelastic.

vent the prolapse of vitreous in the AC and breaking of the hyaloid, which in some cases may be intact. Viscoelastic material must be added constantly to compensate for the material that comes out of the eye when the surgeon enters and exits the chamber with instruments and exerts pressure on the posterior lip of the opening.

Anterior Vitrectomy and Removal of Residual Lens Fragments

Should vitreous be present in the AC, whether free or strands incarcerated in the previous surgical wound, the surgeon should visualize it and begin vitrectomy, as described in the chapter on anterior vitrectomy. Vitrectomy should be performed by using the dry technique (ie, vitrector without infusion), keeping the chamber formed with viscoelastic or by using the two separate way system, which is performed by introducing an infusion line with a shortened 23-butterfly inserted in the paracentesis and keeping the BSS bottle very low—just high enough to keep the AC formed. The surgeon introduces the vitrector through the main opening to dissect and aspirate the vitreous prolapsed in the AC. Then, the surgeon progressively approaches the pupillary plane and continues vitrectomy posterior to the pupillary plane, taking care not to "pull" the vitreous upward.

If the surgeon chooses to perform the dry technique, it is necessary to add viscoelastic continuously as it is aspirated. When performing the dry technique it is best to use an adhesive product such as Viscoat, because it remains in position, controls the vitreous, and is less likely than a cohesive viscoelastic to be removed during vitrectomy. The surgeon then introduces a small spatula in the paracentesis to check for the presence of vitreous strands in the AC and to mobilize or dilate the iris when the vitrector probe goes under the pupillary plane. In this location it is possible to check for the presence of residual lenticular material, which the surgeon will try to remove to permit optimal centering of the IOL, which could be hindered by the lens material and cause postoperative inflammation or secondary IOP rise.

The residual lens material can be removed with the vitrector alone, taking care to open its port as wide as possible, increase aspiration, and decrease cutting frequency. The surgeon should continue replacing the accidentally aspirated viscoelastic when a technique without infusion is being performed. The surgeon can alternate the vitrector with a Buratto's double-way cannula, as the vitrector is straight and its port is positioned so as to make it difficult to aspirate subincisional cortical material.

In effect, the surgeon can perform a double technique, alternating the double-way cannulas with the vitrector, according to the specific need of the moment.

During these maneuvers, posterior synechiae that may not be directly visible at the preoperative examination may become visible. By injecting more viscoelastic material under the iris, adhesions between the iris and capsulolenticular membranous residues can be seen. Creating space with the viscoelastic should enable the surgeon to remove adhesions with the spatula, microscissors, or vitrector itself. The removal of adhesions from the pupillary axis is essential for good visual recovery and to allow IOL implantation.

The surgeon may choose to leave some peripheral synechiae in site to support one of the loops of the IOL. Moreover, in the presence of postcontusive paralytic mydriasis, membranous opacities may be useful to limit postoperative photophobia and to create a sort of "second pupil" behind the iris. Once vitrectomy has been completed, residual lenticular masses removed, and the synechiae hindering implantation resected, the surgeon must inject more viscoelastic to restore correct anatomic relationships as much as possible, to obtain a deep chamber, and to control the vitreous behind the pupil. The surgeon can use a very heavy viscoelastic showing high pseudoplasticity and high viscosity at zero shear rate, like Healon® GV, to best oppose the vitreous push and facilitate surgical maneuvers during implantation of the IOL. If some vitreous persists and the surgeon needs to leave part of the viscoelastic in site, he or she can use Viscoat.

IMPLANTATION AND FIXATION OF THE IOL

There are several techniques that can be used to implant and suture the IOL. The techniques differ based on some fundamental elements:

- Axis of implant positioning in relation to the surgical wound (superior/inferior or temporal/ nasal)
- Use and dimensions of straight or curved needles for suturing
- Direction of the passage in the scleral point (from the inside toward the outside or vice versa) and modalities to allow the suture to pass from one end of the eye to the other and through the sclera

All the techniques are performed with viscoelastic, which functions to keep the AC well formed, protect against accidental contacts between the iris and cornea and the needle, facilitate the passage of the needle in the most atraumatic way possible, and permit the IOL to enter the chamber, pass through the pupillary foramen, and be suspended, centered, and sutured.

A product like Healon® GV is suitable because of its transparency, pseudoplasticity, and high viscosity at 0 shear rate. Alternatively, the surgeon can choose a more adhesive product such as Viscoat, which can be used alone or stratified on Healon® GV to protect the corneal endothelium.

After widening the main incision to permit IOL passage, the application of two different double-armed sutures in 10-0 prolene, performed on one side with a long straight needle and on the other with a short curved needle, is the most effective technique (see Figure 23-1, b and c).

The long needle is passed from the outside toward the inside, entering the sclera under the triangular port 1.5 mm from the limbus. The direction of the needle at the beginning should be perpendicular to the scleral wall, as positioning it parallel may cause contact with the ciliary body and severe bleeding. Once the surgeon is able to visualize the tip of the needle inside the eye, he or she should press lightly on the part of the needle outside the eye so that the sharp end is lifted slightly toward the pupillary plane. Next, the needle tip is rotated toward the main incision, from which it is retrieved by McPherson forceps. The same maneuver is repeated on the other scleral port and a new suture is applied. Then the long needle is withdrawn and prolene is sutured to the hole in the IOL loop. The suture from the sclerotomy on the surgeon's right should be fixed to the distal loop, whereas the other suture should be fixed to the proximal loop.

The surgeon then submits the sutures to tension, particularly the one fixed to the distal loop, and begins to insert the IOL into the AC. As the IOL enters and is placed under the iris, the suture is progressively pulled, keeping it stretched. Once the optic plate has been positioned under the iris, the surgeon grasps the proximal loop and places it under the iris, on his or her left, while pulling on the corresponding suture. Once the IOL has been positioned, both threads are pulled to check whether centering is optimal and the short needle (which remains linked to prolene outside the globe) is passed in the sclera under the scleral port and tied to the suture coming out of the globe, which has been passed previously with the straight needle. This maneuver is repeated with the other suture.

By this point, the IOL is positioned. The main opening is then sutured with 10-0 nylon and, before tightening the suture, the viscoelastic material should be removed (see Figure 23-1e).

If Healon® GV is used, the surgeon should try to remove it as completely as possible to avoid consequent hypertension. If Viscoat is used, partial or complete removal can be accomplished. In cases where vitrectomy has caused some hypotony of the globe, the surgeon can purposefully leave a portion of Viscoat in the eye to achieve a more physiologic postoperative IOP.

At this stage, the surgeon closes both triangular lamellar sclerotomies and the conjunctiva, which serve to cover the prolene knot.

This is a safe technique because it does not cause trauma to the ciliary bodies or potential hemorrhage. In addition, the corneal shape is not deformed, which provides constant control of the needles—the most crucial part of the intervention.

Alternatively, the original technique suggested by Lewis (Figure 23-2) consists of retrieving the straight needle with an insulin needle by entering under the scleral limbus at a point 180° from where the surgeon introduces the long straight needle (Figure 23-2a and b). There are various drawbacks to this technique, such as complicated needle retrieval in the presence of very deep-set orbits or a large nose and difficulty keeping the needle parallel to the iris plane without lifting it as it is being pulled out. If the needle is lifted, the distal part of the needle with the suture attached may sink into the vitreous. Furthermore, in eyes with large corneal diameters, the portion of straight needle remaining outside of the eye is not very large and the bimanual maneuver to push on the armed straight needle as well as the traction exerted on the insulin needle on the opposite side may be invasive.

Another disadvantage to this technique is that on one side of the prolene needle there is a very small and curved needle, which can be used to fix the suture to the sclera, whereas on the opposite side there is a long and straight needle that, although bent slightly by the holder, is more difficult to manage while passing through the sclera.

The final drawback is that the surgeon needs to grasp the prolene, which is passed through the pupil from 3 to 9 o'clock by means of a hook, and, using the hook, carry the folded thread outside through the main incision to tie the two ends of the suture to the respective IOL loops (Figure 23-2, d and e). Then this suture is cut and the loose ends are sutured to the IOL loops.

The only drawback to the technique described previously is that it requires the use of two sutures instead of one. Stark has developed a technique (Figure 23-3) in which a large-sized curved needle is used and passed under the iris, following its posterior surface until it reaches the iris–ciliary recess. In this location the needle is introduced, making it come outside the eye, under the small flap of lamellar sclerotomy prepared previously. This same maneuver should then be performed on the opposite side.

This technique seems to be more disadvantageous, because when entering the chamber with the needle and holder, the corneal dome is inevitably deformed, which causes a decline in the surgeon's visibility and results in poorer control. Furthermore, the contact caused by the needle tip "creeping" behind the posterior surface of the iris may be traumatic.

During such maneuvers, some viscoelastic is always wasted, which decreases the protection it should provide and may reduce spaces, presenting dangerous conditions.

It is preferable to use a curved needle, passing it at 12 o'clock from the inside toward the outside when the axis of the IOL to be implanted is vertical and in the opposite direction whenever capsular remnants are present and provide support for the IOL loops. Thus, one side of the IOL is supported by capsular remnants and the other side fixed with a scleral suture (Figure 23-4). In Table 23-1, our clinical judgment of the various viscoelastic products in the most common surgical situations is summarized.

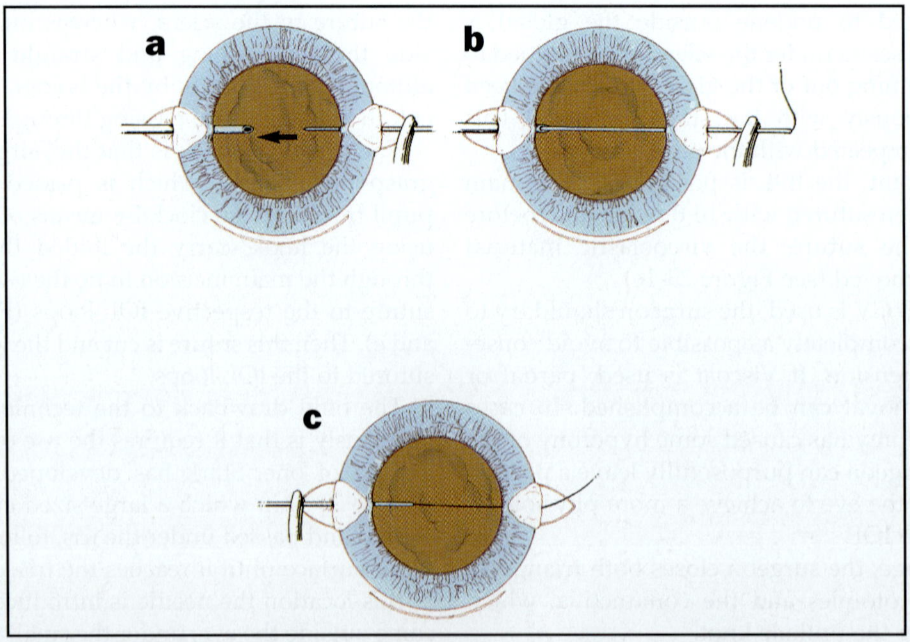

Figure 23-2a, b, and c. Implantation of an IOL with scleral fixation—Lewis' technique. (a) Under viscoelastic protection, the straight needle is inserted from the outside toward the inside, and the same maneuver is performed on the opposite side with an insulin needle. (b) The straight needle is introduced into the insulin needle and the insulin needle is retracted, thus carrying the needle mounted with prolene. (c) The straight needle is retrieved completely by extracting it through the sclerotomy 180° from where it entered.

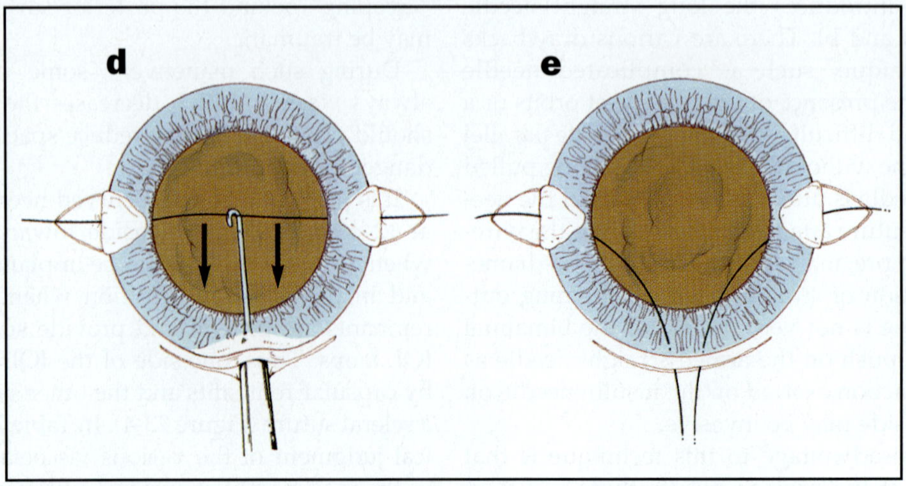

Figure 23-2d, and e. Implantation of an IOL with scleral fixation—Lewis' technique. (d) The prolene thread is retrieved with a hook and taken out through the main incision. (e) Prolene threads are cut with microscissors. Each extremity of the thread will be tied to the respective loop of the IOL.

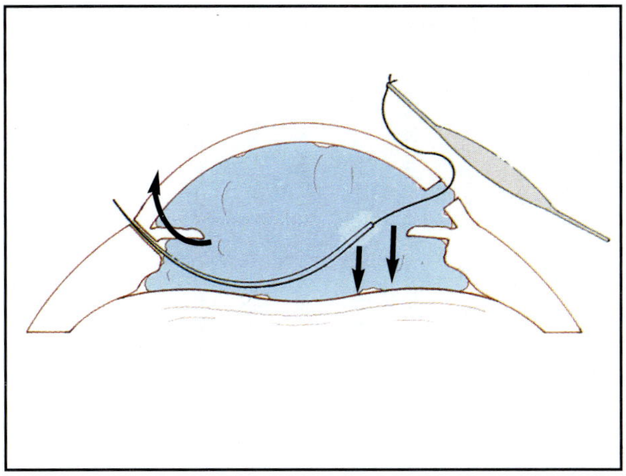

Figure 23-3. Implantation of a scleral fixation IOL—Stark's technique. The suture passes from the inside toward the outside under viscoelastic protection to control the vitreous and create space in the AC.

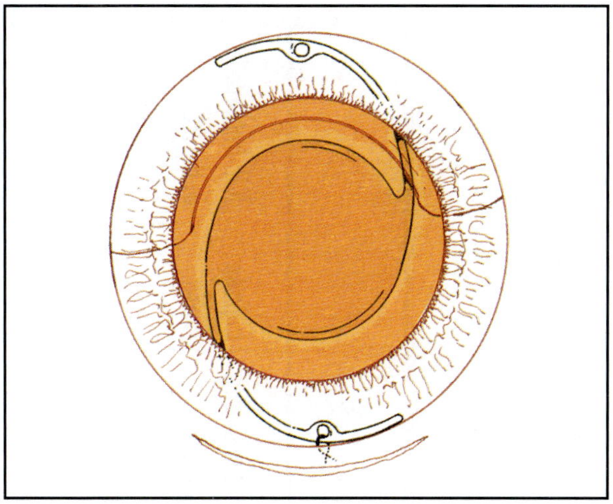

Figure 23-4. Technique of mixed IOL fixing. At 6 o'clock, the loop lies on capsular remnants, whereas at 12 o'clock, scleral fixation has been accomplished.

Table 23-1.
COMPARISON OF FEATURES OF VISCOELASTIC PRODUCTS

Injectability	Space Maintenance and Tissue Stability (Permanent Spatula Effect)	Soft Spatula Action	Phaco	Irrigation and Aspiration	Bag Filling	IOL Implantation	Removal	Demanding Cases	Capsular Breaks	IOL Implantation in the AC
1-Healon® GV	1-Healon® GV	1-Healon® GV	1-Viscoat	1-Viscoat	1-Healon® GV	1-Healon® GV	1-Provisc	1-Healon® GV	1-Viscoat	1-Healon® GV
2-Healon®	2-Healon®	2-Healon®	2-Healon® GV	2-Amvisc Plus	2-Healon®	2-Healon®	2-IAL-F	2-Viscoat	2-Healon® GV	2-Healon®
3-Provisc	3-IAL-F	3-Provisc	3-Amvisc Plus	3-Vitrax	3-Provisc	3-Provisc	3-Healon®	3-Healon®	3-Healon®	3-Provisc
4-IAL-F	4-Provisc	4-Amvisc	4-IAL-F	4-IAL-F	4-IAL-F	4-Amvisc	4-Healon® GV	4-IAL-F	4-Provisc	4-IAL-F
5-Amvisc	5-Amvisc	5-IAL-F	5-Vitrax	5-HPMC	5-Amvisc	5-IAL-F	5-Amvisc	5-Provisc	5-Amvisc	5-Amvisc
6-Amvisc Plus	6-Amvisc Plus	6-Vitrax	6-Amvisc	6-Healon® GV	6-Amvisc Plus	6-Amvisc Plus	6-Amvisc Plus	6-Amvisc	6-Amvisc Plus	6-Amvisc Plus
7-Viscoat	7-Viscoat	7-Amvisc	7-Healon®	7-Healon®	7-Viscoat	7-Vitrax	7-Vitrax	7-Amvisc Plus	7-IAL-F	7-Vitrax
8-Vitrax	8-Vitrax	8-Viscoat	8-Provisc	8-Provisc	8-Vitrax	8-Viscoat	8-HPMC	8-Vitrax	8-Vitrax	8-Viscoat
9-HPMC	9-HPMC	9-HPMC	9-HPMC	9-Amvisc	9-HPMAC	9-HPMC	9-Viscoat	9-HPMC	9-HPMC	9-HPMC

Chapter Twenty-Four

Viscoelastic Materials in Penetrating Keratoplasty and Host Cornea Trephination

Use of Viscoelastic Materials in Penetrating Keratoplasty

Penetrating keratoplasty was the first successful transplant attempted in surgery. The origins of keratoplasty date back to the beginning of the 20th century, when Zirm first transplanted a cornea in a patient with bilateral lime cauterization. Both the theory and application of the surgical aspects of keratoplasty and early successful results took place before corneal pathophysiology was properly understood and the best ways were found to preserve the cornea's delicate structures for transplant. It seems almost incredible that in the 1950s interventions of penetrating keratoplasty were successfully performed, despite imprecise knowledge of corneal endothelial pathophysiology and the absence of liquids suitable for corneal preservation, viscoelastic materials, and often even surgical microscopes.

It is also true, however, that success rates in the past were not the same as those generally achieved today. Penetrating keratoplasty is one of the surgical operations that benefited most from the rapid technical evolution of recent years, achieving standards of quality that were unimaginable some years before. The performance of the intervention is no longer limited to a few well-organized centers, thanks to the simplification of surgical procedures that made it accessible for any experienced surgeon.

Viscoelastic materials had a crucial role in these developments. The first experiences with using hyaluronate in the various phases of penetrating keratoplasty took place in the early 1980s, contemporary with its introduction in clinical practice. The use of sodium hyaluronate is generally considered as a watermark. The first report on the use of Healon® in keratoplasty concerns an experimental study performed in rabbit eyes by Miller and Stegman in 1980. The authors observed a reduced number of complications as well as more transparent grafts in eyes receiving Healon®. Their research was confirmed in a study by Alpar published in 1981. In phakic, aphakic, and pseudophakic eyes, the endothelial cell count on donor grafts, performed before and after surgery, showed significant cell loss in the cases where Healon® was not used. Cell loss was much more limited in eyes receiving a viscoelastic. However, in the same study, Alpar observed that IOP was higher in the eyes treated with Healon® than in the control group, so he suggested removing the viscoelastic at the end of surgery.

The largest study of the early 1980s was published by Polack in 1982. It surveyed 150 keratoplasty procedures, providing data on the time elapsed between donor death and graft harvest as well as on the duration the graft had been preserved in McCarey–Kaufman liquid. The AC was filled with Healon® (up to 0.4 cc) before suturing the surgical flap. When necessary, more Healon® was added during suturing procedures, to prevent endothelial cell loss in the graft due to friction against the receiving ocular structures. The study noted there were no resulting cases of abnormal eye inflammation or defective cicatrization. IOP values also did not significantly increase, due in part to surgical skill.

The advantages of viscoelastics in keratoplasty were so immediately evident that their use spread rapidly among surgeons. In 1991, Goto et al published a survey on corneal transplantation using a viscoelastic in patients with keratoconus. Although Healon® continued to be the most commonly used product, various experiences with other viscoelastic preparations were published later. Hyaluronate from bacterial fermentation, collagen, and methylcellulose achieved results similar to those of cockscomb hyaluronate in animal experiments. However, the data regarding human cornea were controversial. Methylcellulose, a vegetable-derived material, has been successfully used in keratoplasty by Vieira et al, whose report on their work in 1985 noted no complications.

Surgical procedures linked to keratoplasty present a risk of damage to the ocular structures of both the donor (the cornea, particularly the corneal endothelium) and the recipient (the cornea, iris, lens). Consequently, surgical instruments have been devised to limit trauma to donor tissues, such as punch trephines and special forceps. Surgical procedures have been studied in terms of preserving the endothelium of the donor's flap during extraction as well as during grafting.

Viscoelastic materials have been indispensable to the evolution of keratoplasty. In fact, it is unusual, if not impossible, to find a surgeon who does not use them in every intervention. In early phases viscoelastics were helpful in perfecting existing surgical actions, making them easier and safer. Owing to their ability to maintain space, it became possible to perform more complex procedures, which formerly required constant irrigation and resulting decreased visibility. The protective effect on internal ocular surfaces made rapidity of movement less important, while the increased visibility provided by their transparency improved surgical precision.

Later, viscoelastics had a more significant effect on penetrating keratoplasty as well as other types of ocular surgery by making the development of innovative viscoelastic-dependent techniques possible. This group of procedures has been called "viscosurgery."

Viscosurgical Analysis of Penetrating Keratoplasty

Viscosurgical analysis consists of carefully observing surgical procedures in order to define their separate steps. The components of each step are specified: the instruments used, how the surgeon moves them, the force required for such movements, the role of the viscoelastic, and the results achieved.

One important factor is shear rate. This describes the speed of an element present in the operating field (such as a forceps or cannula) compared to the surrounding tissue. In a wider sense, the shear rate also indicates the speed of suspended particles in relation to the fluid containing them, of solute molecules in relation to the solvent, and of a homogeneous solution during injection through a cannula. If the cannula is very narrow, the particles inside it move much more rapidly than through a wider lumen. In the first case the shear rate will be very high, whereas in the second case it will be more limited.

Shear rate is measured in movement rate per second, established in experimental conditions. Its precise definition is outside the scope of the current introduction. For our purposes, it is enough to remember that the shear rate at rest is equal to zero, whereas in dynamic conditions it may reach 1,000 and even higher, as in the previous example of injection through a narrow cannula (Figure 24-1). Viscoelastic materials are non–Newtonian fluids that change their viscosity according to their rate of movement (Figure 24-2).

Most of the main procedures linked to penetrating keratoplasty are performed with very low shear rate. They are mainly static surgical movements, where the most important aspect is that the viscoelastic acts as a cushion maintaining space and preventing contact between tissues. The time required to accomplish antitorsion continuous suturing is an example. It is therefore useful to use a material that has high viscosity at rest and good pseudoplasticity so it is easily injected through a cannula of average diameter. A product with no excessive internal cohesion is also useful to avoid transmitting tangential forces to the surfaces it touches. This aspect is particularly necessary to preserve the endothelial cells of the donor cornea during keratoplasty, which has been studied under experimental conditions by various authors.

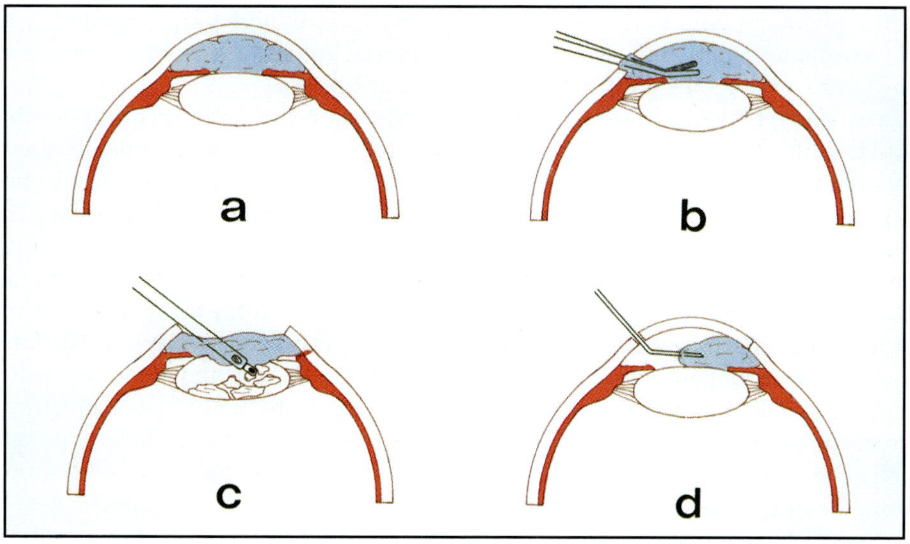

Figure 24-1. Surgical examples of shear rate. The unit of measurement for shear rate is the movement rate (directly proportional to both the number of movements and their speed) divided by time in seconds. Generally this is an approximate number, which expresses the shear rate in 1 second, or per second raised to –1 power. (a) When the AC is filled with viscoelastic and no surgical procedure is performed inside it, the shear rate is 0. (b) The movement of a surgical instrument such as a forceps in the AC creates a shear rate ranging from 1 to 10. (c) During irrigation and aspiration of residual masses during cataract surgery, the shear rate is between 10 and 100. (d) When injecting a viscoelastic material through a thin cannula, the shear rate is presumed to be between 100 and 1000. (e) During phaco, the shear rate at the phaco tip is over 10,000.

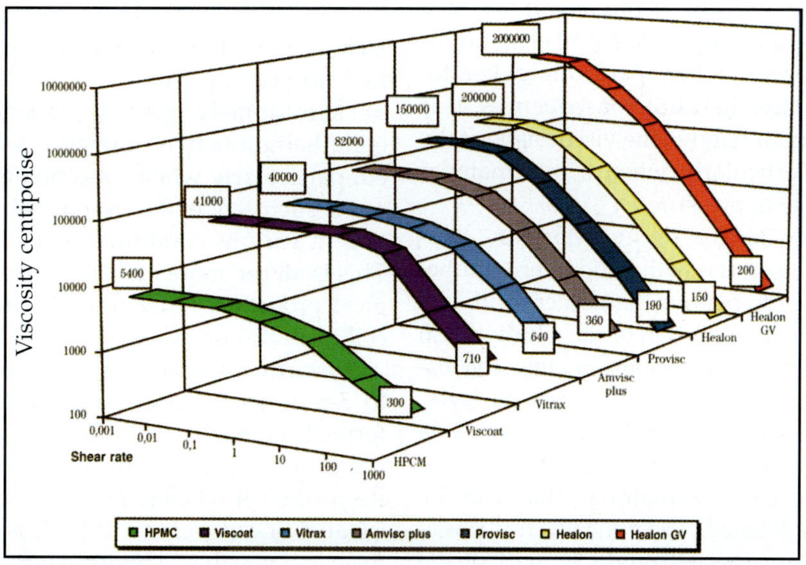

Figure 24-2. Viscosity of various viscoelastics according to their movement rate. Variation of viscosity with changing shear rate is the main feature that makes viscoelastics different from Newtonian fluids.

A viscoelastic with low internal cohesion (see following) is able to adhere better to the structures it comes in contact with, and is labeled dispersive or adhesive. Viscoat and methylcellulose are both adhesive products of this type.

Many additional procedures performed in the AC for surgical reconstruction, iris surgery, and IOL implantation and extraction are performed with very low shear rates, ranging from 1 to 10. In these phases it is mandatory to maintain good visibility as well as surgical space. Pseudoplasticity is either fundamental or irrelevant depending on the need to use thin cannulas. The transparency of a viscoelastic is greatly related to its ability to trap air bubbles, as well as to its tendency to form a homogeneous bubble during injection. Both factors depend on a previously mentioned feature called internal cohesion. Viscoelastics with good internal cohesion tend not to form bubbles when injected, therefore providing the best visibility, and are defined as cohesive. Healon®, Healon® GV, and other preparations with 1% sodium hyaluronate are cohesive products.

Paradoxically, the purity of a viscoelastic is a less important factor in determining its transparency. The purity of the products available is generally excellent. Nevertheless, some preparations of hydroxypropylmethylcellulose may contain particles visible at high magnification that can be confused with vitreous present in the operating field. The need to prevent postoperative IOP elevation is particularly important when performing keratoplasty, as it may have harmful consequences. It is therefore necessary to remove the viscoelastic at the end of surgery, particularly when it is a material causing an increase in pressure.

With the same danger of hypertension, it is preferable to use a material with good internal cohesion, which is easier to remove than others with less cohesion. Unfortunately, high internal cohesion also presents a greater risk of hypertension when the viscoelastic is injected in the AC of phakic eyes. Whether it is preferable to choose a product with a lower risk of hypertension but greater difficulty to remove or a more risky material that can be removed easily is debated. Theoretically, it is possible that with more adhesive products, part of the viscoelastic may remain trapped between the donor and the receiving cornea. Although based on theoretical considerations, this suggests choosing a viscoelastic with high biocompatibility, and therefore a material made of a normal component of human ocular tissues.

Viscosurgical analysis of the mechanical aspects of keratoplasty must not overshadow what is actually the main function of viscoelastic materials: to protect the corneal endothelium. This protection extends not only to the cells of the graft, but also to those of the receiving cornea, which also need careful protection from trauma due to transplant procedures. For this purpose, a substance with good internal cohesion and good viscosity at rest provides good protection from direct trauma, but can be shifted from the surface it is applied to by a force tangent to the surface it should protect. A material that has good adhesiveness—that is, with reduced internal cohesion—protects less from direct trauma but cannot be moved by tangent forces (Figure 24-3). Controlled studies have not found these differences to result in better or worse endothelial protection.

USE OF VISCOELASTIC MATERIALS IN EXTRACTING DONOR CORNEAS

Extracting the donor cornea is the first phase of keratoplasty, often performed some days before the actual keratoplasty, and sometimes in a different facility. Nevertheless, this procedure is considered a real surgical intervention, upon which the outcome of keratoplasty greatly depends. The corneal endothelium may be damaged while being extracted, particularly when collection is performed without a microscope. Recent regulations permit collection in various conditions, even by unskilled staff. This is all the more reason to use safe and easy surgical procedures that provide the best endothelial cell protection possible.

Extracting a donor cornea is performed using a 2 to 3-mm scleral ring. The procedure can be performed manually or with the aid of a specially designed trephine with a 15-mm–diameter blade. Regardless of whether graft extraction is made in an isolated or cadaver eye, the AC is essentially kept as deep as possible. Unfortunately, as soon as it is opened, the chamber tends to empty owing to leakage of aqueous humor, while the absence of blood flow increases hypotony in the posterior segment.

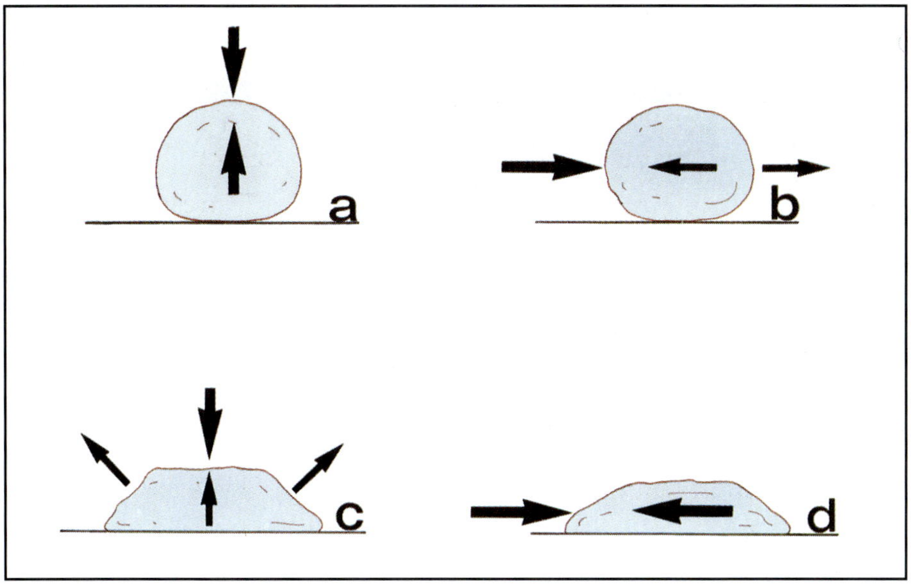

Figure 24-3. (a, b) A viscoelastic with high internal cohesion protects well from direct trauma, but is less effective against tangential forces, which may completely remove it from its injection site. (c, d) An adhesive viscoelastic with reduced internal cohesion protects less from direct trauma but is hardly moved by tangential forces.

Under these circumstances it is difficult to avoid major dangers: not only contact of the corneal endothelium with surgical instruments, but also tangential traction on the cornea, which often causes rough tissue folds. Preventing folds on the corneal stroma is very important, as endothelial cell loss has been shown to occur in the corresponding area.

It has been demonstrated that a viscoelastic can guard against such loss simply by preventing folds from forming. One effective method is to fill the AC of the donor globe with viscoelastic while evacuating all the aqueous humor. Provided that it is able to maintain space, owing to its high viscosity at zero shear rate, the viscoelastic opposes and often prevents the formation of folds. As usual, using a highly pseudoplastic product, which can be easily injected through a small cannula (25 or 27 G), is particularly useful. Less pseudoplastic viscoelastics require larger gauges for injection. In this case, a 19- or 21-G atraumatic cannula, such as Charleaux bow cannula, can be used.

MANUAL SURGICAL TECHNIQUE

The technique we usually use for extraction is as follows (Figure 24-4). Pericorneal conjunctiva is removed after limbal peritomy, thus laying bare 3–4 mm of sclera. With younger patients it is often necessary to push aside Tenon's capsule, which is often exuberant. With a disposable 45° knife, four openings of about 3 mm are cut in the sclera parallel to the limbus and 2 to 3 mm away from it, one for each quadrant. The incisions are deepened to the choroid/ciliary body, taking care not to penetrate the vitreous chamber, as usually happens in cyclodialysis.

A cyclodialysis spatula is introduced through one of the incisions to separate the ciliary body from the sclera. The division is assisted by the injection of viscoelastic, usually 1% sodium hyaluronate in the suprachoroidal space, which helps achieve the largest possible detachment of choroid and sclera. Cyclodialysis is continued until the AC is penetrated. After emptying the aqueous humor, the chamber is then filled with 1% sodium hyaluronate through the sclerotomy and cyclodialysis is performed. We generally use Healon®. Once the AC has been stabilized, the surgeon definitively splits the ciliary body and sclera with a spatula inserted in the scleral incisions. Viscoelastic material is added as required to restore the stability and volume of the AC.

When cyclodialysis is completed over 360°, a silk suture is passed through the corneal rim of a sclerotomy. This thread will be used to move the cornea and hang it inside the conservation bottle. It is important for the surgeon to pass the thread through at this moment of the extraction, when the cornea is still fixed firmly to the sclera and distor-

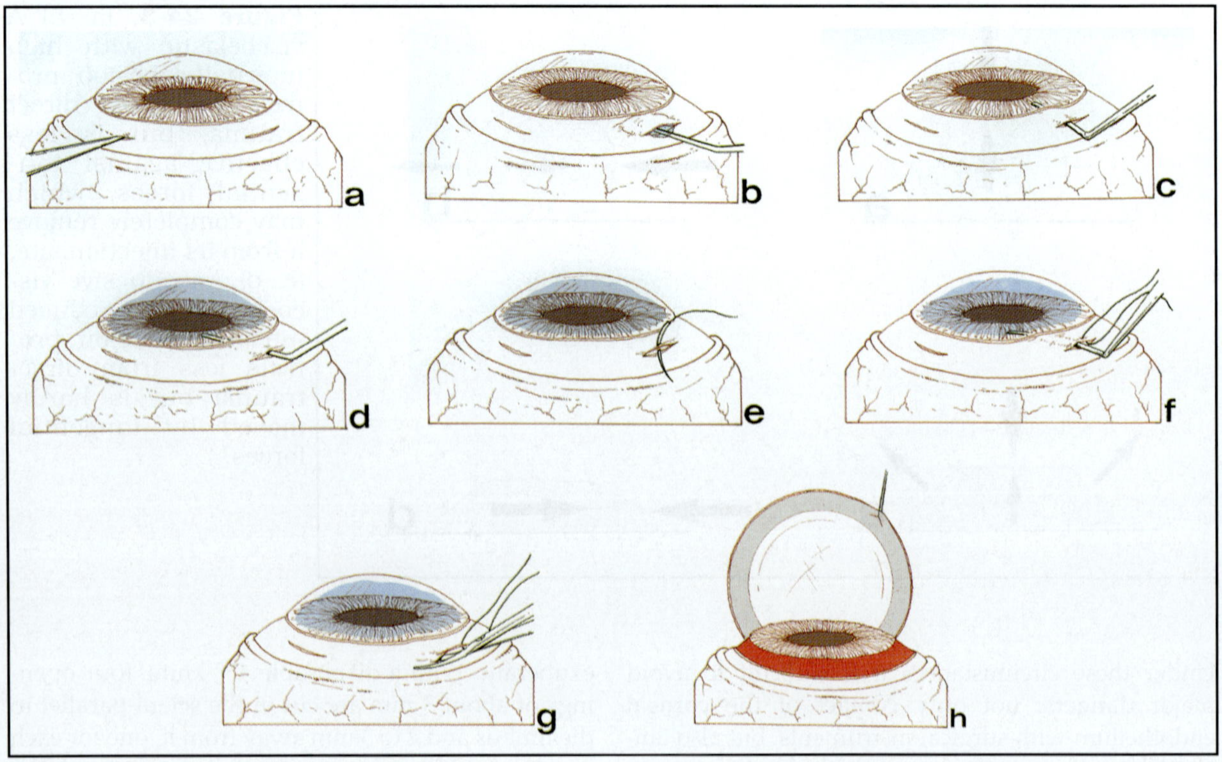

Figure 24-4. Viscoelastic used to extract donor cornea. (a) Once the conjunctiva is detached about 3 mm from the limbus, four sclerotomies each about 3 mm long are cut with a disposable blade parallel to the limbus and nearly 2.5 mm away from it, one in each quadrant. (b) The injection of viscoelastic in the space over the choroid begins cyclodialysis. (c) Cyclodialysis is continued with the spatula commonly used for the procedure, advancing until it penetrates the AC. (d) The AC is stabilized by completely filling it with viscoelastic. (e) The spot is located on the corneal margin of a sclerotomy that will be used to lift and carry the cornea in its means of preservation. Opening the sclera as little as possible and stabilizing the AC with the viscoelastic minimizes distortions of the corneal endothelium during the procedure. (f) The ciliary body and the sclera are separated over 360° with the cyclodialysis spatula and the viscoelastic, using in turn each of the four previous sclerotomies. Procedures should start from the AC rather than move toward it, to avoid any endothelial damage. (g) Cyclodialysis completed, the circumference of the sclera is cut, joining the sclerotomies. (h) Removing the cornea and the scleral ring completes the intervention. If the viscoelastic remains adherent to the endothelial surface of the grafted cornea, it can be gently irrigated or removed later on.

tions of its stroma caused by the needle are very small. Scleral peritomy is completed by curved scissors, with attention to the possibility that residual adhesion of ciliary body and sclera may persist. If so, the adhesions must be gently removed. The presence of viscoelastic in the AC underneath the cornea allows each step of the technique to be performed with safety and reliability, and allows even less-experienced surgeons to achieve a graft with satisfactory technical features.

At the end of the procedure the cornea is lifted by the suspension thread previously introduced and immersed in the conservation bottle. We generally do not wash it to remove any residual viscoelastic deposited on endothelial surface. In the bottle, suspension of the cornea is accomplished by

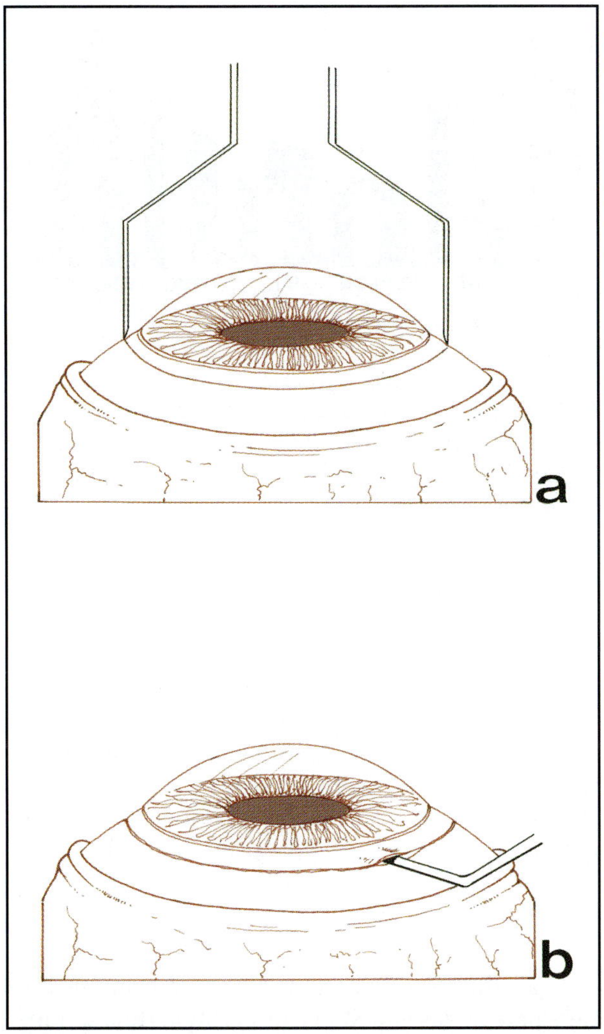

Figure 24-5. Donor cornea taken by trephination. (a) Taking the donor cornea with a 15-mm trephine makes the circumferential cut of the sclera more regular. (b) Once the sclera has been perforated, usually in a limited way at the beginning, the procedure is continued according to the methods already described for manual techniques.

compressing the suspension thread with the screw cap, so that the cornea is kept completely immersed in the fluid, by no means touching the bottom of the container.

SURGICAL TECHNIQUE BY TREPHINE

The extraction procedure by 15-mm trephine is different from that described earlier. Once the conjunctiva around the limbus has been moved away, the trephine is applied and the blade lowered until the sclera is perforated in one or more places (see Figure 24-5). The ciliary body is detached with the technique described above, with the same indications for viscoelastic use. The trephine enables the surgeon to cut a more regular incision than does the manual technique, without any confirmation of difference in the quality of the graft extracted.

EFFECT ON ENDOTHELIUM OF FILLING THE AC WITH VISCOELASTIC MATERIAL

As soon as the extraction is accomplished, the donor corneal graft, with its small scleral ring, is immediately immersed in the conservation fluid. Doubts have arisen about the possible toxic or protective effects of the various viscoelastic materials used in extraction procedures. Specific studies were conducted on cat, rabbit, and even human eyes, with the following conclusions.

In cat eyes, replacing the aqueous humor with 1% sodium hyaluronate did not lead to any alteration in corneal thickness or endothelial cell count, measured 30 days after surgery. A slight increase in corneal thickness and IOP was observed in the first 3 to 4 days after surgery. Similar results were achieved by the same researchers with BSS.

In a second study, various materials (three different preparations of methylcellulose and Type I collagen) were injected in the AC of rabbit eyes. The usual corneal parameters, including endothelial cell count, were observed and the animals were then killed. Sodium hyaluronate was used as a parameter for comparison. The results showed that the other materials tested could be useful in anterior segment surgery.

However, the corneal endothelium of human eyes is much more sensitive than that of animals. Condon observed the effects of chondroitin sulfate, 1% sodium hyaluronate (Healon®), methylcellulose, and a combination of 1% sodium hyaluronate and chondroitin sulfate (Viscoat) on the endothelium of human corneas that had been extracted before grafting. The researcher trephined an 8-mm corneal button from a whole eyeball and immediately fixed the corneal button. In the other eye, the aqueous humor was replaced for 10 minutes with the viscoelastic under observation, and after completion of trephining, more viscoelastic was laid on the button endothelium for an additional 10 minutes before fixation. After fixation, the researcher observed the corneal endothelium, taking into account both the number and the quality of cells (the latter assessed through a morphologic study on mitochondria). Condon observed that the slightest alterations in cell count and endothelial morphology were induced by hyaluronate and chondroitin sulfate when each was used alone. However, the chondroitin sulfate caused marked dehydration of the stroma. The greatest effects, particularly of mitochondria, were caused by methylcellulose and chondroitin sulfate associated with hyaluronate, although the small sample of eyes available did not permit any statistical evaluation of differences (Figure 24-6).

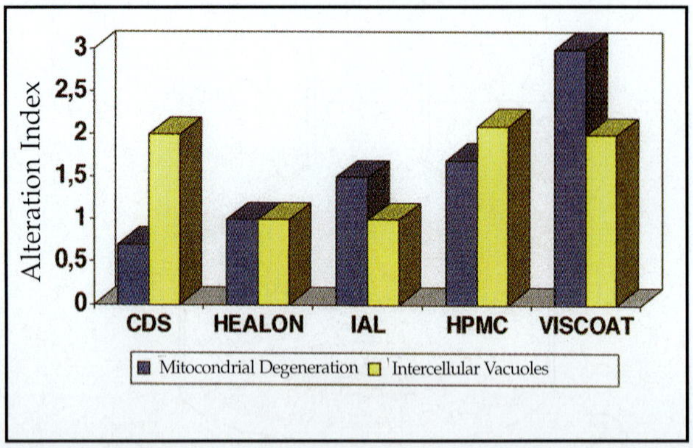

Figure 24-6. Endothelial cell damage when in contact with various viscoelastic substances (from Corydon, 1987). Corneal endothelium alteration with various viscoelastics alteration index.

CONCLUSIONS

Donor cornea extraction has been performed for many years without viscoelastics. The assistance of such materials is invaluable, however, as they make the procedure easier and allow more respect of endothelial cell integrity.

Based on the data in the literature, 1% sodium hyaluronate is the preferred product. Several preparations supplied by various manufacturers now contain material derived from cockscomb or bacterial fermentation. The experimental studies mentioned previously were performed some years ago, and no recent similar studies have been conducted. We do not know whether centers collecting donor corneas have ever recommended using viscoelastics in general for extraction, let alone particular viscoelastic materials.

USE OF VISCOELASTICS IN TREPHINATION PROCEDURES AND PREPARING THE DONOR FLAP

Procedures for trephining and preparing donor flaps are fundamental to successful keratoplasty. They have been greatly improved by the advent of viscoelastic materials. Nevertheless, regardless of their performance, there is always endothelial damage and cell loss near the trephination site that cannot be remedied even by the use of viscoelastics.

TREPHINING BOTTLED CORNEA

Once the cornea has been removed from the bottle where it was stored in conservation fluid, it must be prepared for trephining and subsequent grafting. In the past, the same Franceschetti trephine was used to trephine both the donor flap and the host cornea. In most current cases, trephining is done on the endothelial side with a special "punch" device.

A very sharp disposable trephine descends directly onto the cornea, the vertical movement of the blade generally guided by a guillotine that ensures the upright run of the trephine without deflections. When necessary, this can also be achieved by striking the top of it with a rhinostomy hammer. This punch device is equipped with a hollow silicone or Teflon block that acts as a support to the cornea (Figure 24-7). The hollow has a hole in the middle to drain any possible air or fluid bubbles that were trapped under the corneal epithelium when the donor cornea was placed on the support

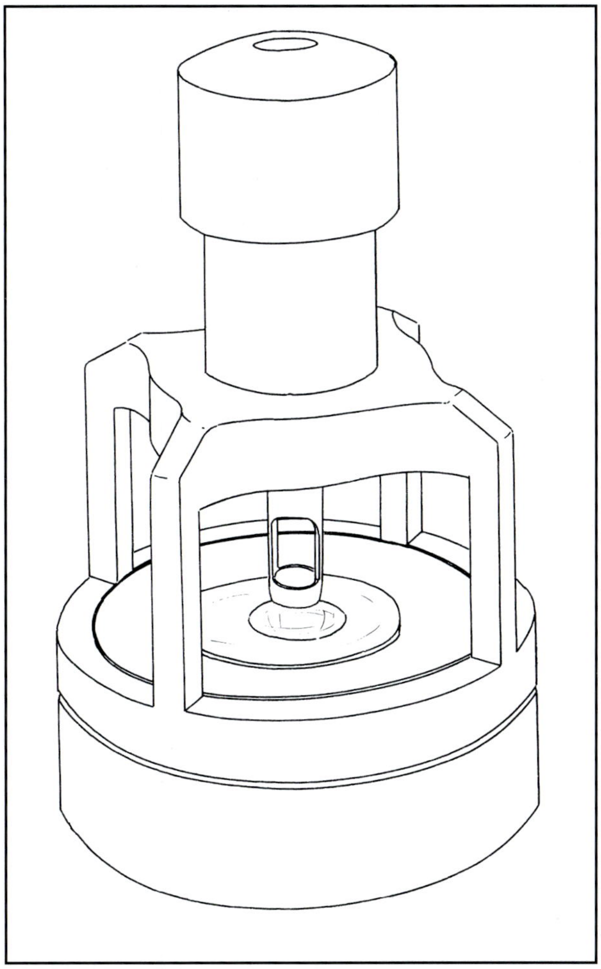

Figure 24-7. A punching device to prepare donor cornea buttons (manufactured by Moria, France). Much simpler machines are also on the market, including some that are disposable.

with the endothelial side up, toward the trephine blade. After properly centering the donor cornea, the surgeon causes the blade to descend like a guillotine, creating a corneal flap with a very regular rim in the desired size. It is also possible to cut on the epithelial side, as in the host eye, but this technique is more invasive and has not had a better practical outcome in grafted eyes. During the performance of such procedures, the cornea should be kept as dry as possible.

Positioning viscoelastic materials under the corneal epithelium should be avoided, as this could allow the donor cornea to move from the site where it has been placed for trephining (Figure 24-8). A viscoelastic cushion on the endothelial side of the cornea is not necessary; in fact, it could make manipulating the flap more difficult.

Conversely, viscoelastics are useful when the trephined button becomes trapped inside the trephine and must be removed. The most suitable technique is to try to make the flap drop without touching it from the endothelial side, which is accomplished by using sodium hyaluronate. A certain amount of Healon® is laid on the flap through the lateral opening of the trephine. The weight of the viscoelastic is often enough to make the flap emerge, to be seized on the epithelial rim by a Pierse forceps. When this cannot be done, a small quantity of BSS dropped on the viscoelastic laid on the endothelial surface of the corneal button increases the load until the button emerges from the trephine. In exceptional cases, a small jet of water is required to free the donor cornea. The presence of a certain amount of viscoelastic absorbs the force of the jet and distributes pressure onto a larger endothelial surface, providing a cushion that protects cells and makes the procedure less traumatic.

In 1985, Insler suggested trephining a donor button by filling the cavity of a trephine similar to Franceschetti device—with a 5-mm retracted piston—with Healon® (Figure 24-9). If the button remains inside the trephine, it feeds the piston exerting force on the viscoelastic, which in turn pushes on the endothelial side of the donor button, allowing it to come out of the trephine in an atraumatic manner.

TREPHINING A WHOLE EYEBALL

Trephining a corneal flap from a whole eyeball can be performed with the same device that can be used later to trephine the host eye. The most commonly used tools are suction trephines such as Hessburg–Barron's disposable device or Hanna's trephine. The donor eye is kept wrapped in gauze or placed on appropriate support enabling good fixation. During the procedure trephine suction exerts such a force that the cornea to be trephined can be deformed.

Controlling IOP during the procedure is important to limit endothelial cell loss on the border of the incision. This can be accomplished easily by injecting viscoelastic material in the AC (Figure 24-

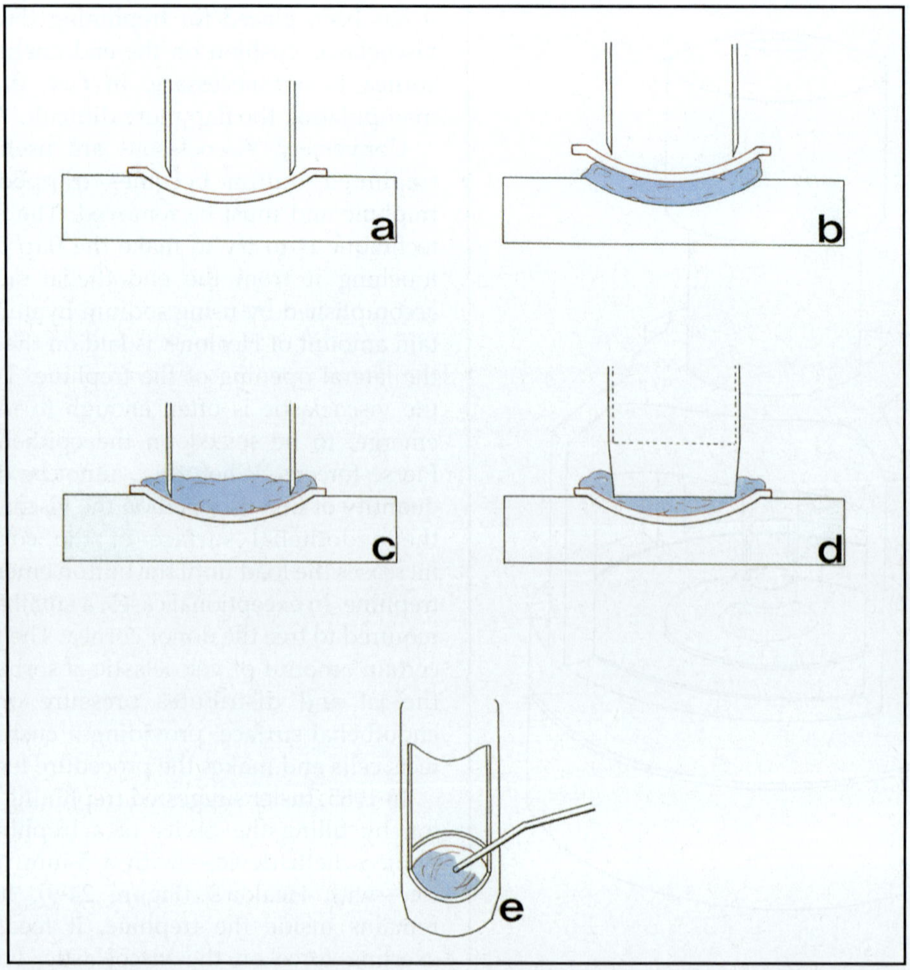

Figure 24-8. Preparing the donor cornea button with the punching device. (a) The procedure consists of dissecting the donor cornea on its circumference, thus obtaining a button for later implantation in the desired diameter. The cornea is cut on the special disposable silicone support with the endothelial surface turned upward, and the punch trephine is sharply driven downward to dissect the cornea, even penetrating the silicone support. (b) Placing a viscoelastic between the corneal epithelium and the silicone support may encourage small movements of the donor cornea during trephination if the punch does not work properly. (c) However, placing viscoelastic on the endothelial side causes no damage. (d) If a nonfenestrated trephine is used and the corneal button remains inside it, it can be expelled by pressing the piston on the endothelial side of the cornea. Viscoelastic must be placed on the endothelial surface of the donor cornea to protect it. (e) When the trephine is fenestrated, a corneal button still adhering to it after trephination can be released with gentle irrigation, drop by drop. The viscoelastic can be placed on the endothelium for better protection. In fact, the weight of the viscoelastic is frequently enough to cause the button to emerge through the lumen of the trephine.

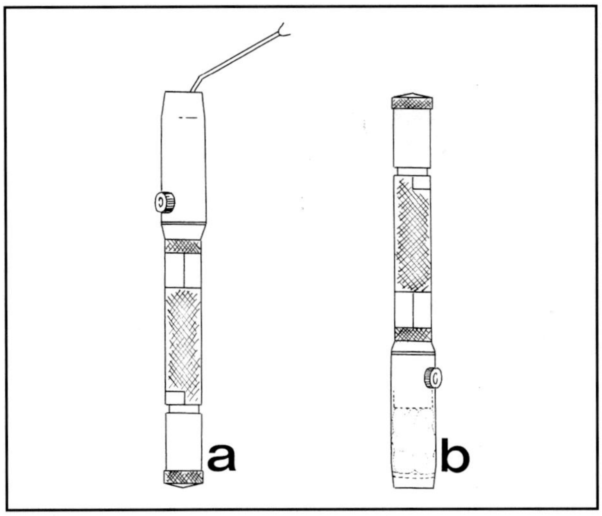

Figure 24-9. Preparing the donor cornea button with Franceschetti trephine, Insler's technique. (a) The cavity of Franceschetti trephine (with retracted piston) is filled with viscoelastic (sodium hyaluronate). (b) After trephination, the pressure applied by the piston onto the viscoelastic causes the donor cornea button to emerge from the trephine.

10). It is necessary to use a product with a high viscosity at 0 shear rate and that is very pseudoplastic so it can be injected through a very narrow needle such as the 30-G cannula. The most suitable material for this seems to be Healon® GV. The narrow lumen of the needle, which can go through the cornea on an oblique pathway, is fundamental for maintaining the integrity of the AC. Once the trephine has penetrated the chamber, the corneal button is removed with Vannas' bent forceps. The viscoelastic that leaks out of the AC during trephination is replenished in order to perform extraction in the most atraumatic manner possible.

PRESERVING THE FLAP BEFORE GRAFTING

However it is obtained, the corneal button is laid on a hollow support and kept on a reversed Petri plate in the moments before grafting. During this time the corneal stroma is in direct contact with the outside of the trephine ring, and the cornea reacts to physical agents in a peculiar way. Contact with air causes stromal dehydration, resulting in a reduced thickness of the flap, which should be avoided. Conversely, immersion in BSS leads to hyperhydration, resulting in thickening of the button and subsequent greater difficulties in transplantation. An important feature of the preservation fluid used is its ability to prevent corneal thickening. That the stromal ring is a crucial area for the sake of the donor button is demonstrated by the fact that possible contact with the preservation fluid even causes a change in the color of the flap, which becomes pink.

All the difficulties mentioned can be avoided by using viscoelastic materials. In this phase it is very useful to cover the flap with a viscoelastic, to avoid both dehydration and hyperhydration and to reduce contact with polluting agents possibly present in the environment. The viscoelastic also continues to protect the endothelium from possible mechanical damage (Figure 24-11), as well as from damage caused by contact with air. For this purpose the viscoelastic must have high viscosity at 0 shear rate along with good adhesion, to keep fastened to the endothelium. Internal cohesion values should not be too high to prevent tangential forces from being conveyed to the endothelium; for example, during irrigation. Perfect isotonicity and absolutely physiologic pH values are necessary when the viscoelastic covers the button of the donor cornea.

The studies focusing on these aspects are rather interesting. Barraquer was among the first to mention the usefulness of sodium hyaluronate to cover the donor button. Liesegang includes this procedure among those mentioned in his review. Bonci and Dal Fiume performed probably the best and most careful investigation.

MANIPULATING THE FLAP BEFORE GRAFTING

In most cases trephination on the donor flap is easy and performed without incident. However, complications may occur owing to instrument malfunctions. In particular, a less than perfectly sharp trephine blade can cut a fringed incision, which may be so irregular that the flap cannot be grafted and another donor cornea must be used. Descemet's membrane may also tear during trephination, which can usually be mended by simple reattachment. This can be accomplished using a viscoelastic material. The same viscoelastic can be

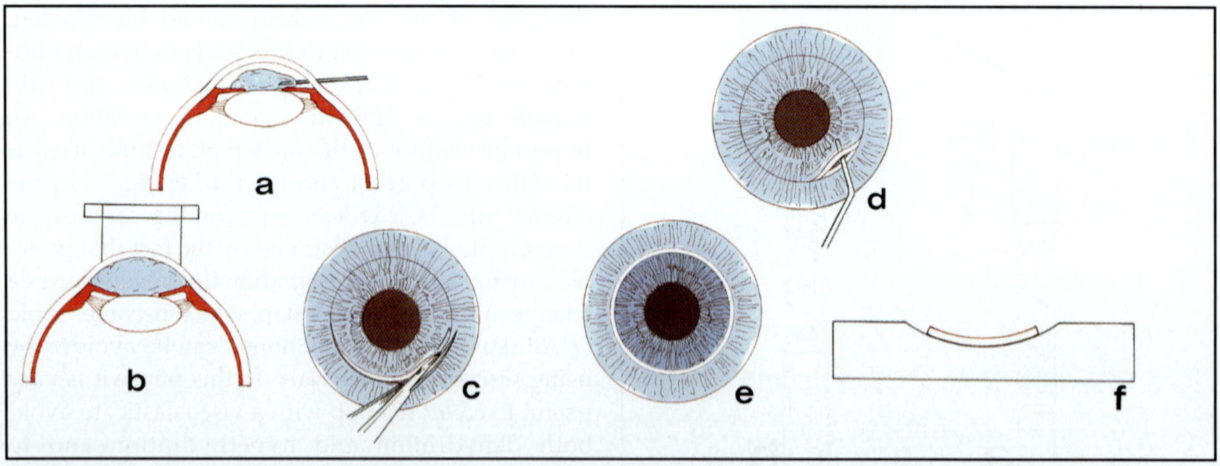

Figure 24-10. Preparing the donor cornea button. (a) Before trephination, the AC is deepened with viscoelastic injected through a 30-G needle inserted in the peripheral portion of the cornea. A highly pseudoplastic product is required. (b) With viscoelastic filling the AC, trephination is more likely to be precise in roundness and depth. (c) Trephination is performed with Vannas' scissors. (d) Any loss of viscoelastic during trephination must be replenished to prevent the eye from losing tone, or the donor button may be damaged. (e) Trephination is completed. The donor button has been taken. (f) The donor button is placed on the special silicone support for further surgical procedures.

Figure 24-11. Preserving the donor cornea button before keratoplasty. (a) The donor button is placed on the concave silicone support, with the endothelial surface turned upward. (b) A viscoelastic is placed around the button, covering the rim of the exposed stroma as well as the endothelial surface. (c) The covered button is protected by a small overturned Petri dish.

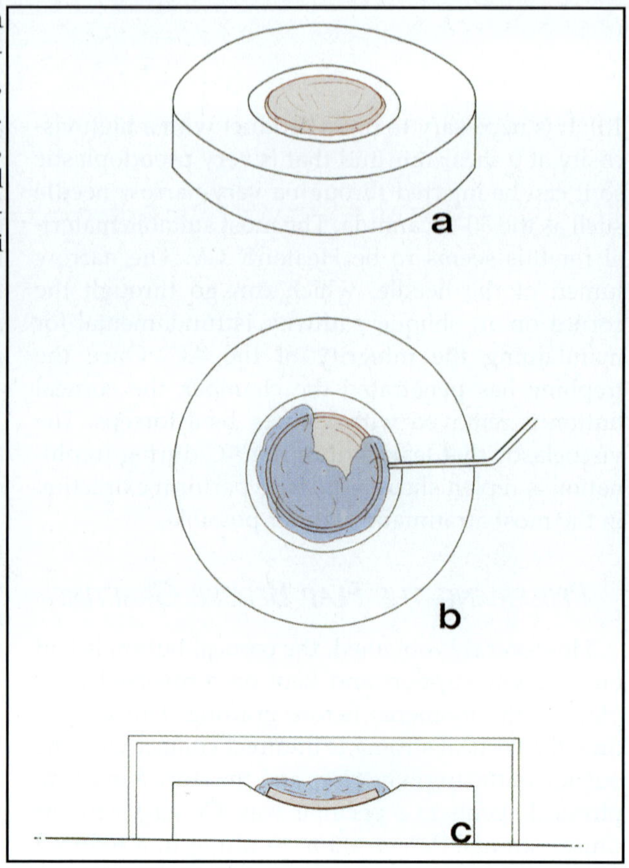

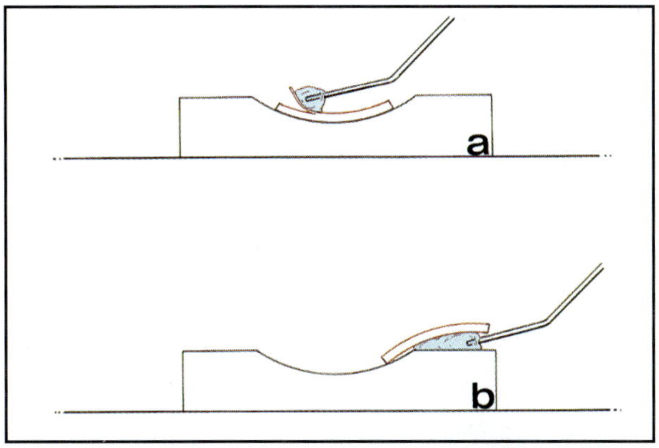

Figure 24-12. Complications in managing the donor button. (a) Limited tearing of Descemet's membrane can be realigned using a viscoelastic. (b) A donor flap that has fallen on the support with the endothelial surface downward can be overturned with a viscoelastic, avoiding any contact with instruments.

used in case of a malpositioned flap (for example, turned with the endothelial surface downward), to correct placement (Figure 24-12).

USE OF VISCOELASTICS IN HOST CORNEA TREPHINATION

Host cornea trephination is a very delicate step in keratoplasty, as highly specific requirements for the precision of the cut must be fulfilled while ocular structures are safeguarded. One possible major complication is inadvertent incision of ocular structures by the blade during the trephination phase. The aqueous humor then rapidly drains from the AC, exposing the iris and lens to the danger of incision. Being made of spongy tissue, the iris is seldom seriously damaged. More serious consequences may occur in the lens, which becomes opaque immediately after incision, thus making removal preferable to any other action. To reduce this risk, the surgeon must attempt to induce the broadest miosis, which allows interposing the iris between cornea and lens in the area where the trephine is going to work. Sometimes, this is impossible—for instance, in the case of irideremia, or in the presence of iris trauma or colobomas that inhibit the iris from protecting the lens along the whole trephined edge.

Intraocular structures can be protected by using viscoelastic materials. In 1984, Gruber reported a new application for viscoelastics in corneal graft surgery. In the host eye, 1% sodium hyaluronate (Healon®) was injected into the AC to protect the underlying structures during trephination and to prevent blood deposits and synechiae. This procedure is useful particularly in eyes with a shallow AC, irideremia, or anterior synechiae. It is necessary to use a highly pseudoplastic viscoelastic, which can be injected into the AC through a 30-G thin needle, obliquely inserted through the cornea. The site of insertion may be peripheral (Figure 24-13), but sometimes it is preferable to pierce the portion of cornea being removed, provided that the central portion is avoided.

The presence of the viscoelastic allows the surgeon to adjust IOP during trephination, which provides some mechanical advantages. The cut is more regular over 360°, making corneal tissue distortions resulting from an irregular circular cut less likely. Eventually, the verticality of the incision is improved, with the external and internal diameters far more similar to one other, exactly like the precise correspondence of the trephine diameter and the diameter of the corneal button extracted. In routine cases, the main advantage of filling the AC with a viscoelastic before trephination is the possibility of performing most of the incision with the keratoplasty trephine, without needing to finish the cut with bent shears, as often occurs for most of the circumference.

According to some researchers, the viscosity rate of the product used must not be high at zero shear rate, so the surgeon can detect any early voiding of the AC through a slow leak of the material. Sodium hyaluronate with low molecular weight seems to be the most suitable for this application. According to other surgeons, using sodium hyaluronate with high molecular weight is preferable, as it remains in the AC even when the cornea is partially opened. A viscoelastic with low molecular weight seems to be most appropriate for routine use in uncomplicated cases, when no particular protection of AC anatomic structures is required. A product with high molecular weight is better when absolute protection is mandatory, as in iridoschisis or keratoplasty in pedi-

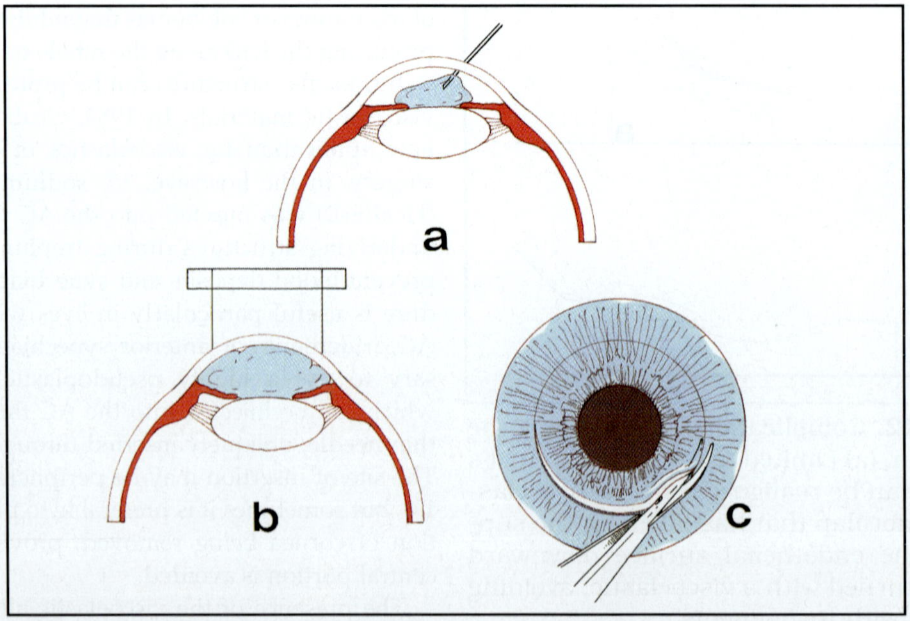

Figure 24-13. Trephination of the corneal button from the host eye. (a) Before trephination, the AC is deepened with viscoelastic injected through a 30-G needle inserted in the central or paracentral portion of the cornea (which will be removed by trephination). (b) With viscoelastic in the AC, corneal trephination is less likely to be asymmetric in depth or imperfectly round, or to damage intraocular structures. A suction trephination with a disposable blade, either Hanna's or Hessburg–Barron's, is used. (c) Trephination usually perforates the AC at a fraction of the corneal button's circumference. It is completed with Vannas' curved scissors. (d) Procedures to complete trephination usually cause the viscoelastic to leak out of the AC, further encouraged by any posterior pressure. It must be replenished to protect the iris and the lens. (e) Trephination is completed. The original button has been removed and the eye is ready to receive the donor button. (f) The host button is laid on a support and carefully preserved, to be used again during the same intervention in case of emergency.

atric patients. This requires a trephine that has a preset blade protrusion (ie, Hanna's trephine).

Only sodium hyaluronate enables the surgeon to accomplish these procedures successfully. Other less pseudoplastic viscoelastics can be used after the cornea has been almost completely trephined and the trephine has made a suitable opening in the periphery of the incision.

Removing the button to be replaced from the recipient cornea is usually completed with Vannas' scissors, which allow the surgeon to follow the incision started by the corneal trephine precisely. The AC is filled repeatedly with viscoelastic during this procedure to protect the iris from possible contact with the scissors. One jaw is introduced in the AC and angled to perform an incision vertical to the iris level. Whenever the incision is cut forward, the movement of the scissors causes the viscoelastic to leak, which must be replenished before continuing the procedure. The product injected must be highly viscoelastic at zero shear rate, as the procedure is performed in an open eye.

When the incision is almost completed and the button almost split, the viscoelastic causes elevation of the host corneal button, which is kept in place by a forceps to provide clear visibility of the trephination to be completed. During this phase it is important to avoid excessive filling with viscoelastic, as it may lift the cornea too much and reduce visibility.

Preparing the Recipient Eye

When trephination is completed, the recipient eye is inspected and prepared for grafting. Further necessary procedures can be performed during this phase of surgery, such as cataract extraction, replacement of an IOL, and reconstruction or manipulation of the iris diaphragm. Viscoelastic materials are useful in improving AC visibility; in splitting and separating structures such as the iris and cornea, which must not lose tone; in guiding dissection of synechiae; and in helping to control bleeding of the chamber angle and iris surface (Figure 24-14). This aspect has been particularly highlighted by Barraquer. He stressed that viscoelastic not only helps control anatomic conditions in cases of complex transplant surgery, but also helps prevent bleeding from angle structures caused by dissected synechiae and possible neovessels on the cornea, deposited on the iris or inside the AC.

In such open-eye procedures, sodium hyaluronate with high molecular weight and high viscosity at rest (such as Healon® GV) is particularly useful, as it can be inserted between the peripheral corneal ring and the iris diaphragm. This type of viscoelastic makes the most of its properties in order to fill the recipient eye, compacting it and protecting it from possible anterior vitreous prolapse. The need to apply Flieringa ring is also reduced by the use of viscoelastics, and the eye seems not to suffer owing to overwhelming use postoperatively. Polack has, however, reported one case of hypertension in an eye filled with 4 mL of sodium hyaluronate.

Preparing the Phakic Eye

Preparing the phakic aye for keratoplasty aims above all to determine the space between iris and cornea. Particularly in small eyes, iris thickness can interfere with placement of the donor flap. In these eyes there is often a certain posterior pressure, due to the relative dilation of the uveal capillary bed once the inside of the eye has been deprived of its physiologic pressure, which leads to zero pressure during corneal trephination (Figure 24-15). The quality of the anesthesia plays a primary role here, as the lower the systemic arterial pressure, the less marked the dilation of uveal capillaries.

A viscoelastic splits the iris and peripheral ring and keeps them separate in the recipient cornea, revealing the posterior pressure through the speed of leakage from the injection site. We find it best to use a product with high viscosity at 0 shear rate, as it is less easily squeezed toward the pupil by the iris–lenticular diaphragm push. High pseudoplasticity is also beneficial, as it allows the surgeon to inject the viscoelastic in the space to be dilated even when access is narrow. A thin cannula also takes up less room, providing better visibility and therefore greater precision.

Based on these requirements, corneal surgeons were immediately interested in a higher molecular weight Healon®. According to Laflamme, Healon® GV represents a step forward. He notes that many surgical procedures in keratoplasty are accomplished with very low shear rates, but also emphasizes the importance of high pseudoplasticity, which enables the viscoelastic to be injected through a thin cannula. The most relevant technical contribution in his study is the possibility of using Healon® GV to deepen the AC even in an eye from which the corneal button needing replacement has already been removed. For this purpose, Laflamme places Healon® GV in a ring shape under the recipient corneal ring, leaving the center relatively empty. Volker-Dieben and Balestrazzi came to similar conclusions. When using products with higher viscosity it is necessary to avoid excessive filling in the middle of the AC, as the clot of material formed may make suturing the flap difficult.

Preparing the Aphakic Eye

The aphakic eye presents special problems for penetrating keratoplasty. The reduced consistency of the globe due to the decreased volume of the vitreous body compared to the space available inside the eye causes normal anatomic relationships to fail once trephination is completed. Excessive hypertension collapses the iris diaphragm, along with that of the sclera and the peripheral corneal ring. Under these circumstances, correctly positioning

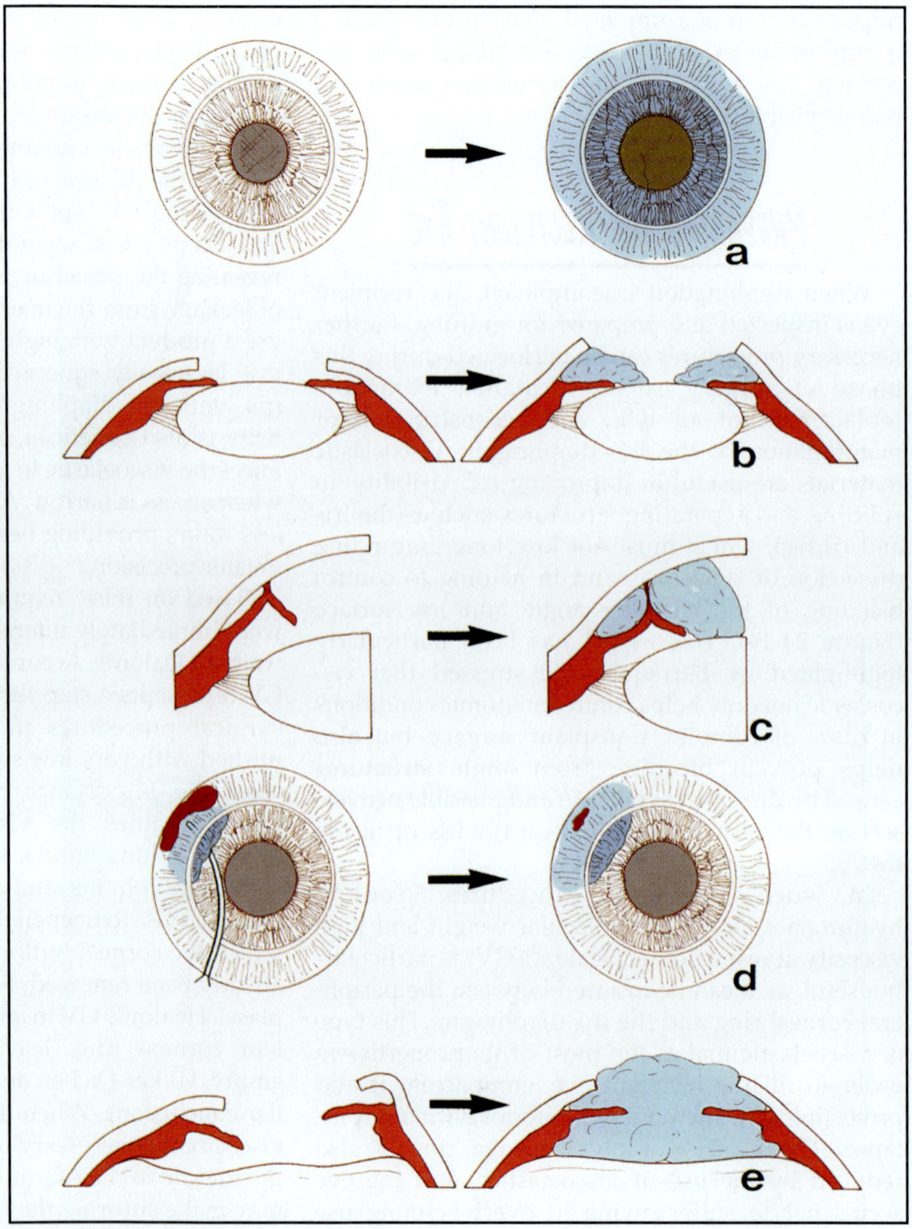

Figure 24-14. Usefulness of viscoelastics in preparing recipient eyes for grafting. (a) Increases visibility by relaxing transparent tissues. (b) Preserves space in both open and closed eyes if viscosity at rest is high. (c) Exposes synechiae, and allows the surgeon to better perceive distorted anatomy. (d) Prevents and stops bleeding. (e) Restores the volume and shape of aphakic eyes.

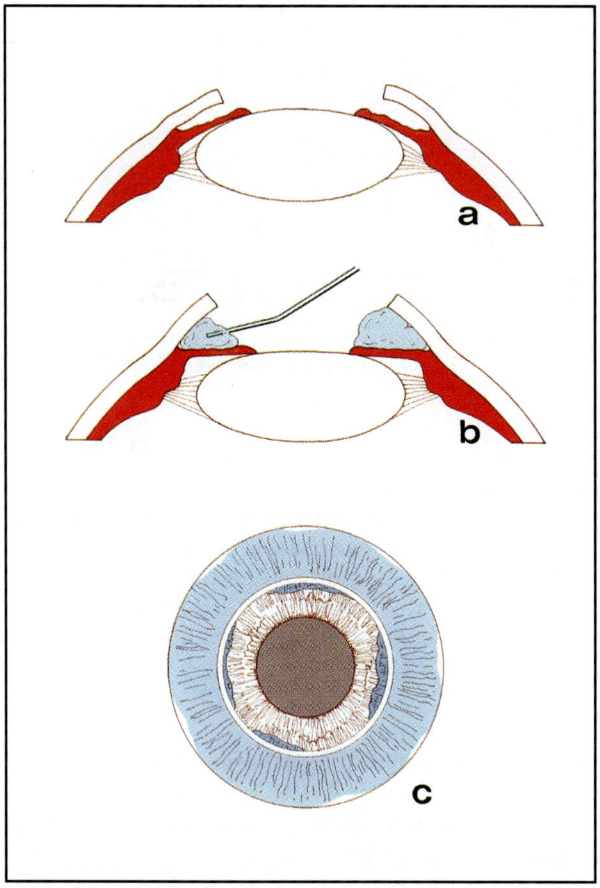

Figure 24-15. Maintaining space in open eyes. (a) Particularly in small eyes, posterior pressure may occur after trephination. (b) A viscoelastic product with high viscosity at rest may contribute to maintaining the space between cornea and iris, even in difficult conditions. (c) Laflamme suggests placing Healon® GV in a ring-like fashion under the peripheral portion of the cornea, but not in the middle of the AC.

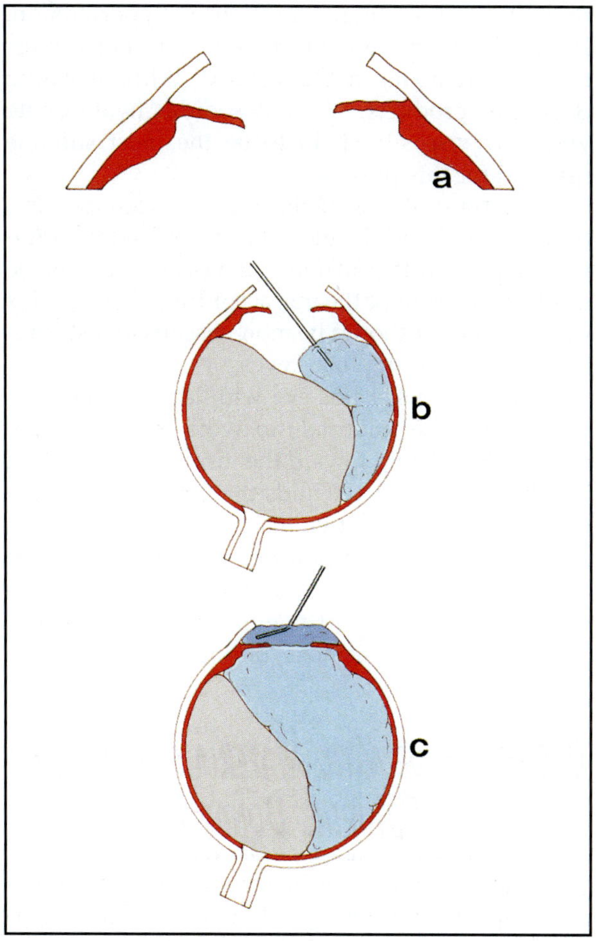

Figure 24-16. Maintaining space in aphakic eyes. (a) After trephination, the aphakic eye may appear hypotonic, with distorted anatomy. Applying a Flieringa ring is useful in these cases. (b) The vitreous chamber can also be filled with a viscoelastic with low viscosity at rest, which is less likely to cause postoperative hypertension. (c) After restoring soundness to the eye, the AC is filled with a viscoelastic having higher viscosity at rest, according to previously described methods. Most of this material must be removed at the end of surgery.

the donor flap—let alone suturing it—is impossible. In the past, attempts have been made to solve this problem with Flieringa ring. This metal ring, available in various diameters and shapes, is sutured to the prelimbal sclera, preventing collapse in the most important area for the grafting suture. Although sometimes invasive and not always effective, the method has become widely used.

More recently, viscoelastic materials have helped to solve problems with grafting in aphakic eyes, recalling viscoelastic's origin as a vitreous substitute (Figure 24-16). A collapsed aphakic eye can be filled with viscoelastic material, which occupies the available portions of the vitreous chamber and restores the soundness of the globe, with no need to apply Flieringa ring. It is necessary to use large amounts of product, which then drains from the eyeball through the chamber angle. The most appropriate material has sufficient viscosity at rest that it is not likely to cause hypertension. Pseudoplasticity and transparency are not important requirements in this context. Without ruling out other products, we find sodium hyaluronate with low viscosity (IAL) to be the most suitable material for this purpose.

Once the volume of the vitreous chamber has been restored and the globe has recovered its original shape, a different kind of viscoelastic can be used on the front of the iris, according to need. This second product should be more viscous at rest, similar to that used in phakic eyes.

In filling the aphakic eye with large amounts of viscoelastic, it is important to avoid creating a consistent flow of fluid toward the inside of a globe that is only partially filled. Fluids that have been in contact with the conjunctiva may seep inside the eye, and therefore risk transmitting infectious chemical and microbiologic compounds present in the conjunctival sac. In this instance the viscoelastic would act as a barrier against toxic or infectious agents.

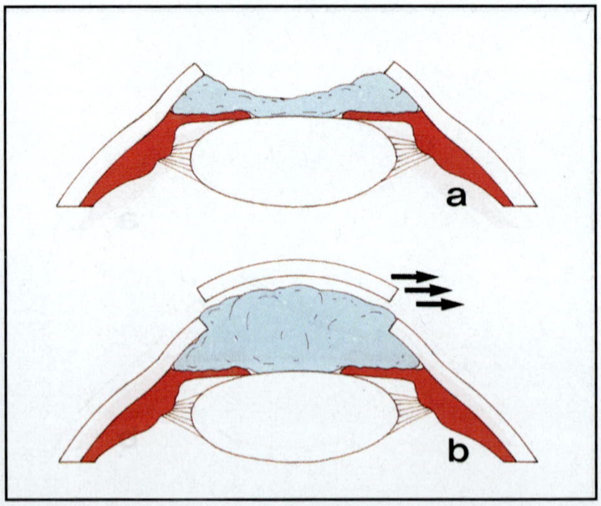

Figure 24-17. Amount of viscoelastic used in penetrating keratoplasty. (a) Viscoelastic inserted in the AC before positioning the donor button must not completely fill it in its middle area. (b) Excessive filling may allow the limbus to shift after placement.

Use of Viscoelastic Materials in Placing and Suturing Donor Flaps

Positioning and suturing the donor flap are the core steps of keratoplasty, taking most of the surgical time in uncomplicated interventions, such as keratoconus surgery. The procedure starts with checking, and adjusting if necessary, the amount of viscoelastic in the center of the AC. The material should fill the AC without reaching the upper rim of corneal trephination. The step formed between the epithelial surface of the recipient cornea and the viscoelastic surface will enable the donor flap to stay in place during the early phases of provisional suturing (Figure 24-17). At this point the donor flap is lifted from its support with a "hollowed jaw" forceps, like a Pierse–Hoskins forceps. The endothelial surface is generally covered with a certain amount of viscoelastic. This amount must not be excessive, to prevent the flap from sliding on the viscoelastic layer, as previously stated.

While the graft is positioned and sutured, the viscoelastic acts as a cushion on which the surgeon can lay the endothelial side of the flap, making sure that cells are protected. The viscoelastic prevents the donor flap from falling inside the AC of the recipient eye where the suture is applied. In addition, it reduces endothelial trauma due to movements of the flap during application of cardinal stitches (Figure 24-18).

The first suture is placed at 12 o'clock. This must not be too tight, or it will be difficult to apply further stitches properly. The AC should not contain an overwhelming amount of viscoelastic, to ensure there is no uncomfortable lifting of the lower portion of the corneal graft. The second suture is placed at 6 o'clock, with care taken to check that it is centered when the needle is still threaded through both the donor and recipient corneas. Should the donor tissue be asymmetrically toward the left or right, the needle can be retracted and passed through again in the proper position with no difficulty. This step is important for the successful outcome of keratoplasty, and is rather difficult to perform when no viscoelastic is used (Fig 24-19). Sutures at 3 and 9 o'clock are placed at the end.

During all these procedures the endothelium of the donor cornea rests on the viscoelastic layer, which protects it from contact with the other intraocular structures owing to forces that may develop both inside the eye (posterior pressure) and from outside (movements by the surgeon or assistant). Particularly in the last phases of suturing, an

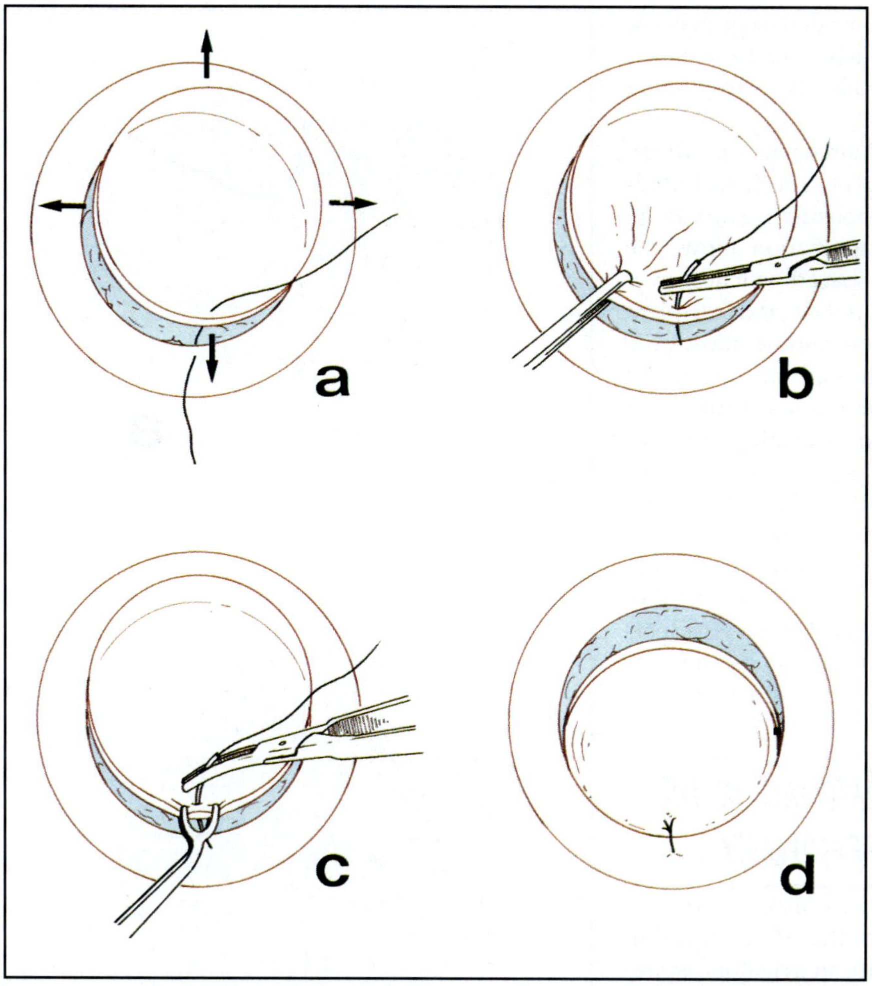

Figure 24-18. Suturing the donor flap in the recipient bed. (a) If the cushion of viscoelastic is too high, the donor flap may move while cardinal sutures are being applied. (b) Using a Pierse–Hoskins one-tooth forceps while applying early sutures can create folds in the corneal stroma. (c) A Polack's double forceps allows placement of cardinal stitches without creating tissue folds. (d) If there is too much viscoelastic, the distal portion of the donor button lifts greatly once the first stitch has been applied.

insufficiently sharp needle may cause distortions of the corneal tissue, with consequent development of forces directed toward the AC. A highly viscous viscoelastic, such as sodium hyaluronate with high molecular weight, is very useful here owing to its resistance to deformation under direct pressure. Nevertheless, the endothelial protection provided by the material during these procedures may be incomplete, as products such as Healon® and Healon® GV, which have high molecular weight and high internal cohesion, may transmit tangent forces that have been shown to be harmful. In any case, the formation of folds on the corneal stroma during this phase leads to endothelial cell loss even in the presence of a viscoelastic.

Studies on the use of sodium hyaluronate with low molecular weight have been conducted mainly in Italy. In 1987, Fruscella et al first reported using IAL in keratoplasty in the framework of a wider study of anterior segment surgery. In that study, conducted on 19 eyes, researchers found that IAL was helpful in keratoplasty, with the only inconvenience being that it required frequent reinjection owing to its tendency to leak out of the AC when large corneal openings were present. About 0.2 mL of IAL was left in the AC at the end of surgery, with no subsequent complications.

The application of definitive suturing completes keratoplasty. In uncomplicated cases, 10-0 nylon antitorsion suture mounted on a 6-mm–3/8 circle needle is perfect. A separate-stitch suture—always 10-0 nylon—is preferable when there is suspicion that the donor or recipient parenchyma may not be resistant, or when rejection or tissue necrosis are short-term threats. As in the completion of trephination, while placing sutures, the viscoelastic level in the AC is replenished when needed to protect the donor endothelium continuously and to separate the iris–lens diaphragm from the area being sutured (Figure 24-20).

Working with the AC full of viscoelastic is advantageous not only for prevention of synechiae, but for better suturing. Correctly juxtaposing tissues along the whole circumference of trephination allows the surgeon to apply regularly spaced stitches over 360°. Partly lifting both the donor and recipient cornea without losing chamber volume allows the surgeon to pass the needle through at exactly the depth desired. Placing the continuous suture with controlled IOP prevents it from becoming too tight postoperatively, which causes myopia, or too loose, causing hyperopia. In particular cases, it is even possible to make use of suture tension and flap dimensions to influence postoperative refraction. All this means better suturing, with greater stability of the AC and fewer corneal defects in the postoperative period. Fewer corneal defects also mean fewer tissue (stromal) folds and reduced astigmatism.

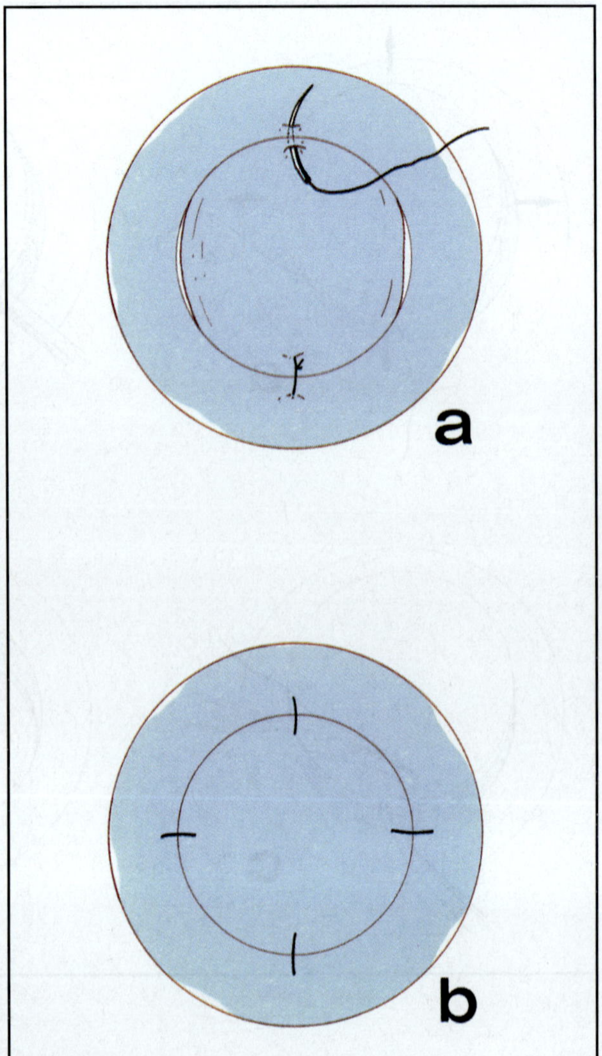

Figure 24-19. Suturing the donor flap in the recipient bed (continued). (a) The surgeon checks the centering of the flap with the suture needle halfway through the site at 6 o'clock. The viscoelastic occupying the AC helps expose possible misalignment, which is corrected by retracting the needle and replacing the suture. (b) When cardinal sutures have been placed, the donor flap lays on a cushion of viscoelastic, which can be correctly sagittally positioned, to prevent tissue footholds from forming in the suture area.

Use of Viscoelastic Materials in the Last Phases of Keratoplasty

At the end of surgery, the viscoelastic is removed as completely as possible from the AC with a thin cannula. We generally do not use an irrigator/aspirator such as the kind used for cataract surgery, in order to avoid exerting any sort of strain on the suture. Instead, we use Sauter's 26-G cannulas, aspirating the viscoelastic little by little, restoring the volume each time with BSS. Here pseudoplasticity is mandatory, because to accomplish this task one should not use a cannula exceeding 25 G. The procedure can be difficult owing to the risk of iris and lens lesions, particularly in the presence of posterior pressure. Should it be impossible to replace the viscoelastic with BSS due to imperfect tightness of the AC, air can be used, although the effects on the corneal endothelium will be more traumatic. If an AC does not hold its shape after air injection, sutures must be repositioned.

Often, total removal of the viscoelastic is too invasive and potentially traumatic. In this case the surgeon leaves a small amount of viscoelastic inside the eye. This residual viscoelastic has some positive effect, as it promotes total tightness of corneal suture and prevents possible microfiltrations (Figure 24-21).

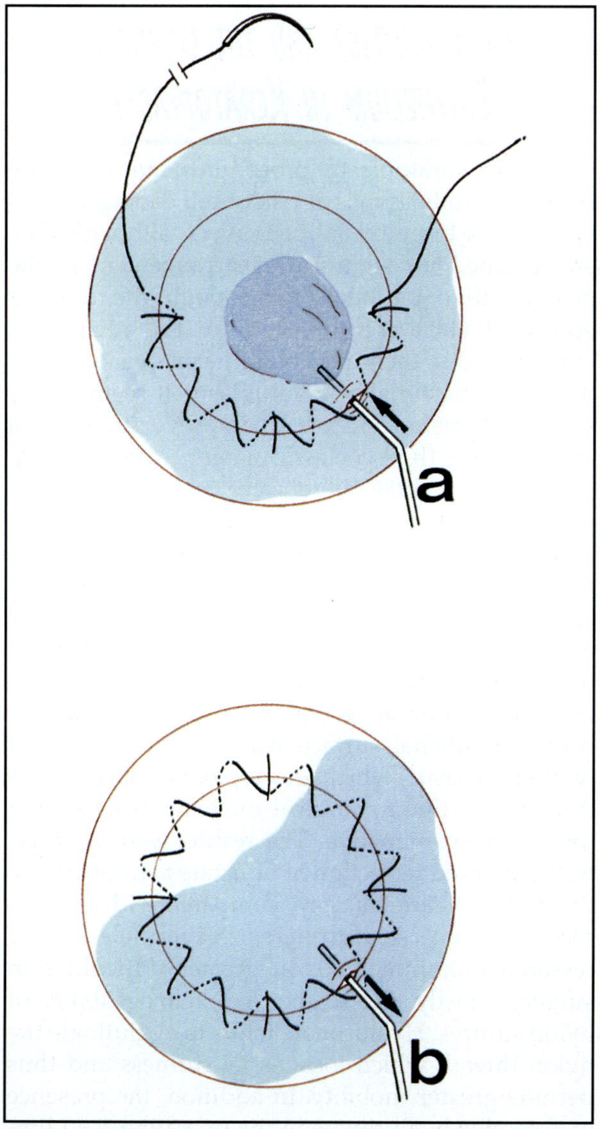

Figure 24-20. Suturing the donor flap in the recipient bed (continued). (a) Any viscoelastic lost during the application of continuous sutures or detached stitches is replenished. Two or three reinjections are usually sufficient if the product used has adequate viscosity at rest. (b) At the end of the suture, the viscoelastic is removed as completely as possible from the AC and replaced with BSS.

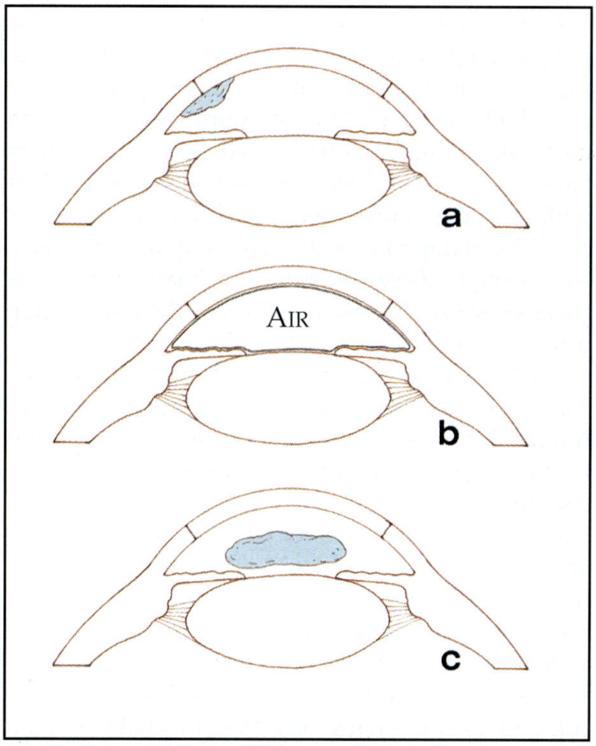

Figure 24-21. Final phases of keratoplasty. (a) A certain amount of viscoelastic remaining in the AC at the end of surgery may help tissues adhere in the area of trephination. A viscoadherent product is the most appropriate here. (b) Air can also maintain the AC, but is more traumatic to the corneal endothelium. (c) According to Barraquer, Lischetti, and Dal Fiume, if a small central cushion of viscoelastic has been placed in the center of the AC, it can be left in the site.

Conversely, the same viscoelastic may increase IOP, a dangerous event after penetrating keratoplasty. This hypertension may be particularly prevalent when sodium hyaluronate with high molecular weight has been used. Some researchers have suggested using viscoelastics only moderately while placing sutures, as they believe removing it could be dangerous to the endothelium and lens. According to these researchers, a small layer of viscoelastic should be used just under the grafted flap during suturing (see Figure 24-21).

This seems to confirm research by Polack in the early 1980s. His study aimed to define tolerance to intraocular viscoelastic injection, determining whether the material had a protective effect on the endothelium of the grafted flap and assessing its effects on postoperative IOP. He injected 30 phakic and pseudophakic eyes with 0.2 cc of Healon® in front of the iris plane prior to suturing the flap. No other viscoelastic was added, whereas the AC was deepened with BSS when necessary during or after suturing. The results were compared with the outcome in eyes receiving BSS only. In phakic eyes, a greater amount of Healon® was injected in the vitreous cavity and AC after vitrectomy. The results showed that Healon® eased the performance of surgical procedures, particularly in aphakic and pseudophakic eyes. Compared with the eyes receiving only BSS, in the Healon® eyes the flap showed better transparency and less thickness in the postoperative period. Ocular hypertension was observed in only one patient, who had received 4 cc of Healon®.

Experimental studies on the pharmacologic effects of sodium hyaluronate remaining in the AC at the end of surgery have achieved controversial results. In 1986, Babin noted that in cat eyes the process of rejection was somehow limited by sodium hyaluronate, a rather interesting effect that was not confirmed by further studies. In 1991, Shimizu conducted a study on the effects of sodium hyaluronate remaining in the AC after cataract surgery, and found that it had a negative effect on the integrity of the blood–aqueous barrier as measured by the flare meter laser. The importance of these studies to corneal surgery has yet to be confirmed.

At present, we can state that, at least in keratoplasty, the advantages provided by the use of viscoelastic materials are far more numerous than the drawbacks.

Viscoelastics and the Corneal Epithelium in Keratoplasty

During keratoplasty procedures, not only the corneal endothelium is at risk of cell damage. Stress also occurs to epithelial cell layers, although they are destined for significant rearrangement in the postoperative period. Even though the donor's epithelial cells are replaced by the recipient's epithelial cells, their quality influences vision in the day immediately after keratoplasty. It seemed reasonable, therefore, to try to improve the corneal epithelium with viscoelastic materials after surgery.

Already in 1986 there were reports about the positive effects of sodium hyaluronate on epithelial regeneration processes after keratoplasty as well as reports of negative effects, although indirect. Reed et al conducted a study to determine whether continued application of 1% sodium hyaluronate on the corneal epithelium during grafting leads to quicker postoperative epithelial regeneration. The corneal epithelial surface was constantly covered with viscoelastic, which was replenished as soon as it dispersed due to surgical movements or sliding toward the conjunctiva. The results were positive, with a marked reduction of punctate keratopathy in the first week after surgery compared with controls receiving no hyaluronate. Nevertheless, the researchers commented on greater difficulties in surgery, mostly due to the poor manageability of nylon sutures. Hyaluronate tends to agglutinate the nylon thread, which loosens its stiffness and thus permits greater mobility. In addition, the presence of excessive hyaluronate in the operating field limited the perception of depth through the surgical microscope (Figure 24-22). Later on, Nishida (1991) and Inoue (1993) confirmed that hyaluronate promoted epithelial proliferation.

It remains to be confirmed whether a product with lower molecular weight can reduce surgical problems without reducing the benefit to the corneal epithelium. A product such as this would leave the cornea more rapidly and would therefore require frequent reapplication. However, hyaluronate mixed with a small quantity of fluorescein would remain stable and even increase the perception of depth during suturing.

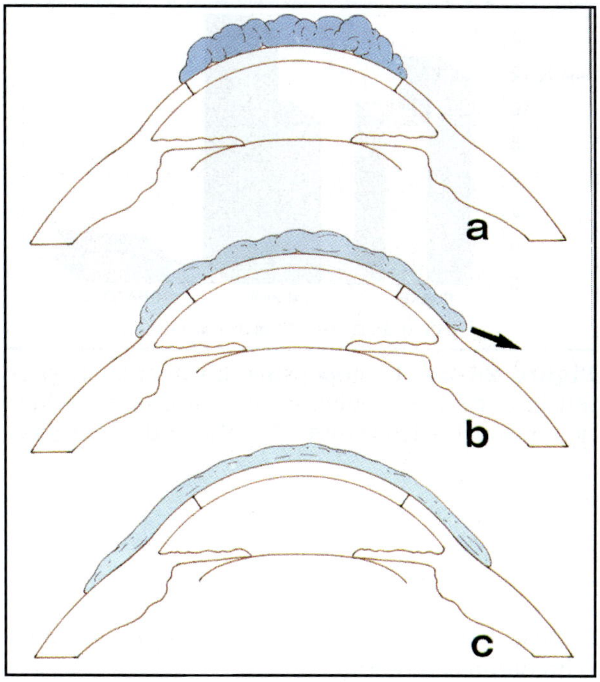

Figure 24-22. Viscoelastics and the corneal epithelium in keratoplasty. (a) Sodium hyaluronate with high molecular weight on the cornea improves the physiology of epithelial cells, but makes managing nylon sutures difficult and reduces visibility of the corneal thickness. (b) Sodium hyaluronate with low molecular weight is more quickly cleared away owing to its poor viscosity at rest, but causes less decrease in visibility. (c) A viscoadherent product may be useful in endothelial protection.

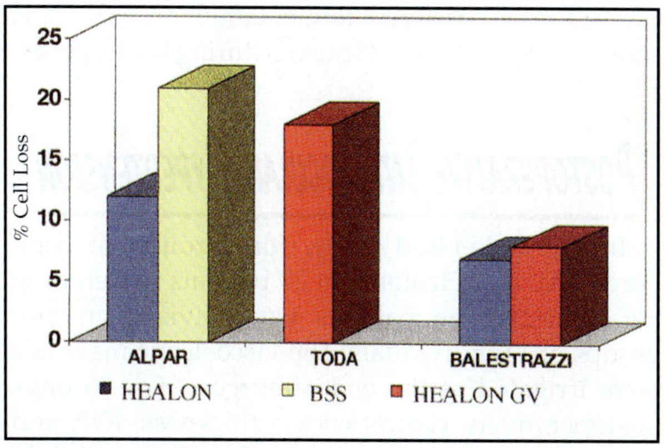

Figure 24-23. Rates of endothelial cell loss after keratoplasty (measured on donor flap).

ENDOTHELIAL CELL PROTECTION PROVIDED BY VARIOUS VISCOELASTICS DURING KERATOPLASTY

In the late 1980s, studies were performed on the results of using Healon® in keratoplasty based on endothelial cell physiology parameters—more refined standards than simple cell counts. Researchers started with the assumption that a thin layer of sodium hyaluronate would adhere to endothelial cells for quite some time, as it bonds to receptors that seem specifically suited for hyaluronate. In 1988, Bazard et al examined a group of 50 eyes undergoing keratoplasty using a specular microscope, among which were 26 that had been surgically treated with the support of Healon®. The researchers assessed the morphology of endothelial cells through a computerized system providing information about the shape and size of each single cell. The outcome emphasized that using the viscoelastic not only led to improved cell count, but also protected normal cell morphology (Figure 24-23).

Another study was published by Toda et al in 1993, who used Healon® GV in 13 eyes receiving keratoplasty. They noted that its high viscosity was greatly helpful in cutting synechiae and in preventing leakage out of the AC during the application of continued sutures following the four cardinal stitches. Postoperative cell count showed a cell loss equal to nearly 18%. The study also reported data on IOP, which remained below 20 mmHg. However, the product was removed at the end of surgery, and all patients were treated with carbonic anhydrase inhibitors in the days immediately following. The researchers concluded that Healon® GV was as safe as Healon® for keratoplasty.

Sodium hyaluronate produced by bacterial fermentation is similar to cockscomb, with a formula similar to Healon®. It was used by Katoh et al to perform keratoplasty in 1992. Researchers observed postoperative endothelial cell density, the cell morphology index, and the amount of cell loss every 3 months after surgery. This showed that the crucial period for endothelial cell loss is between 6 and 9 months after surgery. No differences emerged in the eyes treated with cockscomb-derived hyaluronate and those receiving hyaluronate produced by bacterial fermentation. Researchers concluded that in the preparations they used, the sodium hyaluronate derived from bacterial fermentation provided the same cell protection as Healon® during keratoplasty.

Postoperative Intraocular Hypertension

In a double-blind study, Tomazzoli et al compared IAL and Healon® in 28 patients undergoing keratoplasty. The patients were divided in two groups of 14 individuals. The viscoelastic materials were irrigated at the end of surgery. For 90 days postoperatively, central cornea thickness, IOP, and AC depth were studied. Healon® achieved slightly better, although not statistically significant, values in IOP and AC depth (Figure 24-24).

An interesting comparison of Viscoat and Healon® in keratoplasty was published by Burke et al in 1990. In a group of 62 patients, 31 received Viscoat and 31 Healon®. Neither material was irrigated at the end of surgery. The investigation primarily observed IOP, but in addition found no other complications related to the use of Viscoat. The results concerning IOP are rather interesting, as viscoelastic materials were never allowed to fill the AC of operated eyes after keratoplasty. The researchers did not observe significant differences between the two products; both led to an increase in IOP that even exceeded 40 mmHg in several cases, despite hypotensive treatments administered in each eye having a pressure over 30 mmHg. The only difference was that after 24 hours the Viscoat-treated eyes had recovered their original pressure, whereas the Healon®-treated eyes required longer. Researchers also concluded that Viscoat requires irrigation at the end of surgery, as it appeared to affect IOP after keratoplasty.

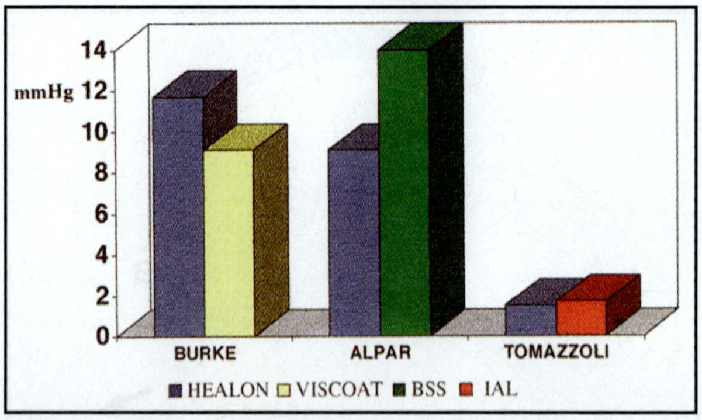

Figure 24-24. Postoperative intraocular hypertension after keratoplasty with various viscoelastics. Viscoelastics removed at the end of surgery.

Keratoplasty Combined With Other Surgical Procedures

Keratoplasty requires a larger opening of the eye's surface than is usual in other types of ophthalmic surgery. All surgical treatments possibly required are worth performing during keratoplasty, after completing recipient cornea trephination. Such procedures may involve the anterior segment (cataract extraction, IOL implantation, iris surgery, reconstruction surgery) and the posterior segment (vitreoretinal surgery).

Keratoplasty Combined With Cataract Extraction Surgery

When correctly performed, keratoplasty may have a negligible risk of causing cataracts, which is why it is not advisable to remove the transparent lens during the main intervention. Nevertheless, cornea grafting is often performed in the eyes of aged patients that already show some lens opacity. In these patients, such opacity may increase as a result of the biochemical decompensation following AC surgery, due to aging or to the administration of common postoperative medications. Cataract surgery performed in eyes previously treated with keratoplasty has the long-term risk of endothelial damage that may induce decompensation of the grafted flap. There is also the remote possibility that careless surgical movements during keratoplasty may eventually cause lens capsule lesions, thus requiring immediate cataract removal. These risks plus the excellent visual rehabilitation provided by IOLs have led to more frequent cataract extractions combined with corneal grafting. Several obstacles particular to the era of intracapsular surgery, when postoperative intraocular conditions after cataract extraction were less controlled, have vanished. Current implant surgery, for example, maintains almost unchanged anatomic characteristics in the iris/lens diaphragm.

Procedures associated with keratoplasty and cataract extraction were also improved by the advent of viscoelastic materials. Polack has published two reports on the viscosurgical results achieved with Healon® in such eyes. The cases he considered include 60 eyes treated with threefold procedure, 13 eyes implanted with an AC IOL, 25 pseudophakic eyes in which the IOL was replaced during keratoplasty, and 65 eyes that received no IOL. The results of these keratoplasty interventions were reported to be excellent, significantly better than those formerly achieved in the same types of surgery without viscoelastic materials. Alpar considered a more limited number of eyes and came to the same conclusion, although he studied endothelial cell count.

Cataract extraction is accomplished during keratoplasty with methods that are both similar to and different from the usual procedures. The main difference lies in the lack of pressure in the AC, which makes several usual procedures invalid. The large opening made by trephination is certainly favorable, but the need to work through it with instruments designed to operate through the limbus may create some difficulty (Figure 24-25).

Capsulorhexis

Once trephination has been completed, anterior capsulotomy can be performed by capsulorhexis, which aims to ensure correct IOL implantation in the capsular bag. In this phase great attention must be paid to the possible presence of posterior pressure, which is difficult to oppose due to trephination. It is therefore better to perform capsulorhexis in small dimensions, to prevent the uncontrolled capsulorhexis from jeopardizing zonular integrity. Particularly in young patients, whose capsule is very elastic and who most frequently have a posterior pressure, the rhexis should start with a very small diameter, even just 4 mm. Generally, no viscoelastics are used in this phase, to allow the surgeon to see both the capsular flap to be gripped and the progression of capsulorhexis. The best visibility is achieved when the capsule is in contact with the air, thus allowing an easier rhexis even in very mature cataracts.

A viscoelastic is useful if capsulorhexis starts to escape toward the periphery, under the recipient peripheral corneal ring. In this case, progress can be restored with a highly viscous material such as Healon® GV, which can be applied in the space between the recipient cornea and the lens with some hope of exerting posterior pressure. Product transparency must be perfect, even though its irregular surface due to the presence of trephination greatly limits visibility in the working field. In open eye capsulorhexis, perfect control of the pressure exterted by posterior structures toward the anterior segment of the eyeball is essential. Because the patient is often anesthetized, the surgeon can rely on the anesthetist for particular conditions of muscle relaxation and arterial hypotension. When the patient is under local anesthesia difficulties are greater, and the possibility of controlling posterior push decreases. If it is impossible to complete capsulorhexis owing to an uncontrolled cut escaping toward the periphery, there is no need to transform it into a can-opener capsulotomy, as advised for cataract surgery. In fact, here the anterior segment will not push toward the vitreous chamber, and the risk of breaking the posterior capsule and scattering lens fragments into the vitreous is rather low. A can-opener capsulotomy should be made only when the posterior pressure is so strong that it causes the posterior capsule to break and the vitreous to invade the operating field, which is exceptionally rare.

Hydrodissection and Viscoexpression

When capsulorhexis is completed, hydrodissection is usually performed. This procedure must be particularly light to avoid premature luxation of the nucleus inside the AC. The nucleus itself is then rotated to ensure its mobility; only then can it be extracted from the capsular bag. The most convenient extraction method is viscoexpression, which consists of inserting a thin cannula under the nuclear periphery at any location on the circumference, then injecting the viscoelastic until the nuclear portion is lifted and then engaged through capsulorhexis. After engaging the equator, the injection of viscoelastic is continued, pushing the whole nucleus outside the capsular bag. The dimensions of the nucleus and its slightly vertical position ease its further passage through corneal trephination to complete removal.

Viscoexpression appears to be preferable to hydroexpression owing to the reduced trauma caused by the cannula injecting the viscoelastic on the posterior capsule. In this case, the most impor-

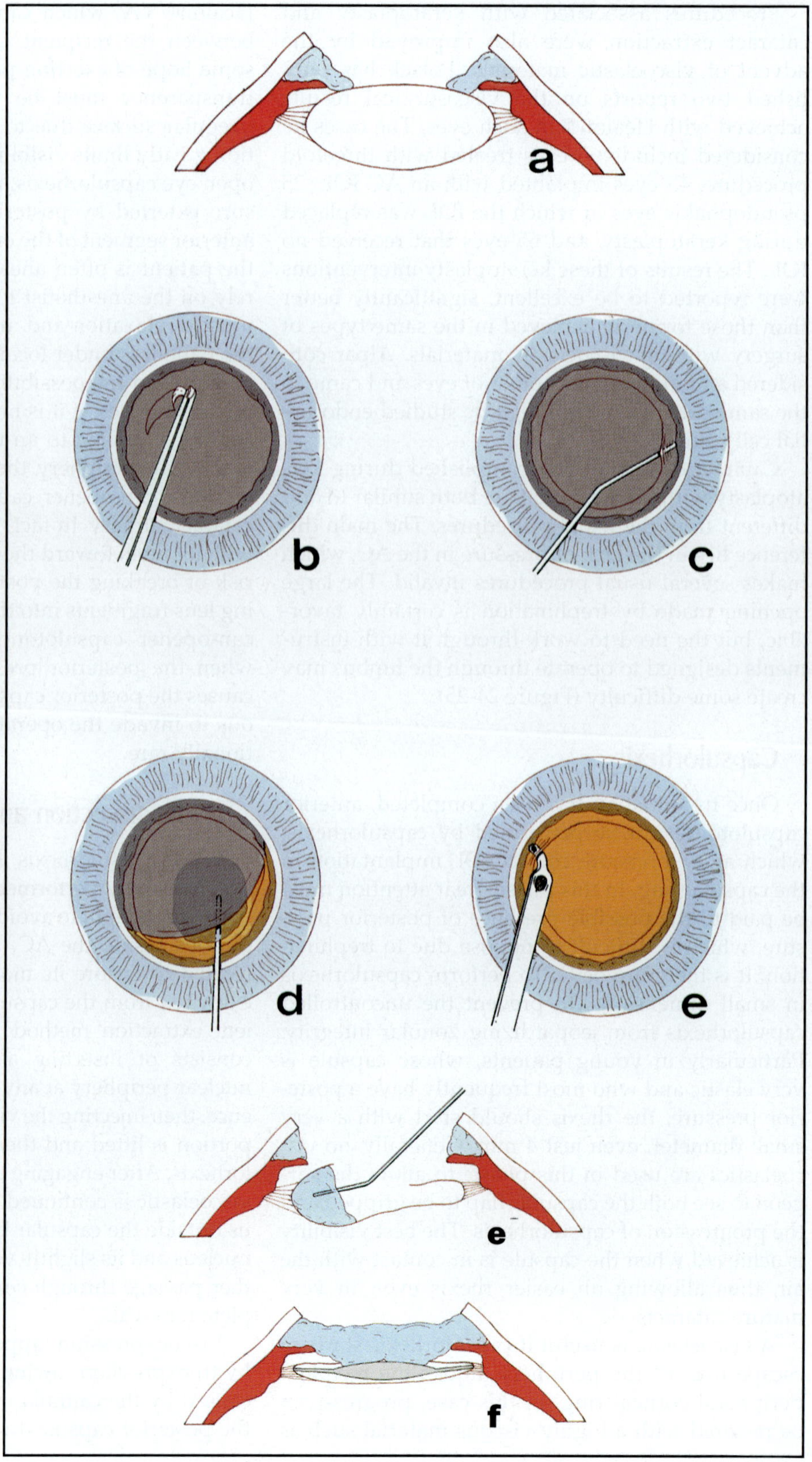

Figure 24-25. Cataract extraction during penetrating keratoplasty. (a) Before capsulorhexis, the viscoelastic may be placed under the corneal ring peripheral to trephination. (b) During open eye capsulorhexis, the rhexis is likely to escape control due to the posterior pressure. A viscoelastic with high viscosity placed under the peripheral cornea keeps the AC deep and opposes uncontrolled capsulorhexis. (c) The capsulorhexis is best made narrower, in order to improve the effectiveness of hydrodissection. (d) Viscoexpression of the nucleus is perhaps the best procedure to extract a cataract during keratoplasty. The nucleus luxated in the AC then emerges through the trephination hole. (e) Irrigation and aspiration procedures are complicated by adherence of the anterior and the posterior capsule, which occurs when the AC remains open. This can only be reduced by using an adhesive viscoelastic with high viscosity. (f) When residual masses have been removed, the capsular bag is reformed. (g) The most appropriate IOL is a capsular implant with 6.5 mm or larger optic and an overall length of 12.5 mm.

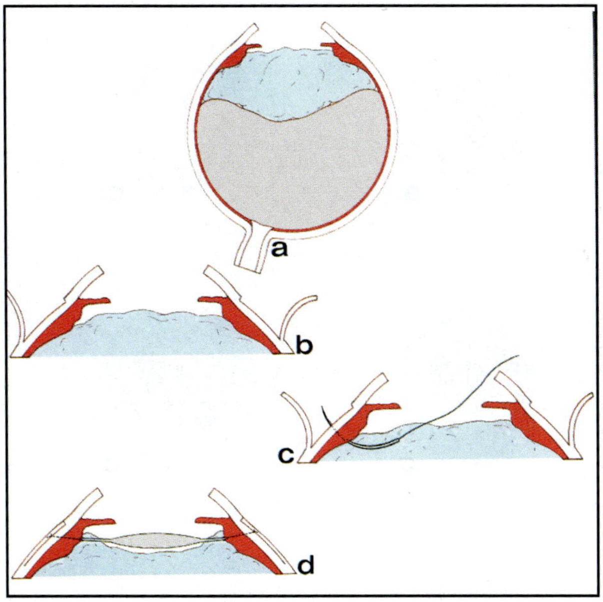

Figure 24-26. Implanting IOL with scleral fixation during penetrating keratoplasty. (a) Scleral fixation of an IOL starts with an extensive posterior vitrectomy, which allows replacement of the anterior vitreous with viscoelastic. (b) Two scleral ports are prepared near the limbus at 2 and 8 o'clock. When scleral fixation of the IOL is planned in the surgical plane, it is best to prepare the ports before performing corneal trephination. (c) The prolene suture that will support the lens is passed from the inside to the outside, to ensure that it passes through the ocular wall corresponding to the ciliary sulcus. (d) At the end of the procedure, the portion of the lens fixed to the sclera is the one usual for this type of implant.

tant requirement of the viscoelastic is good pseudoplasticity, which permits injection through a thin cannula. The cannula must be bent by the surgeon in a particular way, with a sharp bend at the tip, as traditional cannulas designed to work through the limbus are not suitable.

Irrigation and Aspiration and Implantation

Irrigation and aspiration of the residual mass concludes this part of surgery. It is slightly more difficult than usual, as it is accomplished in an open eye. The peripheral flap of the anterior capsule sticks immediately to the posterior capsule, and there is no possibility of separating them, as in standard interventions. On the other hand, the visibility of residual masses is generally good and difficulties of subincisional residual cortex are no greater.

The procedure requires catching and removing each single mass present in the capsulorhexis field, as it is not possible to rely on the aqueous flows to direct them toward the aspiration port. Keeping the irrigation and aspiration tip as tangent as possible to the posterior capsule, the aspiration tip must be slipped under the rim of capsulorhexis to remove equatorial masses. Because there is no actual surgical space between the two flaps, parts of the capsule are very easily trapped during this procedure, causing frequent interruption of aspiration.

When the irrigation and aspiration of equatorial masses is completed, the surgeon inspects the integrity of the capsular bag, then prepares to inject it with viscoelastic. The material is first injected inside the peripheral space between the anterior and posterior capsule to form a ring-shaped cushion, which keeps the bag open. A certain amount of viscoelastic is also placed in the middle of the posterior capsule, to encourage the IOL to slide and rotate. For these eyes we prefer using a lens with a large optic diameter, and haptics shaped for implantation in the bag (capsular lenses). It is generally placed without difficulty. When the capsular bag is intact, the IOL is implanted in it; otherwise, it is placed in the ciliary sulcus. In the latter case we use a slightly larger lens suitable for implantation in the sulcus.

Keratoplasty Combined With IOL Implantation Without Capsule Support

When no support for the artificial lens is available, the implant can be suspended from the sclera or fixed to the iris with sutures that pierce the iris tissue while surrounding the lens haptics. This method of iris fixation differs only in a few details from that accomplished through the limbus.

The posterior vitrectomy must be very extensive. The space free of vitreous is filled with a viscoelastic as densely as possible. Sutures are best placed in the presence of corneal trephination from the inside toward the outside of the eyeball, using small needles introduced in the posterior chamber through the trephination (Figure 24-26). The pupil usually shrinks a bit during the passage of the threads supporting the lens. The lens can then be placed with the optic side in the AC and the haptics in the posterior chamber while stitches are definitively fixed and closed.

A valid alternative to scleral fixation, applied only in keratoplasty, is suturing the IOL to the iris. This surgical technique is performed after achieving pupillary miosis, which allows the surgeon to lay the IOL safely onto the iris, placing the haptics in the posterior chamber. The IOLs of choice have an optic zone of 5.5 mm and the haptics radially separated from the optic body, making the passage of stitches through the iris much easier (Figure 24-27).

The optic zone is then grasped with a McPherson forceps, and lightly lifted so that the haptics to be fixed are visible through the indented iris. At this point, the haptics can be fixed with a suture that clasps it through the iris immediately outside the optic zone. The same procedure is repeated to place the second haptic. These procedures require using viscoelastic materials to stop possible small hemorrhages and to move the blood away from the operating field. The iris is likely to bleed or to go over the haptics, thus hindering its proper visualization. Whenever visibility is reduced, the injection of transparent viscoelastic restores optimal conditions.

In the past, performing implantation in the AC during keratoplasty when no capsular support was available was also recommended. Such an operating choice is no longer justified, owing to high endothelial risks related to AC implantation and to the availability of improved techniques for iris or scleral fixation in the posterior chamber. During keratoplasty, most surgeons replace the IOL present in the AC with one in the posterior chamber. Should the surgeon decide to keep the implant in the AC, great care must be taken that a proper viscoelastic layer fills the AC during placement and suturing of the donor flap.

Removing Lens From the AC

Removing a lens from the AC, in particular an angle fixation lens, is a complex procedure, even when performed in an open eye. The haptics are almost always surrounded by strong iris-angular synechiae, and the traction exerted is likely to cause the iris to bleed and dilate, which hinders the following surgical steps. The procedure usually followed in these cases is to prepare the AC operating field with vitrectomy in front of and behind the IOL

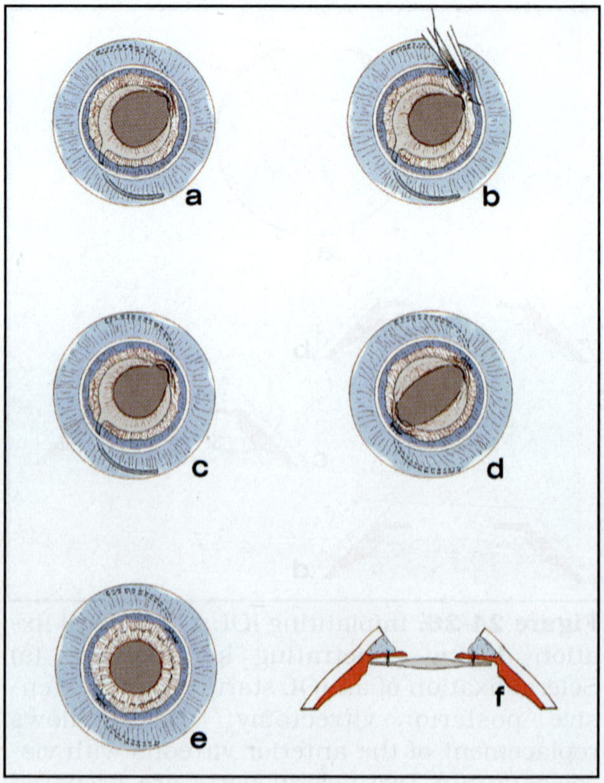

Figure 24-27. Implanting an IOL with iris fixation during penetrating keratoplasty. (a) With corneal trephination, it is easier to fix the IOL to the iris instead of the sclera. It is best to use a self-centering phaco lens, with 5.5 mm optics and loops starting from the optic with a straight angle. The lens is placed on the iris with a small pupil. The loop to be fixed first is passed under the iris. (b) The loop under the iris is sutured by grasping it through the iris with a Pierse–Hoskins hollow forceps, then passing the stitch through, including the loop and the overlying iris tissue. Viscoelastic is very useful to control minor bleeding and to stretch the iris tissue when required. (c) The first stitch is tightened in its site. IOLs with 6.5 or 7 mm optics or with a loop starting tangentially make these procedures very difficult, as the surgeon must then work under the peripheral corneal ring. (d) The second loop is put under the iris, and the optic zone of the lens remains in front of the iris with the small pupil. Now the second loop can be sutured without letting the lens fall into the vitreous. (e) Both iris sutures are in site. The optical body of the lens is placed in the posterior chamber. (f) Cross-section of the finished intervention.

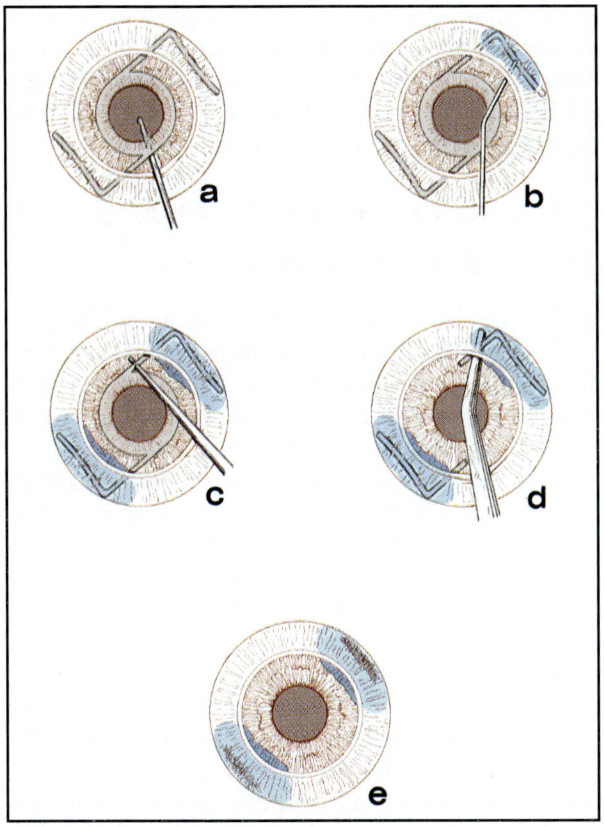

Figure 24-28. Removing AC IOL through trephination during penetrating keratoplasty. (a) The intervention starts with a vitrectomy performed without irrigation, in front of and behind the lens. (b) The peripheral portions of the AC are filled with a viscoelastic having high viscosity at rest. (c) The loops are cut and the optic zone is removed. (d) Protected by the viscoelastic, the loops are slipped off from the synechiae and removed. Minor bleeding and localized iris dialysis may occur. (e) Once the IOL has been removed, the viscoelastic allows the surgeon to assess any damage to the iris.

(Figure 24-28). Vitrectomy should be as complete as possible, keeping irrigation to a bare minimum for mobilizing and extracting vitreous strands with the vitrector. The loops can then be separated from the surrounding tissue with a highly dense viscoelastic.

This procedure allows the surgeon to excise the loops with the special cutter and remove the lens optics first. Further viscoelastic is injected in the chamber angle, corresponding to the supports. These supports must be inspected to confirm their shape when this information is not available preoperatively. The best way to remove lens supports is to draw them out as lightly as possible, adding viscoelastics at each step for better visibility and to minimize iris damage. Any damage to the iris may cause bleeding and jeopardize the ensuing IOL fixation in the posterior chamber. Restoring possible iris dialysis is essential and can be accomplished by suturing the tissue with 10-0 prolene.

Sodium hyaluronate viscoelastics with high molecular weight are basic to the performance of this procedure. They dilate the spaces where surgery will take place; increase the visibility of angle structures, often jeopardized by reduced corneal transparency; and help reposition twisted or even lacerated iris tissue, enabling the surgeon to see the anatomic relationships clearly during the procedure. Once the lens has been removed from the AC, the viscoelastic allows the surgeon to inspect the region behind the iris to check for the presence of capsular residues, as usually occurs during IOL replacement surgery not combined with keratoplasty.

KERATOPLASTY IN THE PRESENCE OF AN ULCER OR PENETRATING WOUND

In the past, wounds penetrating the cornea caused severe loss of vision, as they were repaired without the use of a surgery microscope or viscoelastic materials. A large number of these traumas do not require primary cornea transplant; therefore, we will focus on them more thoroughly in the chapter devoted to trauma. Nevertheless, sometimes the wound is so severe that it requires immediate keratoplasty, owing to lack of tissue or to the particular behavior of the wound. Wound lines involving the cornea and extending to the sclera are the most problematic, as they often cause bleeding.

If an ulcer or wound perforates the whole corneal thickness, the main difficulty is that the AC has collapsed and therefore standard trephination cannot be performed. In the past, complicated procedures were used to solve the problem, sometimes requiring the use of an air pump to maintain the depth of the AC. Viscoelastic materials provided a simpler and more effective solution.

The procedure to repair a corneal wound with keratoplasty starts with an wound suture using10-0 nylon, made while respecting the normal structure of the cornea. When there has been no tissue loss, the cornea can generally be well reconstructed. When tissue loss has occurred, the surgeon must postpone restoring normal corneal structure and keep the area where trephine suction will be applied as untouched as possible, in case it can be used.

A viscoelastic product is always used to repair corneal wounds (Figure 24-29). For instance, Healon® GV can be injected into the AC through the ulcer or the wound, even when it has already been sutured. Owing to its very high viscosity at 0 shear rate, it can keep the chamber deep, keep intraocular structures far from the site of trephination, and restore the consistency of the globe while limiting bleeding. High viscosity at rest enables the viscoelastic to remain in site during the removal of the corneal button being replaced.

The usual trephination methods can seldom be applied in these eyes: trephine suction cannot get a good hold on tissue altered by trauma. The tissue itself twists while undergoing blade rotation, and the resulting cut is not likely to be round. Moreover, the incision of the two borders in a linear wound could turn out to be improperly juxtaposed.

It is not important that corneal wounds are sutured, as the blade cuts sutures first. Because the surgeon has such poor control of the procedure, classic trephination is not advisable in the case of trauma. More often the trephine is used just to mark the line of corneal incision, which is incised by scissors starting from the perforation, then following for the whole circumference of the cut. The resulting trephination is certainly not as regular as that achieved by a round blade in nonperforated corneas, but it allows the surgeon to perform corneal grafting in these difficult conditions.

In this phase the viscoelastic acts as a soft spatula, keeping the underlying ocular structures separate while the scissors are working and pushing the cut corneal portion upward. The amount of viscoelastic leaking out through the corneal wound can be replaced as the removal of the recipient corneal button is performed. Small corneal wounds with viscoelastic leakage—for instance, those made by tips of a certain size—cannot be closed with sutures, owing to excessive tissue distortion that prevents regular incision.

An interesting therapeutic approach to these conditions was suggested by Maguen et al. They sealed the perforation with cyanoacrylate (Figure 24-30) and then deepened the AC with sodium hyaluronate (Healon®) before trephination.

PENETRATING KERATOPLASTY IN CASE OF ADHERENT CORNEAL SPOT

The advent of viscoelastics has made the performance of keratoplasty much easier and safer even in the case of adherent leukoma. In fact, with viscous solutions it is easy to create and maintain space in the AC, resulting in good control of bleeding.

In the first phase of the procedure, the viscoelastic is injected in the AC in order to deepen it. The product should have excellent transparency and high viscosity at rest, along with high pseudoplasticity for injection through a narrow cannula (Healon® GV). The cornea is perforated along an oblique axis by a 30-G needle mounted on the viscoelastic syringe. Great care must be taken to place the tip of the needle inside a deep portion of the AC, but close to the site of adherent leukoma. The injection of viscoelastic deepens the AC and defines the limits of the corneal spot and its relationship with the surrounding structures. The AC should even be filled overwhelmingly, to attempt a first detachment of synechiae via the pressure exerted by the viscoelastic (Figure 24-31).

Corneal trephination follows, which can be accomplished with a traditional suction trephine. The whole circumference can be dissected with no surgical damage to the iris when the adherent leukoma involves only the central area of the corneal endothelial surface. Should the corneal spot adhere to the trephination cutting line, some bleeding will inevitably occur, which can be controlled with the usual devices, including viscoelastics. Once trephination has been performed, the corneal button must not be removed before freeing it from the iris synechiae exposed by the viscoelastic. After cutting adhesions near the leukoma, the surgeon removes the corneal button and assesses iris–lens structure. If the anterior surface of the iris is fringed, the viscoelastic will clearly expose the defects. Even if it is poorly viscous but very transparent, it moves tissues enough to permit the surgeon to see and excise the zones to be removed with scissors. If iris stroma is greatly altered or atrophic,

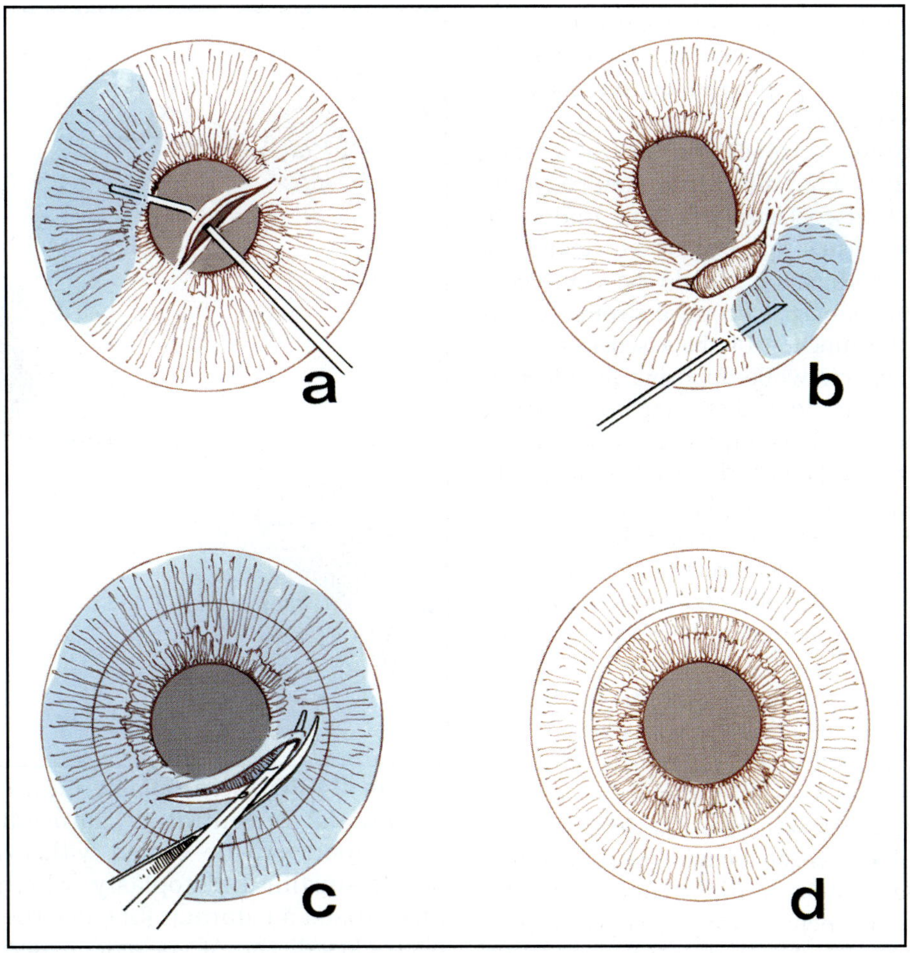

Figure 24-29. Keratoplasty on a corneal perforating wound. (a) In the event of a perforating wound requiring keratoplasty, the viscoelastic can be injected through the wound itself. (b) If the iris is engaged, the viscoelastic can be introduced through the intact cornea with a 30-G needle, in order to reposition the iris. (c) The keratoplasty trephine is often used only to mark the site of future trephination. Starting from the wound, Vannas' scissors are then used to cut the corneal tissue, following along the whole circumference. The outcome will be a slightly irregular trephination. The viscoelastic is injected at various phases to avoid causing further trauma to a damaged and flabby iris. (d) In these eyes performing a regular trephination is greatly assisted by using viscoelastics.

it is better to perform a quadrant iridectomy, guided in dimension by the viscoelastic. Sometimes the iris diaphragm and pupil can be reconstructed using prolene sutures.

When leukoma involves the site of corneal trephination, it is more difficult to remove. In the first phase of viscoelastic injection under the cornea, in the virtual space between it and the corneal spot, trephination should be completed, even with some damage to corneal stroma (Figure 24-32). Here the function of the viscoelastic is to create and fill spaces while opposing the bleeding that always occurs after dissecting vascularized synechiae. Once trephination has been performed, both parts of the leukoma, which has been split by the line of trephination, should be treated as two separate leukomas. When removing them, the surgeon should consider iris structure in the cornea bound for removal, as well as the corneal structure in the peripheral zone where the recipient cornea will rest.

In these phases the viscoelastic moves tissues, limits bleeding, and improves visibility, thus enabling the surgeon to assess both the anatomic damage and the best possible solutions more easily. Neither the molecular weight nor the internal cohesion of the material can be too high, to allow movement of tissue portions in direct contact with the product. A major benefit of using viscoelastic materials in the removal of leukomas adherent to the cornea is their ability to limit or stop bleeding. In case of severe hemorrhage in the AC, the viscoelastic has not much chance of stopping bleeding alone, but can greatly assist in detection of the site. It is important to remember that usual detection by irrigation is less effective when attempted inside a small crater such as that formed by corneal trephination.

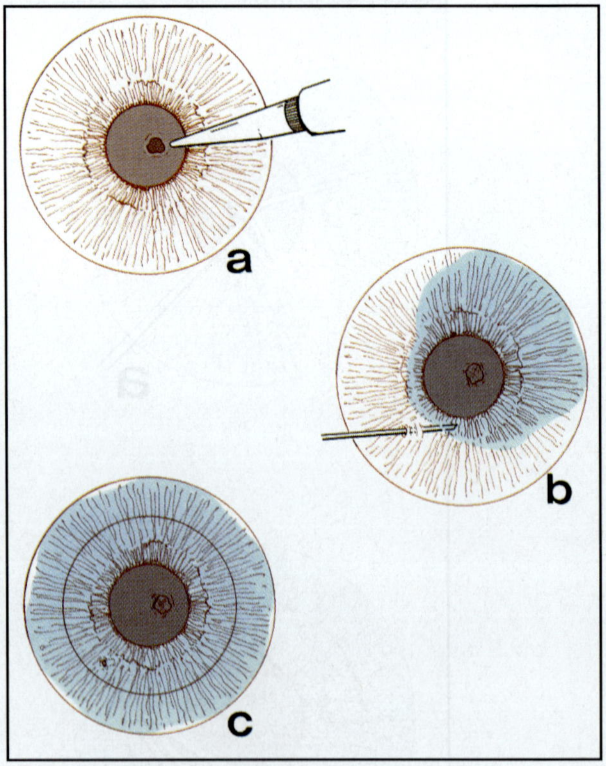

Figure 24-30. Keratoplasty on a corneal stab wound. (a) A central or paracentral corneal perforation can be sealed with cyanoacrylate before starting keratoplasty, whether or not it has caused a cataract. (b) Once the wound has been closed, the AC is redeepened with a viscoelastic injected through the intact cornea. (c) It is now possible to perform corneal trephination with the usual trephine.

Repairing Dialysis and Iris Damage During Keratoplasty

Should iridodialysis be present, it must be repaired in order to allow the iris root to readhere to the chamber angle. This way the anatomic integrity of the eye is restored, and possible negative effects of dialysis on vision are prevented. The iris root cannot be perfectly reattached to the ciliary band, but it is sutured to a portion of ocular wall close to the chamber angle. The surgical procedure generally causes no distortion of ocular hydrodynamic, as the angle distortions it creates are localized and do not always interfere with filtration. The most useful viscoelastic for iris surgery must provide excellent transparency and good, but not excessive, viscosity at rest. For the treatment of phakic eyes, 1% sodium hyaluronate (Healon®) seems to be the most appropriate. A product with less internal cohesion, such as a hyaluronate–chondroitin sulfate mixture (Viscoat), is preferable in aphakic eyes, where there is high risk of contact with the vitreous.

The viscous material is first used to stretch iris tissue and assess the extent and morphology of the damage precisely. During this phase one can stop minor bleeding due to tissue lacerations, but endo-

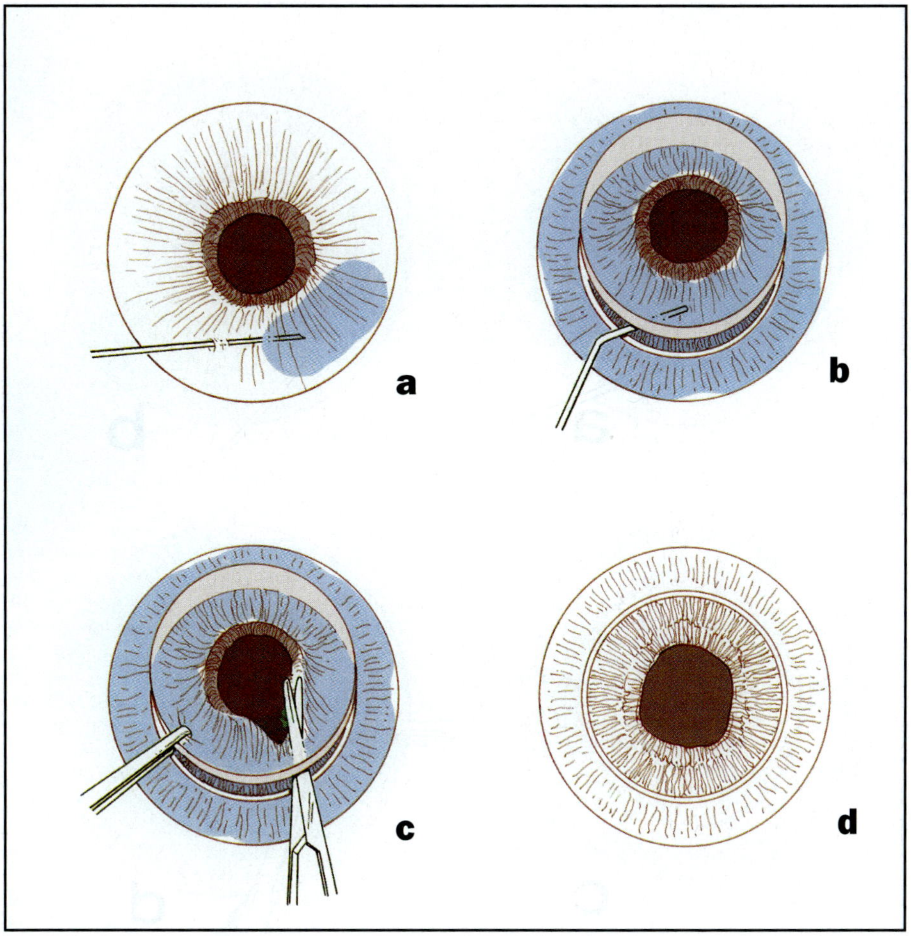

Figure 24-31. Keratoplasty on central adherent leukoma. (a) A highly pseudoplastic viscoelastic having high viscosity at rest is injected through the cornea to move the iris away over 360°, thus permitting trephination. (b) Once trephination has been performed, the viscoelastic enables the surgeon to determine the extent and toughness of the irido-corneal synechia. (c) The synechiae are gently dissected with scissors and spatula. The viscoelastic moves parts of iris away as they are released and keeps them stretched, limiting bleeding. (d) In the most favorable cases, the result of trephination is an almost normal appearance, although with frequent iridopupillary irregularities.

diathermy is seldom necessary (Figure 24-33). At this point it is possible to detect the areas where sutures to correct dialysis should be placed. A circumferential incision nearly 0.3 mm deep is cut at the corneal limbus corresponding to the site of dialysis. Its function is to receive the external portions of the 10-0 prolene thread used for iris sutures. The needle for this thread is bent, short, and very thin. After introducing it in the AC through trephination, the surgeon passes the needle inside the iris tissue in a peripheral position, taking care not to overly damage the adjacent surrounding tissue.

Further amounts of viscoelastic are injected in the chamber angle area, where the thread will pass through the peripheral cornea, in order to widen the angle as much as possible, increasing visibility and therefore precision. If the lens is present, it is better to use a product with high viscosity at rest, such as Healon® GV. The needle is directed out of the AC through the cornea corresponding to the chamber angle inside, and into the incision previously made outside. The other threaded needle passes through in the same way, taking care that the two piercings in the iris are not too far apart inside, and that the two exits in the external incision bed are even closer. The ends of both threads are bound and the knot immersed in the incision. Should it be necessary, the whole procedure can be performed again. At the end the iris root will be positioned back close to its natural seat. In some cases the esthetic and functional outcome will be excellent, and only light pupil distortion will be visible macroscopically. The repositioned iris can be fixed to an IOL following the procedure.

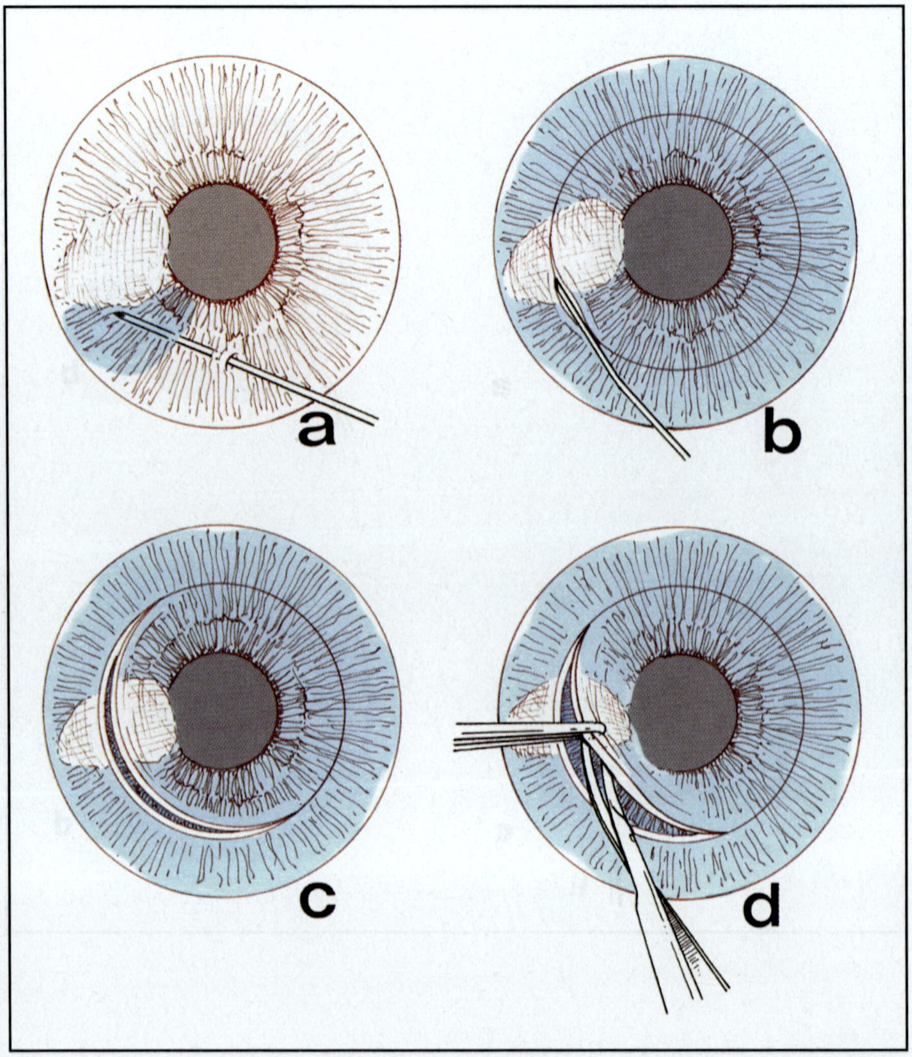

Figure 24-32. Keratoplasty on peripheral adherent leukoma. (a) A peripheral corneal leukoma affects the area of trephination. The intervention starts by injecting viscoelastic into the AC to deepen it, as well as to expose the extent of the leukoma and to move the surrounding iris away. (b) After performing trephination and opening the AC, the cut is completed with corneal scissors, while deepening the AC with repeated viscoelastic injections. (c) The adherent leukoma is split in two parts that must be treated differently. In the center it is easier to respect the iris, whereas on the periphery it is necessary to protect the cornea. (d) Iris tissue is detached from the leukoma with microscissors, replenishing any viscoelastic lost. Bleeding may occur, which the viscoelastic will control.

Repairing iris damage causing no real dialysis is easier, as it is performed completely inside the AC. As in the procedure just described, the viscoelastic is applied to stretch tissue, improve visibility, and stop possible minor bleeding (Figure 24-34). At this point it is possible to assess the damage, then repair it by suturing the iris with 10-0 prolene. Great care must be taken not to exclude iris tissue beforehand, as incorrect stretching can cause the surgeon to assess an exuberant portion that may later turn out to be essential to reconstruct the iris anatomically. The surgeon tries to reconstruct the iris diaphragm and pupil as much as possible, taking into account that if necessary, a quadrant iridectomy causes less visual problems than polycoria.

KERATOPLASTY AND PERIPHERAL ANGLE SYNECHIAE

Inflammation or previous surgery undertaken before keratoplasty may sometimes cause angle synechiae, which contribute to shallow AC depth and increased IOP. The presence of peripheral anterior synechiae is suspect whenever the eyeball is inflamed or there is evidence of prolonged inflammation. They must be removed as fully as possible to prevent chamber shallowing and postoperative hypertension after keratoplasty. Once trephination has been accomplished, it is possible to inspect the chamber angle, even when it was not visible through the opaque cornea.

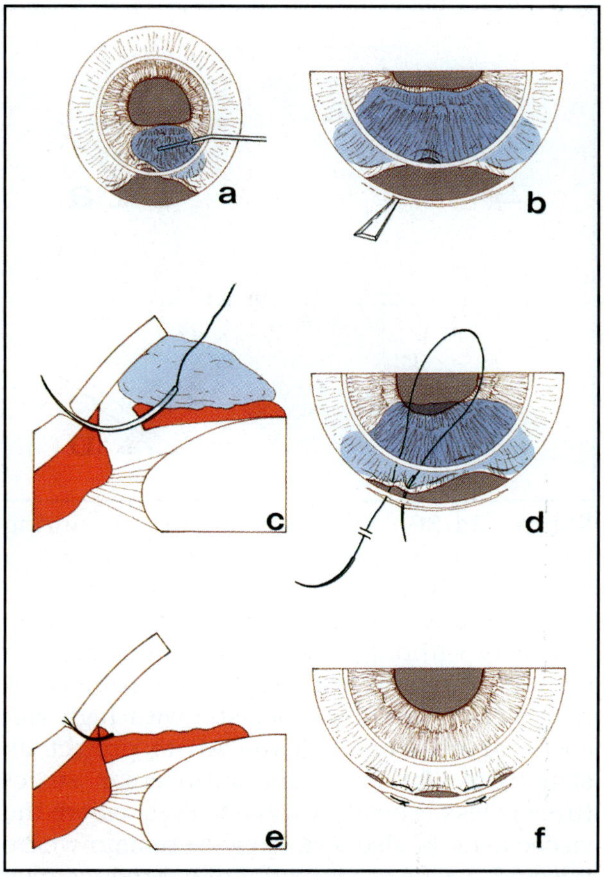

Figure 24-33. Repairing iris dialysis during keratoplasty. (a) Repairing iris dialysis during keratoplasty begins by stretching the iris with a viscoelastic that permits its mobility; that is, a material with low viscosity at rest. (b) The external limbus is freed from the conjunctiva and is incised 0.3 mm deep, following the circumference of the dialysis. (c) A curved needle is used to pass through the iris and the corneosclera, to emerge from the external limbal incision. The 10-0 prolene suture, double-armed, must not be cut. (d) After replenishing the viscoelastic in the area involved, the other needle threaded with 10-0 prolene is passed through in the same way as the previous one. (e) Tightening the suture allows good repair of the iridodialysis. The knot remains submerged in the external limbal incision. (f) More than one U-shaped suture may be required to repair iris dialysis completely.

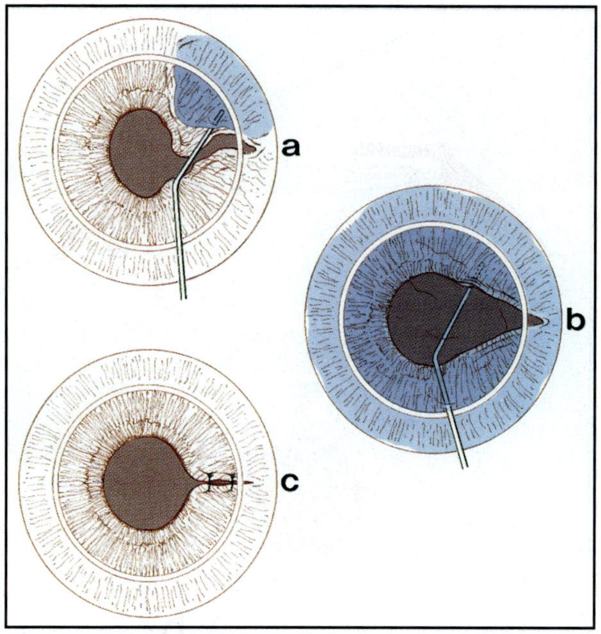

Figure 24-34. Repairing an iris wound during keratoplasty. (a) A viscoelastic with high viscosity at rest and without excessive internal cohesion allows the surgeon to flatten the iris and assess the damage present. (b) The viscoelastic allows the surgeon to separate the iris from the lens or the IOL during iridoplasty procedures. (c) Repairing the iris wound is not difficult to accomplish when the iris is stretched enough by the viscoelastic that it allows the surgeon to suture the right amount of tissue.

The procedure begins with the injection of a small amount of viscoelastic at the angle portion to be assessed (Figure 24-35). At this point the limbus is gently indented from the outside while the corneal ring is lifted corresponding to the indentation. Corneal trephination makes angle synechiae clearly visible, with no need of gonioscopy. They then can be dissected with various methods according to their persistence. The easiest and most common method is to use the viscoelastic as a fluid spatula, which cuts synechiae and acts as a hemostatic agent. Hyaluronate with the highest molecular weight is most appropriate, as it is able to remain in the site even when the AC is kept wide open by trephination.

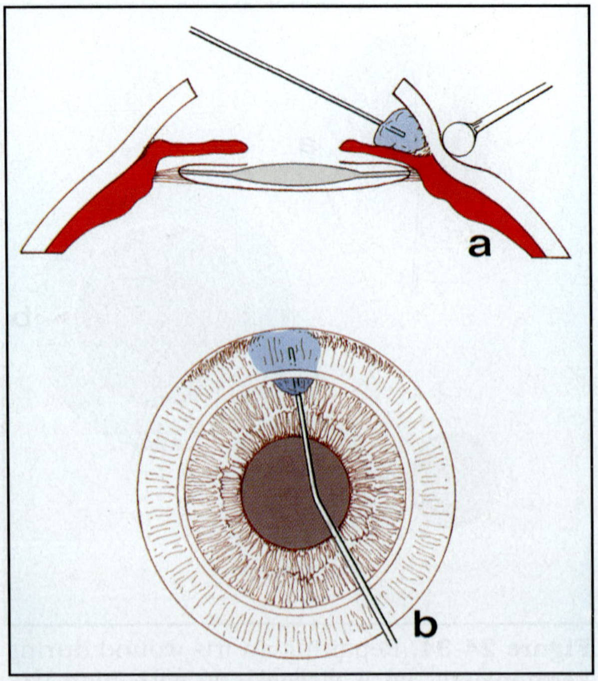

Figure 24-35. Releasing angle synechiae during penetrating keratoplasty. (a) Ab externo indentation and injection of viscoelastic from the inside allow the surgeon to detect angle synechiae. (b) Injecting a viscoelastic with high viscosity at rest corresponding to the synechiae helps to release them. Small movements with a spatula usually cause bleeding, which is effectively opposed by the viscoelastic, ensuring constant visibility.

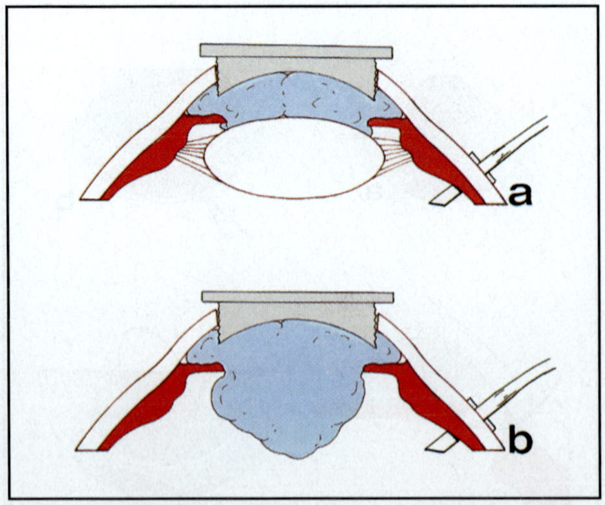

Figure 24-36. Vitreoretinal surgery during keratoplasty. (a) Applying Eckardt's temporary keratoprosthesis allows the surgeon to perform vitreoretinal surgery associated with keratoplasty without causing stress to the donor endothelium and with excellent visibility. A highly transparent viscoelastic with high viscosity at rest must fill the AC to protect its structures. (b) Protecting intraocular structures is less crucial in aphakic eyes, where the viscoelastic is also less likely to remain where injected. Using a viscoadherent product may be beneficial in this case.

According to Campbell and Vela, this procedure is far less effective than when performed with a closed eye (see Chapter 27 on glaucoma). This is performed with a cyclodialysis spatula having a very smooth tip. The spatula is introduced in the space formed by the viscoelastic between the recipient corneal ring and the iris, and the attempt is made to cut synechiae with small movements in order to limit trauma. Each space freed from synechiae is immediately filled with viscoelastic—which stretches tissues, maintains space, and improves visibility—until the whole circumference has been freed.

KERATOPLASTY COMBINED WITH VITREORETINAL SURGERY

When the cornea is not very transparent and vitreoretinal surgery is necessary, a solution must be found that provides good visibility of the posterior segment and does not require waiting for keratoplasty to heal. The solution is to apply a provisional corneal prosthesis, which allows vitreoretinal surgery—usually a long procedure—to be performed without causing damage to the donor endothelium. At the end of vitrectomy, the provisional prosthesis is replaced with the donor flap, sparing it any sort of stress.

The procedure requires using viscoelastic materials, which must fill the AC to avoid any contact between the provisional corneal prosthesis and the lens during surgery in phakic eyes (Figure 24-36).

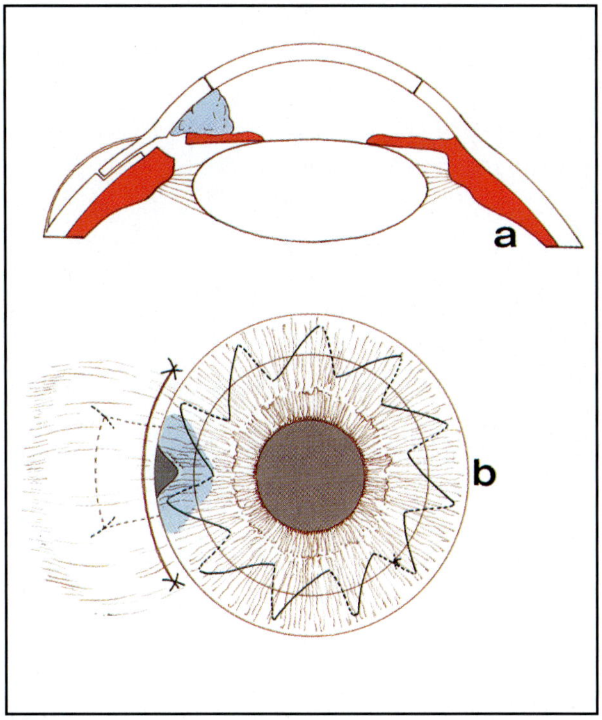

Figure 24-37. Trabeculectomy associated with penetrating keratoplasty. (a) Cross-section of an eye surgically treated with a filtration procedure. Although advised by many surgeons, most ophthalmologists regard the idea of combining a filtrating intervention with keratoplasty with skepticism. (b) An adhesive viscoelastic must be injected near the filtration site. The material will likely remain where injected, tending to limit filtration in the first days following surgery.

In many cases of vitreoretinal surgery, the iris–lens diaphragm moves forward owing to the action of posterior tamponading devices. The need to maintain the AC with viscoelastics is less important in aphakic eyes, where vitreous chamber irrigation can touch anterior segment structures.

KERATOPLASTY COMBINED WITH TRABECULECTOMY

Surgeons do not often consider the possibility of combining keratoplasty with trabeculectomy, generally because they are concerned about changes in IOP during corneal grafting. Nevertheless, Barraquer judged such a combination to be possible owing to the greater safety provided by viscoelastics in case of AC collapse following excessive subconjunctival filtration through trabeculectomy in the postoperative period. He performs trabeculectomy at the end of keratoplasty, leaving the AC filled with Healon® (Figure 24-37).

Leaving Healon® in the AC after trabeculectomy and keratoplasty has not been proven to prevent hypotony or equally dangerous hypertension. We believe combining trabeculectomy and keratoplasty is to be avoided, as grafting in conditions of uncontrolled ocular pressure may cause serious problems. We consider it more suitable to perform trabeculectomy first, and postpone keratoplasty.

CHAPTER TWENTY-FIVE

Use of Viscoelastics in Corneal Refractive Surgery

Refractive surgery is a new frontier of ophthalmic surgery. Performed only occasionally in the late 1970s, it is now more widely performed owing to the improved reliability of a range of procedures.

There are several types of refractive defect interventions. In this chapter we consider the two that have caused the greatest interest among eye surgeons and are the most commonly performed: astigmatic and radial keratotomy and excimer laser applications.

RADIAL KERATOTOMY

The early 1980s saw an extraordinarily rapid expansion in radial keratotomy interventions followed by a phase of reflection.

The results that this technique achieved in mildly myopic eyes were similar to those provided by laser techniques. The relatively low cost of the equipment greatly contributed to its popularity among ophthalmic surgeons. The procedure's immediate results and the absence of complications over the long term also account for ongoing interest.

Radial keratotomy apparently has little to do with viscoelastic products. Nevertheless, they can be useful, resulting in technical improvements. Two types of applications are reported in the literature: during and immediately after surgery.

USE OF VISCOELASTICS DURING RADIAL KERATOTOMY

In a 1986 study, Bolton and Herman observed that during radial keratotomy procedures there are changes in corneal thickness due to dehydration of corneal tissues. The surgeon aims for such dehydration in order to see the incisions more clearly while cutting them. This results in more regular and consistent incisions, and allows for the immediate detection of any microperforations by establishing the source of dripping aqueous humor. Dehydration also occurs independently of the surgeon's will, caused by light from the surgery microscope and the microclimate of the operating room in corneal surfaces not regularly wet by tears or irrigating solution.

A thin layer of sodium hyaluronate with low molecular weight (such as IAL) prevents corneal dehydration and therefore avoids pachymetric alterations during surgery. Thus, the thickness of corneal stroma is not reduced when the procedure takes a bit longer, and the risk of microperforations is lower. Sliding the blade supports is also easier during cutting and the consequent loss of epithelium is theoretically smaller. However, the sodium hyaluronate may have drawbacks. The thin layer of hyaluronate on the corneal epithelium may misrepresent the depth of the blade while cutting incisions (admittedly, the same effect occurs in intraoperative pachymetric measurements, which are used to adjust cutting depth). A thin layer of hyaluronate with low molecular weight placed on the cornea could also make it more difficult to detect optical zone limits and mark radial or curved incisions (Figure 25-1, a and b). Immediate detection of perforations, a basic requirement for safety in this kind of surgery, could be more difficult as well. For these reasons, sodium hyaluronate has not been popular among surgeons performing radial keratotomy.

Nevertheless, a viscoelastic with high molecular weight and high pseudoplasticity should be available when radial keratotomy is being performed. For example, infrequent cases of macroperforation should be immediately treated like a perforating corneal wound with no iris involvement. The AC can be re-formed with a viscoelastic injected through the same macroperforation, which the surgeon can then see clearly at full length and suture (Figure 25-1, c and d). Care must be taken in applying sutures, to avoid excessively opening the nearby incisions. Only a small amount of viscoelastic can be left in the AC once the suturing is completed; most should be removed to prevent postoperative hypertension. Although the eyes treated are young, with no problem of trabecular filtration, excessive pressure increase following radial keratotomy is also a threat, particularly after corneal perforation. A viscoelastic with very high pseudoplasticity is therefore required, that can be injected and aspirated through cannulas of very small diameter.

In 1990, Marchi and Fiormonte published a technique to remedy corneal microperforation during radial keratotomy. As soon as the dripping of aqueous humor is noted, the procedure is suspended to control the width of perforation. If it is less than 1 mm long, Healon® is injected into the AC through the microperforation itself, redeepening and stabilizing the AC. Marchi and Fiormonte checked in particular that IOP then becomes stable according to preoperative values. Surgery can then proceed, ensuring that the incision with corneal perforation is left for last. The researchers found that Healon®'s viscosity is sufficient to prevent it from leaking out through the corneal perforation while keratotomy continues. If this does occur, however, it can be remedied by refilling the chamber accordingly. The surgeons did not remove the Healon® at the end of surgery, in order to prevent lens trauma and to make even partial voiding of the chamber through the microperforation unlikely, taking into account that these patients undergo surgery in ambulatory conditions.

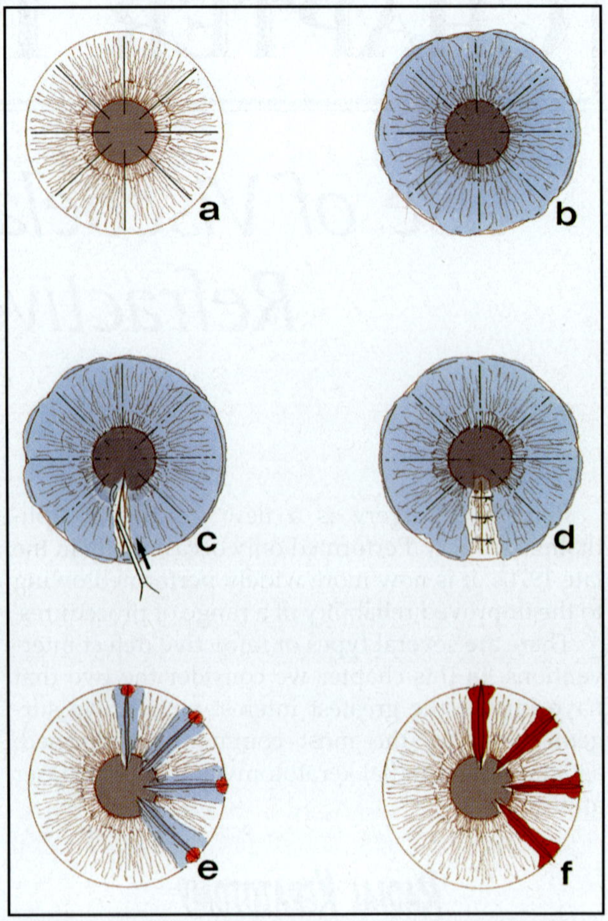

Figure 25-1. (a) When the cornea is dehydrated, the pattern of incisions made by the marker is clearly visible. (b) If a thin layer of viscoelastic is placed on the cornea, the pattern of the incisions made by the marker becomes almost invisible. (c) In the case of macroperforation, injecting viscoelastic in the AC deepens it and allows the surgeon to apply sutures. (d) Sutured macroperforation. The viscoelastic must be removed as completely as possible. (e) The mechanical tamponading provided by the viscoelastic can be useful in controlling perilimbal hemorrhages. (f) Without the use of viscoelastics, hemorrhages are likely to be more prevalent.

Use of Viscoelastics After Radial Keratotomy

Romeo et al have published a technique for using viscoelastics after radial keratotomy that involves injecting sodium hyaluronate with low molecular weight into incisions following surgery, after irrigating them with BSS. The main advantage of this procedure is in the mechanical tamponading effect of the viscoelastic, which stops limbal bleeding and thus prevents blood from infiltrating incisions and delaying the migration of epithelial buds (Figure 25-1, e and f). The researchers also believe that the biological effects of sodium hyaluronate on tissue repair and inflammation suggest it can be beneficially applied after each intervention of radial keratotomy.

Refractive surgeons widely support the use of this technique, although with different purposes, as the technique has evolved and the cuts now do not reach the limbus. Surgeons can now use collyres containing sodium hyaluronate with low concentration, applied repeatedly in the postoperative period for lubrication and re-epithelialization.

EXCIMER LASER AND VISCOELASTIC MATERIALS

There are two primary procedures in laser treatment. Refractive photokeratectomy (PRK) aims to correct myopic refractive defects. Therapeutic photokeratectomy (PTK) aims to ablate corneal opacities that limit vision or to make an uneven corneal surface regular.

Whereas there is currently no role for viscoelastics in the performance of refractive surgery, the application of these materials is important in PTK interventions. Included in this group are "leveling" or "smoothing" procedures, accomplished during excimer retreatment of refraction in eyes showing regression. Therapeutic photokeratectomies can be divided into two basic groups according to whether the original corneal surface is regular or not.

When the surface to be treated is regular despite some astigmatism, the purpose of laser treatment is to remove epithelial or subepithelial opacity, reforming a corneal surface that is "lower" than the original, but showing the same refractive characteristics. This involves creating a small "crater" in the optic zone of the cornea. When the corneal surface is uneven, a simple excimer laser treatment would ablate the surface in a uniform way over juts and depressions, thus reproducing "on a lower level" the same irregular features of the original cornea. To obtain a smooth and uniform corneal surface, it is necessary to perform special viscoelastic-dependent procedures.

THERAPEUTIC PHOTOABLATION OF SMOOTH-SURFACE CORNEA

Performing therapeutic photoablation of normally surfaced cornea usually requires a laser spot with a large diameter (5 mm or more), with no adjustable diaphragm. The laser forms a crater in the anterior corneal portion, the bottom of which reproduces the original corneal surface.

Early on, the procedure achieved far less than the refractive precision required, and a large number of treated eyes became hyperopic. The equipment and software currently available are much better and effectively prevent this effect. While studying the causes of such hyperopia, various remedies were hypothesized, such as epithelial hyperplasia close to the crater walls or a capillary effect such that any fluid on the corneal surface during treatment adhered to the crater walls, reducing the effects of the laser on that area. As a result, no fluid or viscoelastic agents are usually used to perform this type of therapeutic photoablation (Figure 25-2a).

The problem of different ablations induced by the same laser radiation on parts of corneal tissue with varying thicknesses remains. Starting from a smooth surface and covering scars or corneal calcifications, it is possible to achieve an irregular surface once the opacities hindering vision have been ablated. The resulting irregular astigmatism can be treated by excimer laser following the smoothing procedure, or can be corrected with a contact lens.

THERAPEUTIC PHOTOABLATION OF IRREGULARLY SURFACED CORNEA

Applying excimer laser energy directly to an irregular corneal surface simply results in thinning the cornea without improving its smoothness. Various more or less viscous fluids, able to fill topical depressions to improve homogeneity of the ablation bed, have been used as surface modulators. The basic requirements of these fluids are:

- the ability to spread all over the cornea to create a homogeneous surface
- the ability to remain in site for at least some dozen seconds
- an ablation rate close to that of the corneal stroma

Viscoelastic materials were among the first tested, with various experiments performed to determine the most suitable kind and concentration of product. Among the first materials studied were viscoadherent products such as methylcellulose-based preparations, which were tested in 2% and 0.3% concentrations. Higher concentrations turned out to be unsuitable (Figure 25-2b), as they form too thick a layer, altering the conformation of ablation craters as they are created by laser action. The best results were achieved with a 1% concentration at the beginning of surgery and 0.5% at the end, after main irregularities had been removed. It is advisable to perform the procedure step by step, using slit-lamp microscopy and corneal topography to check the results gradually achieved.

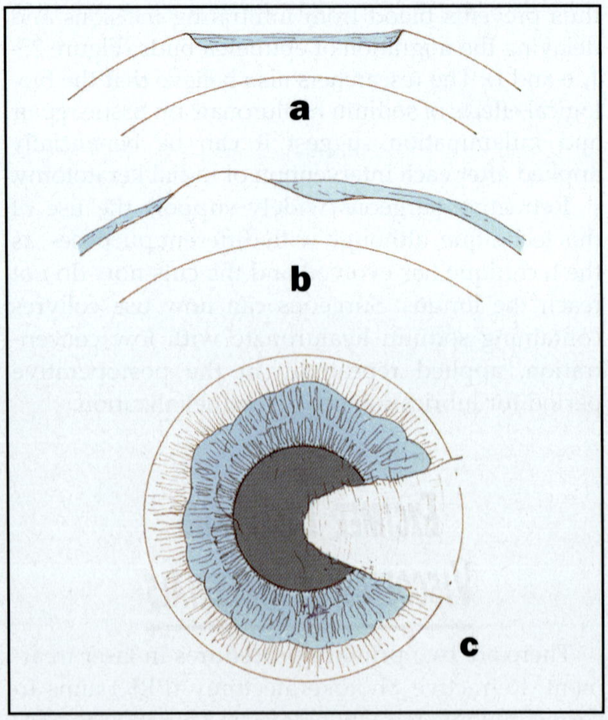

Figure 25-2. (a) Any fluid present on the cornea during PTK creates a meniscus near the margin of ablation due to capillarity. This alters the following ablation. (b) The ideal masking agent for PTK must be deposited in the depressions, but not on the unevenness of tissue to be made regular. (c) During PTK, less viscous viscoelastics may be useful as masking agents, but only for marked alterations of the corneal surface, such as pterygia.

Some studies compared a variety of materials, such as 0.3% hydroxypropylmethylcellulose, 1% carboxymethylcellulose, 0.1% dextran 70, and physiologic solutions. Other materials proposed include various types of gel and collagen. Sodium hyaluronate seems poorly suited for this use, particularly the kind with higher molecular weight at concentrations typically used in ophthalmic surgery. Usual formulations of Healon® and Viscoat are not appropriate. IAL would be helpful in correcting gross surface irregularities, such as those caused by removing a pterygium involving the corneal central portion (Figure 25-2c). When more diluted, the same materials can be used successfully to modulate smaller irregularities.

An important feature of these modulating agents is the homogeneity of ablation compared to the corneal stroma, with the same incident radiation. The problem is not easy to solve. A corneal stroma with irregular thickness due to scars of calcification, for instance, reacts in an irregular way to excimer laser light. A study conducted in Italy found that sodium hyaluronate with low molecular weight and 0.4% concentration has the same ablation rate as normal corneal stroma. This then could be the first modulating agent used in normal PTK. Nevertheless, the procedure needs fine-tuning, and further research is necessary to better define its usefulness and limits.

However, from a theoretical point of view, it seems that the deeper the depressions, the higher the unevenness of corneal surface, and therefore the greater importance of a specially selected modulating agent. In the smoothing that follows normal refractive surgery procedures using excimer lasers, the choice of the modulating agent could be less crucial, as irregularities of the stromal surface after PRK are very small and the ablation rate of corneal stroma is well-known. For this application we prefer very diluted sodium hyaluronate solutions, such as those normally present in artificial teardrops.

MYOPIC KERATOMILEUSIS

Myopic keratomileusis is an intervention that aims to reduce corneal refraction power while thinning the central portion of the corneal stroma. This so-called in situ technique, proposed by Ruiz, is an evolution of the original technique developed by Barraquer, which had already been modified by Krumeich and Swinger. The procedure used at present is called automated lamellar keratoplasty. The intervention consists of cutting a corneal flap with a microkeratotome, attached on one side, with a 7 to 8-mm diameter and 130 to 160-micron thickness. The flap is then turned over on one side. From the uncovered stromal bed, the same microkeratotome removes a disk of cornea thick enough to correct myopia in the operated eye. The first flap is turned back over onto the cornea and the intervention is completed.

Viscoelastic materials are not generally used during myopic keratomileusis, as they could interfere with adhesion of the corneal flap to the stromal bed at the end of surgery.

EXCIMER LASER–ASSISTED KERATOMILEUSIS (LASIK)

Proposed several years ago by Buratto and Pallikaris, excimer laser–assisted keratomileusis (LASIK) has rapidly risen to a prominent place in corneal refractive surgery. The intervention aims to correct the corneal refractive power acting on the corneal stroma, which is thinned by excimer laser.

Access to the stroma is not achieved by mechanically removing the epithelium and then Bowman's membrane with the laser, as happens in superficial photokeratectomy. Here the cornea is dissected horizontally by a microkeratotome, which cuts a superficial flap attached on one side. The corneal flap is then turned over to allow the excimer laser to treat the exposed stromal bed. After completing photokeratectomy—myopic, hyperopic, or astigmatic—the corneal flap is put back in place and caused to adhere to the bed through dehydration. At the end of the procedure, the surgeon checks whether the flap has been correctly placed on the stromal bed modified by the laser.

Laser keratomileusis is generally performed without viscoelastics. It is important that the stromal bed is kept dry during application, whereas the use of a viscoelastic would require rinsing for removal. At the end of surgery, no viscoelastic is applied to the corneal surface.

Chapter Twenty-Six

Viscoelastics and Anterior Segment Perforating Trauma

The therapeutic and surgical treatment of ocular perforating trauma has changed dramatically over the last 30 years. The choice to enucleate, which occurred at a 20% rate in the 1960s, is now rare owing to better antibiotic and anti-inflammatory treatments and improved surgical techniques. Viscoelastic materials were already indispensable in the treatment of ocular perforating trauma in the early 1980s. They have greatly assisted advances in the solutions of many formerly difficult problems.

Viscoelastics improve visibility of the anatomic structures injured, thus allowing the surgeon to assess relationships and immediate repair needs. They also permit "soft" manipulation of tissues, avoiding any contact with surgical instruments that could intensify trauma or jeopardize optimal recovery. Viscoelastics also can reduce intraocular bleeding and dissect newly formed synechiae. Any foreign bodies present in the AC can be moved or removed with the help of viscoelastic products as well.

Viscoelastic Requirements in Trauma Surgery

Ocular trauma includes a complex range of pathologic events that are unlikely to be standardized. In delineating the general criteria guiding the use of viscoelastics, it is best to start with their physicochemical properties.

Viscosity at Rest

A product with high viscosity at rest is fundamental in the performance of trauma and reconstructive surgery. It is unlikely to leak out of the eye, thus assisting in repair surgery. Highly viscous sodium hyaluronate provides unquestionable and very useful advantages.

Transparency

One of the main factors in trauma surgery is visibility: the selected material should be crystal-clear, without the tendency to trap air bubbles during injection. When air bubbles reduce the product's transparency, the visibility of anatomic structures, which are already damaged and out of place, becomes very poor and prevents optimal results. Viscoelastics with high internal cohesion are preferable in such cases, particularly the various preparations of sodium hyaluronate. Should it be necessary to use a less cohesive material, which tends to trap air bubbles while being injected, great care must be taken to minimize this complication. One preventative method is to eliminate any residual air from the syringe containing the product. Another is to use syringes with noncompressible pistons; that is, those with no "feedback effect" of sucking air inside the cannula during pauses in injection, and eventually injection into the viscoelastic itself once the application has been started (Figure 26-1).

Internal Cohesion

When internal cohesion is not excessive, the surgeon can better control the vitreous that is on the iris plane or AC as a result of the accident. Similar to procedures used in cataract surgery in case of posterior capsule rupture with vitreous leakage, a viscoelastic with high molecular weight and low internal cohesion allows the surgeon to greatly limit the loss of vitreous.

PSEUDOPLASTICITY

Pseudoplasticity should be very high in viscoelastics used for trauma surgery. It is often necessary to introduce the viscoelastic into the AC through a corneal wound, in a very small space. Sometimes the wounded cornea must be pierced to penetrate the AC and re-form it with viscoelastic, which can be done only with a 30-G cannula through which the viscous product passes. Once in the AC, the material must be highly viscous in static conditions to provide the advantages mentioned in often very difficult conditions.

BIOCOMPATIBILITY

Contact with lacerated and often hard-to-detect tissues means that viscoelastic products used for this type of surgery must be highly biocompatible. Nearly all surgical experience with viscoelastics in trauma has been with sodium hyaluronate. Another factor requiring high biocompatibility is the large amount of viscoelastic often used in the treatment of severe trauma, where significant amounts of viscoelastic often remain inside the eye at the end of surgery.

Despite this, no contraindications have been reported in the literature on the use of other less-biocompatible products, such as hydroxypropylmethylcellulose.

ADHESION

Adhesive properties are unnecessary and even undesirable in cases of perforating wounds, as an adhesive product could jeopardize rapid removal at the end of surgery. Nevertheless, this feature can be useful when the vitreous body must be treated, as it is better managed by adhesive materials than by cohesive products.

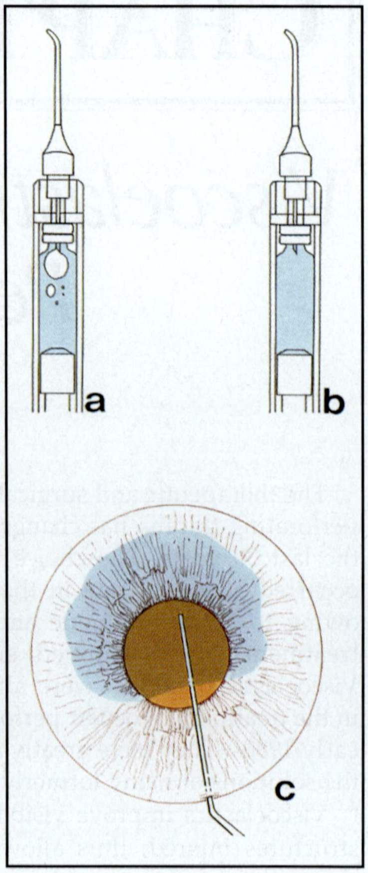

Figure 26-1. Precautions with poorly pseudoplastic and poorly cohesive viscoelastics. (a) To improve the transparency of these materials it is best to first eliminate any air bubbles present in the syringe. (b) Other air that must be eliminated penetrates the cannula when injection of poorly pseudoplastic materials is temporarily interrupted, due to the backward expansion of the syringe's rubber piston. (c) A poorly cohesive product must be injected inside itself in the AC.

COLOR

The surgeon often needs to discern between the viscoelastic and the vitreous body, another gelatinous and transparent element often present in the AC after trauma. One solution is to use a viscoelastic that has been mixed with a small amount of fluorescein. A yellow-dyed sodium hyaluronate preparation with high molecular weight, made available in recent years, is suitable for this purpose. Its effectiveness and tolerability were not reduced by the dye.

SURGICAL TECHNIQUES

Repairing an anterior segment perforating wound starts with corneal assessment, almost always accomplished when the patient is already

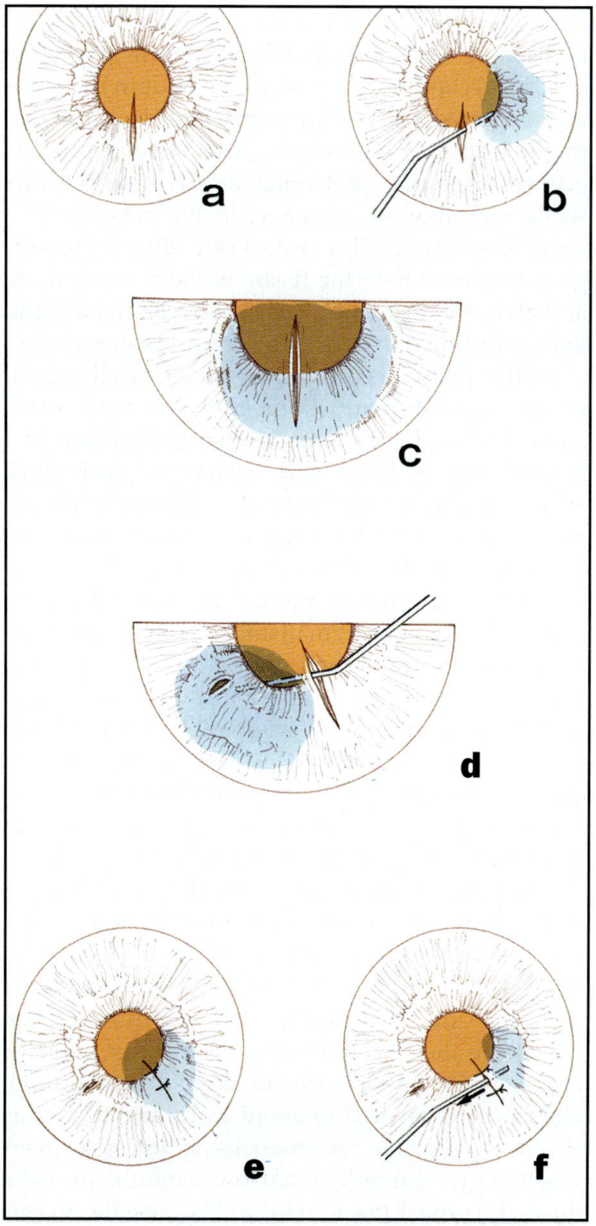

Figure 26-2. Corneal wound with no iris engagement. (a) A small wound perforating the cornea may not be complicated by iris engagement. (b) The viscoelastic material can be injected into the AC through the wound itself, and permits accurate inspection of the ocular structures. (c) A product with high viscosity at rest stretches the iris in the area of injection, separating it from the wound and enabling its examination. (d) In the event of a small iris wound, the viscoelastic can be injected between iris and lens with no damage to the lens. (e) With the viscoelastic in the AC, it is easier to apply sutures with the correct tension. (f) At the end of surgery the viscoelastic must be removed from the AC through a thin cannula.

under general anesthesia. The inspection allows the surgeon to assess the shape and extent of the wound, the conditions of the margins, any material loss, and whether the suture will interfere with the visual axis. Very often, corneal wounds are perforating only in part, and injecting a viscoelastic in the AC allows the surgeon to see their nature clearly. Without a viscoelastic the assessment becomes more difficult, and partial suturing is required to reform the AC before the surgeon can assess repair requirements accurately.

SMALL CORNEAL WOUNDS

The AC can be filled with viscoelastic through the wound site when it is not extensive and does not involve the iris (Figure 26-2). The action of the viscoelastic is enough to deepen the chamber, particularly when the material used is highly viscous at rest, such as Healon® and similar products. When it is certain that the underlying structures (iris and lens) are not severely damaged, the AC can be overwhelmingly filled with viscoelastic. Any leakage of product out of the wound partly cleans its borders. With a deep chamber, clear inspection of corneal continuity is easier. The underlying iris is also explored for synechiae or small wounds that might trap a foreign object. The viscous product acts as a spatula, stretching the iris little by little while revealing any damage. In the presence of a small iris wound, the viscoelastic allows the surgeon to manipulate the tissue without touching it, and above all to create a space between the iris and lens, avoiding damage from surgical maneuvers.

At this point it is possible to assess the alignment of the wound margins precisely. A very small corneal wound may remain unsutured, whereas a corneal lens is fixed with Hennekes' technique. When suturing is necessary, the alignment of margins achieved with viscoelastic injection allows the surgeon to apply a suture that will result in good stitching of the tissue, minimizing corneal distortion and ensuing astigmatism. A base is thus created for better reconstruction, and refractive restoration, of the corneal surface—a further advantage of viscosurgery in anterior segment trauma. This is possible only when the AC is deep and ocular consistency is restored. Viscosurgery also makes it possible to place stitches under the correct tension, also contributing to good and rapid refractive results.

The same method can be used to suture more extensive wounds that have caused hypotony without iris involvement. After filling the AC with Healon®, we apply a first stitch in the center of the corneal wound, in order to approach tissues. Then we suture the two parts of the wound separately, taking care to pass the thread alternatively through one or the other half to avoid distorting tissues as much as possible. A viscoelastic injected overwhelmingly through a narrow cannula or even through corneal tissue with a 20-G needle reveals any suturing defects. When pressure in the AC is increased, it exposes possible folds in corneal tissue. When the product leaks out through badly stuck areas, it indicates where further stitches are needed.

At the end of surgery, the viscoelastic should be removed with the utmost care, depending on the kind of material used. Aspiration must be more complete when sodium hyaluronate with high molecular weight is used owing to the risk of postoperative hypertension, but this material is the easiest to remove completely. Viscoadherent products may have a lower risk of causing postoperative hypertension, but they are almost impossible to remove after corneal suturing when the irrigation and aspiration handpiece cannot be used, and only small, one-way cannulas are appropriate. When the surgeon wants to remove the whole viscoelastic, a very pseudoplastic product should be prepared, which can be aspirated through a narrow cannula and used through a corneal suture with no wound diastasis.

Sometimes it is best to leave a small amount of viscoelastic inside the AC at the end of surgery, as it can "tamponade" areas of poorer cohesion between the flaps of the corneal wound, thus reducing or eliminating leakage of aqueous humor in the postoperative period. In this case a viscoadherent product is preferable, which remains in the site of injection longer.

CORNEAL WOUNDS WITH IRIS INVOLVEMENT

When the iris has been involved through the wound, the AC is not completely eliminated, and in many occasions can appear to be deep. The involved iris is often traumatized, lacerated, or atonic, and generally covered with fibrin membranes that must be removed with great care. The prevalent remedy in the past was to excise all the membranes protruding from corneal wounds, probably owing to the enormous difficulty of replacing them and assessing anatomic alterations caused by trauma. With the advent of viscosurgery, it is now possible to replace the iris discharged from the corneal wound and even restore its anatomy as much as possible to minimize photophobia and esthetic discomfort in the postoperative period.

Once the operating field has been cleaned, clearing it in particular from any fibrin membranes present, the iris can be replaced through the same wound. If the wound still has a certain tonicity, involvement is limited and iris anatomy is fairly preserved. Pharmacologic mobilization of the iris is often helpful. Prolapse of the central portion can be reduced by mydriatics, whereas peripheral prolapse is controlled by miotics. The iris can be pushed gently toward the AC by the cannula injecting the viscoelastic, then by the spatula effect of the viscoelastic itself while it is forming the AC (Figure 26-3). During these procedures great care must be

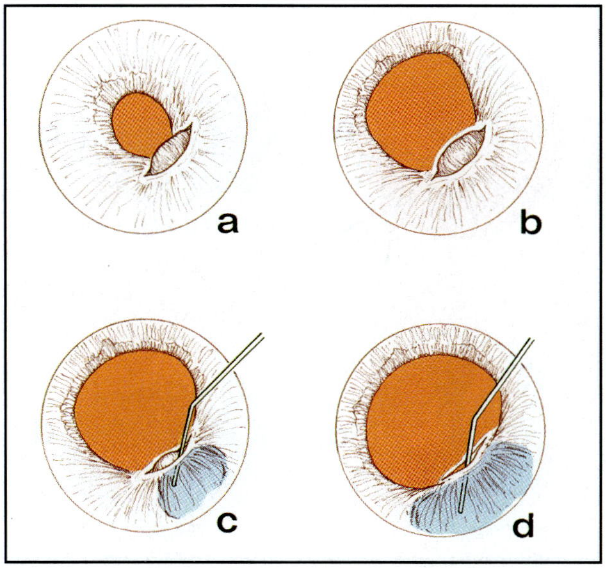

Figure 26-3. Corneal wound with iris engagement. (a) This often occurs without collapse of the AC, as the iris tissue obstructs the opening and prevents the aqueous humor from leaking out. If the engagement is moderate and the iris tonic and mildly damaged, it can be repositioned through the wound. (b) Pharmacologic mobilization of the iris is often very helpful. A prolapse in the center (as illustrated) can be opposed by mydriatics, and miotics can oppose prolapse in the periphery. (c) Once fibrinous synechiae have been released, the iris can be gently pushed toward the AC by the same cannula used to for the viscoelastic. (d) Repositioning is completed with a viscous spatula that stretches the iris. If the surgeon injects too much viscoelastic, it could cause recurrent prolapse of the iris if it flows back from the wound.

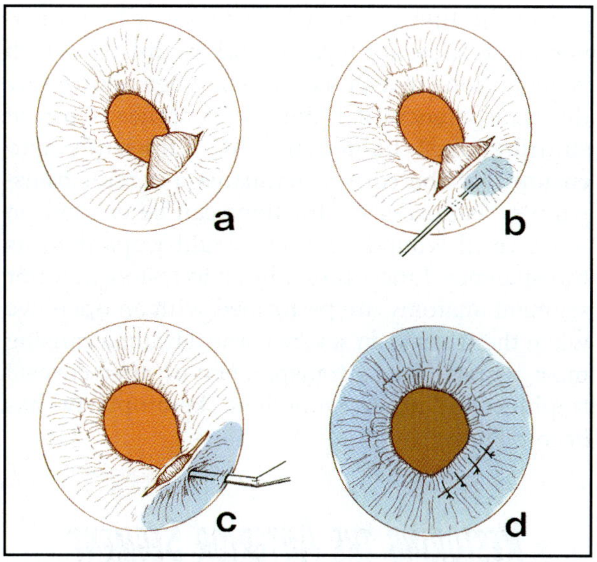

Figure 26-4. Corneal wound with severe iris engagement. (a) When the iris protrudes markedly, it is better not to try repositioning it through the corneal wound. (b) A viscoelastic product is injected in the AC through a 30-G needle. The chamber deepens again, eye tone is restored, and the iris is stretched toward its site by the spatula effect of the viscoelastic. (c) A spatula introduced through a limbal opening completes iris repositioning. (d) After replacing the iris, the surgeon can examine and suture the corneal wound, thus permitting optical recovery of the anterior segment.

taken not to inject too much viscoelastic into the AC, as it could push the iris outside again through the wound or aggravate iris involvement.

When iris protrusion is greater owing to a more extensive wound or to the amount of tissue discharged, it is better not to try repositioning it through the corneal wound. The AC is pierced with a thin (30-G) needle mounted on a syringe containing viscoelastic, which penetrates a peripheral portion of the cornea (Figure 26-4). Best suited for this procedure are products with high pseudoplasticity, such as the various preparations of sodium hyaluronate, including those with high viscosity (Healon® GV). The viscoelastic injected in the AC allows the surgeon to assess the condition of the iris before any manipulation of the protruding tissue. The viscoelastic acts as a viscous spatula, allowing the surgeon to replace the prolapsed tissue. The iris is generally repositioned with a small spatula introduced through a 1-mm paracentesis near the limbus, or acting directly on the prolapsed iris as described.

Once the discharged tissue has been replaced in the AC, the chamber is filled with viscoelastic, and first repairs of the corneal wound can proceed. The aim of the first suture, which may not be permanent, is to allow for further work in the AC, which is better done in a closed system when allowed by the transparency of traumatized cornea. Corneal suturing must tighten the AC sufficiently and ensure that the cornea maintains a certain transparency. No excessive tractions can be exerted on the corneal wound, as they would jeopardize its transparency. Procedures aiming to restore anterior segment anatomy are performed with an open eye when there has been severe corneal trauma causing most tissues to lose transparency or after corneal trephination when immediate keratoplasty has been planned.

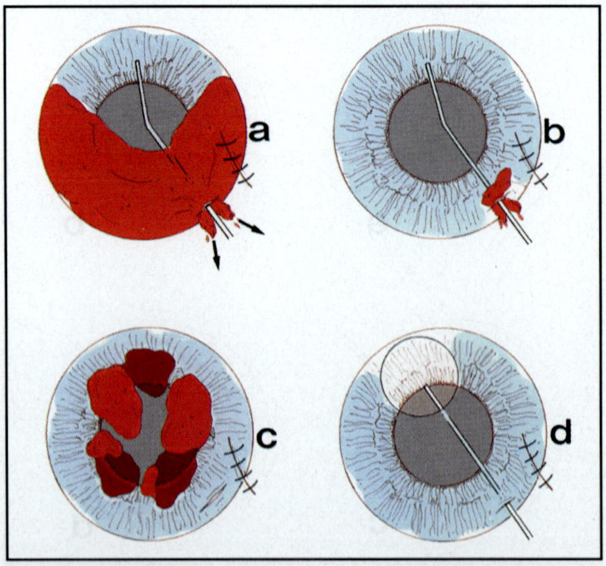

Figure 26-5. AC bleeding. (a) Blood present in the AC due to a wound can be removed by viscoelastic injection, then directed out through a paracentesis close to the site of bleeding. (b) Further oozing of iris or ciliary body bleeding spontaneously leaks out of the AC if it is filled with viscoelastic and the paracentesis is next to the wound. (c) If the viscoelastic gets mixed with blood, visibility is greatly reduced. It is better to replace the whole injection with another product with higher internal cohesion. (d) Part of the viscoelastic can be replaced by air to limit the risk of postoperative hypertension.

Restoring the Anterior Segment

Anterior segment reconstruction procedures range from relatively simple iris surgery to rather complicated surgery involving the iris, lens, and vitreous. In most severe cases the AC is filled with iris, lens, and vitreous material mixed with blood. The most complex of these situations are beyond classification, but it is possible to describe some procedures that are often performed. As a rule, we perform these procedures through small openings of the AC at the limbus, never through the original corneal wound. This way tissue damage is not increased and visibility is optimal, as distortion of corneal tissue is minimized. In any case, most ocular surgery instruments are designed to work in the AC through limbal surgical openings, so procedures performed through central or paracentral openings are rather difficult to accomplish.

Anterior Chamber Hyphema

The presence of blood in the AC may be due to leakage from iris vessels or the ciliary body. Total hyphema usually causes marked hypertension, with possible blood staining of the cornea, and must be removed surgically. Blood clots must also be removed, as they may contribute to the formation of peripheral anterior synechiae.

Fluid blood can be removed from the AC by injecting a viscoelastic, with minimal if any damage to the endothelium, iris, and lens. Most suitable in this case are cohesive viscoelastics such as Healon® and Healon® GV, which are unlikely to mingle with the blood even when it is fluid. The advantage of viscoelastic injection is that it does not remove any small blood clots that prevent further bleeding (Figure 26-5). Active bleeding can be reduced and even stopped by the mechanical action of the viscoelastic or the increased pressure in the AC. As in posterior segment surgery, pauses in hypertonic conditions can be greatly helpful. Nevertheless, when blood comes from a breakage in the ciliary body it is difficult to stop dripping without direct diathermy, and sometimes even this treatment may be ineffective. The prognosis for possible functional recovery is then far less positive.

Mixture of viscous material and blood must be avoided as this greatly reduces visibility. When this occurs, all the viscoelastic mingled with blood must

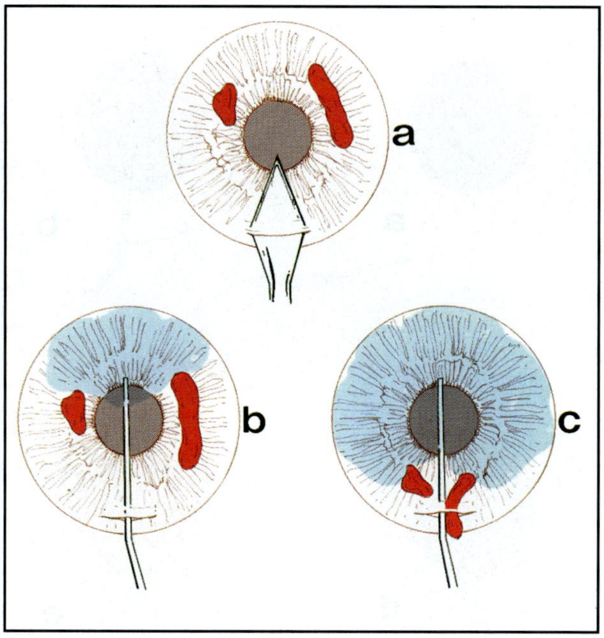

Figure 26-6. Removing blood clots from the AC. (a) Blood clots in the AC must be treated like foreign objects and can be manipulated by viscoelastics. First, a 3.0-mm valve incision is created with a calibrated blade. (b) The surgeon starts injecting a viscoelastic having high viscosity at rest and high internal cohesion. (c) The viscoelastic pushes the blood clots toward the corneal incision, thus accomplishing their viscoexpression. Minimized anatomic abnormality, persistent tone of the eye, and the mechanical effect of the viscoelastic on blood vessels reduce the risk of further bleeding.

be replaced with newly injected material, which mechanically removes the old product. In this case the opening at the limbus must be large enough to permit this replacement without consequent high pressure in the AC, which might dislocate tissues that, although damaged, have remained in place.

The same viscoelastic procedure can be accomplished to treat a hyphema not likely to resorb in the days following repair surgery. Using a viscoelastic with low molecular weight to replace a blood clot in the AC allows the surgeon to restore a certain amount of visual function immediately, and at the same time avoid the risk of corneal blood staining. The material can be left in the AC when it is beneficial to maintain some postoperative hypertension to help stop further bleeding, or can be removed when bleeding is presumed not likely to recur. In our experience, we have not found any other method of removing blood clots, such as injecting an enzymatic activator of thrombolysis into the AC, to be beneficial. Clots tend to thaw in a few dozen minutes but re-form over the following hours, or bleeding may recur.

Clots of blood or fibrin in the AC must be treated like foreign objects. That is, they are susceptible to viscoelastic procedures but retain a certain plasticity. For removal, an opening, not necessarily large, is required in the AC, to which the clot is guided (Figure 26-6). When the surgeon chooses to perform viscoexpression, a viscoelastic with high internal cohesion such as Healon® GV is most appropriate, even though pseudoplasticity is not a relevant feature in this case. The material is injected under and over the clot, and then overwhelmingly behind it to push it out of the AC. The viscoelastic material thus forms a sort of "slide" that enables complete removal of the clot. When viscoexpression cannot be performed, the clot must be removed by a vitrector, for which the corneal opening can also be minimal. The viscoelastic of choice should be a product with low internal cohesion, so it can immobilize the clot despite the fluids flowing in the AC, as in vitreous removal. Viscoat seems to be the most appropriate in this case.

LENS DAMAGE

In the presence of lens damage, even only anterior capsule laceration, it is better to remove the lens during the first intervention of reparation surgery. After filling the AC with viscoelastic, more material is gently injected alongside the capsular opening to reveal its configuration (Figure 26-7). The capsulotomy started by the agent that also caused the wound is easily completed with a needle or scissors; sometimes it is even possible to accomplish capsulorhexis.

Before cataract extraction it might be necessary to separate the iris, which is often lacerated, from the lens material. A viscoelastic is very useful in dissecting early posterior synechiae gently, and produces the best mydriasis possible in such difficult conditions.

A phacoemulsificator is seldom helpful in cataract removal, as it requires irrigation and pressure in the AC that are excessive for a traumatized eye. Aspiration is also not particularly gentle in the case of lack of tone or iris trauma, and causes damage to structures already suffering from trauma. If the cataract presents a formed nucleus, it can be expelled from the AC by viscoexpression, which exerts an equal and opposite force toward the vitreous chamber. A very pseudoplastic viscoelastic (such as Healon®) is injected through a narrow, bent cannula under the nucleus or the lens material to be expressed, directing it first into the AC, then outside the eye. During the procedure trauma to the cornea must be prevented by injecting another viscoelastic immediately underneath it. In theory, a viscoadherent product such as Viscoat seems to be best for corneal protection, as it is more effective in reducing tangential forces acting on the endothelium. A product with high internal cohesion is a must for viscoexpression, as it produces a bolus that exerts an expulsive force on lens material.

If the nucleus is not formed, as happens in young patients, viscoexpression is always useful, but irrigation and aspiration procedures must be started beforehand, always taking great care that excessive pressure is not induced inside the AC. The occurrence of hypertension during these procedures may cause iris discharge, or even direct lens material inside the vitreous chamber through the posterior capsule or zonular breaks. In view of these threats, a highly viscous viscoelastic with low shear rate is appropriate, provided that its internal cohesion is not so high that it controls corneal pearls or iris fragments, thus preventing them from being caught by the aspiration tip. Although they remain in the AC just a bit longer than materials with high internal cohesion, these viscoelastics may require reinjection during irrigation and aspiration. In addition, there is also the drawback that they cannot be completely removed at the end of surgery.

After removing the cataract, an IOL can be implanted when preoperative refraction is known, following the biometry of the other eye. This IOL is fixed in the ciliary sulcus or with scleral suture, and in exceptional cases only, in the capsular bag.

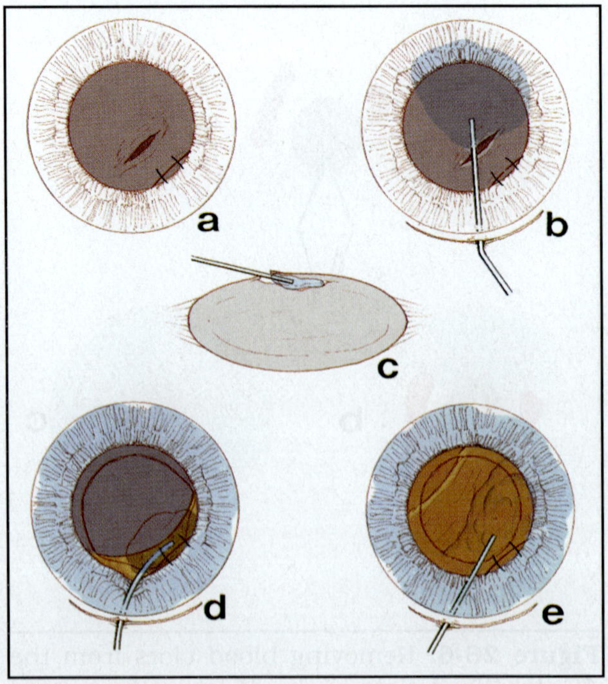

Figure 26-7. Immediate removal of traumatic cataracts. (a) With an anterior capsule wound, particularly when the anterior cortex of the lens is damaged, it is best to remove the cataract at once. (b) A very transparent and cohesive viscoelastic is injected until the AC is filled to make the capsule clearly visible. (c) In some cases, injecting another product with poor viscosity at rest above and below the capsular flap allows the surgeon to assess the damage and complete capsulotomy as desired. (d) Viscoexpression of the nucleus exerts minimal pressure on the vitreous chamber during cataract extraction. (e) If the vitreous appears through the unevenness of the posterior capsule, it is necessary to use a poorly cohesive viscoelastic, which can better control vitreous prolapse.

VITREOUS IN THE ANTERIOR CHAMBER

The presence of vitreous in the AC makes the performance of anterior vitrectomy mandatory, which must be as complete as possible. The presence of vitreous is typically revealed by air bubbles or by absorbing sponges that adhere to it and "stretch" it when withdrawn. Its visibility is not improved by

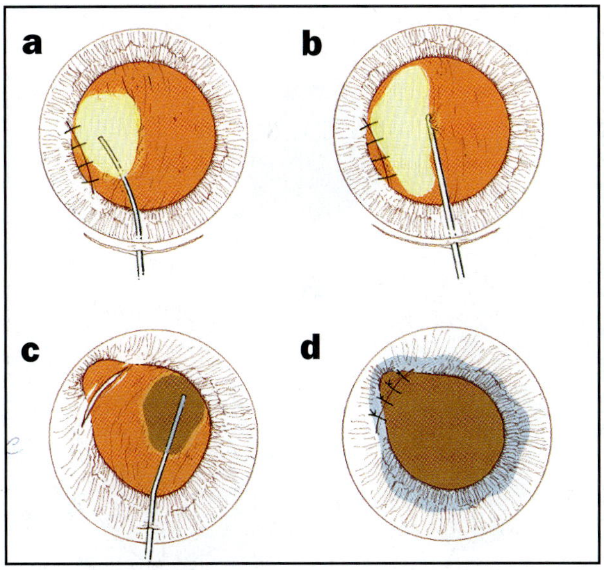

Figure 26-8. Managing vitreous in the AC. (a) Using a viscoelastic dyed with fluorescein allows the surgeon to distinguish the vitreous present in the AC from the viscoelastic. (b) Anterior vitrectomy can then be more selective and complete, as it is possible to avoid the postoperative presence of residues and vitreous strands in the AC. (c) Even when it is already present in the AC, the vitreous can be fairly well-controlled by a an adherent viscoelastic. For optimal visibility, this material must be injected inside itself. (d) A viscoelastic with poor internal cohesion absorbs the nonhomogeneous push of the vitreous and allows the surgeon to work in the AC again without difficulty.

using the usual viscoelastics, which cannot be distinguished from it. Thus the advent of sodium hyaluronate mixed with fluorescein (Healon® Yellow*) was a significant achievement, allowing surgeons to distinguish the colorless vitreous from the dyed-yellow viscoelastic (Figure 26-8, a and b).

Vitrectomy can be accomplished as completely as possible, replacing the vitreous gradually removed with yellow viscoelastic. Coaxial infusion is very seldom used in anterior vitrectomies, in order to avoid increasing the mobility of vitreous fragments that are difficult to detect. Owing to the use of dyed viscoelastic, there is lower probability of leaving residual vitreous strands in the AC, which cause pupillary stretching. It must be remembered that the permanence of vitreous strands in the wound, whether surgical or not, often leads to postoperative cystoid macular edema.

It is sometimes necessary to keep the vitreous material behind a diaphragm, made for instance of capsular or iris residuals. In these cases a viscoelastic with low internal cohesion is particularly useful, as it is not moved by the vitreous pressure but instead absorbs it. The surgeon can thus maneuver safely close to the vitreous (Figure 26-8, c and d).

Viscoat seems to be the best viscoelastic for this application, as it provides good pseudoplasticity and viscosity at rest, even with the mild internal cohesion required. It is a bit less transparent, but sufficiently so if the surgeon follows the precautions for injection described at the beginning of this chapter.

While performing vitrectomy with the help of a viscoelastic, the utmost care must be taken to save as much of the lens capsule as possible, both anterior and posterior, for immediate or future IOL implantation. When the lens–vitreous material has been cleaned, the newly injected viscoelastic can push into the vitreous chamber other transparent vitreous that tends to enter the AC while surgery is being completed.

REPAIRING IRIS DAMAGE

Repairing iris tissue damaged by trauma follows AC cleaning and lens diaphragm reconstruction. When iris damage is moderate and tissue is tonic, the procedure is easy to accomplish (Figure 26-9). However, when iris structure is greatly disarranged, mobile tissue fragments in the AC are rather intrusive, and are therefore moved away and stabilized by a viscoelastic. In these cases early repair may also be required, which prevents further iris damage during lensectomy and vitrectomy. A viscoelastic with high molecular weight and low internal cohesion is preferable in this phase, as previously mentioned.

Once the AC has been cleaned and an eventual IOL implanted, iris repair is best accomplished

**Healon® Yellow is no longer being manufactured.*

under a viscoelastic with very high molecular weight, which stabilizes tissues while creating the space required for surgical movements. A dense product like Healon® GV is not likely to leak out of the AC through surgical wounds where instruments are introduced. It will also exert enough pressure toward the vitreous chamber without being rapidly sucked in, as no aspiration procedures are performed at this point. Movement rate during the repair of an iris wound is rather low—less than 10.

IRIS COLOBOMA

Iris coloboma can be repaired with a prolene 10-0 suture mounted on an STC-6 straight needle (manufactured by Ethicon), which must be long enough to pass through the whole AC. This technique can be performed even through a single 1-mm opening in the corneal tissue, whereas on the opposite side it is sufficient to make the needle come out by passing it through the whole cornea (Figure 26-10). The thread is withdrawn from the side of the incision and the knot is made outside the eye, then taken inside it and closed. The whole procedure is accomplished by using a viscoelastic, which allows the surgeon to determine the places in the iris where the threads must pass and keeps the procedure perfectly visible. As occurs in all iris structures, tissue is stretched with a highly viscous viscoelastic, which prevents the tissue from curling up inside the knot.

Less invasive techniques involve making two small openings through which a small Vannas' forceps can be introduced to cut the thread after tying it (Figure 26-11). Viscoelastics must fill the AC during this procedure, as in repairing iridotomies performed during cataract surgery in the presence of closed miosis. Only when the iris has been stabilized by a viscoelastic with high viscosity at zero shear rate is it possible to pierce it in the desired place and to take the needle through the AC without touching tissues that do not need further trauma.

If the coloboma is too large, performing real surgery on the iris may be necessary. Less complicated cases can be solved by mobilizing an area at the base of the iris with small relaxing incisions. More complicated situations can involve mobilizing a portion of the iris and suturing it to the corneal limbus according to the technique for iridodialysis reparation (Figure 26-12). The utmost care must be taken to achieve a round and preferably centered pupil, considering that postoperative laser treatment can correct overly small pupils without problems, but not overly large pupils. Once again, without viscoelastics, performing these procedures would not be possible.

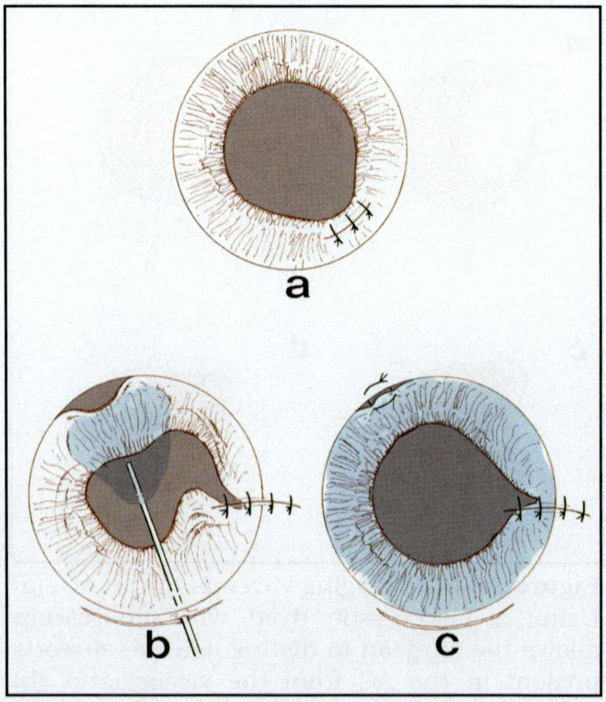

Figure 26-9. Repairing less important iris damage. (a) In the presence of slight iris damage, procedures can generally be performed in the AC without difficulty, such as cataract extraction. (b) When iris structure is disturbed, the viscoelastic product enables the surgeon to move and keep iris fragments far away from the pupillary field during lensectomy. A product with low internal cohesion and high viscosity at rest is most appropriate in this case. (c) Initial repairs to the iris may be necessary to accomplish lensectomy and vitrectomy.

IRIDODIALYSIS

Sometimes contusions and perforations may cause iridodialysis. Repairing a small iridodialysis

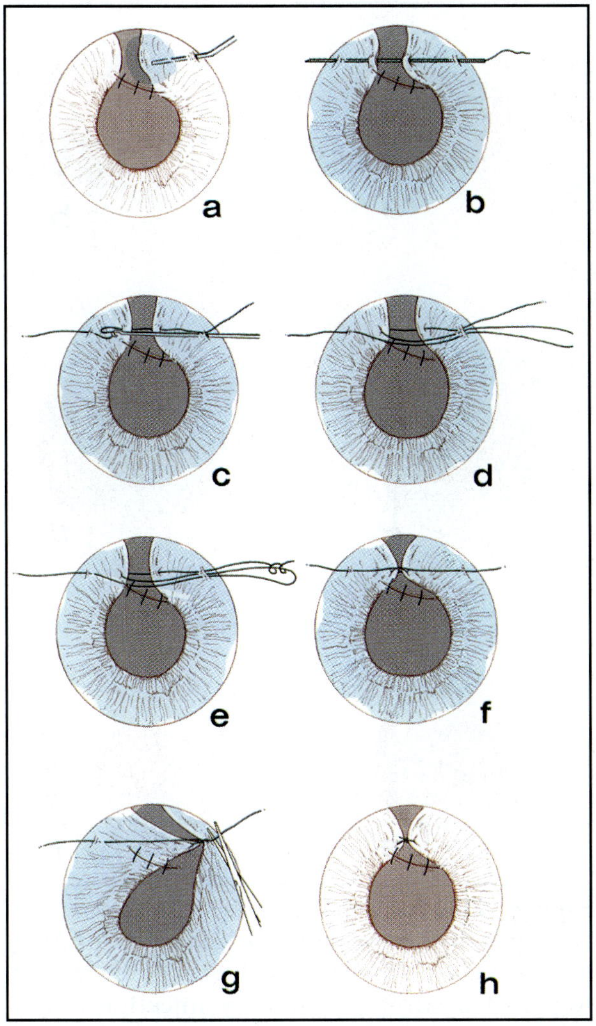

Figure 26-10. Repairing iris wounds in a closed eye. (a) A 1-mm corneal incision is cut on the right of the wound, in a suitable position for sutures. Through it the AC is filled with a viscoelastic, which stretches the iris and allows the surgeon to determine the most suitable area for sutures. (b) The same incision is used to introduce a straight STC-6 needle with 10-0 prolene. The needle is directed through the iris tissue in proper position, then out through the cornea on the opposite side. (c) A hook introduced in the 1-mm incision pulls the prolene thread outside the eye through the incision. The viscoelastic filling the AC immobilizes the thread, allowing the surgeon to catch it. (d) A long portion of the thread is extracted from the chamber. (e) Outside the AC, the surgeon prepares a knot tied with both threads. The viscoelastic is replenished to prevent the iris tissue from curling during the application of sutures. (f) The surgeon slides the knot inside the AC and tightens it. When necessary, the procedure can be repeated. (g) The thread is cut close to the knot, pulling the iris toward the corneal incision on one side and toward the corneal puncture on the other. (h) The outcome achieved with this procedure is generally very good, and the AC has not been actually opened to a large extent.

may be useless, but repositioning the iris root in case of large dialyses is useful to avoid monocular diplopia, to free the pupillary field invaded by the iris, and for esthetic reasons. The procedure developed by Eisner completely depends on the use of viscoelastics, particularly when the lens is intact, and requires more piercing than real openings in the AC (Figure 26-13). At the beginning a scleral flap is made at the limbus next to the dialysis. Then a viscoelastic with high viscosity at rest and high internal cohesion (Healon® GV) is injected next to the site of dialysis in order to move any vitreous pearls protruding through the damaged zonulae back to their original place, and also to prevent bleeding. In the second phase the viscoelastic is injected into the center of the AC to stretch the iris and start moving it toward the ciliary body in the area of dialysis. More product is placed under the iris to detach it from the lens, particularly when it is intact.

At this point the surgeon passes 10-0 prolene sutures through the dialysed iris near the root, applied according to preference. Eisner has described a technique using a single long, bent needle (Figure 26-13, d–f). We prefer performing a simpler but more extensive procedure, using various 10-0 prolene double sutures on a straight STC-6 needle. This needle can be maneuvered through small corneal incisions. Both suture needles are introduced in the AC through the same incision, passing through the iris near the detached root, and emerge at the corresponding limbus, in the bed for-

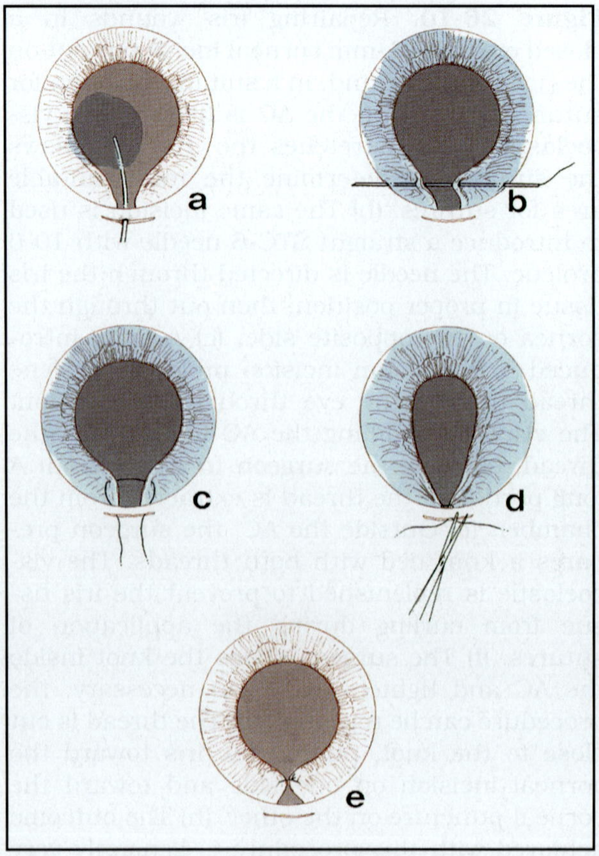

Figure 26-11. Repairing iris wounds in an open eye. (a) A small limbal incision is created next to the iris wound. The AC is filled with viscoelastic through this opening. (b) The STC-6 needle penetrates the AC through the cornea, then passes through the iris tissue stretched by the viscoelastic, to eventually emerge from the corneal tissue opposite to the site of introduction. (c) The thread is cut and the two ends retracted through the limbal incision with McPherson forceps. (d) The knot is tied outside the AC, while slightly stretching iris tissue and pupil. Then the thread is cut next to the knot. (e) The outcome achieved is good, and the technique used minimally invasive. However, the corneal incision must be sutured.

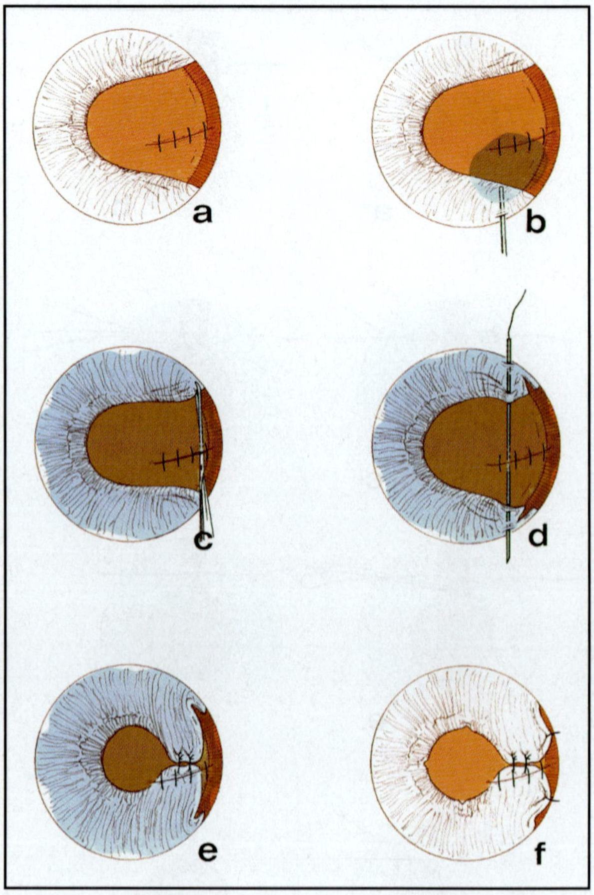

Figure 26-12. Repairing iris coloboma. (a) One possible consequence of a perforating wound may be an extended iris coloboma. (b) Reparative surgery starts by injecting a viscoelastic with high viscosity at rest, filling the whole AC. (c) The iris must be incised close to the base on both sides of the coloboma. The viscoelastic helps the surgeon accomplish the procedure and limits bleeding. When possible, it is better to enter the AC through the wound or to use vitrectomy scissors. (d) After mobilizing two iris portions, one for each side, the coloboma is sutured in the usual way. (e) The result is that the coloboma is transformed into a small or medium-sized iridodialysis, which can in turn be repaired. (f) Small multiple sphincterotomies, assisted by the presence of a viscoelastic, can prevent pupil decentration.

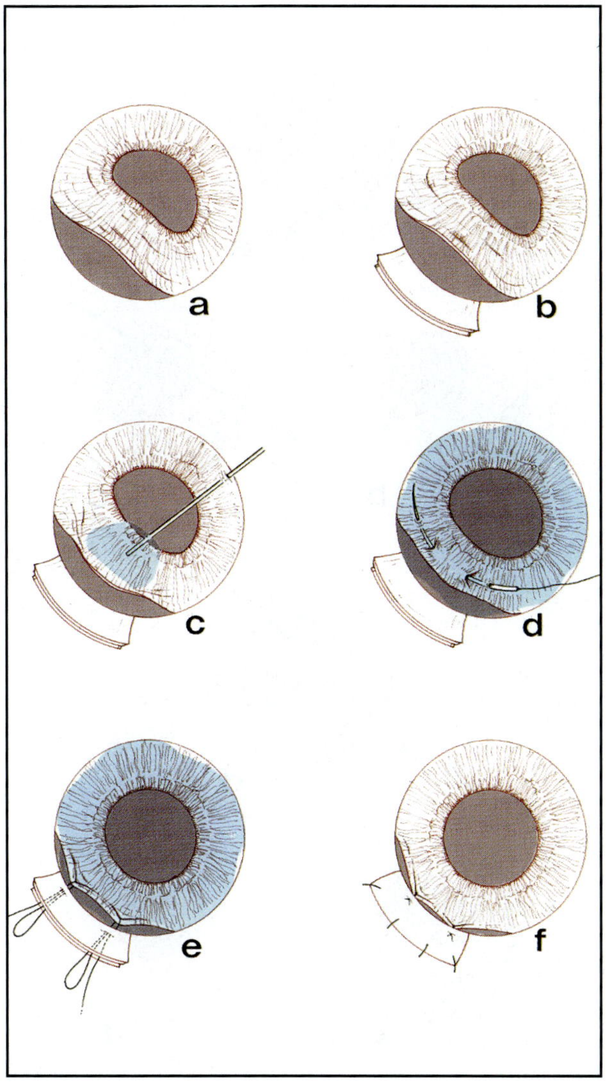

Figure 26-13. Repairing iridodialysis in a closed eye, Eisner's technique. (a) Extensive iridodialysis needs to be repaired with nonresorbing sutures, which are applied on the inside of the sclerocorneal wall. Vitreous is often present in the AC, resulting from zonular dialysis. (b) A scleral flap is prepared posterior to the limbus next to iris dialysis, which covers the knots of prolene thread. The viscoelastic used in this case is a viscoadherent product that can best control the vitreous. In a closed eye, a cohesive product could trap vitreous bands in the AC, on the side of the viscous bolus. (c) The viscoelastic injected in the AC pushes the vitreous back, stretches the iris, and separates it from the lens. The AC must not be filled overwhelmingly, as some of the viscoelastic may pass into the vitreous chamber through the zonular dialysis and increase IOP, besides causing a posterior pressure that shallows the AC and renders many procedures dangerous for the lens and the corneal endothelium. (d) A curved, large needle mounted on a 10-0 prolene suture is passed through the cornea and iris, producing two anchorage sites in the dialyzed portion of the iris. (e) The thread is pulled out through two small limbal incisions made in the bed of the scleral flap, then fixed to the same flap bed in the two sites. (f) After the flap is closed, the knots are in intrascleral position and iridodialysis is repaired.

merly prepared in the scleral flap (Figure 26-14). The needles are drawn until the thread makes the iris root adhere to its original seat. At this point the suture is tied outside the eye so as to remain completely inside the sclera without extruding under the conjunctiva. Two or three stitches of this kind are usually enough to repair iridodialyses. In practice the technique is not particularly difficult to accomplish, owing to the help provided by viscoelastic materials, yielding good results in the cases published.

FOREIGN OBJECTS IN THE ANTERIOR CHAMBER

Perforating trauma is often caused by a foreign object being present inside the eye. Glass or wood fragments are often found in the AC as well as cilia, whereas the force of metal fragments is often enough to project them right through the anterior portion of the eye to finish their travels in the posterior segment. When present in the vitreous chamber, a foreign object must be removed via vitrectomy, generally performed after early wound reparation. When the foreign object is in the AC, extraction must occur immediately. Injecting a cohesive, transparent viscoelastic with high viscosity at rest

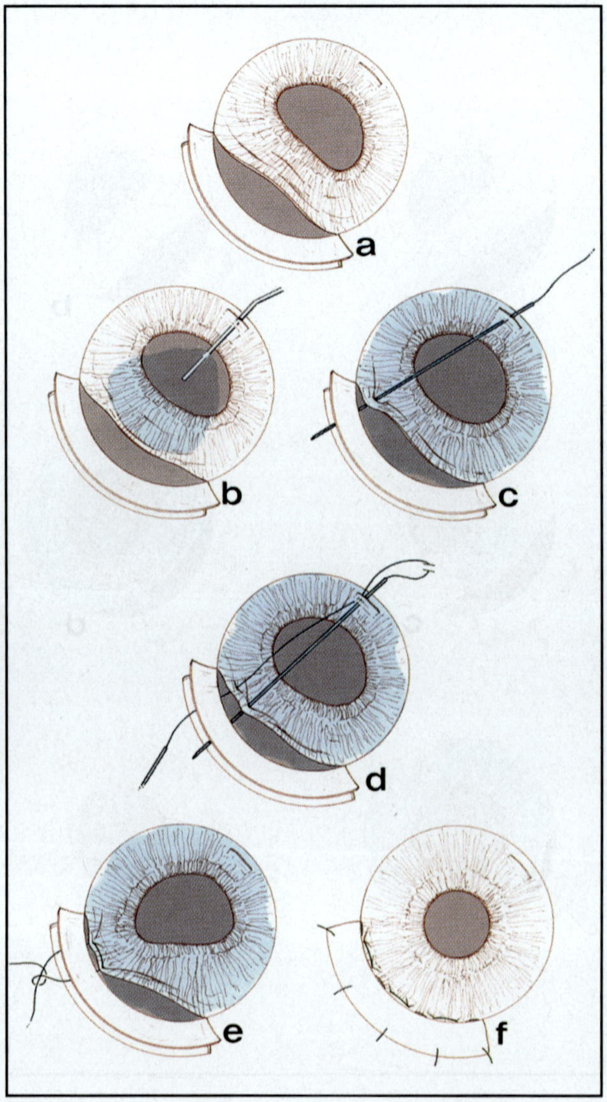

Figure 26-14. Repairing iridodialysis, alternative technique. (a) A half-thickness corneal flap is prepared (2 mm thick), which extends to the limbus until it nearly covers the site of dialysis. In full peripheral cornea, opposite to the dialysis, a 2-mm valve incision is cut. (b) A viscoelastic product that is highly viscous at rest and highly cohesive or adherent in the presence of vitreous is injected in the AC, taking precautions against excessive filling. A large amount of liquid vitreous requires an anterior vitrectomy. (c) A straight STC-6 needle mounted on 10-0 prolene is introduced in the AC through the incision. The needle goes across the iris near the root and emerges under the scleral flap. (d) In the same way, the other needle of the double-armed suture is introduced near the previous one, at a suitable distance. (e) After retrieving both needles, the surgeon knots the thread outside the eye. The iris is brought near to the limbus, with the surgeon tying the prolene and keeping the knot under the flap. (f) If the dialysis is large, several sutures must be applied to achieve a good result.

(such as Healon®) into the AC is very helpful. The viscoelastic allows the surgeon to detect the foreign object while separating it from any blood, thus easing its removal (Figure 26-15).

Foreign objects are removed from the AC by different techniques according to size, shape, and precise location of the object in relation to the surrounding anatomic structures. Sometimes the rate of inflammation determines the technique used for removal.

Foreign Objects Protruding Into the Anterior Chamber

Foreign objects lodged in the cornea and protruding into the AC can be complicated by chamber shallowing during removal attempts. When the foreign object cannot be extracted at the first attempt, lens damage is likely to occur. Lens opacity or endothelial damage are also likely to occur as a result of repeated surgical manipulations to attempt extraction. Viscoelastic materials are fundamental to preventing such additional damage.

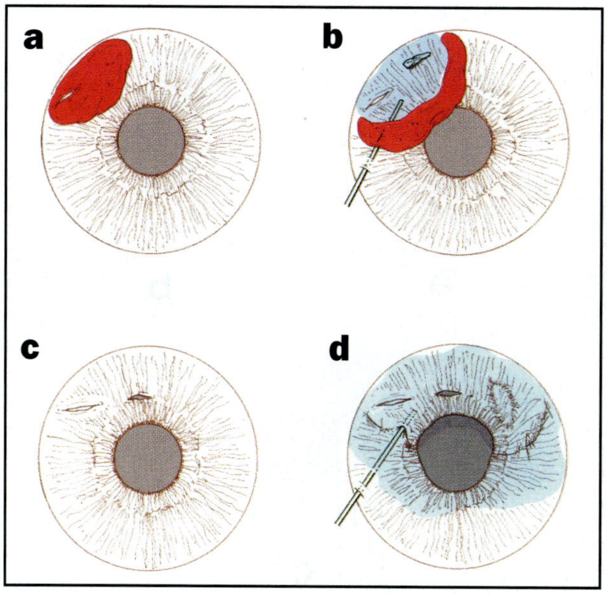

Figure 26-15. Penetrating corneal wounds caused by foreign objects. (a) Penetrating corneal wounds causing AC hematoma have often injured the ciliary body. The presence of a foreign object under the hematoma is exposed by radiologic or echographic examination. (b) Using a viscoelastic product allows the surgeon to move and extract the hematoma, thus exposing the foreign object. (c) When the wound involves both cornea and iris, the foreign object may be present between the iris and the lens/zonule. (d) Viscoelastic widens the space behind the iris and moves soft tissues, thus allowing detection of the foreign objects lodged between the iris and lens.

Before beginning to extract the foreign object, the aqueous humor in the AC is replaced by a viscoelastic. A product with high viscosity at rest and high pseudoplasticity is necessary, as it can be injected through a small cannula. Its transparency must be very high to permit detection and extraction of the object and its fragments. Healon® GV appears to be the most suitable material. The replacement can be accomplished by discharging the aqueous humor through a small limbal incision while injecting the viscoelastic through a 30-G needle passed obliquely through the cornea (Figure 26-16).

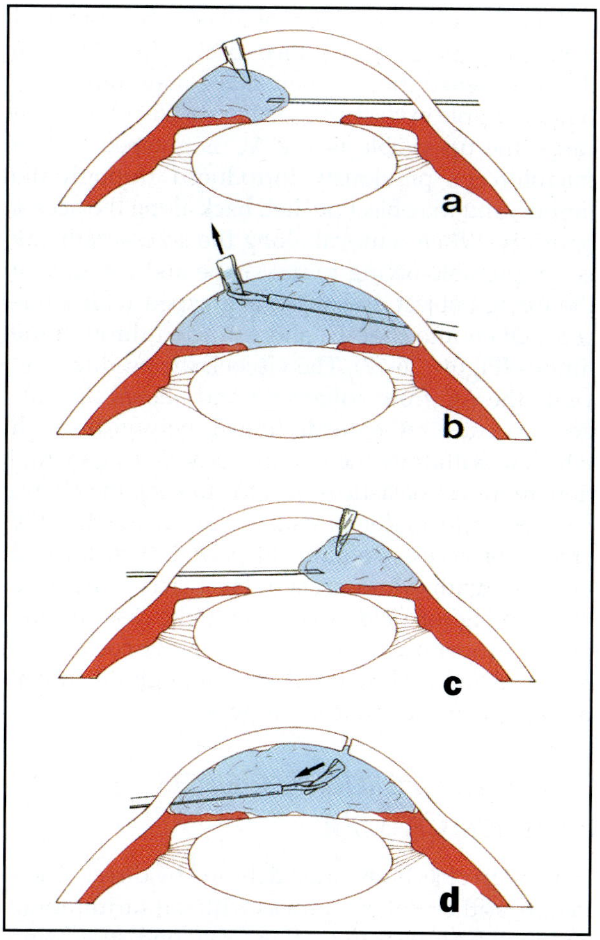

Figure 26-16. Foreign objects sinking into the cornea. (a) A foreign object that sinks into the cornea and projects into the AC is initially treated by filling the chamber with viscoelastic, which keeps it deep during the removal and protects the corneal endothelium, iris, and lens. (b) The surgeon removes the object by pushing it back, toward the outside. The viscoelastic prevents the AC from emptying, allowing the surgeon to manage the corneal wound. (c) Other foreign objects jutting into the AC cannot be pushed back. (d) After viscoelastic injection, the object is grasped by a forceps, pulled into the AC, and extracted via the limbus. A viscoelastic product with high viscosity at rest allows even glass fragments to be removed.

Foreign objects are best removed when grasped from the outside and pulled back. However, the depth of penetration or their shape may sometimes hinder simple extraction (see Figure 26-16). In such cases, the tip visible in the AC is grasped with a microforceps previously introduced through the limbus, and the object pushed back along the access pathway. When removal along the access pathway is not possible owing to the shape and fragility of the foreign object, the object is grasped with a forceps, taken into the AC, and extracted through the limbus (Figure 26-17). The viscoelastic product prevents the AC from collapsing and allows the surgeon to cut a rather wide limbal incision through which to withdraw the foreign body. During extraction, more viscoelastic is injected to keep the chamber deep and under pressure. After extracting the object, the access wound is inspected, then sutured or sealed with cyanoacrylate (Hystoacryl, one drop after drying the field) according to the case. To prevent postoperative hypertension, the viscoelastic is removed and replaced with BSS through the limbal incision, which completes surgery.

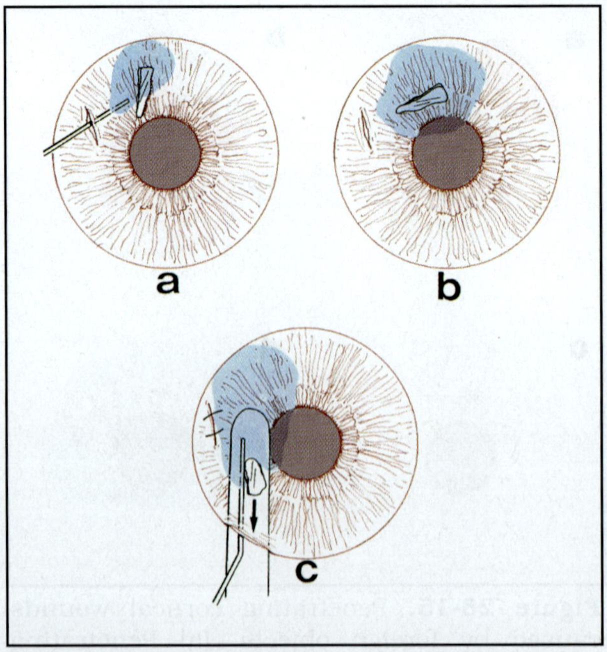

Figure 26-17. Corneal wound with free foreign object in the AC. (a) The foreign object is positioned for extraction with the viscoelastic, which is injected through the same entrance. (b) The correct positioning for objects undergoing extraction is longitudinal. Very often the entrance is smaller than the foreign body, so the opening must be widened or even abandoned for the extraction. (c) A suitably placed corneal incision and an advantageously cut Sheet's glide enable the surgeon to remove the foreign object while preventing it from getting stuck to the chamber angle.

MOBILE FOREIGN OBJECTS IN THE ANTERIOR CHAMBER

Foreign objects are often detected by direct observation, as their color contrasts with the surrounding structures. At other times they are found after being suspected and searched for. In special cases detection may be difficult, due to reduced visibility caused by fringed wound rims or the small dimensions and color of the object itself. The places where a foreign object can migrate in the anterior segment may also render its detection almost impossible. There have been cases where glass fragments placed under the iris were extracted after many months when they appeared again in the entrance, with neither lens lesions nor uveal inflammation.

A cohesive viscoelastic with high viscosity at rest (Healon® GV) allows the surgeon to search for, detect, and manipulate any foreign objects present in the AC without trauma (see Figure 26-17). Viscoelastic injection stretches tissues and creates spaces free from blood where foreign objects can be detected and mobilized. Sometimes the failure of spaces to dilate after injection of a highly viscous viscoelastic leads the surgeon to suspect the presence of a foreign object or an anatomic alteration that is worse than initially expected.

Foreign objects can also be manipulated by a viscoelastic, which can immobilize them in a particular area or move them toward a suitable site for removal. When ready for removal, foreign objects can be guided by the viscoelastic for extraction through small incisions. More compact fragments are grasped with McPherson forceps, whereas fragile ones require slightly larger incisions. A Sheet's glide, cut on the spot from a sterile plastic sheet, helps prevent the foreign body from being trapped in the corner of the chamber during these procedures.

Some removal techniques are particularly appropriate to remove vegetable or animal fragments

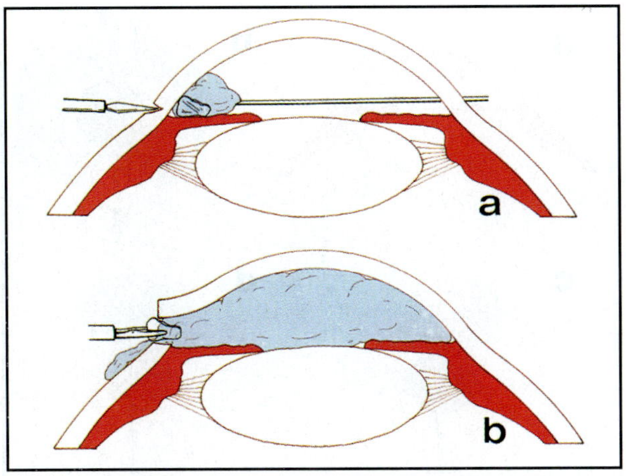

Figure 26-18. Foreign objects in the chamber angle. (a) When its shape is not sharp, a foreign object in the chamber angle can be surrounded and immobilized by viscoelastic. (b) Continued injection of viscoelastic creates a pressure gradient that directs the foreign object toward the corneoscleral incision applied for removal. The viscoelastic leaks out through it, at the same time removing the foreign object.

that are sometimes found in the AC. One particular kind of foreign object that often penetrates the eye with no wound is caterpillar setae. Sometimes a cilium is completely inside the AC and others project from the cornea toward the AC. A perfectly transparent viscoelastic is crucial for the extraction, as it allows the surgeon to detect the largest number of cilia. These can be grasped with McPherson forceps, but might also break in fragments, thus increasing problems. When possible, they must be guided only by the viscoelastic, which can incorporate them and thus permit removal by aspiration or push them outside through an opportunely cut incision. Despite the assistance provided by most transparent viscoelastics (such as Healon®), removing caterpillar setae or other animal fragments from the AC can be very difficult.

Foreign Objects on the Iris

If the foreign object is lying on the surface of the iris, removing it can be difficult, as it often adheres to the iris tenaciously. Once the AC has been filled, the needle injecting viscoelastic can split the foreign object from the iris by lifting one corner and injecting the viscous product between it and the iris. Then the foreign body can be grasped by the forceps and extracted through the limbal incision. In selected cases it will be necessary to perform a small anterior iridectomy, removing a small portion of the anterior iris membrane along with the foreign body.

Foreign Objects in the Chamber Angle

When the foreign object lies in the chamber angle, it is better to inject a viscoelastic to mobilize it and help extract it through a limbal incision made near the object. Sodium hyaluronate with high molecular weight is injected with a thin needle through the opposite limbus, while a suitably sized limbal incision with the inside rim immediately above the foreign object is cut next to it. Viscoelastic injection eases the expression of the foreign body, which can be grasped with the forceps as soon as it is outside the eye (Figure 26-18). There is no danger of hypotony, as the material keeps the chamber deep, even though the extraction wound is slightly widened during the procedure.

Special Cases

Fluid, liquid, or gaseous bodies may be present in the AC as a consequence of posterior segment surgery. Viscoelastic materials can direct silicone or gas bubbles out of the AC, even though they tend to reabsorb spontaneously. Materials with lighter weight than viscoelastic solutions are voided through a corneoscleral incision, kept elevated by the surgeon (Figure 26-19, a and b). Because they have poor viscosity, residuals of heavy fluids such as perfluorocarbons can be immobilized by the viscoelastic while the patient is inclined, then extracted through a cannula (Figure 26-19, c and d). In this procedure the viscoelastic is also useful to prevent a heavy residual from moving to a place where its detection could be difficult—for instance, at the back of the iris through the pupil or an iridectomy. Performing these procedures is most comfortable under a slit-lamp microscope, with self-closing limbal incisions made in the upper portion for light materials and in the lower portion for heavy materials.

CICATRICIAL OUTCOME

When recent, perforating wounds can be treated as described above. However, when the cicatricial phase has already started, they create special difficulties. Overwhelming amounts of viscoelastic help the surgeon understand anatomy that has been altered by previous trauma, besides protecting the injured structures. It also maintains space well in these eyes, which have frequently lost vitreous. The viscoelastic can also expose the presence of synechiae in the AC, which can be excised while bleeding is controlled by further viscoelastic injection (Figure 26-20). A material with high molecular weight (such as Healon® GV) is greatly helpful in moving tissues and creating suitable spaces for scissors and blades, thus allowing surgery to be performed as desired.

Despite careful performance, dissecting iris–corneal synechiae often causes excessive bleeding and is not always beneficial. When adhesions occur in a central area and therefore interfere with vision they must be released, whereas they can remain in place when peripheral portions of the cornea are involved and keratoplasty is not necessary. For example, the frequent occurrence of pupillary stretching with ectopia caused by the presence of a scar with synechiae in the chamber angle is best solved with simple corepraxia under viscoelastic, which is in practice risk-free (Figure 26-21, a and b). Debridement of iris/angle synechiae would almost certainly cause immediate bleeding, and perhaps more severe consequences to the posterior segment, such as cystoid macular edema. However, cosmetic requirements must also be taken into account. These are perhaps more evident in eyes with a pale iris, where sometimes a cicatricial outcome requires iris surgery. Functional needs such as monocular diplopia are occasionally present, which require "cold" manipulation of the traumatized iris (Figure 26-21, c and d).

Anterior adherence of the iris to the corneal stroma is exposed by injecting viscoelastic all around the area. When the synechia is in a central position, it can be easily detected and requires no further treatment. The surgeon checks its consistency with a small spatula, which in very fortunate cases can alone release it. Tough synechiae are cut with microscissors, taking care to leave as little iris residue as possible adhering to the corneal endothelium. A highly viscous viscoelastic allows the surgeon to perceive the precise location of the cut with consequent minimal risk of a sudden shallowing of the AC.

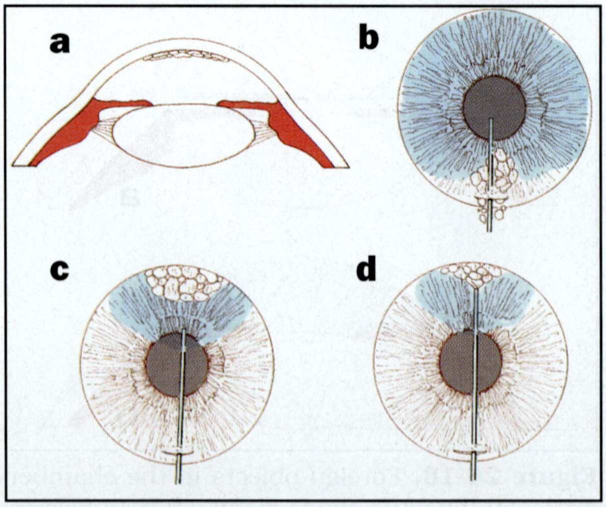

Figure 26-19. Removing silicone oil and liquid perfluorocarbonate from the AC. (a) Residues of silicone oil as well as partial silicone emulsion in the AC adhere to the cornea when the patient is prone. (b) A viscoelastic material filling the AC permits the surgeon to remove all the oil present. (c) Residual liquid perfluorocarbon tends to adhere to the iris when the patient lies down. These can be im-mobilized with a visco-elastic product. (d) The immobilized residues can be aspirated through a Charles cannula introduced in the AC.

Precise movements are mandatory to limit iris damage and consequently the expansion of the coloboma requiring repair. If the synechia reaches the periphery, the whole extent is often not visible. Sometimes a viscoelastic passing beyond the synechia can expose its extent toward the chamber periphery. A dyed viscoelastic such as Healon® Yellow is helpful in this instance, which can be used in addition to a previously injected colorless product.

After addressing anterior synechiae, the surgeon turns his or her attention to posterior iris adhesions occurring between iris tissue and lens residues (Figure 26-22, a–c). If only the capsule remains or a real traumatic cataract persists, separating the iris plane from the lens plane is a crucial phase of repair

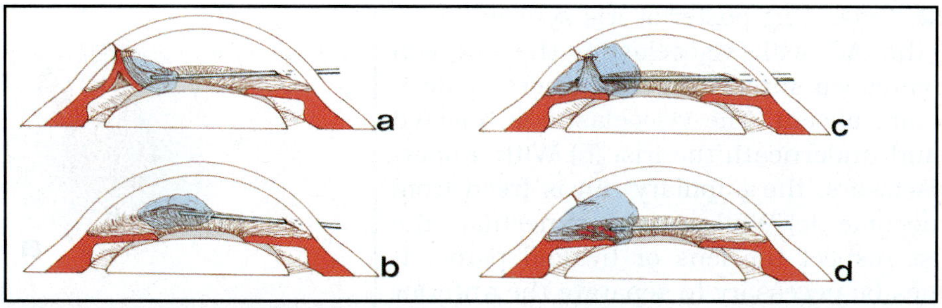

Figure 26-20. Repairing resulting scars. (a) Anterior synechiae of cicatricial origin are clearly exposed by a transparent viscoelastic with high viscosity at rest. (b) The viscoelastic also effective in exposing the angle synechiae. (c) Although sharp, the tool releasing adhesions produces the least damage, as all the tissue not involved by synechiae is moved far away by the viscoelastic. (d) Further injection of viscoelastic in the AC limits possible bleeding.

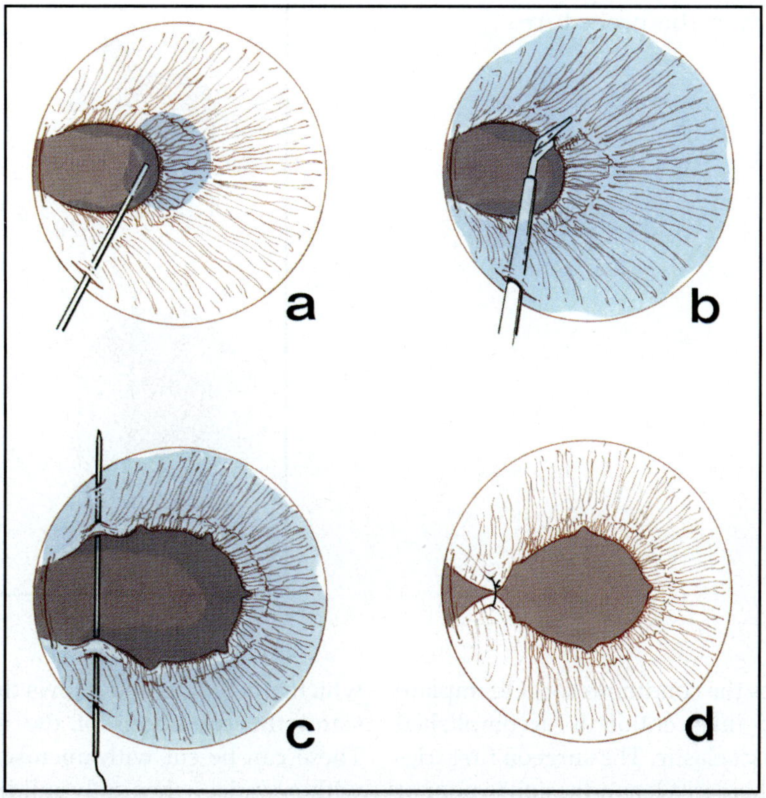

Figure 26-21. Cicatricial pupillary ectopia. (a) Tough adhesions of the iris to a corneal wound may cause pupillary ectopia. Viscoelastic injection over and under the pupillary portion immobilizes the iris away from the lens and cornea. (b) With vitrectomy scissors, the surgeon performs sphincterotomies through a 1.5-mm incision, through which the viscoelastic is not likely to flow back. (c) The iris can be sutured to reduce pupillary dimensions. (d) The outcome can be good, with no iris adherence to the wound.

Figure 26-22. Dissecting posterior iris synechiae. (a) After filling the AC with viscoelastic, the surgeon detects or creates via surgery an area where posterior synechiae are absent. The viscoelastic is injected in that site and underneath the iris. (b) With a spatula or microscissors, the pupillary rim is freed from posterior synechiae. (c) While cutting synechiae, the surgeon must respect the lens or hyaloid plane. It may sometimes be necessary to separate the anterior and the posterior iris membrane in various places. (d) Little by little, the pupillary portion of the iris is cleared from synechiae and lifted by the viscoelastic, which helps control bleeding and maintain fair visibility. (e) The implant may be slightly decentered owing to the synechiae that could not be removed. (f) Regularizing the pupil under viscoelastic concludes the intervention. (g) The surgical outcome usually confirms the worth of the procedure.

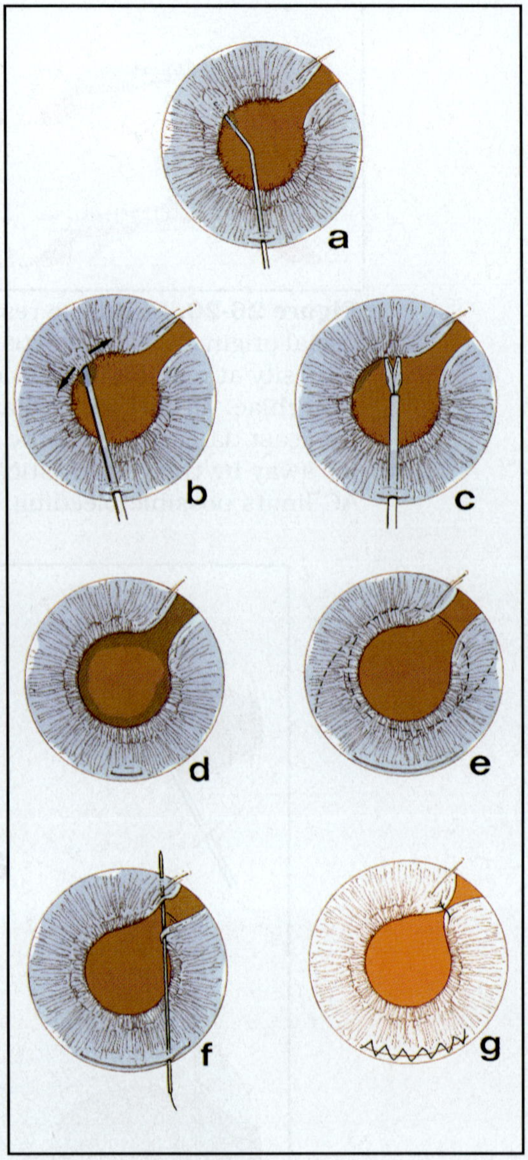

surgery, as it creates the conditions for IOL implantation. The whole intervention is accomplished with the use of a viscoelastic. The surgeon first tries to detect an area where iris–lens adhesion is poor or absent. This zone is more favorable when it occurs at the pupillary border, but an iris coloboma can also be used. After releasing adhesions in this area, the viscoelastic material is injected under the iris, enlarging spaces and creating a passage under the iris that possibly reaches the border of the lens. This first assessment of posterior synechiae is completed by injecting highly viscous sodium hyaluronate, which lifts the iris and allows the surgeon to understand the conditions of the posterior synechiae. These can be cut with microscissors, or unbridled with spatulas when only mildly resistant. Limited bleeding usually occurs during these procedures, which is easily controlled by additional viscoelastic injections.

If possible, the whole iris is freed from posterior synechiae. Sometimes this cannot be done owing to the risk of damaging the anterior hyaloid or the membrane replacing it. In this case only an indispensable part is freed for the sake of IOL implanta-

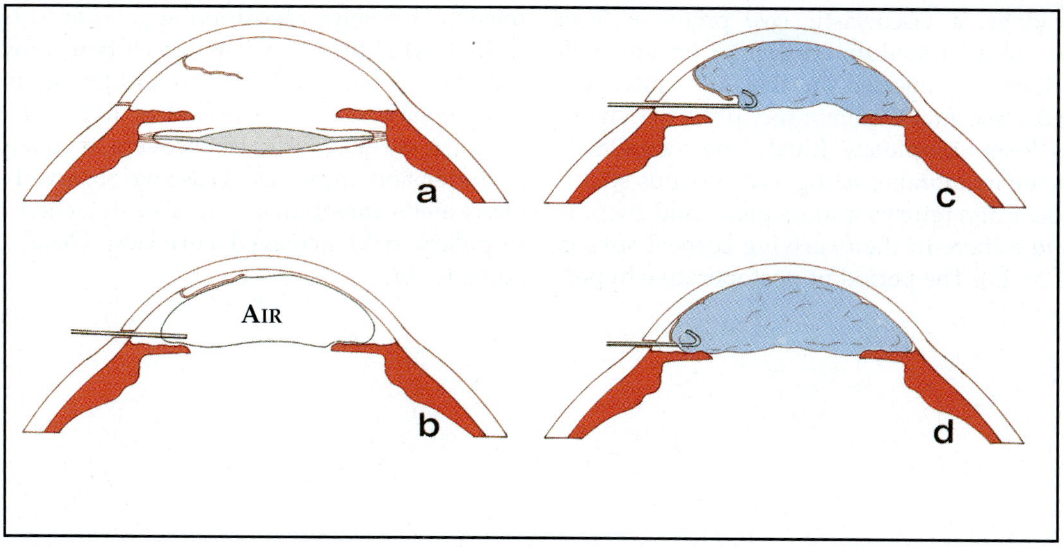

Figure 26-23. Reattaching Descemet's membrane. (a) During cataract surgery, a portion of Descemet's membrane can be accidentally detached. (b) The air introduced in the AC flattens the detached membrane against the endothelium, preventing it from being reattached. (c) A viscoelastic product injected in the middle of the detachment stretches the membrane, encouraging its reattachment. A hooked cannula provides further maneuverability, but the membrane can also be manipulated by injecting the viscoelastic on the opposite side of the cornea, using a straight cannula. (d) The membrane is correctly placed and kept in site with the viscoelastic. The danger of postoperative hypertension must be assessed.

tion, considering that paracentral synechiae may turn out to be useful when the surgeon can trap the lens loops in the iris–lens periphery. In our experience, the presence of posterior synechiae has prevented scleral fixation of the implant on several occasions. The cleavage plane is sometimes inside the iris, and only separating the anterior from the posterior layer can achieve a certain lens support.

Once posterior synechiae have been unbridled, surgery continues with the extraction of lens material, at least in the central portion. A dense, fibrous coat is often present, like a second pupil in a white-colored diaphragm, which is cut with scissors in the middle. This diaphragm is an excellent support for the implant (Figure 26-22, d and e). Surgery continues with the repair of iris damage (Figure 26-22, f and g). At the end of surgery it is not necessary to aspirate all of the viscoelastic used in the AC, as frequent vitreous loss and communication of the AC and vitreous chamber make the development of postoperative hypertension unlikely.

DETACHED DESCEMET'S MEMBRANE

The detachment of Descemet's membrane is a special kind of trauma, often following intraocular surgery. Sometimes it is caused by inappropriate injection of viscoelastic material, and other times by incautious maneuvers undertaken without the use of a viscoelastic. Some eyes seem to be predisposed to detachment of Descemet's membrane, particularly those of young patients in whom the AC is less deep.

This latter condition is probably one of the most suitable examples to demonstrate the usefulness of viscoelastic materials in ocular surgery. Restoring a detached Descemet's membrane was traditionally performed with air bubbles that pushed the membrane in place and allowed suturing with 10-0 or 11-0 nylon. The drawback of the air bubble was that it could not stretch a furled membrane, which therefore had to be manipulated by a spatula sliding directly on the corneal endothelium. The procedure was not always successful.

Nowadays, a viscoelastic (we prefer sodium hyaluronate with medium molecular weight such as Healon®) is injected in the AC under the detached Descemet's membrane, until the chamber has been completely filled. The viscoelastic unfolds the membrane, acting as a "viscous spatula" if necessary, returns it to its place, and encourages it to adhere to the overlying corneal stroma (Figure 26-23). The period of postoperative hypertension also helps repositioning, and must be controlled with beta blockers or carbon anhydrase inhibitors when too high. No additional suturing is necessary. Once the period of hypertension is over, the cornea gradually recovers its transparency and vision improves. A case we observed where Descemet's membrane was also detached in the pupillary field achieved corrected visual acuity equal to 0.8.

Chapter Twenty-Seven

Use of Viscoelastics in Glaucoma Surgery

Glaucoma surgery has undergone a remarkable technical evolution in the last 30 years, following the extraordinary advances achieved in ophthalmic surgery. As in other types of ophthalmic surgery, glaucoma interventions benefited from the development of new procedures and from the modification of established procedures stimulated by enormous interest in cataract microsurgery. In this respect, research in cataract techniques yielded benefits far beyond expectations, involving a variety of other ocular pathologies. Descriptions of and innovations in glaucoma surgery are difficult to summarize owing to the wide range of glaucomas and possible surgical treatments. However, the main developments in glaucoma surgical treatments during the early 1990s can be considered to be the following:

- The use of trabeculectomy as the intervention of choice in uncomplicated cases. It has been stated—with good reason—that trabeculectomy is probably not a good antiglaucoma intervention. Nevertheless, it is the best currently available for the ophthalmologist.
- The wide use of antimetabolite medications in surgical cases at risk of cicatrization, with large-scale use of mitomycin C and 5-FU.
- More frequent lens extractions during trabeculectomy, due to the procedure's tendency to cause cataracts. This effect is particularly evident in subjects with well-established cataracts, particularly those over age 70. The trend has increased after the advent of phacoemulsification, which limits postoperative inflammation and astigmatism.
- The obsolescence of simple iridectomy interventions, now replaced by Nd:YAG laser iridoclasis.
- Knowledge of the aspects particular to congenital glaucoma, now treated with goniotomy or ab externo trabeculotomy.
- The establishment of surgical interventions for a limited number of special cases, such as cyclodialysis and cyclodiastasis interventions or cyclodestructive procedures, now also accomplished endoscopically.
- The acceptance by most surgeons of seton surgery as the means to treat refractory glaucomas, formerly treated through multiple operations.
- Attempts to use laser energy to create antiglaucoma fistulas, in order to reduce surgical trauma and complications. These appear to be far from successful.

In most recent evolutions of glaucoma surgery, viscoelastic materials have played a primary role, even though they are not as widely used as they are in cataract surgery. At present, a large number of antiglaucomatous procedures are performed without viscoelastics, even though their usefulness has often been demonstrated.

The Use of Viscoelastics in Glaucoma Interventions

The main goal of glaucoma interventions is to create a fistula between the AC and the subconjunctival space, through which the aqueous humor must be discharged from the eyeball. Less frequently, the intervention may also aim to restore the patency of normal outflow structures (goniotomy) or to increase the outflow through unusual structures (cyclodialysis). One must also consider cyclodestructive procedures, which aim to reduce the production of aqueous humor.

VISCOSITY AT REST

The observation that a viscoelastic has to maintain space during the performance of surgical procedures may seem obvious. Nevertheless, it is important to remember that in glaucoma surgery, nothing but the viscoelastic is usually available to create the volume in the AC necessary for surgical procedures. There is no liquid infusion as in cataract extraction surgery or air injection as sometimes happens in retinal surgery. When a glaucomatous eye is being operated on, the ability to create the necessary space is rather limited, yet the need to do so is great owing to the common presence of a transparent lens, which can by no means be damaged (Figure 27-1a). The main requirement of a viscoelastic used in glaucoma surgery is that the degree of viscosity at rest be high in order to implement a "space tactic" rather than a "surface tactic." The importance of this is clearer for eyes with a shallow AC and a narrow chamber angle, which are at higher risk of lens damage during fistulization.

Whatever filtering procedure is chosen, the immediate consequence is usually marked bulbar hypotension, which can last some days and have harmful effects on the eyeball. In particular, excessive filtration may cause AC collapse, and often choroidal detachment, which prevents chamber reformation (Figure 27-1b). As a result, inflammation can develop between adjoining ocular tissues, which does not occur under normal conditions. Iris–corneal adhesion is likely to cause the formation of peripheral anterior synechiae, observed in a large number of cases after several days of hypotony. For this reason, if hypotony persists longer than 5 to 6 days, the current trend is to surgically drain choroidal detachments while reforming the chamber.

A product that can be left in the AC at the end of the filtration procedure and that can reduce the risk of hypotony appears to be a remarkable advance for the ophthalmic surgeon. In fact, virtual elimination of hypotony could reduce both trauma following filtration surgery and postoperative complica-

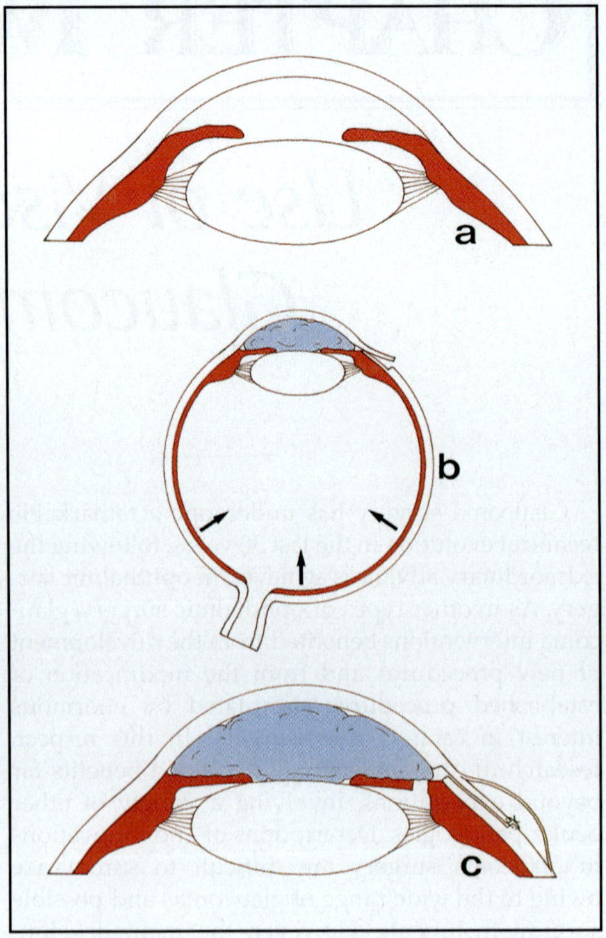

Figure 27-1. Principles of viscoelastic use in glaucoma surgery. (a) In glaucoma surgery it is particularly important to protect the lens, which is often transparent. Because viscoelastic materials can hold space, they consequently play a central role in such protection. Another structure to be protected is the corneal endothelium, particularly in view of possible further interventions. (b) Once the AC is opened, IOP suddenly drops to nearly zero. The choroidal bed may dilate, thus contributing to a reduction in AC depth. Viscoelastics with high viscosity at rest keep the AC deep. (c) When left in the AC at the end of surgery, the viscoelastic could oppose excessive filtration and formation of a serous choroidal detachment, at least in the early postoperative hours. Because it is often injected through thin needles crossing the cornea, the viscoelastic must have excellent pseudoplasticity.

tions. Even though such considerations are mostly theoretical, the main requirement of a viscoelastic for application in glaucoma surgery is the ability to maintain space when the movement rate is zero, in order to enable the choroidal vascular bed to adapt postoperatively to new IOP. Products with low viscosity at 0 shear rate would not be useful for this purpose, as they would not be able to counterbalance even slight posterior pressure. Newer products with very high viscosity are better suited to this application.

BIOCOMPATIBILITY AND ENDOTHELIAL PROTECTION

Biocompatibility is an equally important feature for a viscoelastic to be used in glaucoma surgery. The fact that the viscoelastic will likely not be removed from the AC at the end of surgery and will be cleared by the eye in the days following implies that it must be absolutely biocompatible. That is, it must not cause inflammatory or degenerative problems in eyes with a rather delicate morphofunctional balance. Moreover, the product should provide excellent protection to the corneal endothelium, whose integrity is at risk in glaucoma surgery (Figure 27-1a). Very often, eyes operated on for fistulization will undergo surgery again sooner or later (ie, for cataract extraction) or will have been previously treated for glaucoma or some other pathology. Generally, patients undergoing glaucoma surgery are relatively young, and their life expectancy requires the most careful preservation of endothelial cells.

Some studies on the effects of viscoelastics on trabecular cells have been conducted by Miyazaki et al, who demonstrated the superiority of sodium hyaluronate versus chondroitin sulfate or methylcellulose. In 1992, Wirt studied various hyaluronate preparations in animals, and concluded that the product he used showed good biocompatibility.

EASY REMOVAL

Viscoelastics are removed from nonfistulized eyes through the corneoscleral meshwork, with possible hypertension when the quality and quantity of the product temporarily obstructs the filtrating structures. Actually, in glaucomatous eyes, filtering structures are already compromised, and therefore cannot be relied upon for postoperative filtration. Injecting viscoelastics in the AC during filtering operations should not cause any increase in IOP, owing to the presence of the fistula.

Nevertheless, it would be better to use a viscoelastic product that is able to go through the trabeculum without obstructing it even temporarily, or alternatively, to use a material that is rapidly degraded in the AC before it passes through trabecular structures. This conflicts with the need for a highly viscous product, so this is not the optimal solution. However, when the patency of the fistula is uncertain in the days immediately after surgery, it may be better to avoid using most viscous viscoelastics.

It must be noted that even in aphakia, a condition that was often associated with the need for glaucoma interventions, there is a risk that the viscoelastic will cause postoperative hypertension. Despite the larger space available for the diffusion of the injected material, the viscoelastic can occlude the filtering structures, through which it should be discharged in aphakic eyes.

PSEUDOPLASTICITY

There are specific procedures for injecting the viscoelastic easily in filtering glaucoma surgery. When eyes are affected by nonsevere open-angle glaucoma, with no intraocular hypertension at the moment of intervention, surgery can be accomplished without complications or posterior pressure. However, the eyes being treated are often small, with a shallow AC and no posterior vitreous detachment that would allow reduction of the posterior pressure through preoperative oculopressure. During surgery, systemic hypertension in the patient, caused by stress and the possible effect of general and topical medications administered, may cause dilation of the choroidal vascular bed, with consequent development of a posterior pressure that greatly reduces the surgical space in the AC. Under these conditions, the viscoelastic used must be pseudoplastic (Figure 27-1c). A very pseudoplastic viscoelastic can be injected through a cannula of small diameter, or even better, passed through the same 30-G needle used to create a limbal paracentesis, inclined very obliquely. In our experience, we have never had leakage of the AC contents, or worse, iris involvement in the presence of such paracentesis, even with IOP exceeding 40 mmHg.

Poorly pseudoplastic viscoelastics need a real paracentesis opening for injection—similar to that routinely made for cataract extraction—that is not suitable for eyes undergoing glaucoma surgery, owing to its large dimensions and sometimes reduced effect.

Hemostatic Effect

An important feature of viscoelastics in general, although with remarkable differences among products, is their ability to control and stop the bleeding that frequently occurs in ocular surgery. Bleeding is even more frequent in filtering operations performed in eyes showing some congestion of the episcleral circulation. Hemorrhages can appear in scleral regions that have been dissected and cannot be reached for cauterization, unless the cautery is applied blindly under the scleral flap—a rather hazardous procedure with little effect. Sometimes blood leaks out of a lesion in the ciliary body, a possible occurrence during trabeculectomy or peripheral iridectomy that is almost always combined with filtering procedures. Air is often ineffective in controlling such bleeding, as it cannot provide enough pressure to achieve adhesion to the bleeding vessel. However, a viscoelastic product can produce the pressure necessary to stop bleeding.

The effectiveness of the viscoelastic is proportional to its viscosity at rest. The greater the viscosity, the greater pressure it exerts on the blood vessel in a narrow space such as the AC. It is also directly proportional to the internal cohesion, which prevents blood from infiltrating the viscoelastic, and to the adhesiveness of the viscoelastic product, which enables it to remain longer in the site of injection. Based on these observations, Healon® GV appears to be the most suitable material.

Internal Cohesion and Adhesiveness

Almost always in filtering operations, at least one part of viscoelastic is left in the AC after surgery. Therefore, easy removal seems not to be a determining factor in the choice of the material. The rate of internal cohesion is relevant only for the sake of transparency. We can likewise state that greater or poorer adhesion is not important in many respects, as all procedures are accomplished at low shear rate and with no development of tangent forces that may damage more delicate ocular structures, such as the corneal endothelium. In the postoperative period, an overly rapid discharge of the viscoelastic by the normal ocular physiology or a shifting from the site where it was placed are generally undesirable. It is therefore important that the product is able to provide a certain adhesion, so that it can remain exactly on the spot where it has been placed without being moved by aqueous flow. In this case, preparations like Viscoat are generally effective.

Trabeculectomy

Currently, trabeculectomy is the most performed glaucoma intervention. Cairns' original idea was to restore the normal outflow through Schlemm's canal, where the aqueous humor could have access through the open ends after excising a portion of corneoscleral meshwork. The formation of a conjunctival bleb was not deemed necessary for the success of trabeculectomy; on the contrary, it was regarded as a side effect. Now we know that the intervention is effective because it accomplishes filtration of the aqueous humor in the subconjunctival space. In fact, it should be called "protected partial sclerectomy."

Accomplished through several technical variations, all equally effective, the technique consists of the following steps:

- Creating a conjunctival flap, with the base at the limbus or fornix
- Creating a scleral port of partial thickness, with variable shape and size
- Removing a portion of the port bed in contact with the aqueous humor
- Performing a peripheral iridectomy, which prevents the iris from occluding filtration
- Suturing the port
- Suturing the overlying conjunctiva

The intervention is far from perfect. Results range from 60% to 80% success, depending on the practitioner and the type of glaucoma being treated. We must point out that trabeculectomy yields poor results in a large number of glaucoma pathologies, particularly in young patients. Nevertheless, it is the glaucoma intervention with least tendency to result in complications. Therefore, ophthalmologists are constantly trying to find means to improve it and extend its effectiveness to

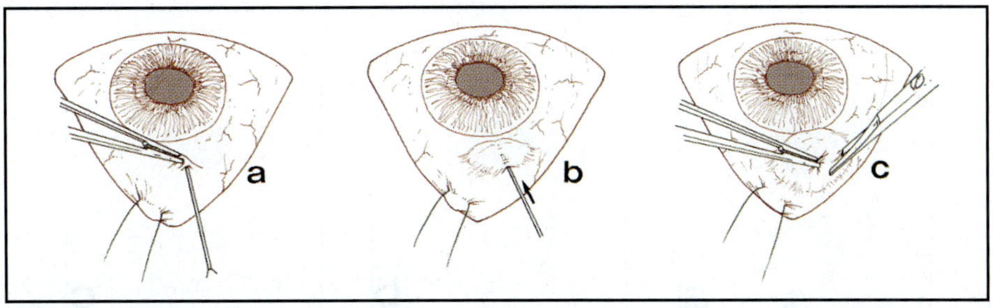

Figure 27-2. Dissecting the conjunctiva using a viscoelastic. (a) Conjunctival dissection using a viscoelastic begins by injecting a highly viscous viscoelastic under the conjunctiva and Tenon's capsule, while these are being lifted by a forceps in the episcleral space. (b) The viscoelastic lifts the conjunctiva and Tenon's capsule, forming a "balloon." (c) The lifted conjunctiva can be incised at the fornix, as shown in the illustration, or at the limbus, to create access to the episcleral space.

the treatment of formerly insensitive glaucomas. This is why viscoelastic materials have been used in glaucoma pathologies since the beginning, although with contradictory results. The most frequently used product is sodium hyaluronate, because it was the first available and based on observations concerning safety and biocompatibility. Some experiments have recently been conducted with a mixture of 3% sodium hyaluronate and 4% chondroitin sulfate (Viscoat), but supporting data from numerous trials have not yet appeared in the international literature.

In general, surgeons' experiences over the last 10 years have shown that the best way to improve the results of trabeculectomies, while reducing the rate of intra- and postoperative complications, was by using viscoelastics.

DISSECTION OF THE CONJUNCTIVA

Dissection of the conjunctiva is a routine but debated step of trabeculectomy. It is thought that detachment of the conjunctiva from the episclera is a mandatory phase to create access to the sclera and space for the formation of the filtering site. Conversely, it is well known that the cicatricial reaction induced by surgical procedures causes greater postoperative adhesion of the conjunctiva to the episclera. Consequently, manipulations should be limited or even abolished. Some trabeculectomy techniques have been developed that do not involve dissection of the conjunctival flap.

DISSECTING UNTOUCHED CONJUNCTIVA

Few surgeons currently use viscoelastic materials to make a conjunctival flap for trabeculectomy of eyes that have never been operated on before. The surgical technique consists of injecting the viscoelastic through a thin needle introduced into a conjunctival fold lifted by a forceps, corresponding to the site where the flap is going to be made (Figure 27-2). The viscoelastic gently detaches the conjunctiva, which is lifted in the form of a bubble or a balloon up to the limbus, where it can be cut at the fornix. The advantages of this procedure as opposed to dissection by scissors and forceps are remarkable:

- The whole thickness of the conjunctiva is maintained, undamaged by inadequate movements of scissors or blunt dissection procedures.
- Bleeding is minimized, owing to the features of conjunctival detachment and the hemostatic effects particular to the viscoelastic.
- (As a result of the above, the cicatricial stimulus is minimized.)
- The ensuing conjunctival incision providing access to the sclera is more precise.
- The surgical field is free from blood, providing excellent visibility of the conjunctiva and the underlying anatomic structures.

Drawbacks seem to be limited to possible inaccurate needle positioning during injection. If the position is too superficial—for instance, over Tenon's capsule—the detachment cannot reach the

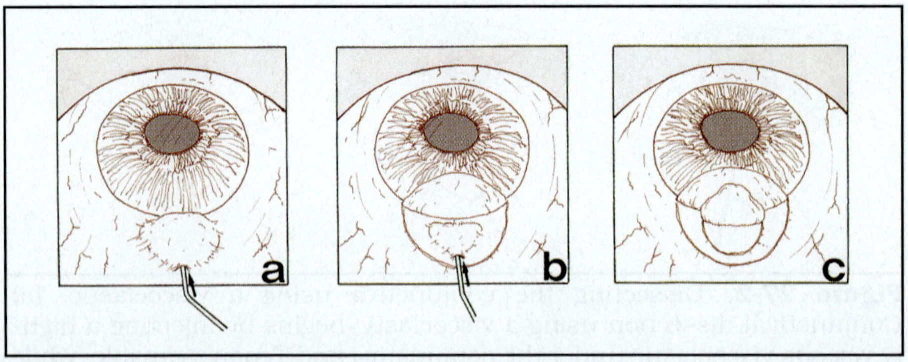

Figure 27-3. Dissecting the conjunctiva and Tenon's capsule using a viscoelastic. (a) In young patients it is better to dissect the conjunctiva and Tenon's capsule separately. The dissection begins by injecting the viscoelastic material under the conjunctiva only, in order to detach it from the Tenon's capsule. (b) The conjunctiva is incised and reflected onto the cornea, while more viscoelastic is injected under Tenon's capsule. (c) At the end of dissection there are two flaps, one consisting of the conjunctiva and the other of the Tenon's capsule.

episclera. Because of the transparency of the viscoelastic material, however, the surgeon can easily see such inaccuracies and reposition the needle, this time a bit closer to the episclera.

To accomplish these procedures, the practitioner needs a product with high viscosity at rest, which can form a "balloon" under the conjunctiva that is able to detach it from the underlying planes. High biocompatibility seems not to be mandatory, as the viscoelastic injected in the subconjunctival space is removed during subsequent procedures, unless an appreciable amount reaches intraocular structures. Pseudoplasticity must be moderate, as it is possible to use a medium-sized cannula needle without problems. Both adhesive and cohesive materials seem to be suitable for the purpose.

Viscoelastic products are also helpful in dissection of the conjunctiva in young patients where Tenon's capsule is represented. A large number of surgeons dissect the conjunctiva of pediatric patients based at the limbus, separating Tenon's membrane from the real conjunctiva (Figure 27-3). Then both membranes undergo separate treatment, and are even sutured on different planes, so antimetabolite medication can be applied directly onto the episclera without touching the conjunctiva. When required, injection of viscoelastic can separate the conjunctiva from Tenon's membrane, which makes surgery easier.

Dissecting Cicatricial Conjunctiva

Dissecting the conjunctival flap is simple to accomplish in eyes with untouched conjunctiva, but may present some difficulty when the tissue has already undergone surgery; for example, previous filtering operations. In that case, cicatricial retraction hinders good detachment of the conjunctiva from the underlying layers, and the conjunctival tissue is at risk of laceration, which would make it unusable for the formation of the filtrating bleb. The problems linked to the fragility of previously treated conjunctiva are even greater when surgery has recently been performed and tissue appears friable even at the lightest touch. Moreover, bleeding often occurs, which makes it difficult to continue with the dissection, particularly when a "club-like" blade is used instead of scissors to prevent laceration of the conjunctival tissue.

A viscoelastic is able to accomplish conjunctival dissection even under these difficult circumstances. Viscoelastics are injected 10 mm away from the limbus, corresponding to the limbal zone to be reached. At that distance, one can find a portion of conjunctiva that is easy to detach, where a needle mounted on the syringe can penetrate without problems (Figure 27-4, a–c). It is best to avoid a conjunctival buttonhole, which would allow a fair amount of the viscoelastic to flow back out and

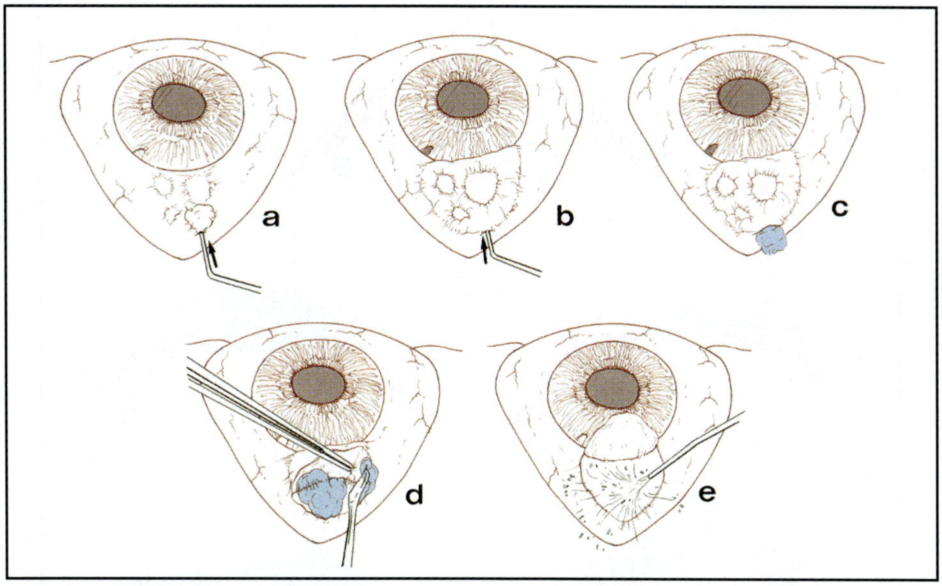

Figure 27-4. Dissecting the conjunctiva in previously operated eyes. (a) Dissection of the conjunctival flap using a viscoelastic begins 10 mm from the limbus, where it is easier to find an area of conjunctival tissue free from adhesions. (b) Injection of viscoelastic detaches the conjunctiva from the episclera and allows the surgeon to detect the areas of adhesion. (c) Once the conjunctiva has been opened, the viscoelastic tends to leak out. It is therefore even more important that it has high viscosity at rest. (d) With the help of the viscoelastic material, which reveals adhesions, preserves transparency, and controls bleeding, conjunctival dissection can be extended to the whole area. (e) At the end of conjunctival flap dissection, the operating field is cleared from the viscoelastic, then dried after diathermal hemostasis and application of an antimetabolite drug.

would not generate enough force to facilitate good dissection. The needle should be turned toward the sclera to reduce scleral damage and therefore bleeding, and if possible should be made to penetrate under Tenon's capsule. As the viscoelastic injection proceeds, the conjunctiva is detached from the episclera and a bleb of transparent material is formed. This allows the surgeon to detect the areas of greatest cicatrization, which then can be treated in turn with a suitable blade. High viscosity at rest is a very important factor in this procedure; Healon® GV is probably the most suitable product.

Once the desired bleb has been formed, the conjunctiva is opened at the fornix or at the limbus, according to the surgeon's experience, and the dissection of adhesions can begin. It is best for the opening to be small, to allow pressure to develop inside the conjunctival bleb following further injection of viscoelastic. During this procedure bleeding is likely to occur, which can be controlled by the viscoelastic, owing to its hemostatic properties (at least of sodium hyaluronate) and to the pressure exerted on the bleeding vessel. Remember that diathermy is contraindicated, as it may cause further shrinking of a conjunctival tissue already showing cicatricial retraction. Another advantage of the viscoelastic is its ability to form a balloon of transparent material, which removes blood from the crucial zone, greatly increasing visibility during surgery and reducing the risk of conjunctival perforation. Once dissection of the conjunctiva has been completed, the original opening is widened and the conjunctival balloon is transformed into a conjunctival flap (Figure 27-4, d and e). The viscoelastic is rinsed with cold solution and the sclera is ready for application of antimetabolite medication, usually mitomycin C, which we also advise using in difficult cases of previously treated eyes.

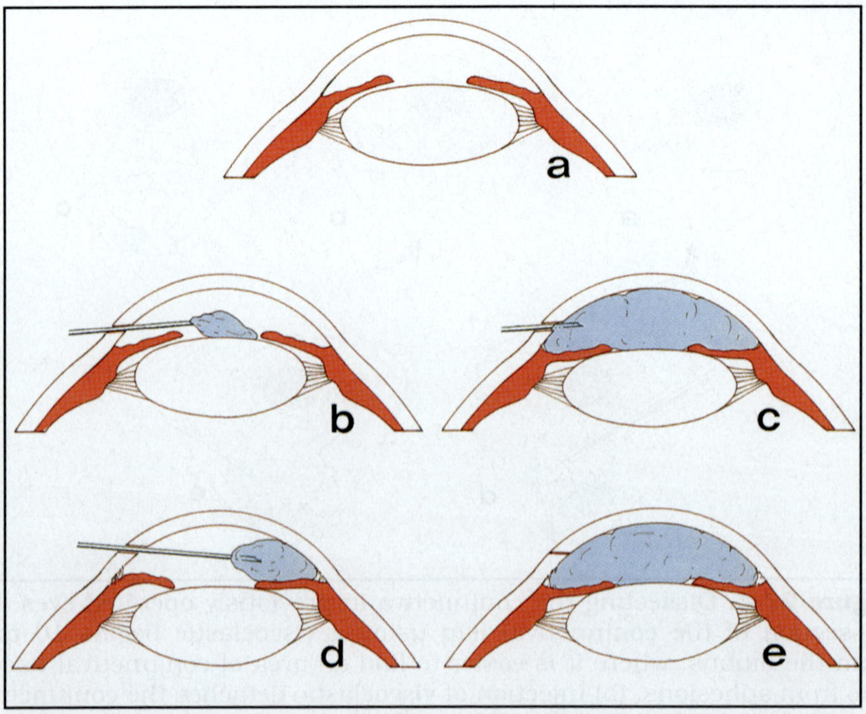

Figure 27-5. Viscoelastic injection in the AC before its opening. (a) Eyes planned for glaucoma surgery often have a shallow AC. (b) According to Barak, it is always worth injecting the viscoelastic before opening the AC, through a paracentesis performed with a thin needle or a blade. (c) Sodium hyaluronate with a high molecular weight deepens the AC and keeps it formed. (d) The injection is particularly useful in the presence of angle synechiae detected during preoperative gonioscopic examination. (e) A viscoelastic with high viscosity at rest is able to release the adhesions and deepen the AC.

DEEPENING THE ANTERIOR CHAMBER BEFORE OPENING

Trabeculectomy is a surgical procedure implying some manipulation of structures in contact with the AC or even inside the chamber. The intervention is far more easily performed when the AC has been deepened by viscoelastics injected even before the chamber is opened. In fact, many eyes that have undergone glaucoma surgery have had a shallow AC, and surgical procedures risk being too traumatic for the cornea on one side and for the lens on the other. Sometimes angle synechiae are already present, which may contribute to the failure of surgery. All these are valid reasons for early injection of viscoelastics in the AC.

The technique proposed by Barak et al consists of injecting sodium hyaluronate through a paracentesis after creating the scleral port, but before the distal incision of sclerotomy (Figure 27-5). The paracentesis is made with a blade that creates a self-sealing incision. This prevents any collapse of the AC due to excessive hypotony, in compliance with Wand's guidelines. Surgery continues while the viscoelastic is maintained in the AC, even at the end of the intervention. In Barak's study, the AC remained formed during the whole intervention in 10 out of 11 eyes studied. With the AC filled with viscoelastic, peripheral iridectomy is more difficult to accomplish, as the iris does not spontaneously appear in the site of sclerostomy but must be grasped with a forceps and pulled outside to be cut. This did not cause any complications in the study mentioned. The results of such early injection of sodium hyaluronate during trabeculectomy were rather good, especially in terms of endothelial pro-

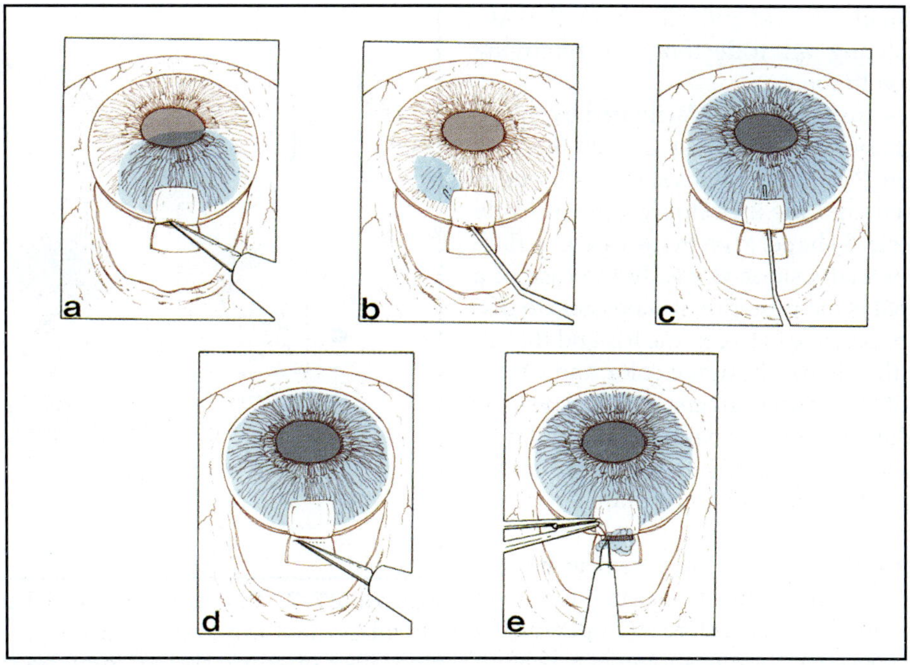

Figure 27-6. Viscoelastic-assisted trabeculectomy. (a) The presence of a viscoelastic in the AC makes trabeculectomies safer from the point of anterior corneoscleral incision onward. (b) After opening the AC, it is always beneficial to inject a viscoelastic or refill the amount that has leaked out in case it has already been introduced through a paracentesis. (c) A product with high viscosity at rest seems to be preferable, as it is less likely to leak out through the port of trabeculectomy. (d) Posterior sclerocorneal incision is at higher risk of iris or ciliary damage, as in that area the AC is less deep, and is reduced further by its surgical opening. (e) A viscoelastic with high viscosity at rest is also able to keep the chamber deep during sclerotomy.

tection. Cell loss after 3 months was equal to 7 +/- 9% in eyes receiving Healon® versus a loss rate of 17 +/- 11% in the control eyes receiving BSS. These data are relevant, taking into account that many eyes that undergo trabeculectomy are destined to undergo other open eye interventions in the future.

DEEPENING THE ANTERIOR CHAMBER AFTER OPENING

The AC is most commonly deepened with viscoelastic after it is opened in the site of sclerectomy. The chamber may collapse owing to excessive posterior pressure or incautious movements by the surgeon. Completion of sclerectomy also becomes difficult in conditions of excessive hypotony, as the position of the tissue to be removed is more difficult to access and the iris is interposed. The maintenance of ocular tone and space achieved with the viscoelastic allows the surgeon to perform all the incisions required to create a filtering fistula, starting from the proximal corneoscleral incision (Figure 27-6). After opening the AC, the highly viscous viscoelastic remains in its intraocular place, allowing the surgeon to perform the distal scleral incision and complete the sclerectomy.

Sometimes it is necessary to fill the AC with viscoelastic intraoperatively to control excessive posterior pressure originating from the choroid (Figure 27-7) or to limit small hemorrhages that often present themselves in the AC but originate in the zone of sclerostomy. More seldom the viscoelastic is used to perform small surgical procedures in the AC, such as perfecting an iridectomy or removing scraps of scleral tissue.

Iridectomies are also greatly facilitated by injecting a small amount of viscoelastic over the area selected (Figure 27-8). The removal of iris tissue is more controlled, and the iridectomy is more likely to have the desired shape, even in the case of a flabby, atrophic, or malpositioned iris. In the case of a sclerectomy that is too posterior, it is possible to discern the area of passage between the iris and the ciliary body by the change in tissue color and different position of the muscle fibers. The viscoelastic then allows the surgeon to spare the ciliary body, avoiding the onset of hemorrhages that would be difficult to control and uncomfortable for the patient.

Nevertheless, these procedures seem to be less effective in protecting corneal endothelium than when the injection is given before AC opening. In addition, postoperative complications such as hemorrhage, hypotension, and choroidal detachment appear to be greater. Facilitation of surgical procedures is also out of the question, particularly in very difficult cases, where the availability of viscoelastics may make a great difference.

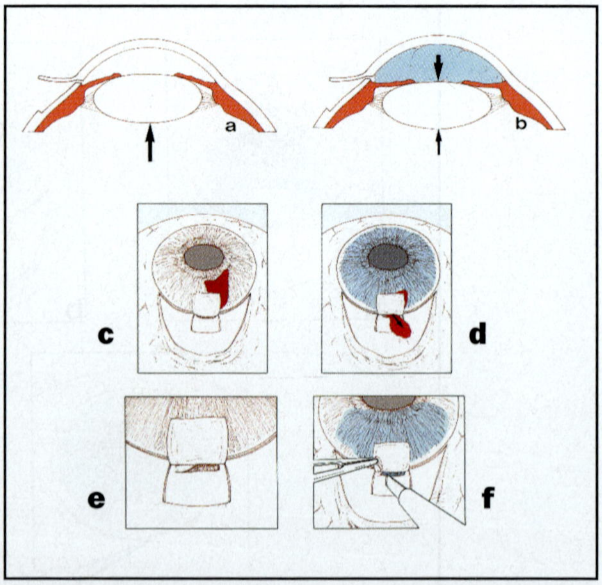

Figure 27-7. Viscoelastics and the difficulties of trabeculectomy. (a) Posterior pressure occurring after opening the AC may be due to a dilation of the choroidal vascular bed. (b) The viscoelastic tends to counterbalance this pressure with a force dependent on its viscosity at rest. Surgery can then be continued with greater safety. (c) Some bleeding often occurs, originating in the area of sclerectomy, and tends to invade the AC. (d) The viscoelastic material can increase pressure in the AC, filling it completely and exerting a direct hemostatic effect on the bleeding vessel. A small hemorrhage thus stops or tends to be discharged outside the eye. (e) Sometimes it is still necessary to remove some fragments of scleral tissue that tend to migrate into the AC. (f) The viscoelastic material permits the surgeon to catch and remove these fragments without damaging the iris or the ciliary body.

DEEPENING THE ANTERIOR CHAMBER AT THE END OF SURGERY

Early use of sodium hyaluronate in glaucoma surgery aimed to deepen the AC at the end of trabeculectomy surgery. The technical reasons for this application are easy to discern. The presence of sodium hyaluronate in the AC at the end of surgery should prevent the possible onset of postoperative hypotony, enabling the eye to heal without trauma under the new hydrodynamic conditions. Choroidal detachment, a threatening complication for its effects on anterior segment anatomy, primarily the lens, should also be less frequent, as should postoperative blood effusion in the AC, which often originates from small vessels close to the ciliary body that do not bleed during surgery. Finally, there is the hope that in the long run, filtration will turn out to be a better choice than not using a viscoelastic.

The best technique to fill the AC with viscoelastic at the end of trabeculectomy is to use a paracentesis made at the beginning of the procedure, when the eyeball still has tone (Figure 27-9). It is better not to inject the material through the scleral port. There is a risk of damaging the lens, as well as deforming the port and allowing some of the injected material to leak out.

The product used in this case is almost always sodium hyaluronate. According to some surgeons, it is not necessary to fill the chamber completely if one chooses a viscoadherent product, which remains longer in the site of injection because it is less likely

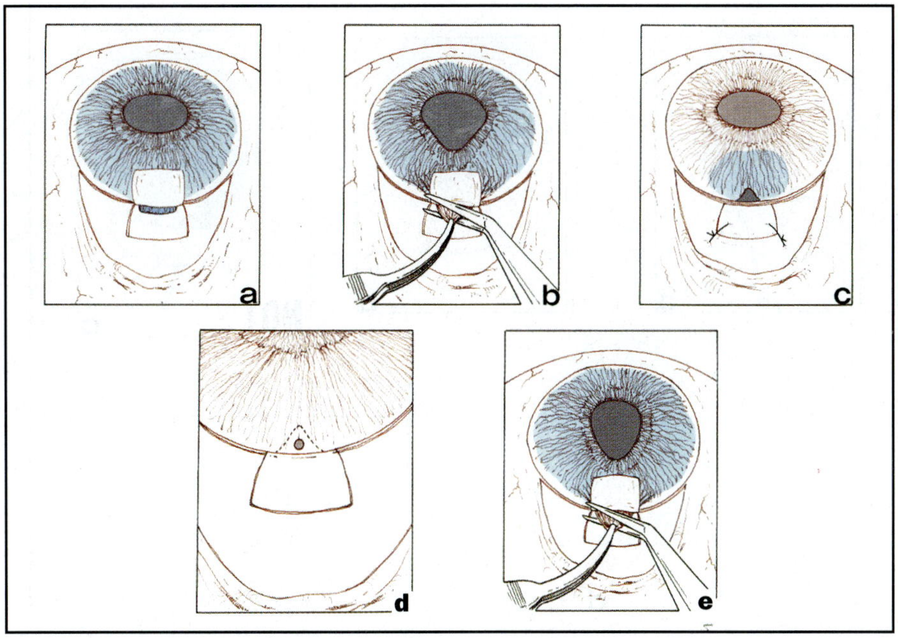

Figure 27-8. Viscoelastic-assisted trabeculectomy: iridectomy. (a) The presence of a viscoelastic in the AC prevents the iris from prolapsing spontaneously on the threshold of sclerectomy. When the amount of viscoelastic introduced is excessive, it will instead encourage iris prolapse. (b) The iris must be grasped by a thin-toothed forceps and extracted in order to be cut. (c) Iridectomy has been completed. Additional viscoelastic injected through the sclerectomy in the area of iridectomy stretches the iris and allows the surgeon to see the extent of the surgical iridectomy. (d) The iridectomy may turn out to be incomplete, particularly when the iris is thick and very tonic. In the illustration, the posterior layer has been pierced in only one spot. (e) Injecting viscoelastic in the AC allows iridectomy to be repeated without affecting the lens.

to be removed by aqueous flows (Figure 27-9). They state that injecting 0.05 to 0.1 mL of Viscoat near the fistula ensures the required tissue separation for a period of time comparable to that achieved when filling the chamber with sodium hyaluronate alone. The possibility that in this case a limited amount of viscoadherent product has the same effect as a larger amount of cohesive product is a consideration accepted by most surgeons. The presence of the fistula should prevent the increase of postoperative pressure, which generally occurs when a viscoelastic is left in the AC at the end of cataract surgery. Some hypertension does occur in control eyes that received no injection. However, the hypertension is never high, seldom exceeding 30 mmHg over 1 to 2 days. Some studies deny the danger of such tension peaks for the optic nerve; nevertheless, it seems reasonable to use this procedure cautiously in eyes with a severely diminished visual field. Viscoelastics more prone to stimulating hypertension must be used very cautiously.

Among the objectives that injecting viscoelastics at the end of trabeculectomy aims to achieve, only one has been undeniably accomplished: the control and reduction of hyphemas. Wilson's study of 119 cases compared with 122 controls demonstrated that postoperative hyphemas were reduced from 20% to 3%, an extraordinary outcome that alone supports using sodium hyaluronate for this purpose in trabeculectomies.

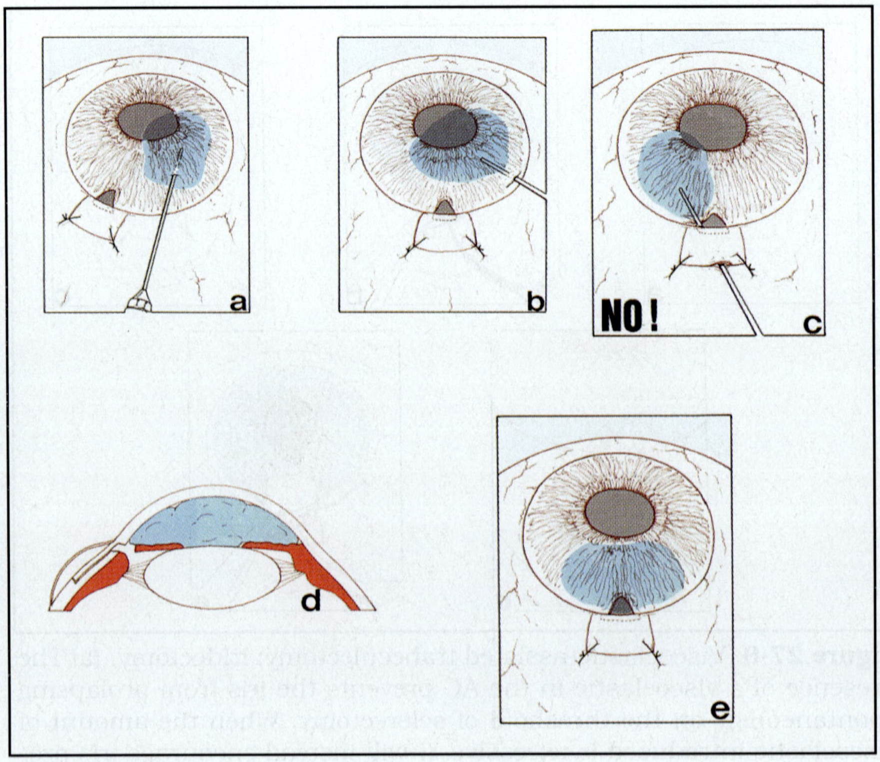

Figure 27-9. AC re-formed by a viscoelastic at the end of trabeculectomy. (a) At the end of surgery, particularly in the presence of hypotony, a viscoelastic can be injected in the AC through a thin needle inserted very obliquely into the central cornea. The product chosen must be very pseudoplastic. (b) A viscoelastic product with lower pseudoplasticity requires creating a paracentesis at the beginning of surgery that allows the insertion of a 21-G or 19-G cannula. (c) Owing to the risk of possible anatomic distortion and lens damage, it is not advisable to pass the viscoelastic cannula through the sclerectomy. The material injected is likely to flow back out through the site. (d) Leaving the AC full of viscoelastic at the end of surgery reduces postoperative hyphema and is likely to reduce excessive filtration. (e) Some researchers have noted that postoperative hypotony is reduced when some viscoelastic is left in the chamber, but exhaustive studies have produced no findings to confirm this observation.

Other postoperative features appeared not to differ between the group treated with Healon® and the control group. The number of cases of hypotony with choroidal detachment did not decrease, nor did the number of scleral draining procedures, and anatomic and tension results were not better in the long run. Such results led to the conclusion that filling the AC at the end of trabeculectomy is useful primarily for patients who are likely to experience postoperative bleeding. Further studies confirmed these early impressions about the prevention of bleeding, despite some disagreement, and also showed that eyes receiving sodium hyaluronate were less likely to develop cataracts 1 year after surgery. Researchers also found that the presence of the viscoelastic in the AC inhibited filtration in the hours immediately after surgery, with beneficial effects on the anatom-

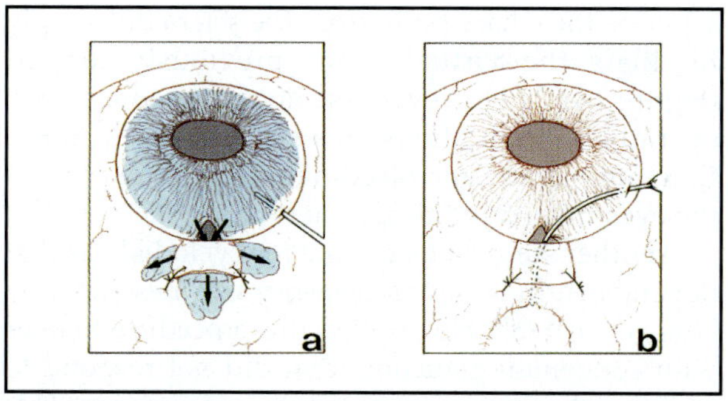

Figure 27-10. Conjunctival bleb filled with viscoelastic at the end of trabeculectomy. (a) Wilson's technique: The AC is overwhelmingly filled through the paracentesis, and the viscoelastic spontaneously flows into the subconjunctival space through the sclerectomy. (b) Boles-Carenini's technique: The subconjunctival space is filled through the sclerectomy by a cannula inserted in the AC through a lateral paracentesis.

ic integrity of ocular structures. More recently, viscoelastics have been noted to reduce postoperative hypotony.

SUBCONJUNCTIVAL INJECTION AT THE END OF SURGERY

Nearly all surgeons who leave the viscoelastic in the AC at the end of surgery also fill the conjunctival bleb, hoping on one hand to contribute to filtration control in the early postoperative period, and on the other to keep the conjunctival bleb more evident in the late postoperative period. Wilson's technique consists of overwhelming AC filling through the paracentesis, so as to induce the viscoelastic to leak through sclerectomy until the subconjunctival space is filled. Boles-Carenini instead prefers injecting Healon® in the subconjunctival space through the AC paracentesis, passing with a cannula through sclerectomy (Figure 27-10).

Regardless of the technique used, the immediate result is encouraging, with evidence in the first days after surgery of a larger bleb than without the use of viscoelastics. The long-term outcome is likely to be the same, as there are no anatomic differences between blebs filled with viscoelastic and those left to spontaneous filling.

DISCUSSION

The application of viscoelastics to trabeculectomy made several surgical procedures easier and safer, especially when performed on eyes with a shallow AC or in the presence of posterior pressure. The whole surgical procedure has become much safer in general, with a great reduction in complications linked to hemorrhage. Nevertheless, the advantages provided by viscoelastics are probably relevant only in cases that otherwise would have severe complications during surgery.

The best routine use of viscous products seems to be early injection, as maintained by Barak. The most suitable material seems to be sodium hyaluronate with high molecular weight, such as Healon®. The viscoelastic can remain in place at the end of surgery, unless the optic nerve is not able to bear several hours of hypertension, in which case it is better to inject an adhesive product such as Viscoat. One should not expect positive effects on filtration or the risk of hypotension with choroidal detachment.

In filtration surgery, viscoelastic-dependent techniques have not yet been developed, in contrast to other surgical fields such as cataract surgery and keratoplasty.

CYCLODIALYSIS

Developed by Heine in 1905, cyclodialysis is a glaucoma intervention that aims to facilitate the outflow of aqueous humor in the superchoroidal space, using a specially designed instrument to perform a limited detachment of the ciliary body. This instrument, the cyclodialysis spatula, is now commonly used in ophthalmic surgery. The intervention both increases filtration and reduces the production of aqueous humor induced by ciliary detachment.

SURGICAL TECHNIQUE

The traditional technique begins by making a conjunctival incision 7 to 8 mm away from the limbus, uncovering a portion of sclera. The sclera itself is cut 4 to 5 mm away from the limbus, 3 to 4 mm wide, leading the incision to the choroidal plane. A spatula bent in the shape of the eyeball is then used to split the ciliary–choroidal complex from the sclera. The spatula is moved forward until it appears in the AC, then rotated to the right and the left to increase the portion of ciliary body detached from the sclera. After the spatula is withdrawn, the scleral incision is sutured. The closure of the conjunctiva ends the intervention.

Cyclodialysis is not very popular among ophthalmic surgeons owing to the frequency of complications. While performing this technique it is easy to cause significant bleeding, or worse, inadvertently perforate the choroid and thus damage the zonule and lens. In addition, its ability to control IOP in cases of decompensated glaucoma appears to be limited over time. This intervention can be difficult to titrate, with the possibility of prolonged hypotension leading to marked anatomic and functional damage. For these reasons, cyclodialysis is a seldom used intervention. However, using viscoelastic materials can greatly improve cyclodialysis, clarifying its surgical actions and reducing complications, which has led to a new assessment of this old operation.

The most common technique is to dissect the choroid and ciliary body by injecting sodium hyaluronate (Healon®) through a smooth cannula oriented toward the limbus (Figure 27-11). The cannula is directed toward the angle while the Healon® is being injected, so that the viscoelastic separates the tissues. In fact, Healon® appears in the AC before the tip of the cannula. The injection of viscoelastic continues as the cannula is moved to the right and left, in order to create a tunnel filled with viscoelastic, which will actually be a bit larger than the width of the cannular movements. The intervention ends by suturing the sclera and conjunctiva. By using this procedure, Alpar achieved a remarkable reduction in intraoperative complications, hemorrhages, and hyphema, to 21% of the eyes treated. When cases were checked over a year after the procedure, they showed that glaucoma had been successfully controlled in all 24 instances. All the operated eyes underwent gonioscopy to assess the cyclodialysis opening, which was 4 mm wide in most cases, and in others as wide as 6 and 7 mm. The conclusion was that the use of viscoelastic to separate tissues in cyclodialysis increases the safety and probably the efficacy of the operation.

One technical variation is to inject the viscoelastic material only at the end of cyclodialysis, not to separate the ciliary body from the sclera but simply to dilate the virtual space previously formed (Figure 27-12). However, this does not reduce postoperative complications. In a study done by Boles-Carenini, significant bleeding occurred in 50% of the eyes treated in this manner.

Another surgical technique for cyclodialysis that depends entirely on viscoelastics was described by Draeger in 1985. He applied the procedure to eyes with congenital glaucoma that did not respond to traditional surgery; in particular, goniotomy. This "ab interno cyclodialysis" was performed under the microscope with the aid of Barkan's silicone lens. The AC was filled with sodium hyaluronate, and goniotomy accomplished as usual. Hyaluronate enabled Draeger to continue dissecting the ciliary body and sclera in a limited area, maintaining the perfect visibility required by this delicate procedure (Figure 27-13). After cyclodialysis, the relative tunnel was filled with viscoelastic material, which kept it patent in the early postoperative period, when the risk of closure is higher. At the end of the procedure, some air was left in the AC to control bleeding and limit a hypertensive response to the hyaluronate. The surgical procedure was accomplished in a very controlled manner owing to the properties of the viscoelastic, which allowed the surgeon to widen the chamber angle and discern the details of the ciliary body while avoiding touching large vessels. This new ab interno technique reduced the instance of hemorrhages from 41% (in traditional cyclodialysis) to 25%—according to Draeger, the main advantage of using viscoelastics.

In all the various techniques of performing cyclodialysis it is important to have a suitable viscoelastic available. Biocompatibility must be absolute, as the material is left inside the eyeball in a crucial position. Viscosity at zero shear rate must be very high, because the product has to keep cyclodialysis open. Adhesiveness must also be high to prevent the material from being moved. Pseudoplasticity must be excellent as well, as the cannula used for cyclodialysis cannot have a large diameter yet must be flat like a cyclodialysis spatula. These are somewhat conflicting requirements, which makes it impossible to recommend a product most suitable for this application. Most recent sodium hyaluronate preparations with high molecular weight seem appropriate, but no specific experiences with them have been published.

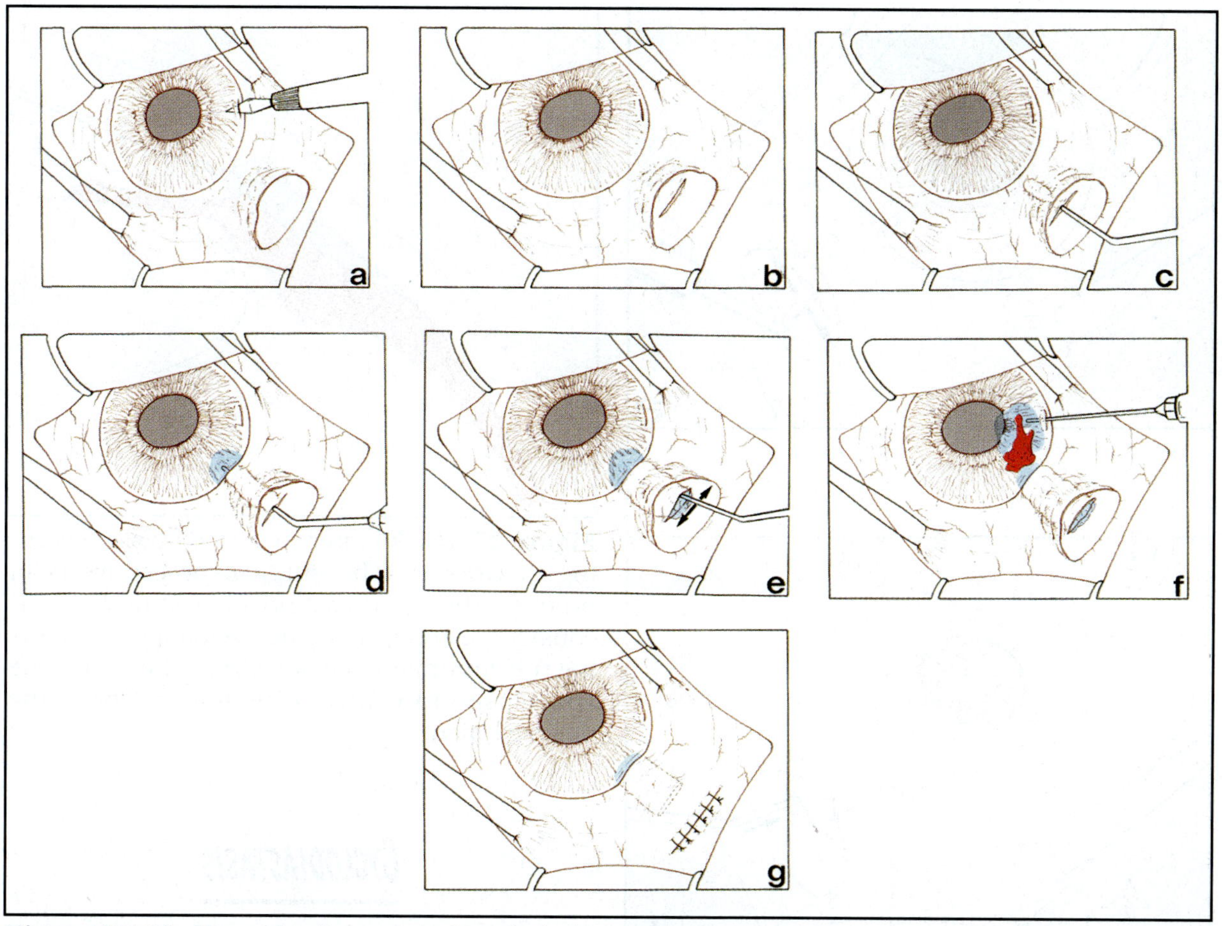

Figure 27-11. Viscoelastic-assisted cyclodialysis: Alpar's technique. (a) In a quadrant found to be free from goniosynechiae at gonioscopy, the conjunctiva is incised 7 mm away from the limbus and parallel to it. When possible, it is better to choose the superotemporal quadrant. The sclera is exposed (the right eye is depicted in the illustration). A corneal paracentesis is made near the temporal limbus. This will be used during surgery to check AC depth. (b) A 4-mm scleral incision is prepared about 4.5 mm from the limbus. The incision is deepened until the choroid is reached and cauterized when required. The outer portion of the incision is wet with 1:1000 adrenaline, applied with a sponge, to ensure vasoconstriction. (c) A small amount of 1% sodium hyaluronate (Healon®) is injected between the sclera and the underlying tissues through a blunt cannula directed toward the limbus. (d) While the viscoelastic is being carefully injected, the cannula is pressed against the sclera and advanced toward the AC. The ciliary–choroidal detachment must be accomplished by the viscoelastic, not by the cannula. (e) After being withdrawn, the cannula is moved away from both sides of the incision and advanced again to reach the limbus, while continuously and gently injecting the viscoelastic material. (f) The paracentesis is used to control possible small hemorrhages by injecting air or viscoelastic through it into the AC. Air, viscoelastic, or blood can also be cleared through this opening. (g) The scleral wound can be sutured or not, according to the surgeon's preference. The conjunctival incision must be sutured with great care, far away from the scleral wound, to avoid any exposure of the scleral incision.

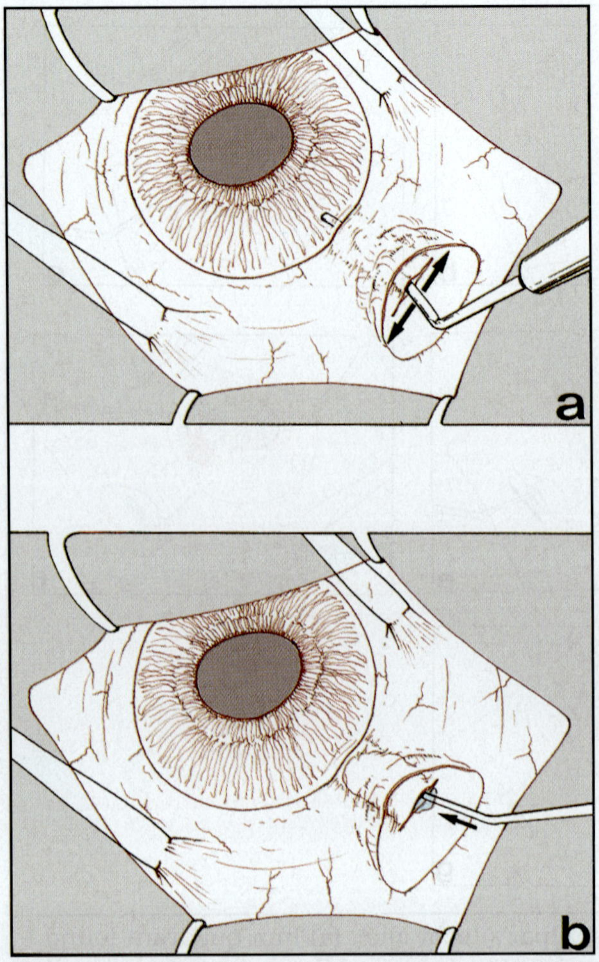

Figure 27-12. Viscoelastic-assisted cyclodialysis: Boles-Carenini's technique. (a) Cyclodialysis is accomplished following traditional methods, using a cyclodialysis spatula. (b) At the end of surgery, Healon® is injected in the superchoroidal space until it disappears into the AC, and is then left in place. In this technique the viscoelastic is not intended to control intraoperative bleeding.

Viscoelastic solutions are also useful in managing complications of cyclodialysis, in particular hypotony occurring in the early postoperative period. Injected in the AC, they restore the consistency of the eyeball, thus enabling reasonable therapeutic treatments to continue. As for all injections done with thin needles into a closed eyeball, both high pseudoplasticity and great transparency are necessary.

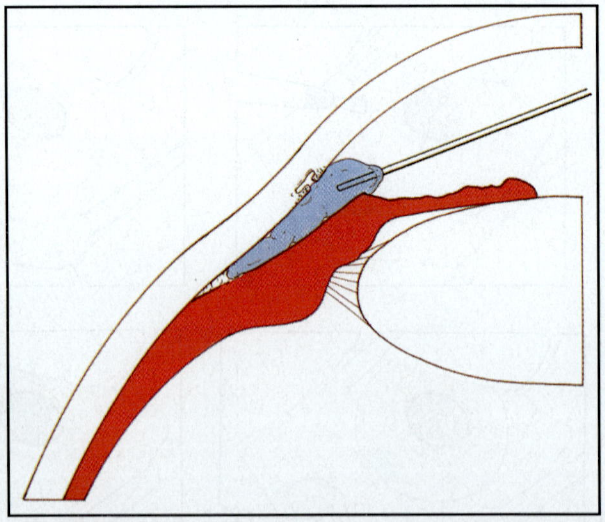

Figure 27-13. Ab interno cyclodialysis according to Draeger. The surgical procedure is in practice the continuation of a goniotomy. It consists of creating a true cyclodialysis following the circumference of a circle, then injecting viscoelastic to control bleeding and keep the dialysis open.

CYCLODIASTASIS

According to Strampelli, cyclodiastasis is to practice a cyclodialysis strengthened by a prolene thread, which aims to keep the passage between the AC and the suprachoroidal space constantly open. The intervention can be most usefully applied in cases of secondary glaucoma, in glaucoma in aphakic eyes, and in glaucomatous eyes that have been operated on previously, even several times, without success. However, the procedure's tendency to cause high and persistent astigmatism greatly limits its use in eyes with limited visual function. The creation of rhegmatogenous retinal lesions is a further complication.

To be performed correctly, cyclodiastasis requires keeping the AC deep and transparent when the fistula has already been created and collapse is a typical threat. Strampelli created a special device to keep the chamber deep by continued air injection, which he called a "pneumatizer." At present this is one of the best applications of viscoelastic materials.

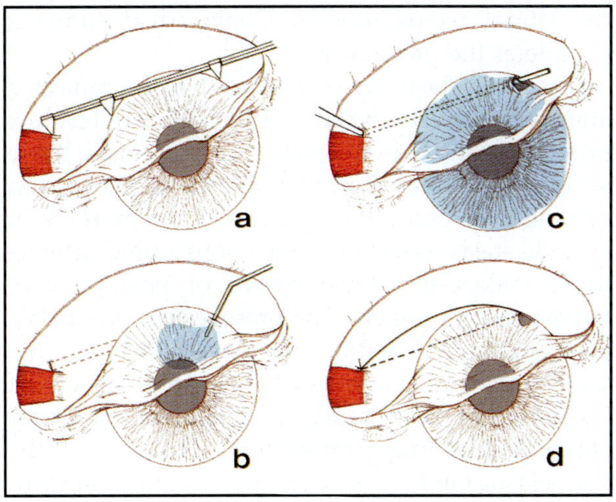

Figure 27-14. Viscoelastic-assisted cyclodiastasis. (a) The intervention starts by detaching a wide portion of conjunctiva and using a special marker to mark the three points of reference, one under the lateral rectus muscle for cyclodialysis incision and two at the limbus. (b) After preparing cyclodialysis, the AC is cleared of any vitreous and filled with viscoelastic. (c) A long L-shaped cannula allows the surgeon to pass the thread through the scleral opening into the AC, then out through the limbal incision. (d) When the thread has been positioned, the knot must be submerged under the lateral rectus muscle.

SURGICAL TECHNIQUE

To perform cyclodiastasis, the conjunctiva is opened in the lower temporal sectors by a large flap with a limbal base. The conjunctival flap must also expose the insertion of the lateral rectus muscle, under which the knot of cyclodiastasis is made. To accomplish this, one can use viscoelastic materials according to our previous instructions regarding trabeculectomies, taking into account that a conjunctival scar is almost always present as a result of previous interventions, often extending to the areas to be involved in the cyclodiastatic procedure.

After cauterization, which is always necessary in eyes that have undergone multiple surgeries, Strampelli's triangular compass is used to plot three reference points:

- A scleral point under the lateral rectus, 8 to 10 mm away from the limbus, where a sclerotomy is performed and cyclodialysis is to begin
- A point at the limbus, where the spatula performing cyclodialysis will enter the AC
- A point at the opposite limbus, on the same line of the former two points, where paracentesis will help the surgeon perform a basal iridectomy and allow the 6-0 prolene thread to emerge from the AC (Figure 27-14)

While performing the sclerotomy under the lateral rectus muscle and during detachment of the ciliary body toward the AC, it is necessary to move the muscle away with a hook. The ciliary body can be detached with the cyclodialysis spatula alone, according to the original technique, or detachment can be induced by injecting highly viscous viscoelastic, as it has been described in the previous section on cyclodialysis. If a spatula is used, then when cyclodialysis has almost reached the AC, corresponding to the spot previously marked, it is better to withdraw to avoid prematurely opening the eyeball. This would cause the chamber to collapse, with subsequent corneal folds, possible involvement of the vitreous (which is often present in the chamber), and risk of hemorrhage. When a viscoelastic is used for detachment, it is possible to reach the chamber with the least damage, provided that the ciliary dialysis is not widened too much.

At this point, paracentesis of the AC is performed at the third reference point. The position of paracentesis is crucial. If it is too far forward, it will allow the prolene thread to be exposed on the corneal plane, and if it is too far back, it will likely fall in a zone of angular synechiae. This is why it is always better to perform a rather angled paracentesis—for instance, through a gauged blade designed for phacoemulsification. Angled paracentesis has the ability to open the AC almost like a valve, without causing immediate collapse. In fact, it allows any potential hypertension to decrease gradually, which cannot be corrected postoperatively, and permits the surgeon to perform the following procedures safely.

The main function of viscoelastic materials in cyclodiastasis starts here. The first procedure is to free the AC from any vitreous present. The presence of vitreous on the front of the iris has been considered a contraindication to cyclodiastasis. The technique is the one usually performed with anterior "dry" vitrectomy—that is, without irrigation, followed by air injection that allows the surgeon to see any vitreous residues still to be removed. Then air is replaced with a suitable viscoelastic to keep the vitreous clear of the AC. Products with reduced internal cohesion and good viscosity at rest, such as Viscoat, are very useful for working close to the vitreous, and can be placed beneath products with high internal cohesion, such as Healon®, which are more transparent.

The viscoelastic with high viscosity at rest allows the surgeon to detect and resolve any peripheral anterior synechiae, which are often present in eyes that undergo cyclodiastasis. This in turn facilitates further procedures, such as iridoplasty, that were not able to be performed in the past. The internal cohesion of the viscoelastic tends to prevent both hemorrhage and mixing of the viscoelastic with blood. The transparency of the material also improves visibility, which is already limited by other factors, particularly those related to the corneal condition. Above all, viscoelastic products are useful in giving the eyeball the consistency needed to continue surgery, and in significantly reducing postoperative hypotony, which is a potential source of problems. It is also important to use a material with high viscosity at rest, which can maintain space despite the presence of large openings in the AC.

Once a peripheral iridectomy has been accomplished and the eyeball has recovered its consistency (owing to the viscoelastic), it is possible to conclude cyclodialysis by penetrating the AC with the spatula to widen the opening laterally, or by widening the former opening. The 6-0 prolene thread, which keeps the cyclodialysis open, is positioned with a blunt cannula bent in an "L" shape, where the thread itself is made to pass through (Figure 27-14). The cannula is inserted in the sclerotomy, travels along the tunnel of cyclodialysis, passes through the AC, and emerges through the paracentesis. After the cannula is retracted the thread is retrieved outside the eyeball, and the ends are tied together near the sclerotomy, with enough tension to keep the ciliary dialysis open. This should not be too high, to avoid excessive deformation of a very hypotonic eyeball. The viscoelastic is particularly useful in this delicate phase, as it provides the eyeball with the tension needed to complete the procedure successfully. Both ends of the thread are shortened (and preferably cauterized, so they do not cause irritation), then hidden under the tendon of the lateral rectus muscle. Conjunctival suturing completes the procedure.

The viscoelastic does not need to be removed after cyclodialysis, as the eyes usually manifest low pressure in the days following surgery, and achieve a consistency allowing optimal restoration of vision only after several weeks. Moreover, the presence of cyclodiastasis associated with nonsutured sclerectomy makes the development of postoperative hypertension unlikely. The presence of a viscoelastic filling the AC, and in some cases also part of the vitreous chamber, limits the negative effects of excessive hypotony, especially intraocular or suprachoroidal bleeding complications. However, as the viscoelastic tends to be reabsorbed rapidly, one cannot expect complications to be reduced until 3 to 4 days after surgery. Likewise, bulbar and corneal deformation mean that visual function will not be recovered for many weeks.

GONIOTOMY

Along with ab externo trabeculotomy, goniotomy is one of the main interventions available to treat congenital glaucoma. It is the treatment of choice in cases involving a transparent cornea because it does not involve the conjunctiva or the limbal zone. These then remain available for further procedures, which are often necessary with this form of glaucoma. The purpose of goniotomy is to dissect anomalous mesodermic tissue, which prevents the aqueous humor from entering trabecular structures. Success of the treatment is based on filtrating structures being normal or relatively normal. It differs from the ab interno trabeculotomy in that the latter also aims to dissect the meshwork, thus linking the AC with Schlemm's canal.

During goniotomy, tissue incision at the chamber angle must be kept as superficial as possible. Before surgery, it is necessary to observe the chamber angle carefully with a three-mirror gonioscopic lens. This allows the surgeon to choose the area to cut at the circumference and to detect Schwalbe's line, so that the incision can be made immediately behind it.

SURGICAL TECHNIQUE

To facilitate the procedure, the head of the young patient is inclined about 45° opposite the entrance site of the goniotome. The eyelids are kept open by a blepharostate. An assistant holds the eyeball with two strong forceps at 12 o'clock and 6 o'clock, so it can be turned according to the surgeon's instructions. The surgeon uses the gonioscopic lens to establish the anatomic ratio of the lens to be treated. After lifting the lens, the surgeon inserts the goniotome, passing it through the cornea 1 mm from the inside of the limbus. The goniotome is simply a very sharp needle, with the tip shaped according to the surgeon's preference. The needle is connected to a bottle of BSS placed at a suitable height to keep the chamber deep during surgery and to wash away any possible blood.

The irrigating goniotome must have a somewhat oblique direction of penetration to oppose aqueous outflow from the incision during the following procedures. However, the incline should not hinder the movements of the goniotome itself. The surgeon replaces the lens, then directs the goniotome forward to the part of the chamber angle opposite to the site of corneal penetration, and with gentle but firm movements, superficially makes an incision in the tissue immediately beneath Schwalbe's line. The surgeon must feel no opposition to the goniotome, but must also be aware that he or she is cutting a tissue only through what he or she sees. As the incision continues, the root of the iris retracts and a white Barkan's line typically becomes visible at the angle. The incision is usually extended to a third of the circumference. Beyond this it is not possible to continue with visual control, so it is better to stop in order to prevent damage compromising the outcome through induced inflammation. Even so, severe bleeding is likely to occur, which heals in a few days after the operation. The goniotome is retracted and the AC filled with air. When necessary, the entrance of the goniotome is sutured with a stitch of absorbable material. When the AC is not deep enough, the performance of goniotomy is more difficult and dangerous to ocular structures. The goniotome is introduced into a hypertensive eye, and the BSS flow is frequently barely sufficient to hold the space. In addition, early hemorrhages often reduce visibility during goniotomy, which may also cause interruptions.

All these complications indicate that viscoelastics can be useful in goniotomy. In fact, sodium hyaluronate has been used several times. Healon® was chosen because it was the first product available, but also because it is apyrogenic and absolutely biocompatible. Goniotomies are greatly eased by viscoelastics, which allow the surgeon to work without haste, within a constantly deep chamber, and with perfect visibility of the angle structures. Unfortunately, eyes scheduled for goniotomy are sensitive to the presence of viscoelastic residues in the postoperative period, and develop marked and long-lasting hypertension, along with equally significant inflammation. As a result, viscoelastic materials have been largely rejected for goniotomies, except as a teaching tool in enucleated globes, where their help is indispensable.

Whenever one wants to use a viscoelastic in goniotomy, it is best to choose a material made of sodium hyaluronate, which shows fair viscosity at zero shear rate and good pseudoplasticity to be introduced through a narrow cannula. Another fundamental feature is internal cohesion, which must be high to allow for complete removal at the end of surgery. Complete removal is so important that it is a good idea to use dyed material, so that possible residue can be detected at the end of surgery. These considerations make Healon® Yellow* the most suitable product available.

After making a small valve paracentesis, the aqueous humor is discharged and replaced with a viscoelastic injected through a 27-G or 30-G cannula (Figure 27-15). Once the AC has been deepened, it is possible to perform goniotomy without irrigation, as possible angle hemorrhages will be controlled by the viscoelastic. The viscous product can always be replaced or restored in case of more severe hemorrhage or leaks through paracentesis (see Figure 27-15). Goniotomy is easier not only owing to the depth and stability of the chamber, but also to the width of the valve incision, which eases goniotome movements while reducing the tasks of the assistant surgeon. Nevertheless, at the end of surgery the viscoelastic must be completely aspirated—for example, through a miniaturized irrigation and aspiration cannula. In doubtful cases, air can help to detect the viscoelastic, particularly when blood makes its yellow color less visible. At the end of surgery, paracentesis must be sutured, for example with 10-0 nylon. Although the technique is interesting, there is some

**Healon® Yellow is no longer being manufactured.*

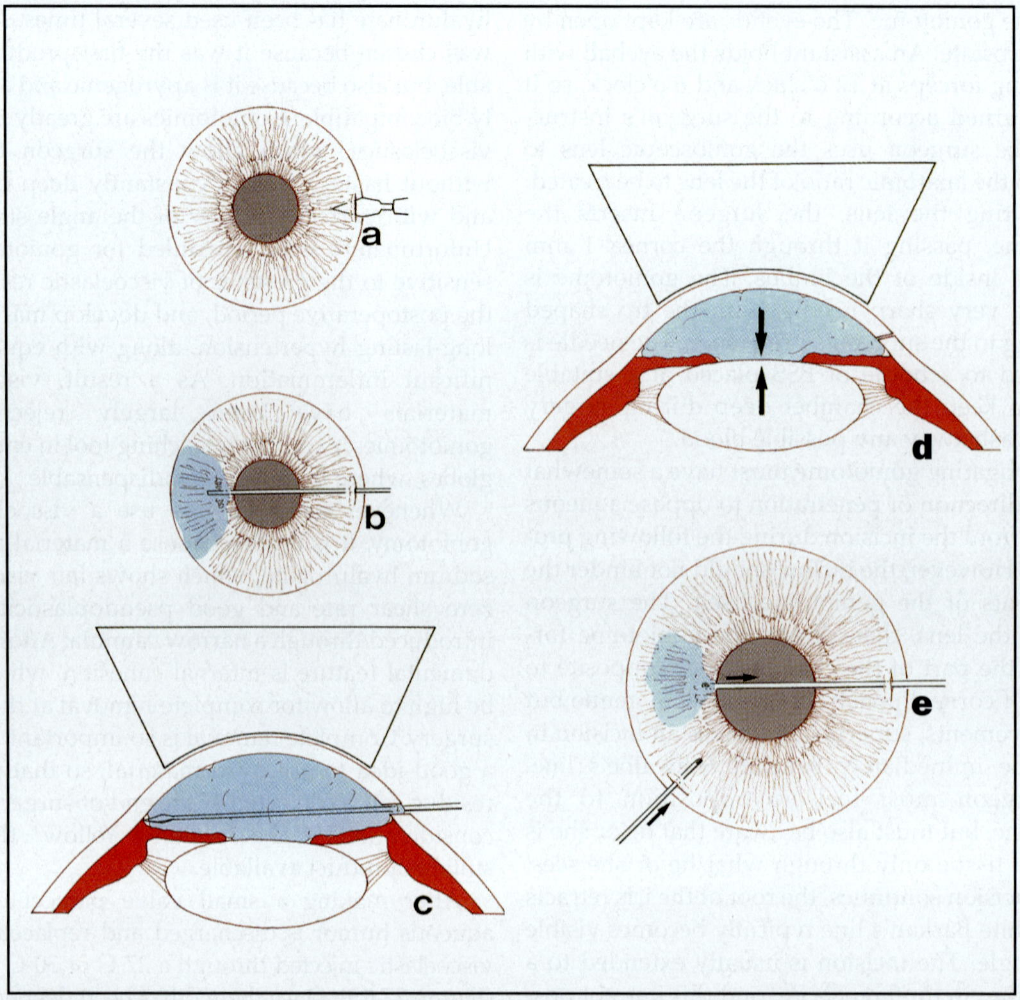

Figure 27-15. Viscoelastic-assisted goniotomy. (a) In a suitable site, the surgeon creates a valve paracentesis, which allows the aqueous humor to drain. (b) The aqueous humor is replaced by a very transparent viscoelastic, which can be easily removed. However, some surgeons do not use viscoelastics in goniotomy, due to risk of hypertension, which has been reported to occur in eyes with very distorted or absent drainage systems. (c) Using a viscoelastic in goniotomy allows the surgeon to detect the area to be incised precisely. Should its transparency be reduced, for instance by blood, the viscoelastic material can be replaced. (d) The viscoelastic is able to counterbalance posterior pressure, always significantly elevated in these eyes, without flowing back out through the paracentesis. (e) A two-way cannula can be used at the end of goniotomy to drain the viscoelastic completely. Each paracentesis should be sutured when the eye being treated has congenital glaucoma.

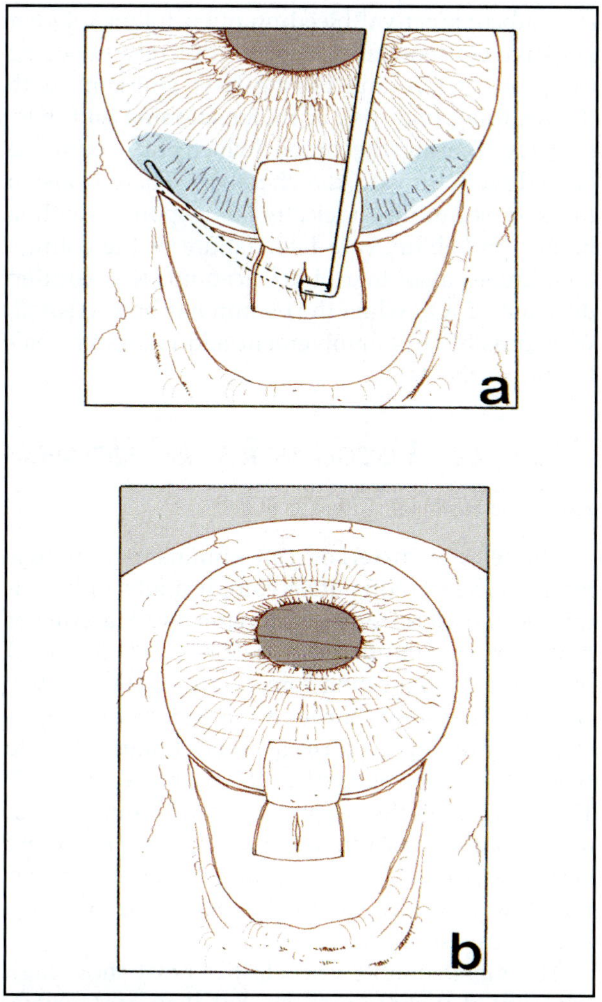

Figure 27-16. Viscoelastic-assisted ab externo trabeculotomy. (a) Viscoelastic materials can be useful in ab externo trabeculotomy to control AC depth. (b) Using viscoelastic products in the AC is contraindicated in the presence of vitreous opacities, which hinder their correct detection and removal at the end of surgery.

doubt about the real amount of endothelial trauma, also taking into account that many goniotomy interventions will need to be repeated eventually.

AB EXTERNO TRABECULOTOMY

Like goniotomy, ab externo trabeculotomy is a surgical intervention designed to treat congenital glaucoma. Surgeons currently favor this procedure because of its greater respect of AC structures, its feasibility in the presence of corneal opacities, and its slightly better results in controlling IOP. On the other hand, ab externo trabeculotomy alters the conjunctiva in the areas involved, thus creating conditions for cicatricial reaction, which may cause problems in subsequent surgeries.

SURGICAL TECHNIQUE

The operation consists of forming a conjunctival flap based at the fornix or the limbus and carving a scleral flap of partial thickness, as in a trabeculectomy. Dissecting the sclera must be led to the limbus after cutting the bed radially and deepening the incision little by little until a small amount of aqueous humor appears, showing that Schlemm's canal has been dissected. Once the canal has been detected, a trabeculotome—a bowed probe with a 90° handle—is introduced inside it. A double probe is also available, which helps the surgeon follow the movements of the part introduced in the lumen of the canal. The trabeculotome is turned until it appears in the AC, in front of the iris, in order to lacerate the angle tissue covering Schlemm's canal toward the chamber (Figure 27-16). The same procedure is repeated on the opposite side of the radial incision. Like the conjunctiva, the scleral port is sutured at the end of surgery.

An effective variation on this procedure, called diathermotrabeculotomy, was suggested by Maselli. It involves using a diathermic trabeculotome, which partly cicatrizes the lacerated tissue. In ab externo trabeculotomy, a small space is left for the use of viscoelastics. These materials are sometimes used to re-form the AC when BSS and air are not enough. In congenital glaucoma interventions that are not real filtering operations, the use of viscoelastics has special constraints. The surgeon must be extremely careful to avoid the possibility of postoperative hypertension.

During surgery, the AC can be deepened at any time by viscoelastics, provided that they are highly biocompatible, show good viscosity at rest, and are easily injected (ie, they have good pseudoplasticity). Above all, they must be able to be easily detected and removed (dyed and with good internal cohesion). Although they do not contraindicate a trabeculotomy, the presence of corneal opacities may be a contraindication for using viscoelastic materials.

HOLMIUM LASER THERMOSCLEROSTOMY

A recent type of glaucoma surgery, holmium laser thermosclerostomy, consists of making a full-thickness fistula between the AC and the subconjunctival space. Sclerostomy is accomplished with thermal laser energy, about 2-mm wavelength, applied by a specially designed probe.

SURGICAL TECHNIQUE

According to Hoskins, the technique is performed under local or even topical anesthesia. The eyeball is turned in a suitable position and a conjunctival buttonhole is formed far away from the limbus, taking care to contact the sclera directly. The laser probe is introduced through the buttonhole and directed forward on the scleral plane until the tip touches the limbus. It is necessary to do this carefully so that the probe is placed tangentially to the limbus before starting laser emission. The thermal pulse is directed to the AC by the angle of the final portion of the probe. In a few seconds it makes a sclerostomy, 200 to 300 µm in diameter. Once sclerostomy has been accomplished, one may notice subconjunctival aqueous leaking, movement of pigment in the AC, reduced chamber depth, and iris movement. Then the probe is withdrawn and the conjunctival buttonhole closed with a stitch of absorbable material.

The results of holmium laser thermosclerostomy have not met the expectations that arose for this new technique at its début. This is partly due to postoperative problems, related to the fact that this is a full-thickness technique, comparable in early times to Elliot's trephination. In the long run, the fistula tends to close, probably due to its small initial dimensions. Furthermore, although limited in duration, thermal coarctation of the nearest corneal tissue makes laser treatment less advantageous than trabeculectomy.

There are also intraoperative problems related to various phases of the intervention. In many operated eyes that have previously undergone filtering surgery a number of times, the trauma caused by subconjunctival shifting of the probe is too great, and subconjunctival bleeding often follows. Other negative consequences include difficulty in seeing the probe before and during laser emission, with the resulting high risk of malpositioning and inaccurately rotating the probe (which must emit the laser directly toward the chamber). There is also a marked stimulus to cicatricial response, with a higher probability of a later failure of the ostium. One must also take into account the sudden decrease of IOP when the ostium has been created, with possible iris involvement and excessive shallowing of the AC.

USE OF VISCOELASTICS IN HOLMIUM LASER THERMOSCLEROSTOMY

Viscoelastic materials can eliminate or reduce many of the intraoperative complications of holmium thermosclerostomy. Schumann and MacAllister have already modified the basic method conceived by Hoskins, suggesting forced introduction of viscoelastic (Healon®) through the conjunctival–episcleral buttonhole to form a tunnel linking the site where the probe entered to the limbus (Figure 27-17). As a result, the conjunctiva can be detached in an absolutely atraumatic way while respecting cleavage planes, even cicatricial, minimizing and possibly preventing both the risk of hemorrhage and fibrosis stimulus.

The most suitable viscoelastics must show high viscosity at 0 shear rate, so that they can achieve and maintain conjunctival detachment in the same manner as trabeculectomy. Pseudoplasticity seems not to be important, because the caliber of the cannula can be medium–large. In 1994, La Torre et al proposed using a gonioscopic lens to aim the laser probe precisely. A perfectly transparent viscoelastic (hyaluronic acid with high viscosity at rest and medium viscosity at low shear rate) is placed between the gonioscopic lens and the eye in order to maintain the viscous meniscus, thus also allowing the movement of the gonioscopic lens. A product with high internal cohesion seems preferable here, as in other conditions where viscoelastics are used under diagnostic contact lenses. According to La Torre, the increased precision of the laser reduced thermal distortion of the corneal tissue. Pain is controlled by adding most hydrosoluble anesthetics, ie, 0.5 cc 2% mepivacaine in 2 cc of product (Figure 27-17d).

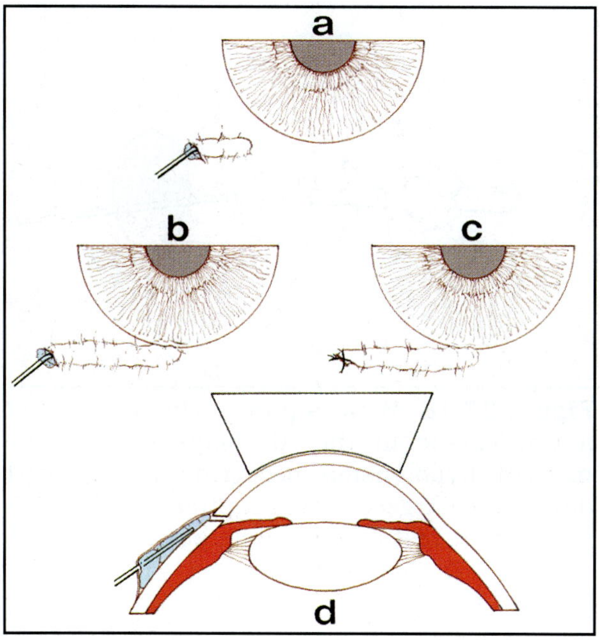

Figure 27-17. Viscoelastic-assisted thermosclerostomy with holmium laser: MacAllister and La Torre's technique. (a) Forced insertion of a viscoelastic under the conjunctiva in the episcleral space creates a conjunctival tunnel through which the probe will be passed. Conjunctival bleeding, often present in eyes that have had previous surgery, is thus greatly reduced. (b) The fiber optic probe delivers the laser pulse that creates the ostomy. (c) The presence of viscoelastic in the subconjunctival space controls the rapid outflow of aqueous humor that occurs when the probe is withdrawn. (d) According to La Torre, using a gonioscopic lens with a very transparent viscoelastic acting as a coupling agent to the cornea allows the surgeon to see the site of sclerostomy clearly.

The presence of viscoelastic in the subconjunctival space somehow tamponades the sudden outflow of aqueous humor from the AC, which occurs when ostium has been completed and the probe is withdrawn. As a result, consequences such as iris involvement in the ostium and hypotony, which may induce choroidal detachment after this kind of surgery, become less likely. The product is left in place at the end of surgery. It is now certain that the presence of subconjunctival sodium hyaluronate after filtrating surgery does not cause failure of the cicatricial bleb; on the contrary, it may have beneficial effects.

SETON AND VALVULAR IMPLANTS

In the attempt to control IOP in cases of refractory glaucoma—that is, glaucoma that resists the most common therapies and interventions—one can consider implanting a foreign material that may encourage the aqueous humor to drain. Devices that attempt to facilitate aqueous humor outflow without controlling its direction are called seton implants, and have been used since the 1900s. Nowadays, their interest is merely historic, except for Molteno's prosthesis. A special kind of seton, Molteno's prosthesis is a small silicone tube connected to a silicone plate, whose task is to ensure maintenance of the outflow in sub–Tenon's space. The substantial distance between the site of the plate and the limbus should avoid late cicatricial closure of filtration.

Devices that attempt to facilitate aqueous humor outflow by a valve mechanism are called "valvular implants." These are the type most commonly used. Among them are Krupin's valve, White's shunt pump, and the more recent device by Ahmed. These prostheses all have a valvular mechanism that ensures unidirectional flow of the liquid. The valve should open when IOP exceeds 13 to 14 mmHg, and close when pressure is 2 to 3 mm lower.

SURGICAL TECHNIQUES

Surgical techniques used to implant these prostheses require carving a large conjunctival flap based in the fornix in a suitable quadrant, usually the superior nasal quadrant, undermining the conjunctiva beyond the equator. After uncovering the sclera, the surgeon sutures the main part of the device to it, taking care that the body of the valve does not touch anatomic parts such as oculomotor muscles. The small tube projecting from the body of the prosthesis, which links the AC to collect the aqueous humor, is cut to a suitable length to be inserted in the AC, penetrating it about 3 mm. Insertion in the chamber is accomplished through a calibrated incision, directed under a scleral flap, which in turn will cover the small tube and prevent its extrusion. Suturing the scleral flap and the conjunctiva concludes the procedure.

The role of viscoelastics in seton and valvular surgery is limited to the main phases of intervention. Sometimes viscoelastics can turn out to be useful in dissecting the conjunctiva at the perilimbal level, as the eyes being treated have often undergone repeated interventions and have a cicatrized, fragile conjunctiva, with many vessels bleeding at the lightest touch. The main use of viscoelastics, however, is to prevent the severe hypotension generally occurring after seton or valvular implant positioning, which may cause severe choroidal detachment in the immediate postoperative period and bulbar phthisis in the long term. For this purpose, Boles-Carenini fills the AC with sodium hyaluronate at the end of surgery (Figure 27-18). In the series of eyes he studied, postoperative shallowing of the AC occurred in 66% of the cases after using Healon®, whereas the rate was 83% in eyes receiving no viscoelastic.

This use of viscoelastics differs from that after trabeculectomy, as eyes receiving a filtrating prosthesis are not supposed to have any filtration activity through the meshwork. Hence, the viscoelastic can be discharged only through the filtering valve. Highly pseudoplastic products with medium viscosity at rest seem to be the most appropriate. Those with low pseudoplasticity might congest the valve, with negative effects on IOP. The adhesiveness of most viscoelastics could also turn out to be useful in this intervention. There are no definite data on how useful viscoelastics are in valvular implant surgery. Late failure (frequent in this type of surgery due to fibrotic occlusion of sub–Tenon's or subconjunctival filtration) occurs such a long time after surgery that it cannot be influenced by viscoelastics.

RECENT ANGLE CLOSURE

Diffused synechial closure of the angle due to the formation of peripheral anterior synechiae persisting on the corneoscleral meshwork may cause severe glaucoma. When angle closure exceeds 270°, medical therapy for glaucoma is often ineffective, and it is necessary to resort to surgery, even though the results of filtering operations in these eyes are often inadequate.

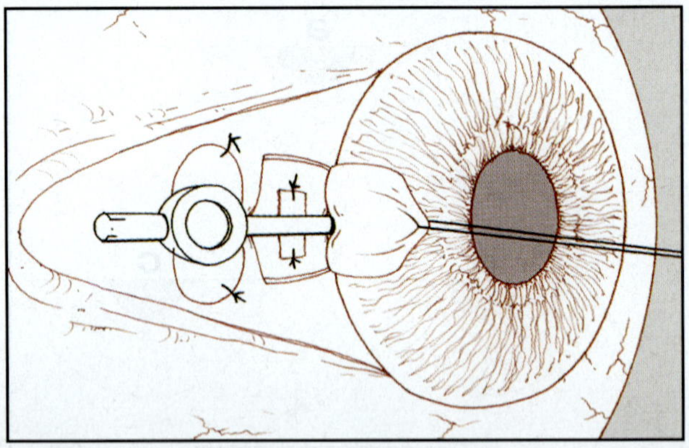

Figure 27-18. White's pump. The presence of a viscoelastic in the AC helps prevent the marked hypotension occurring in the first days after surgery. Using a product with high viscosity at rest is most preferable.

A more satisfactory treatment of these adhesions would be synechiolysis, which exposes the meshwork again and opens the way for filtration. To be feasible, the intervention requires normal or near-normal filtering structures. It is known that overly prolonged angle closure may cause anatomic alterations to the meshwork, inhibiting restoration of filtration, even after dissecting the synechiae. There is no agreement, however, on how long the closure can be before permanent alterations will develop, especially considering the differences from case to case depending on the amount of inflammation present.

One of the main problems up to now with reopening chamber angles obstructed by goniosynechiae has been the inaccuracy of the surgical technique. Until the advent of viscoelastics, the procedure involved inserting cyclodialysis spatulas in the AC without being able to control the depth of the insertion, with consequent risk to the cornea, iris, and lens, and frequent bleeding, which further reduced visibility. Most of these problems have been overcome with the availability of viscoelastic materials, which make it possible to reopen the chamber angle more safely in cases of recent synechial closure.

SURGICAL TECHNIQUE

The surgical technique was described by Campbell and Vela, who reported on the treatment of five eyes with synechial angle closure that exceeded 270° and had persisted for 1 year or less. The patients were treated under local anesthesia. A paracentesis was prepared at the temporal limbus, a bit lower, directed toward 6 o'clock. Anterior chamber fluid and posterior chamber fluid that had been forced into the AC was drained through the paracentesis by compressing the limbus over the whole circumference with a muscle hook. The AC was shallowed to the thickness of two corneas in the central portion (Figure 27-19). This procedure permits subsequent deepening of the chamber, which the researchers accomplished by injecting sodium hyaluronate with a high molecular weight (Healon®). The same outcome can now be more easily achieved with a heavier product having higher viscosity at rest (Healon® GV). The AC was overwhelmingly filled with sodium hyaluronate, in the central portion up to 6 to 8 times the corneal thickness, through a short 30-G cannula (Figure 27-19).

During this procedure one must be careful that IOP is not elevated so much that it causes corneal edema, and that the peripheral portion of the iris can be observed while the chamber is progressively deepening. In very small eyes that have no posterior vitreous detachment, this may be difficult owing to the lack of space inside the eyeball. In selected cases, limited posterior vitrectomy, accomplished by a single sclerotomy at the pars plana, reduces the vitreous contents of the eyeball, enabling the chamber to deepen without causing hypertension.

Using a viscoelastic product is preferable to using BSS or air for detaching peripheral anterior synechiae because it:

- Protects intraocular structures, reducing trauma (especially to the endothelium), and limits damage caused by surgical instruments
- Keeps the AC deep without leaking out through the paracentesis
- Helps stop bleeding that often occurs during dissection of synechiae
- Limits the spread of blood through the AC, ensuring that visibility is close to optimal
- Keeps the chamber deep even in the presence of open iridectomy, which could trap BSS behind the iris

For these reasons using viscoelastic products is considered mandatory. The most suitable seems to be highly viscous sodium hyaluronate, which provides the required transparency and pseudoplasticity.

At this point in the procedure, the diagnosis of synechial angle closure can be confirmed under the surgical microscope with the help of a gonioscopic lens, and the intervention can begin. With a Ziegler's blade, Campbell and Vela cut two limbal incisions in clear cornea, one at 3 o'clock and the other at 9 o'clock. The endothelial side of the incision must be wider than the epithelial one 1) to improve the mobility of the instruments introduced and to permit their rotation up to nearly 180° without corneal folds occurring and 2) to limit the possible leakage of sodium hyaluronate out of the chamber through the same incision (see Figure 27-19).

An irrigating cyclodialysis spatula, long and thin with a blunt tip, is then introduced through an incision and moved forward to almost reach the opposite chamber angle. The researchers preferred to perform irrigation to improve AC control. This can be substituted with repeated Healon® GV injections when necessary.

To visualize the following goniosynechiolysis directly, Campbell and Vela used a Barkan's gonioscopic lens, but any sort of gonioscopic lens can be used. Synechiae are dissected by an anteroposterior movement of the cyclodialysis spatula, repeatedly performed over 160 to 170° for each entrance, through which one attempts to see the ciliary band. The movement of the spatula must be very gentle and strictly controlled, to avoid damaging the lens and the iris and to avoid inadvertently causing iris dialysis. Lateral movements of the spatula must be avoided, as they appear to be far more traumatic to the meshwork and can lacerate iris tissue. The whole procedure is assisted by a suitable rotation of the eyeball, handled by the assistant surgeon as in goniotomy procedures. The assistant must also inform the surgeon about any complications occurring during the intervention. In Campbell and Vela's study, this occurred in only one case, when a hemorrhage not immediately controlled through elevation of the infusion bottle required a momentary suspension of surgery to reinject sodium hyaluronate in the AC.

After dissection of the peripheral anterior synechiae is completed, the main causes of synechial angle closure will have been removed. In case of progressive closure caused by repeated glaucoma crises, peripheral iridectomy will be sufficient, whereas more complicated cases could require more complex procedures. At the end of

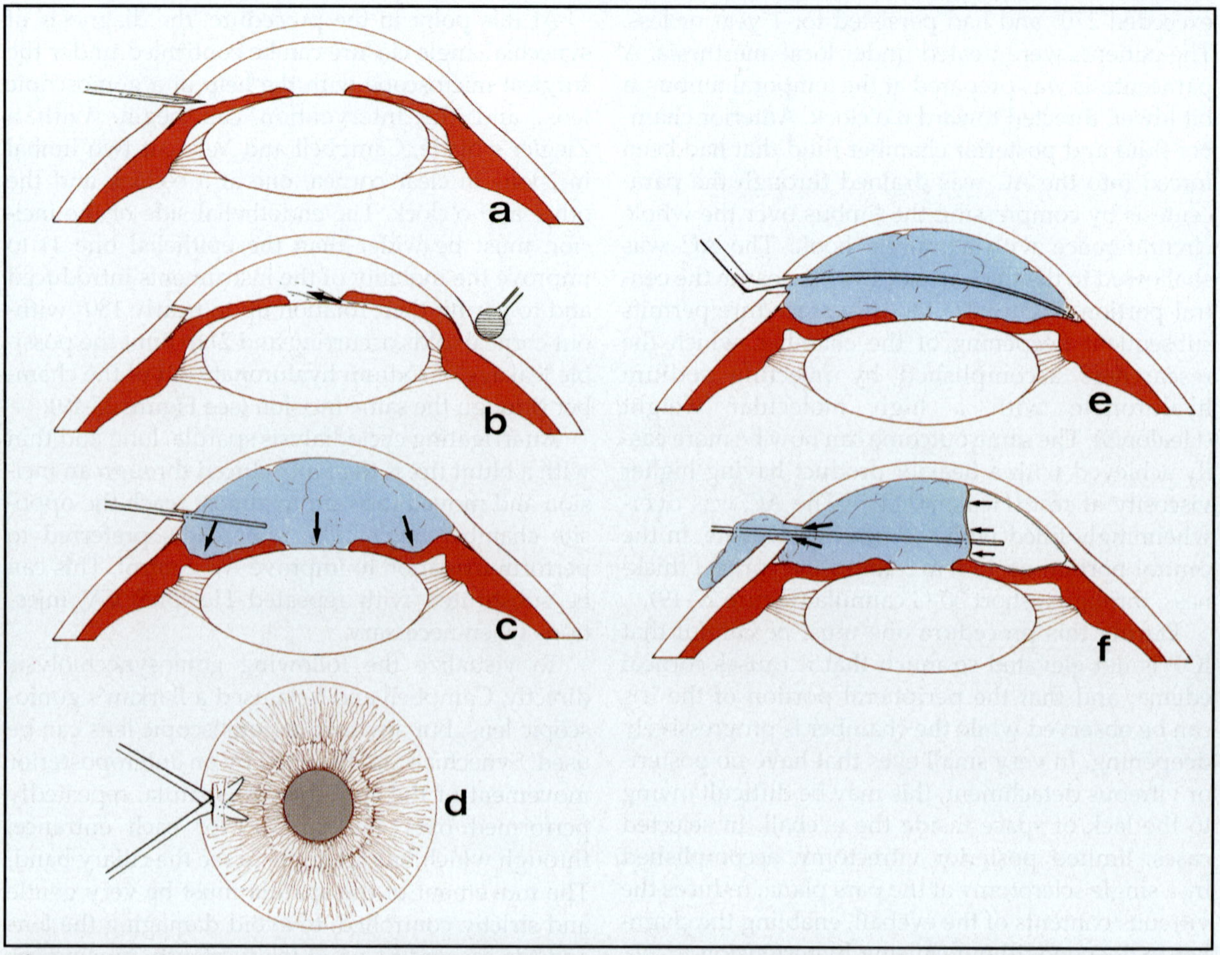

Figure 27-19. Viscoelastic-assisted goniosynechiolysis according to Campbell and Vela. (a) The intervention is started with a paracentesis that enables the aqueous humor to leak out, thus reducing AC depth. (b) Pressure applied at 360° to the ciliary body forces the liquid to pass from the posterior to the AC, where it is evacuated through the paracentesis until the AC has been shallowed to two corneal thicknesses. (c) The AC is then filled with 1% sodium hyaluronate until its depth is 6 to 8 times the corneal thickness. Gonioscopy is repeated to confirm the diagnosis of glaucoma due to goniosynechiae. (d) Two incisions are made at the temporal and nasal limbus for the cyclodialysis spatula, rotating the knife in such a way that the internal incision is wider than the external one. (e) Using a curved cyclodialysis spatula with thin and blunt tip equipped with irrigation, the surgeon separates synechiae from the corneoscleral meshwork in an anteroposterior movement, exposing the ciliary body. (f) The viscoelastic is removed by the forced injection of BSS through the temporal incision. Very cohesive sodium hyaluronate usually comes out as a whole bolus. Because two incisions are present, the viscoelastic can also be removed by irrigation and aspiration.

surgery, hyaluronate is removed from the AC by irrigation and aspiration through both paracenteses, through which Buratto's cannulas can be used as well. Aspiration of the viscoelastic is beneficial, as it tends to hinder the outflow of aqueous humor in the first days following surgery, which is more marked when highly viscous sodium hyaluronate has been used. Closing the paracentesis with single nylon 10-0 sutures completes the intervention.

DISCUSSION

Before the advent of viscosurgery, unbridling the peripheral anterior synechiae causing angle closure was attempted, but with poor results. Surgeons' dissatisfaction with this technique are mainly that:

- It is difficult to accomplish without damaging other ocular structures
- Visibility is poor during surgery
- Synechiae tend to recur easily, particularly due to bleeding
- The advantage of filtration in cases with a long history is limited, due to the damage to the filtering meshwork underlying synechial angle closure

Viscoelastics enable the surgeon to open the chamber angle, providing safe access to the peripheral anterior synechiae. It seldom happens that the force exerted by the viscoelastic alone is able to dissect old synechiae, but their transparency permits further surgical treatment without collapsing the AC. The crucial aspect of the procedure is to control bleeding, which is achieved by preventing it via the use of a viscoelastic and the resulting increase in intracameral pressure, or by removing the blood from the area. Sometimes very thin drops of blood are trapped in the viscoelastic, but these do not significantly decrease visibility. Controlling bleeding also results in an improved postoperative prognosis, when recurrence of synechiae is to be avoided. Taking action to prevent their recurrence is a determining factor for long-term success. Synechiolysis alone would produce only temporary results.

Good candidates for this kind of surgery seem to be eyes where the synechial angle has not been closed for so long as to cause significant and permanent alterations of the meshwork. In the original work by Campbell and Vela, an angle closure of 1 year was the outside limit at which one could hope for success. In one case reported, anatomic success was coupled with failure to maintain low pressure in an eye with an almost 6-year-old angle closure. The cause of this failure was found to be excessive trabecular damage. The time limit for successful intervention probably varies from case to case, depending on factors such as the cause of synechiae formation, the severity of concomitant glaucoma, the rate of retinal ischemia present, and the rate of previous and present intraocular inflammation. Viscosurgical goniosynechiolysis appears to be a technique to try in these eyes, which are often doomed to a bad prognosis even when they undergo filtering surgery, valvular implantation, or cyclodestructive procedures.

Eyes that have undergone vitrectomy involving the use of tamponading methods may also experience conditions that lead to synechial angle closure. When the method is gas, the angle closure is not likely to be permanent, and can be solved by placing the patient in a suitable position following surgery. When the tamponading method is oil, overwhelming filling of phakic eyes may lead to the formation of peripheral anterior synechiae, which can be unbridled by the technique described above, while removing some tamponading oil. Many surgeons try to prevent the development of peripheral anterior synechiae in these circumstances by introducing viscoelastic in the AC at the end of the vitrectomy. This prevents angle closure in the first hours following the intervention, when correct positioning of the anesthetized patient is difficult. For this kind of application, we prefer using hyaluronic acid with a low viscosity, which keeps the space closed without excessively congesting filtering structures during elimination. Pseudoplasticity must be very high, as the material is introduced through a 30-G needle inserted very obliquely in the cornea.

POSTSURGICAL HYPOTONY

Often after filtering surgery the surgeon is confronted with a threatening complication: delayed AC formation. The immediate result of the operation may be excessive (overfiltration), or prolonged use of beta blocking agents may have reduced the

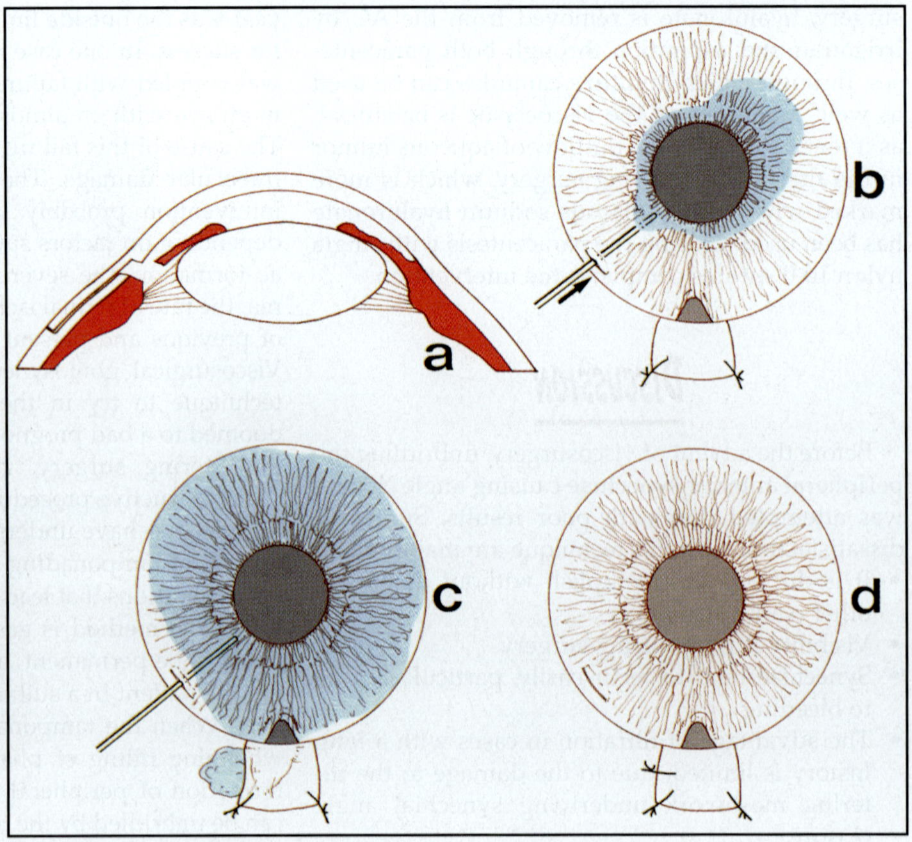

Figure 27-20. Correction of excessive filtration. (a) Correction of excessive filtration after glaucoma surgery that has caused hypotony is easy to accomplish when assisted by a viscoelastic product. (b) The AC is filled with viscoelastic through a paracentesis or by piercing the cornea obliquely with a 30-G needle. (c) The chamber is overwhelmingly filled with material. The site where the viscoelastic leaks out marks the zone of excessive filtration. (d) Excessive filtration is corrected. The AC is left full of viscoelastic.

production of aqueous humor. In such cases, choroidal detachment is frequent, and more often serous than hemorrhagic. This leads to hypotony, and requires special surgical treatment.

Viscoelastic materials have radically changed both the treatment and the prognosis of postsurgical hypotony, which must be corrected if it persists longer than 5 to 6 days. After that time, permanent effects develop, including peripheral anterior synechiae, corneal endothelial damage, and lens damage. The product used must be highly pseudoplastic, as it is frequently injected through the cornea by a 30-G needle inserted obliquely, to prevent the viscoelastic from flowing back through the incision. The viscoelastic must also cause moderate hypertension when left in the AC. We commonly use sodium hyaluronate with a molecular weight that is not too high, at 1% concentration.

Surgical Technique

When hypotony is not associated with choroidal detachment, or detachment is limited and flat so that drainage is not advisable, it is generally adequate to inspect filtration in order to limit it when excessive, or to correct a defect in the conjunctival suture that is preventing the formation of the filtering bleb. Under local anesthesia, the AC is overwhelmed with viscoelastic to deepen it and allow the surgeon to check for a possible leak of the product through a site of excessive filtration (Figure 27-20).

We prefer closing the chamber well with 10-0 nylon sutures, which can be cut later with laser and Hoskins' lens in case of ocular hypertension.

At the end of the intervention, a portion or the whole of the viscoelastic is left in the AC to prevent it from shallowing again, which is bound to occur if the cause of hypotony has not been completely removed. For example, untreated choroidal detachment will almost certainly cause reshallowing of the chamber, even when a viscoelastic with high viscosity at rest (Healon® GV) has been introduced. Occasionally, the procedure can be accomplished at the slit lamp. In the more frequent instance when hypotony is caused by a ciliary–choroidal detach-

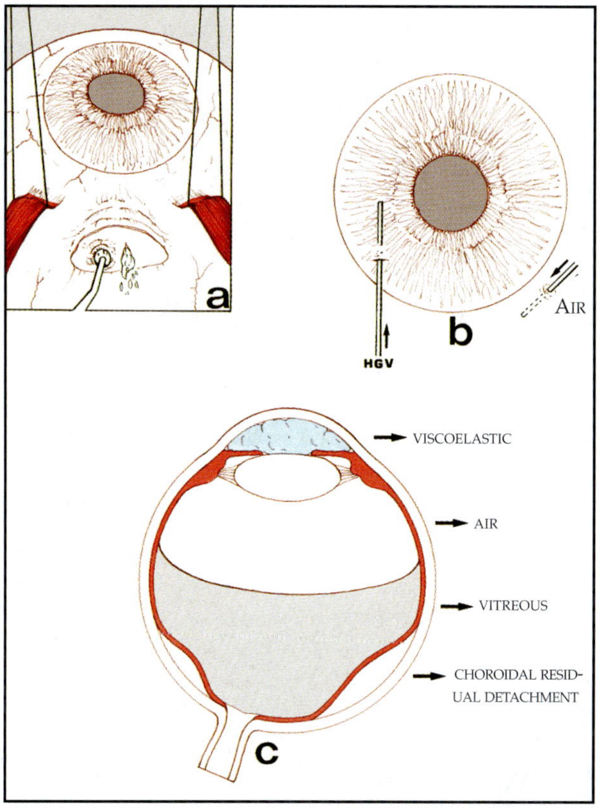

Figure 27-21. Management of choroidal detachment. (a) The fluid causing the choroidal detachment is first drained through a sclerotomy made corresponding to the site of detachment, which the surgeon has detected by echographic examination. (b) To restore the consistency of the eyeball and prevent recurrent hypotony, the AC is filled with viscoelastic, and the vitreous chamber is re-formed with air injected by a 30-G needle inserted 3.5 mm away from the limbus. (c) At the end of surgery, a residual choroidal detachment often persists, but this spontaneously resorbs. In the vitreous chamber a large air bubble will be present, and the AC can be left full of viscoelastic.

ment confirmed by echography, a simple anterior approach will not solve the problem; it is necessary to perform drainage. Under local anesthesia, the conjunctiva is opened in the space between the two rectus muscles, and retracted on 2-0 silk threads to expose the zone planned for intervention. The sclera is exposed and cut with a 30° blade between both rectus muscles, 4 to 5 mm behind their insertion (Figure 27-21).

As soon as perforation has been accomplished, a liquid comes out that can be citrine yellow (serous detachment) or blood red (hemorrhagic detachment). Choroidal detachment is drained as much as possible, the AC restored with viscoelastic soon after starting drainage, and the vitreous chamber re-formed with air in case of excessive hypotension. To inject the viscoelastic, the cornea is pierced by a 30-G needle directed rather obliquely, even though developing sufficient IOP may be difficult. To inject air in the vitreous chamber, the sclera is pierced by a 30-G needle 4 mm away from the limbus, with care taken to check that the position of the lens is not too far posterior in phakic eyes. After voiding the detachment and filling the AC and the vitreous chamber, the sclerotomy and the conjunctival incision are closed. At this point the surgeon focuses on the first filtrating intervention, trying to correct the condition that caused choroidal detachment. It is usually necessary to close excessive filtration by suturing the scleral opening of trabeculectomy or closing the overlying conjunctiva more securely.

The relationship between the viscoelastic in the AC and the air in the vitreous chamber is rather relevant. In our experience, using gas in the AC—even sulfur hexafluoride, which is relatively short acting—causes more severe damage to the lens, which then has to be removed sooner. Using air causes no cataract, but the superficial tension of the bubble hinders the starting of filtration, which is important in the days immediately after surgery. The viscoelastic protects the corneal endothelium, which is always at risk in the presence of hypotony. In the vitreous chamber, gas must be used very carefully and in nonexpanding mixtures, to avoid causing excessive pressure on the lens, which in turn may cause the AC to shallow once again.

Viscosurgery has allowed drainage of choroidal detachment to become much more gentle. It also helps the eyes recover function and is effective for eyes that have previously had a bad prognosis. Drainage repeated two or three times with the help of viscoelastics has not caused bullous keratopathy or any other irreversible damage to AC structures. The only consequences seen in most complex cases are those involving the lens, which suffers from complications and surgical trauma depending on the patient's age.

MALIGNANT GLAUCOMA

Malignant glaucoma, or glaucoma due to ciliary block, occurs postoperatively in 2 to 4% of eyes with angle-closure glaucoma, depending on the type of surgery performed. Actually, the disease has a much wider clinical presence, as it can be detected in many other clinical conditions, both surgical and nonsurgical. Early treatment of these types of glaucoma is essentially medical, and is mainly accomplished with mydriatic and cycloplegic drugs. The resistant forms must be treated surgically to prevent damage to the corneal endothelium and angle structures, which occurs after 5 to 6 days of ocular hypertension with a shallow chamber.

SURGICAL TECHNIQUE

Awaiting success of medical therapy and trying to minimize damage before surgery, Juzych et al attempted reformation of the AC with 1% sodium hyaluronate under slit-lamp microscopy, injecting Healon® through the cornea with a 28-G needle (Figure 27-22). This technique was applied in six eyes, three formerly operated with filtering surgery (in one case associated with cataract extraction) and three operated with Molteno's valvular implant. The time elapsed between diagnosis of malignant glaucoma and viscoelastic injection was 0 to 7 days. One eye had remarkable pressure increase (64 mmHg) 24 hours after injection that was treated by removing part of the viscoelastic. Three eyes required a second injection 4 to 7 days after the first. In all cases glaucoma was cured, with AC deepening and IOP below 20 mmHg. Mydriatic therapy with atropine was continued for a long period.

Some suggested hypotheses to explain the mechanism that accounts for the positive effect of intrachamber sodium hyaluronate injection and for the reduction of IOP. By deepening the AC and moving back the ciliary processes and the vitreous, the viscoelastic may alter the pathologic dynamics of fluids. It is also possible that injection of sodium hyaluronate has been effective only in the prevention of damage to ocular structures, and that the resolution of malignant glaucoma, at least in some eyes, is due to late effects of medical therapy. In either case, AC injection of sodium hyaluronate in cases of malignant glaucoma should be attempted before starting more complicated surgery.

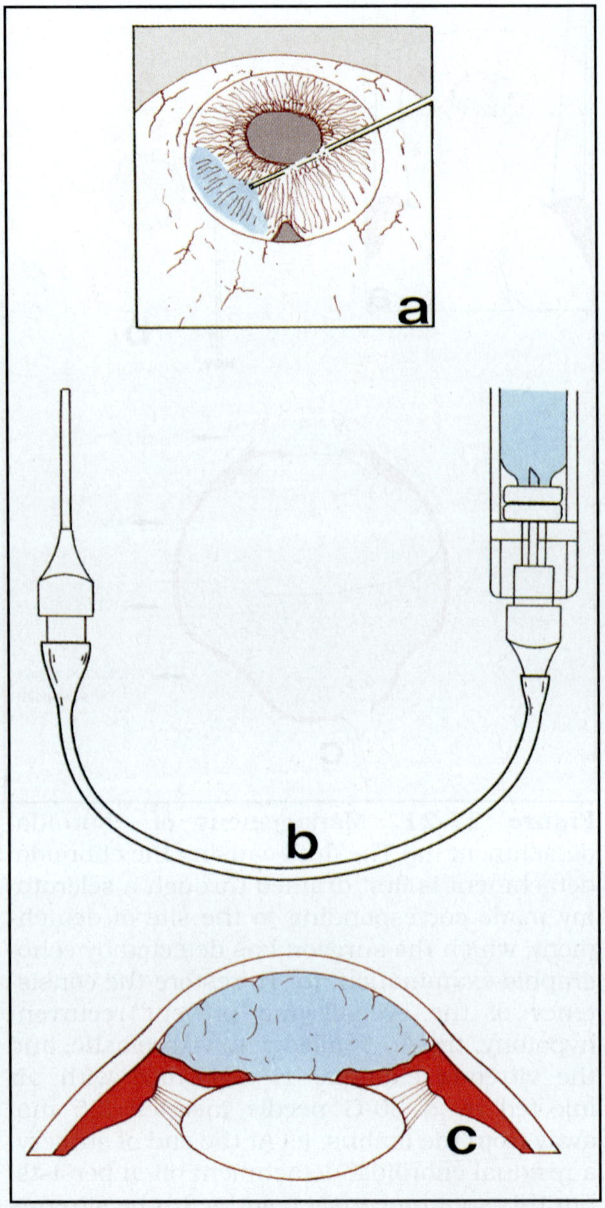

Figure 27-22. Management of malignant glaucoma according to Juzych. (a) In the event of glaucoma due to ciliary block (malignant glaucoma), Juzych suggests injecting viscoelastic in the AC before vitrectomy. The procedure is done under the slit lamp with a 30-G needle directed obliquely into the cornea to reach the AC. (b) A short silicone connection allows an assistant to push on the piston of the syringe, while the surgeon concentrates on its position. (c) The AC is forcibly deepened with viscoelastic, possibly pushing the ciliary bodies back. This way the pathologic pathway of the aqueous humor can be corrected, thus resolving malignant glaucoma.

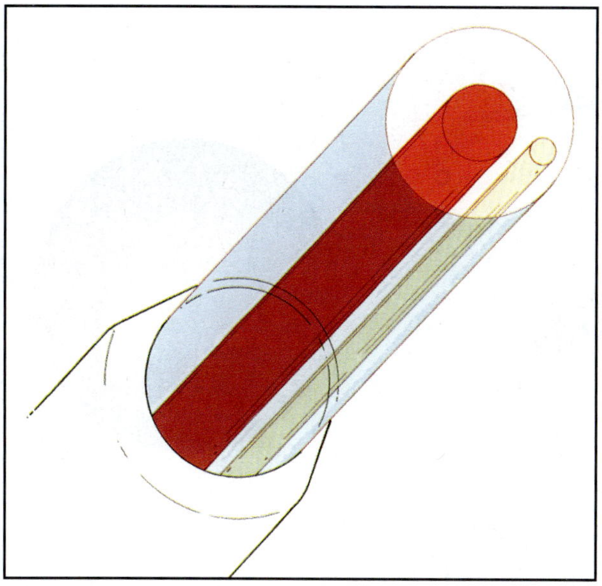

Figure 27-23. The probe used for laser endocyclophotocoagulation contains three groups of fibers: for lighting, for collecting images, and for aiming the laser beam.

ENDOPHOTOCOAGULATION OF CILIARY BODIES

Developed in recent years, cyclodestructive techniques aim to weaken the ciliary body in order to reduce the production of aqueous humor permanently. The main drawback of such procedures is difficulty in titrating the dosage. Consequently, treatments are often either insufficient or excessive. Uram has suggested a new procedure, proposing to perform photocoagulation of the ciliary bodies not ab externo, through the scleral wall, but ab interno, using an endoscopic probe. The procedure is almost completely viscoelastic-dependent—probably the first procedure designed based on the possibilities provided by viscoelastics. The probe used is 1.1 mm in diameter and contains three groups of fiber optics: those that carry light, those that collect images, and those that carry the laser and aim the beam. The wavelength used is that of the diode—810 nanometers (Figure 27-23).

SURGICAL TECHNIQUE

Most commonly, photocoagulation of the ciliary bodies is done through the AC and is completely dependent on corneal transparency, as observation occurs through the endoscopic probe rather than a surgical microscope. A small paracentesis is made in the peripheral portion of the cornea, about 1.5 mm wide (Figure 27-24). Viscoelastic is injected through this paracentesis. The material is generally sodium hyaluronate with high viscosity at rest and high pseudoplasticity (Healon® GV), which provides the transparency required. The viscoelastic fills the AC and permits the surgeon to perform a second paracentesis almost opposite to the former one. A new injection of viscoelastic allows the surgeon to lift the iris and keep it lifted, expanding the space in the posterior chamber to permit the endoscopic probe to access the region behind the iris. The presence of mydriasis is a favorable but not mandatory element of surgery.

The endoscopic probe is introduced inside the AC through one of the paracenteses and directed forward until its tip is near the ciliary bodies, behind the iris. At this point the surgeon stops observing through the microscope and starts watching the monitor, where the image from the probe appears. The surgeon detects and photocoagulates the ciliary bodies one by one to the extent required, adjusting laser power to whiten the processes, avoiding the crackling sound that signifies excessive power.

When photocoagulation of the accessible processes is complete, the probe can be moved in the second paracentesis to access other processes. A new injection of viscoelastic may be necessary to maintain the space between the iris and zonular–capsular complex. Although more easily performed in aphakic and pseudophakic eyes, endocyclophotocoagulation can also be applied to phakic eyes, provided that ocular pressure is lowered by osmotic agents. After completing the procedure, the viscoelastic must be removed to avoid intense and prolonged postoperative hypertension, which would certainly occur following a procedure that does not act on the outflow but on aqueous humor production. Two separate Buratto's cannulas, one for irrigation and one for aspiration, are introduced in both paracenteses and the viscoelastic removed by irrigation and aspiration. At the end of surgery, none of the product should be left inside the eyeball. It is thus best to use a material that is

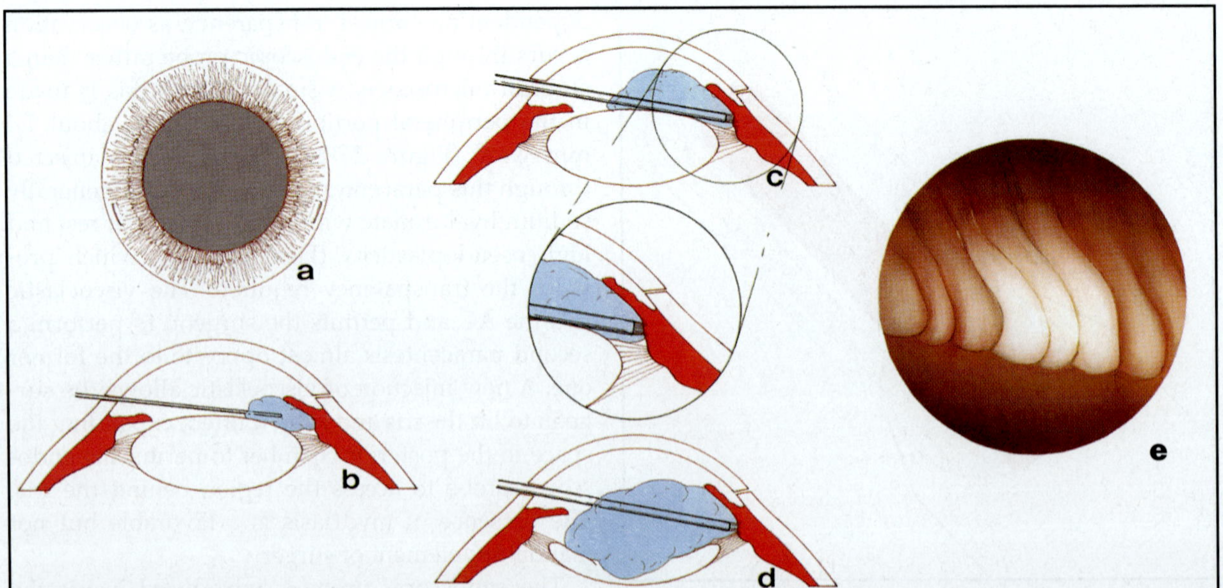

Figure 27-24. Endocyclophotocoagulation of ciliary bodies: Uram's technique. (a) The intervention, which greatly depends on corneal transparency, starts with the creation of two paracentesis of 1.5 mm in the AC near the limbus, at about 10 and 2 o'clock. (b) A very transparent viscoelastic with high viscosity at rest (Healon® GV) is injected through these paracenteses into the AC, with care taken to lift the iris from the lens as much as possible. (c) The endocyclophotocoagulation probe contains three groups of optic fibers, designed for lighting, endoscopy, and laser direction. This is introduced through a sclerotomy and directed forward under microscopic or endoscopic control until it gets close to the ciliary body opposite to the site of introduction. (d) The 810-nm diode laser is directed through the zonules without damaging them. The desired number of ciliary bodies are photocoagulated. At the end of the procedure, the probe is retracted. The viscoelastic is removed by irrigation. (e) In aphakic or pseudophakic eyes, the procedure is eased by the absence of the lens, which provides easier access to the ciliary bodies.

easy to remove rather than a viscoadherent product. Requirements such as space maintenance, transparency, and easy removal make Healon® GV the most appropriate for this use.

Chapter Twenty-Eight

Use of Viscoelastics in Vitreoretinal Surgery

Viscoelastic materials were first used in ophthalmology during retinal detachment surgery. Sodium hyaluronate, the only viscoelastic available at that time, was used to manipulate the detached retina without touching it with surgical instruments. Later it became clear that hyaluronate was too quickly absorbed when not enclosed inside a bubble of vitreous gel and in direct contact with the detached retina.

These studies led to attempts to replace the vitreous body in order to internally tamponade the retina into its natural place. It seemed reasonable to use two components close to the natural vitreous elements: collagen and sodium hyaluronate. The outcome of this early research was a vitreous substitute that caused inflammation, like the collagen preparations that were also tested. Sodium hyaluronate with low molecular weight was used with some success in complicated cases of retinal detachment, but interest in it waned during the 1960s and early 1970s, mostly due to insufficient knowledge of vitreous body pathophysiology in retinal detachment. In the 1980s, interest in using viscoelastic materials in posterior segment surgery increased, and studies were published periodically by prestigious schools in various countries.

We now know that sodium hyaluronate persists in the vitreous much longer than in the aqueous humor, the duration depending on its concentration, viscosity, and amount, as well as degree of inflammation present in the vitreous. Other factors affecting the absorption rate of hyaluronate include density and the structural integrity of the cortical vitreous gel. The most important factors, however, are the presence of the lens capsule and the integrity of the zonules. It has been demonstrated that the primary means by which sodium hyaluronate is reabsorbed from the vitreous is via the chamber angle through the corneoscleral meshwork. Sodium hyaluronate is reabsorbed very slowly when the vitreous is well-shaped, but when the gel is more fluid, sodium hyaluronate is discharged completely within 1 week or less.

The tolerability of sodium hyaluronate introduced in the vitreous chamber is excellent when the product is purified, which is generally the case, but can be poorer when the product contains polluting elements. Other less biocompatible viscoelastics, such as HPMC, have been used in vitreoretinal surgery with varying degrees of tolerability, as outlined in various studies.

Even though viscoelastics were first used and studied in vitreoretinal surgery as vitreous substitutes, recent developments in viscosurgery have attracted greater attention from surgeons. Sodium hyaluronate and other materials have been used in the dissection of epiretinal membranes, in the removal of foreign bodies from the vitreous chamber, in cases of trauma or intraocular hemorrhage, and more generally in almost every step of vitreoretinal surgery. Before the advent of liquid perfluorocarbons, viscoelastic materials were the only means available to assist surgery in particular conditions; for instance, the dissection of membranes adherent to a very mobile retina. Since 1990, their importance has been decreasing. Nevertheless, their usefulness persists, based on their biocompatibility and similar weight to aqueous solutions, which contrast with the toxicity and high weight of liquid perfluorocarbons.

REQUISITES OF VISCOELASTICS FOR USE IN VITREORETINAL SURGERY

The posterior segment of the eye is a particular anatomic–surgical area that differs from the anterior segment in form and, above all, in dimension and volume. In most surgical interventions, the large vitreous chamber is emptied of its contents, and the surgeon's attention is entirely devoted to a thin membrane, such as the retina. Thus, there are none of the space problems that occur in the AC, and it is usually not necessary to oppose pressures that tend to induce collapse of the space available for surgical procedures. The pressure inside the chamber is adjusted by rate of infusion, accomplished by gravity or assisted by a pump that maintains pressure at values preselected by the surgeon. Even so, the features that make a viscoelastic suitable for use in vitreoretinal surgery are not very different from those already described regarding anterior segment surgery.

VISCOSITY AT REST

High viscosity at rest is not an absolute necessity in vitreoretinal surgery. There are conditions where low viscosity at rest is required; for example, in assessing the site and dimensions of the opening in an epiretinal membrane. In some other conditions, greater viscosity at rest is required, as when lifting a portion of membrane to continue dissection. Whereas use of a product with low viscosity such as IAL is not likely to be dangerous, injecting a highly viscous material such as Healon® GV in a narrow space may cause excessive stretching of tissues, followed by iatrogenic retinal lacerations in particular cases. The surgeon should choose the most useful product on a case-by-case basis, taking into account that high viscosity at rest requires active suction to remove the viscoelastic when it is no longer necessary or when it must be replaced with a permanent tamponading device. At least three types of viscoelastic products must be available for use in vitreoretinal surgery: materials with low, medium, and high viscosity at rest.

PSEUDOPLASTICITY

Most surgical procedures on the posterior segment are accomplished through sclerotomies that are calibrated to receive instruments with a 0.9 mm diameter. That is also the maximum diameter of the cannula introducing the viscoelastic. Therefore, high pseudoplasticity does not appear to be relevant in the introduction of viscoelastics in the vitreous chamber. However, in retinal viscosurgery, the viscoelastic needs to be placed in very small spaces and in contact with very delicate structures. The cannulas selected for this use must have very small diameters. In this case, high pseudoplasticity is important, perhaps even more so than in anterior segment surgery. The various preparations of sodium hyaluronate available are suitable for this use.

VISCOELASTICITY

The "soft spatula" effect attributed to viscoelastics is probably best demonstrated in vitreoretinal surgery. We can consider the retina to be as delicate as the corneal endothelium, but even more important, owing to its irreplaceable nerve tissue. It is often necessary to manipulate the retina to move it from the place where it lies. Viscoelastic materials are mostly suitable for this purpose, both when unrolling the retina near a giant tear and creating space between the two adherent parts of the retina. During such operations, the viscoelasticity of the product is an important factor. Usually it should be high, in order to detect residual traction without causing excessive mechanical push on a retina that is still adherent. On other occasions the viscoelasticity should be lower to underline any residual lack of mobility of the retina itself.

TRANSPARENCY

Transparency is perhaps the most relevant feature of viscoelastics for use in vitreoretinal surgery. Through a transparent viscoelastic, one can observe and manipulate even the most delicate tissues, whereas when transparency is insufficient, visibility may become so poor as to prevent continuation of the procedure. It is also best to avoid viscoelastics containing optical polluters, even nontoxic ones, which might cause the surgeon to confuse the viscoelastic with the vitreous, or which could simulate released membrane fragments. However, perfect transparency of the viscoelastic may sometimes make detecting it difficult during surgery, especially in relation to the transparent vitreous. When this situation must be avoided, it is best to use a dyed viscoelastic. The only one currently available is Healon® Yellow.

INTERNAL COHESION

The degree of a viscoelastic's internal cohesion determines whether it is likely to trap air bubbles inside it, and consequently is a main factor influencing transparency of the material after injection. A poorly cohesive viscoelastic is also more difficult to remove. For these reasons, internal cohesion should remain high in vitreoretinal surgery, where transparency and easy removal are fundamental features for any product used, including air, silicone, and liquid perfluorocarbons as well as viscoelastics.

ADHESIVENESS

The ability of the viscoelastic to adhere to the tissues with which it comes in contact may be a favorable feature in some conditions and problematic in others. As a general rule, the use of adhesive viscoelastic is to be avoided when adherent vitreous gel is still present, owing to the possibility of confusing the materials. Conversely, when the retina is completely free from vitreous, a product with good adhesiveness such as Viscoat can protect it from certain kinds of surgical trauma better than can a nonadhesive material.

BIOCOMPATIBILITY

Injecting a poorly biocompatible chemical product into the vitreous chamber causes severe histopathologic and functional alterations of the retina. A study on the tolerability of different antibiotics at various dosages shows how important it is that any material in contact with the retina is biocompatible with it. This is not as relevant when the product is intended to be completely removed, as with liquid perfluorocarbons, but it is fundamental when using viscoelastics, which cannot be removed completely owing to their solubility in water and their lower gravitational gradient compared with liquids and vitreous gel.

The biocompatibility of some viscoelastic materials has been investigated under experimental conditions using cell cultures and animal eyes. The results achieved have been consistent for the most part, but have occasionally conflicted.

In 1984, Vidaurri-Leal et al determined which vitreous component was responsible for metaplasia of pigment epithelium cells once they came into contact with the vitreous body, using cell cultures obtained from cadavers. They found that contact with the collagen component induces alterations in cell polarity, thus jeopardizing the function of the cells themselves and, more importantly, rendering the "pump" effect ineffective. This pump effect is crucial in maintaining retinal reattachment. Such phenomena occurred both with Type I collagen, extracted from the flexor tendon of bovine adults, and with Type II collagen, extracted from the septal cartilage of bovine noses. When the same cells were exposed to sodium hyaluronate extracted from cockscomb, no alterations of cell polarity occurred. Investigations of the morphology and migration of cells, studied by direct observation at the microscope, resulted in similar conclusions. Collagen stimulated alterations and mobility, in contrast with sodium hyaluronate, which did not. In addition, cell proliferation, observed through tagged thymidine absorption, was evident when the pigment epithelium came in contact with collagen, whereas it was absent when it contacted sodium hyaluronate.

In a similar experimental study, Verstraeten et al tested Healon®, Amvisc, and Viscoat to discover which product was most biocompatible for intravitreal use with pigment epithelium cells. The results were that cell polarity was best preserved with Healon® (Figure 28-1), whereas no differences among the products emerged concerning the integrity and morphology of cells. Proliferative activity, shown by tagged thymidine absorption, was equal to that observed in control cells exposed to BSS for all the viscoelastic preparations studied, whereas it was rather high in those exposed to silicone oil (Figure 28-2).

Other investigations of intraocular tolerability concerned HPMC, which was injected in small amounts in the vitreous chamber of rabbit eyes without vitrectomy to simulate posterior capsule rupture following cataract surgery. An amount equal to 0.3 mL at 2% concentration did not cause any ophthalmoscopic or histopathologic alterations compared with controls receiving BSS. Riss et al filled rabbit eyes with HPMC after vitrectomy and lensectomy, leaving the material in the anterior and posterior chambers. In this study, 7 out of 10 eyes had severe inflammation, whereas in the remaining

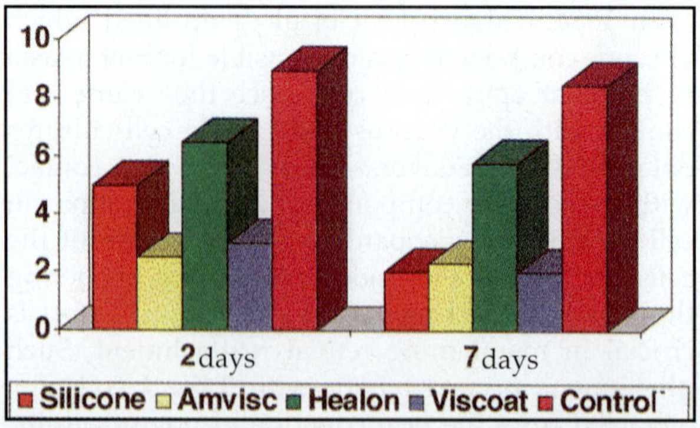

Figure 28-1. Apical/basal activity of gamma-glutamyl transpeptidase of rabbit pigment epithelial cells when in contact with various viscoelastic substances. The test maintains an index of cell polarity. (The results were better with Healon®.)

(Reprinted with permission from Verstraeten TC, Wilcox DK, Friberg TR, Reel C. Effects of silicone oil and hyaluronic acid on cultured human retinal pigment epithelium. *Invest Ophthalmol Vis Sci.* 1990;31:1761-1766.)

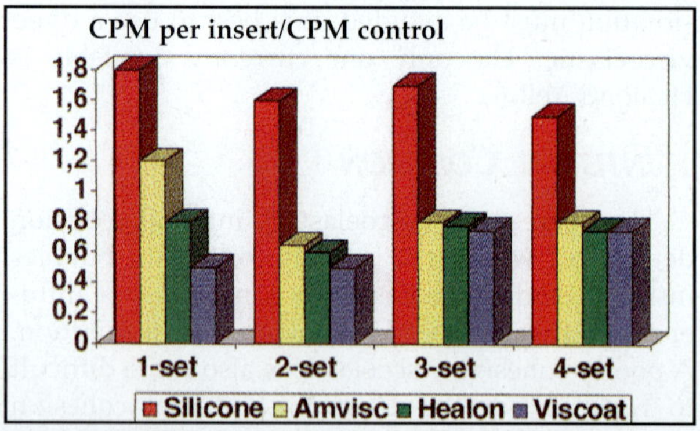

Figure 28-2. Incorporation of 3H thymidine into pigment epithelium cells in rabbit's retina in contact with various viscoelastic substances. The test is an indicator of mitotic activity, that should be as high as possible. (Results are better for viscoelastics than for silicone oil.)

(Reprinted with permission from Verstraeten TC, Wilcox DK, Friberg TR, Reel C. Effects of silicone oil and hyaluronic acid on cultured human retinal pigment epithelium. *Invest Ophthalmol Vis Sci.* 1990;31:1761-1766.)

3 eyes, a reaction developed that was attributed to the viscoelastic. The researchers identified the large amount of product left inside the eye at the end of surgery as the main cause of failed biocompatibility.

This study shows that preparations of sodium hyaluronate provide the best biocompatibility. No data are available on the differences between sodium hyaluronate derived from cockscomb and that obtained from bacterial fermentation. All findings on the biocompatibility of viscoelastics in vitreoretinal surgery must take into account how long they will remain in the vitreous chamber, which could make even poorly biocompatible products more or less acceptable if left in place for a short period.

Duration in the Vitreous Chamber

Rapid resorption of viscoelastics from the vitreous chamber depends on the amount of vitreous gel present as well as on the integrity of the zonule–lens barrier. The rate of intraocular inflammation appears not to be an important factor. No data are available concerning the influence of patient age. Resorption is least when the vitreous chamber is full of well-formed vitreous and the viscoelastic has been injected inside the vitreous gel. Resorption is highest in aphakic eyes, particularly when the vitreous is disaggregated and the viscoelastic can be easily dispersed by movement of liquids and by natural diffusion to contact with the chamber angle.

Experimental research on animals has been conducted by Fernandez-Vigo et al to study in particular the metabolism of 1% sodium hyaluronate and 2% HPMC. The experiment involved 116 eyes of 58 rabbits, all submitted to complete pars plana vitrectomy, sparing the zonule–lenticular diaphragm. At the end of surgery, the vitreous chamber was filled with a nonexpandable SF6 mixture. Three days after the intervention the gas was removed, and the vitreous chamber was filled with the viscoelastic under observation. The amount of viscoelastic present at various time intervals in the postoperative period was detected by diphenylamine reaction technique. Measurements were taken at 0, 7, 14, 30, and 180 days. One week after filling the vitreous chamber with viscoelastic, 100% of the sodium hyaluronate and 60% of the HPMC was still present inside the eyeball. The rate decreased to 62% and 38%, respectively, after 2 weeks (Figure 28-3). The results of this study demonstrate that both products have a short duration inside the eyeball, which as a rule is not sufficient to accomplish any sort of internal tamponading, even temporarily. This is particularly true in the case of HPMC. Paradoxically, the complications caused by the poorer biocompatibili-

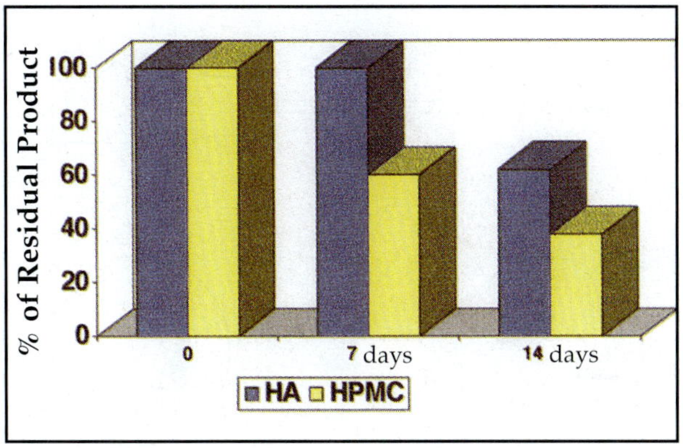

Figure 28-3. Duration of sodium Hyaluronate and of methylcellulose in rabbit eyes after vitrectomy sparing lens and zonule.

ty of this material could be compensated by its rapid metabolism, thus allowing it to be used as a surgical tool with no requirement of accurate removal, as occurs with liquid perfluorocarbons.

Based on their reduced duration in the vitreous chamber, the use of viscoelastics as tamponading devices does not seem practical, even in the long term in retinal detachment surgery. Once again, their main use is as a surgical tool to allow manipulation of posterior segment tissues with a precision and care that could not be achieved otherwise while ensuring and improving the visibility of procedures.

EASY REMOVAL

Should it be necessary to undertake internal tamponade of the vitreous chamber with a nonexpandable tamponading device such as silicone oil, it is crucial to remove the viscoelastic completely at the end of surgery. Easy removal is of basic importance in choosing which product to use, as only some of the viscoelastics available can be easily removed from the retinal surface. Sodium hyaluronate with low molecular weight, which is poorly adhesive and poorly viscous at rest, enters the opening of Charles' cannula more easily than does a more viscous material. On the contrary, methylcellulose, which is adhesive and poorly pseudoplastic, is more difficult to remove.

HEMOSTATIC EFFECT

Viscoelastic materials, particularly sodium hyaluronate, provide hemostatic features not only in anterior segment surgery but also when retinal bleeding occurs. In a 1985 study of 10 diabetic patients undergoing vitrectomy with Healon®, Klemen et al found a far lower prevalence of postoperative bleeding in patients treated with Healon® compared to the control group. The same observation was made by Packer in 1985. In the attempt to explain the mechanism of procoagulating action, Packer also did some experimental research that found that hyaluronate has no direct effect on coagulation factors.

Packer hypothesized that the hemostatic effect was due to the viscoelastic creating a barrier at the site of bleeding, which concentrated the coagulation factors normally present in blood. A prospective study was subsequently performed that highlighted the usefulness of viscoelastics in reducing bleeding in diabetic eyes undergoing vitrectomy. Small amounts of sodium hyaluronate were placed on the bleeding sites of the retina in phakic eyes at the end of surgery with no direct retinal lesions. A total amount of Healon® equal to 0.5 to 0.75 mL was used. Patients were made to rest for 48 hours postoperatively. The results of the study showed that Healon® remarkably reduced hemorrhages in the vitreous chamber in the first 2 days after surgery, thus providing better visualization of the fundus and safe residual photocoagulation. No difference was evident after 7 and 14 days compared to the control group. Researchers found that the short duration of the beneficial effects of using Healon® permitted better postoperative assessment of ocular conditions, enabling surgeons to apply laser photocoagulation to complete the laser treatment already performed during surgery.

SURGICAL PROCEDURES ON THE POSTERIOR SEGMENT WITH VISCOELASTICS

Viscoelastic materials can be beneficial in a range of posterior segment surgical procedures. The fact that they weigh about as much as water and vitreous make viscoelastics preferable to other surgical instruments such as liquid perfluorocarbons in many conditions. In addition, as viscoelastics and liquid perfluorocarbons do not mix, it is possible to use them together. In such cases, adhesive products will remain in the site of injection better than non-adhesive products, which tend to float on the liquid perfluorocarbon bubbles.

Under certain conditions, perfluorocarbon exerts excessive force on the detached retina, which may contribute to reattachment or cause trauma or lacerations. The viscoelastic occupies space, also stretching the retina, but in a more gentle way, without compressing the retina downward and without exerting excessive force on it. It is then possible to estimate retinal mobility and fold more accurately.

VISCODELAMINATION OF EPIRETINAL MEMBRANES

Viscodissection of epiretinal membranes offers various advantages over conventional vitrectomy techniques. Viscodissection distributes the forces that accomplish separation of membranes from the retina over a large surface instead of on a limited area, as happens when hooked scissors or forceps are used. Consequently, the risk of causing iatrogenic retinal holes is reduced, although they can still occur. The viscoelastic material also maintains tissue separation. Once it has been injected, it is then possible to perform the procedures required to solve the specific problem, such as dissecting synechiae or removing a membrane fragment with a forceps.

Although the following procedures are valid for viscodissecting all epiretinal membranes, we first discuss cases of intraocular proliferation due to diabetic retinopathy. The complexity and toughness of membranes encountered in eyes with diabetic retinopathy, let alone the difficulty and risks of removal, best illustrate the advantages of applying viscosurgery to the posterior segment.

INSTRUMENTS

After the first reports of the 1980s and studies by Stirpe and Orciolo (1985–1989), it was clear that the best method of viscoelastic injection was through a specially designed metal cannula with a 20-G external diameter, tapering to a smaller 30-G external diameter. The tip of the cannula is flat and bent to form an angle of nearly 90° (Figure 28-4). The aim of such a shape is to allow the viscoelastic to be injected beneath epiretinal membranes. This cannula is linked to a silicone tube, 0.02 mm internal diameter, which is connected at the opposite end to a syringe containing the viscoelastic. During injection, the syringe is handled by the assistant according to the surgeon's instructions.

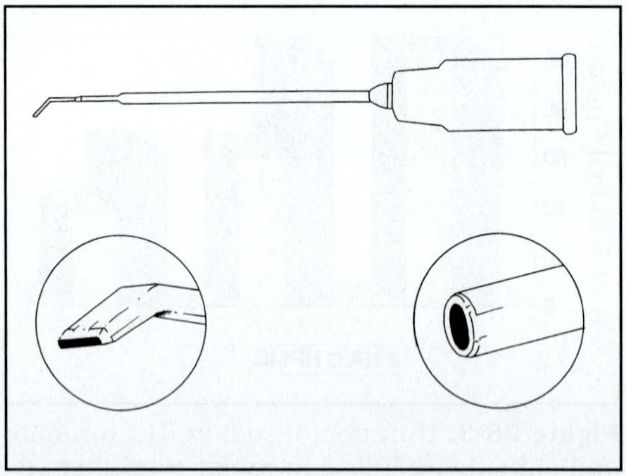

Figure 28-4. A common cannula used for viscoelastic injection into the vitreous chamber. The cannula body has an external diameter of 21 G (0.9 mm), thinning to 30 G at the tip. The opening at the tip can be round or flat.

A pneumatic system has also been developed for the injection of liquids with average viscosity such as viscoelastic products, using lower pressures than those used for silicone oil, but this innovation has had limited practical application to date. An infusion cannula equipped with fiber optics has been used by Ryan for viscodelamination of membranes in diabetic eyes.

TYPE OF VISCOELASTIC

When one uses thin cannulas, such as the one described previously, it is necessary to use a viscoelastic with very high pseudoplasticity. In practice, only preparations of sodium hyaluronate have the properties for use with this device, whereas other viscoelastic materials require cannulas with a larger diameter. Viscodissection of membranes has also been performed with 1% methylcellulose, seemingly without problems of ineffectiveness or toxicity. The sodium hyaluronate used can have low (IAL), medium (Healon®), or high (Healon®

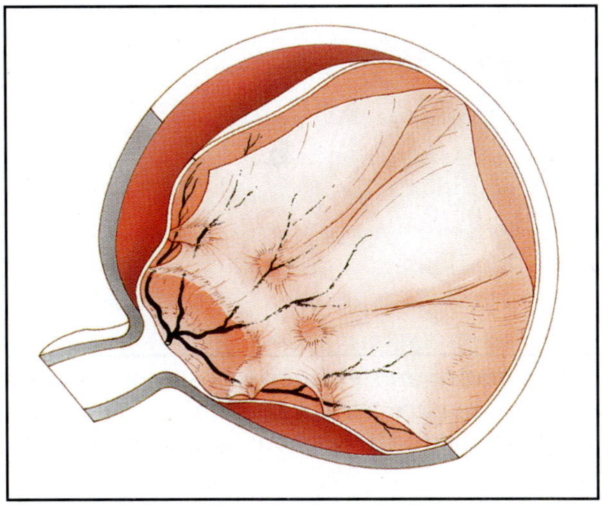

Figure 28-5. In diabetic retinopathy, retinal detachment is caused mainly by tractions parallel and perpendicular to the retinal plane. They are initially due to vitreous retraction between the vitreous base anteriorly and the area interested by fibrovascular proliferation posteriorly. Often areas of vitreous detachment from the retina develop. At first, retinal lacerations are usually absent.

GV) molecular weight, with different indications according to the various products. In many situations it is useful to use hyaluronate dyed with fluorescein, which makes it easier to detect in the presence of the vitreous and the other elements occupying the posterior segment.

A hyaluronate with low molecular weight will exert a limited force on the membrane, allowing any other solutions present to flow through unimpeded. In most situations hyaluronate with low or medium molecular weight will be suitable, as it exerts a viscoelastic force that is not excessive for the membrane. In special cases it will be necessary to use a product with higher molecular weight, taking care that its greater force in creating spaces and separating tissues does not cause retinal tears. Because most of the works published used sodium hyaluronate with medium molecular weight, in our discussion of various surgical techniques we consider the use of that product as a standard, emphasizing different requirements when necessary.

PROLIFERATIVE DIABETIC RETINOPATHY

Retinal detachment is one of the most severe complications of proliferative diabetic retinopathy. It is caused by retraction of the posterior surface of the vitreous and the fibrovascular proliferative tissue, which create both antero–posterior and tangential forces, leading to a tractional retinal detachment. Retinal tears are secondary occurrences and may occur after detachment. In eyes with proliferative diabetic retinopathy and retinal detachment, there is usually a partial posterior vitreous detachment. The vitreous remains adherent to the base and the peripheral margin of more posterior areas of fibrovascular proliferation (Figure 28-5). The dimension of the areas where the fibrovascular tissue grows is partly determined by the time of onset and the extent of the posterior vitreous detachment. Because the posterior vitreous cortex is the necessary framework for the growth of extraretinal fibrovascular tissue, when complete detachment of the vitreous occurs relatively quickly, the eye does not develop typical proliferative diabetic retinopathy. On the contrary, when the vitreous is not separated from the retina, posterior fibrovascular proliferation may become quite extensive.

Incomplete posterior detachment of the vitreous usually develops between the peripheral margin of the posterior proliferative tissue and the vitreous base, but the vitreous cortex may remain adherent to the retina in the equatorial and postequatorial portions, particularly in the upper quadrants. According to McLeod, carefully observing the extent of posterior vitreous detachment is important to determine in which eyes viscodissection of membranes en bloc has the greatest potential of success.

Eyes with tractional retinal macular detachment and those with tractional detachment along with retinal tears but with limited posterior detachment of the vitreous appear to require viscosurgery for anatomic–surgical success. Eyes with extended posterior detachment may also benefit from viscodelamination, but do not need it as much. Furthermore, much greater amounts of viscoelastic must be used in these eyes (Figure 28-6).

Vitreoretinal surgery for tractional retinal detachment that complicates diabetic retinopathy aims to eliminate antero–posterior and tangential tractions, removing the posterior vitreous surface along with

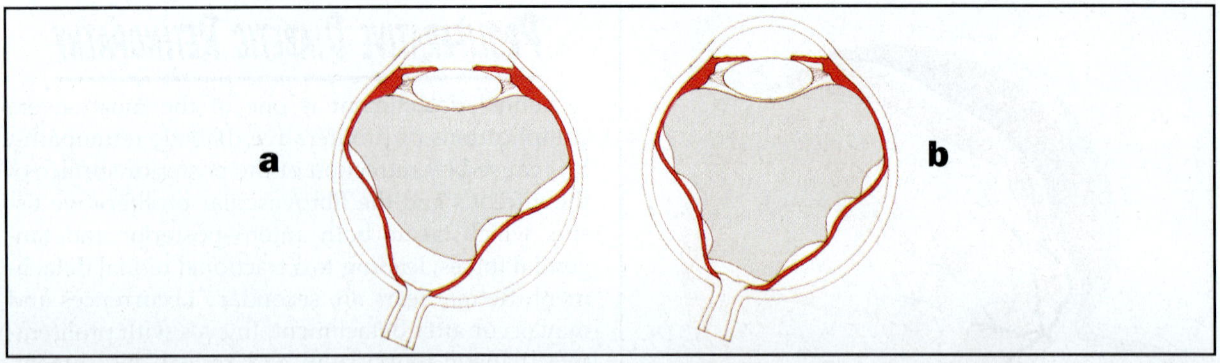

Figure 28-6. a) Section of an eye with diabetic retinopathy and extensive posterior vitreous detachment: areas of adherence between vitreous and retina are few. b) Section of an eye with diabetic retinopathy and limited posterior vitreous detachment: the vitreous is adherent to the retina in many areas of fibrovascular proliferation.

the greatest amount of fibrovascular tissue possible. The intervention starts by removing the central portion of the vitreous, according to the usual three-way technique. The subsequent phases of the intervention depend on the surgical method chosen.

EN BLOC TECHNIQUE

Once vitrectomy has proceeded to the site corresponding to the posterior vitreous cortex, the surgeon locates an opening in it through which to inject the viscoelastic. This opening must be placed corresponding to a zone of vitreous that is already detached. Should such a suitable opening be absent, the surgeon can incise the posterior cortex with a sclerotome or the vitrectomy cutter—always in an area where the vitreous is expected to be detached—and then inject the viscoelastic through the hole opened (Figure 28-7, a and b). When posterior vitreous detachment is not present, surgical difficulties greatly increase, as in these conditions it is more difficult to start viscodelamination. The viscoelastic (IAL or Healon®) is injected through a 20-G cannula, bent on the tip like a hockey stick. During injection in the space between the posterior vitreous cortex and the retina, the infusion fluid that is moved forward is made to flow out through the sclerotomies or through the infusion cannula. The assistant adjusts the speed and amount of viscoelastic injection according to the surgeon's instructions.

Viscodelamination is performed along with limited mechanical separation of the vitreous cortex, achieved with the same bent cannula used for viscoelastic injection. In some eyes it is necessary to make other holes in the posterior vitreous cortex to separate the vitreous over 360° posterior to the vitreous base (Figure 28-7) while minimizing traction on persisting adhesions between retina and epiretinal membranes. This en bloc technique tries to avoid or minimize local circumcision of vitreoretinal adhesions as well as segmentation of proliferative membranes by the scissors. These procedures are performed only in cases where they are necessary, during and after viscoelastic injection, while the "cone" of cortical vitreous remains essentially intact, as the cortical vitreous is not too mobile inside the eyeball owing to the presence of the viscoelastic.

After completing viscodelineation of the membrane, the surgeon uses the vitrector again to excise and aspirate the whole posterior cortical vitreous, dissecting it at the optic nerve and along the circumference of the vitreous base. Epiretinal membranes that were lifted above the retinal plane by the viscoelastic are also removed (Figure 28-7d). Most of the injected viscoelastic is aspirated as well, but a small amount may remain in contact with the retina, particularly when the material used is not sodium hyaluronate, but a more adhesive material such as 1% methylcellulose. The residual viscoelastic touching the retina becomes evident when diathermy is performed, producing a small whitish halo around the spot where heat was applied.

The intervention continues with the assessment and treatment of retinal holes formerly present or occurring during surgery. Internal tamponade follows, always mandatory in the presence of holes.

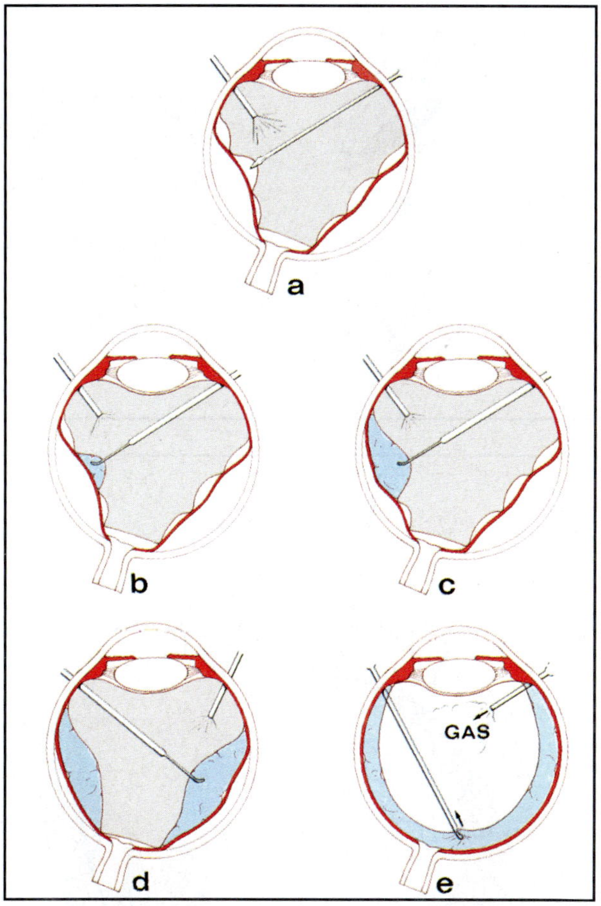

Figure 28-7. Viscodelamination of diabetic epiretinal membranes: the 'En Bloc' technique. a) After core vitrectomy, the posterior hyaloid membrane is incised in an area where it seems detached from the underlying retina. Incision of a posterior hyaloid adherent to the retina is more delicate and dangerous for retinal integrity. b) Viscoelastic is gently injected between posterior hyaloid and retina. c) Viscoelastic injection is continued, separating posterior hyaloid from the retina. The retina itself begins to flatten as soon as vitreous adherences are broken. (Firm adhesions are not eliminated by this method.) d) More than one injection site can be necessary to detach membranes over 360°. e) After membrane removal by vitrectome, the internal tamponade can take place. When gas is employed, it is not necessary to remove all the viscoelastic.

This can be accomplished with gas or silicone oil. When silicone oil is used, it is necessary to remove all the viscoelastic from the vitreous chamber to achieve the best conditions for correct internal tamponade.

COMPLICATIONS

The intervention of en bloc delamination of membranes due to diabetic retinopathy is not only elegant, but also demonstrates good clinical effectiveness. Compared to traditional surgical treatment, the use of viscoelastics allows surgery to be completed more quickly while increasing safety. Viscoelastic use has been found to be very useful in dissecting multiple epiretinal membranes as well as vascularized membranes in the midperiphery of phakic eyes. However, viscoelastic use is not free from complications, the major one being accidental injection under the retina (Figure 28-8a). Viscoelastics, especially sodium hyaluronate, are not particularly toxic to the retina, but the material may alter the subdivision planned by the surgeon for the end of surgery, influencing the outcome. Its presence may also keep the retina lifted for a long time postoperatively.

Another complication is bleeding, which often occurs in the preretinal space during viscodelamination. The cause of such bleeding seems to be the removal of vascularized synechiae between epiretinal membranes and the retina. The procoagulative effect of viscoelastics, which are intended to act primarily as a barrier to the diffusion and dilution of leaking blood, is not always enough to oppose bleeding. Bleeding is more marked when the vessel is torn instead of being cut with scissors (Figure 28-8, a and b). Therefore, viscodelamination must not be excessive in case of very vascularized membranes.

The technique of viscodelamination carries the significant risk of creating retinal breaks, which follows excessive filling of nonexpandable spaces with the viscoelastic. The risk increases with viscoelastics having a higher viscosity at rest and higher pseudoplasticity, as they can be rapidly injected in large amounts through very narrow cannulas (Figure 28-8c). Epiretinal membranes are very likely to occur when the attempt is made to lift extremely adherent fibrovascular membranes that should instead be cut with scissors. Good communication between the surgeon and the assistant is also mandatory to avoid retinal breaks, as in many cases the assistant has the task of injecting the viscoelastic.

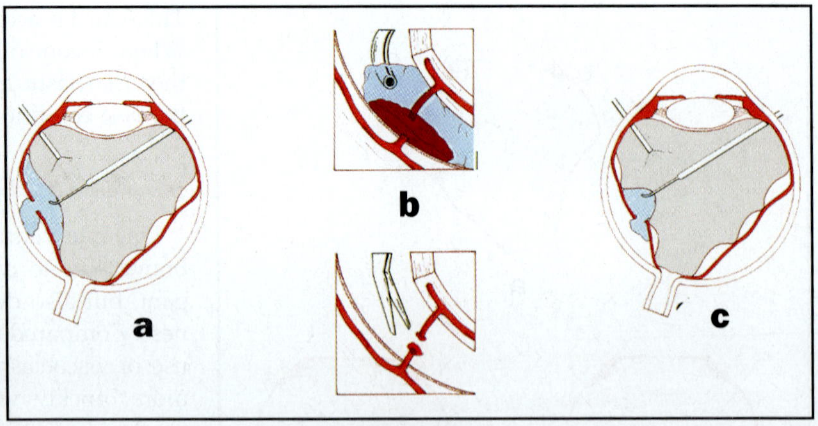

Figure 28-8. Complications of viscodelamination of diabetic epiretinal membranes. a) The viscoelastic can go under the retina through an existing or iatrogenic hole. b) New vessels can be broken in the areas of proliferation, with some bleeding. The bleeding is reduced when major vessels are cut by microscissors. c) The retina can break when a heavy viscoelastic is injected into a narrow space surrounded by firm adherences.

The possibility of recurrent proliferation seems not to be a complication of the technique or the viscoelastic used, but rather appears to be a characteristic of the patient's disease. Similarly, development of neovascularization at the retina or extending to the anterior segment is not influenced by viscoelastics positively or negatively.

Technique of Segmentation

Segmentation is an alternative to the en bloc technique that seems more appropriate in cases of fibrovascular proliferation where bleeding is likely and where large posterior vitreous detachment is present. Once central vitrectomy has been completed, the real intervention can be started, preparing the peripheral vitreous for removal. For this purpose a circular incision is cut in the posterior hyaloid surface, in the portion shaped like a cone (Figure 28-9). The circular incision is made easily when the posterior surface of the vitreous is very far away from the retina, but can be impossible when the vitreous is attached to the equatorial and postequatorial retina (Figure 28-10a). In the latter case, a hole is made in the vitreous cortex, at a site where it appears detached from the retina. A viscoelastic with low viscosity at rest (IAL) is then injected between the two structures to separate the vitreous from the retina and improve visualization of the remaining vitreoretinal adhesions (Figure 28-10b). The viscoelastic moves the vitreous toward the center of the eyeball, thus making its removal by vitrector easier. Little by little, the whole vitreous, already detached or detachable by viscodissection, is fragmented and aspirated by the vitrector (Figure 28-11).

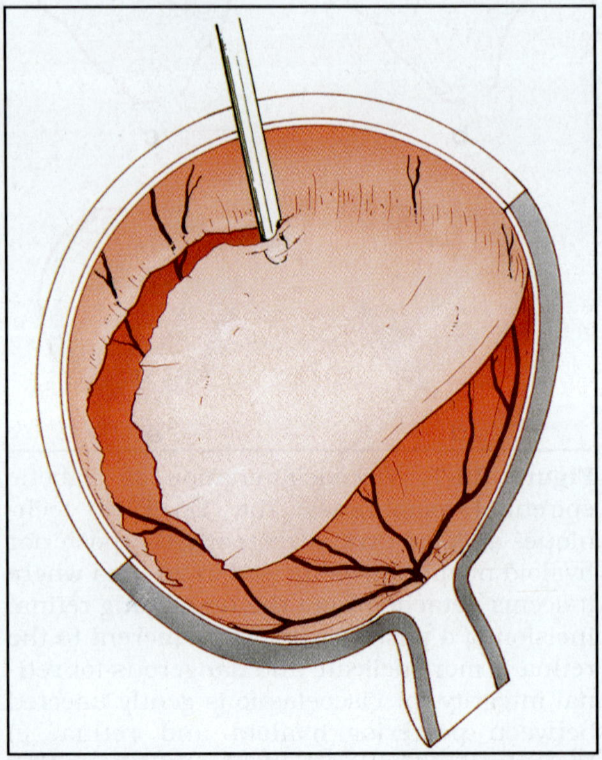

Figure 28-9. Viscodelamination of diabetic epiretinal membranes: the technique of segmentation. Following core vitrectomy, the posterior hyaloid membrane is cut around 360° anteriorly to the zones of fibrovascular proliferation.

Extracting extensive fibrovascular membranes from the posterior retina after removing the surrounding vitreous poses particularly difficult problems (Figure 28-12). The epiretinal tissue may be

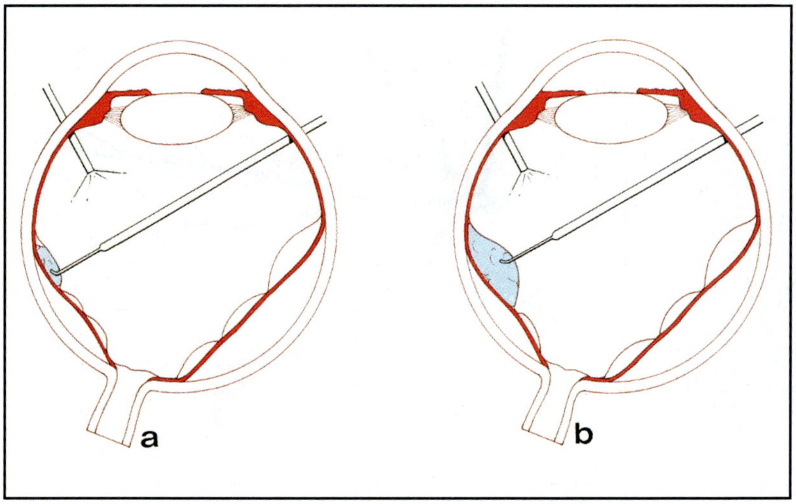

Figure 28-10. a) Even when retinal adhesions are extended, delamination begins by viscoelastic injection where the vitreous is partially detached. b) The viscoelastic substance injected underneath the posterior hyaloid surface further elevates the vitreous, makes some adhesions free, and shows those to be surgically cut.

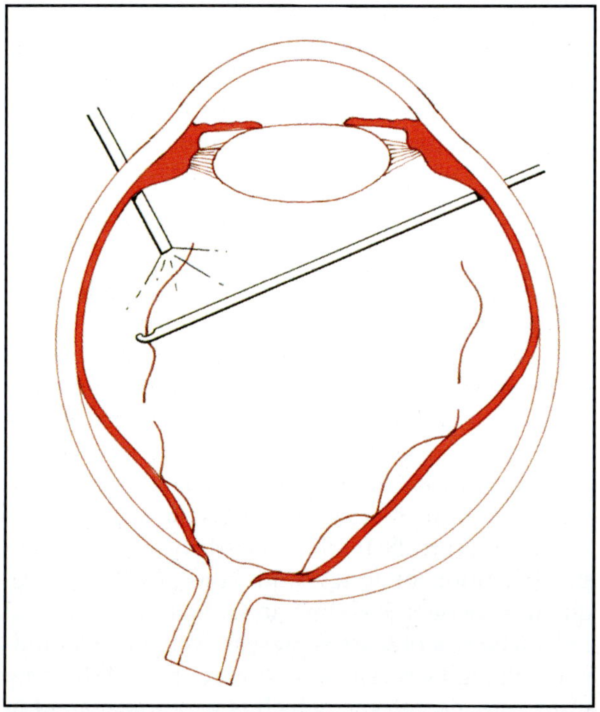

Figure 28-11. Membranes delaminated by viscoelastic and surgically cut are removed by vitrectomy step by step.

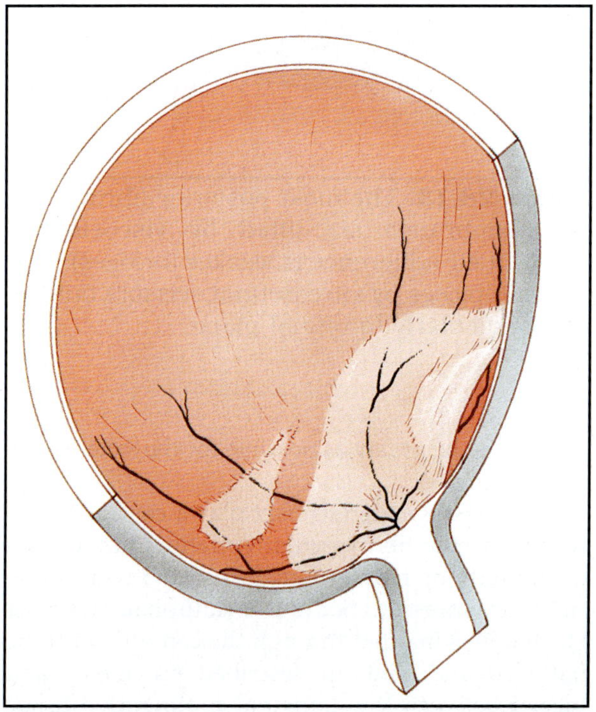

Figure 28-12. Near the posterior pole, the adhesions between retina and proliferative membranes are stiffer and more extended. Wide proliferation areas can remain after removal of more peripheral membranes.

widely adherent to the underlying retina or can pass like a bridge over some areas of the retina. The technique of segmentation consists of dissecting each portion of the fibrovascular tissue surrounding a zone of adhesion with scissors, then removing as many membranes as possible with the vitrector (Figure 28-13). Usually most of the fibrovascular tissue can be removed, but there may be areas where adhesions of the fibrovascular tissue to the underlying retina are too strong. Some "islets" of proliferated tissue may therefore need to be left in place, but

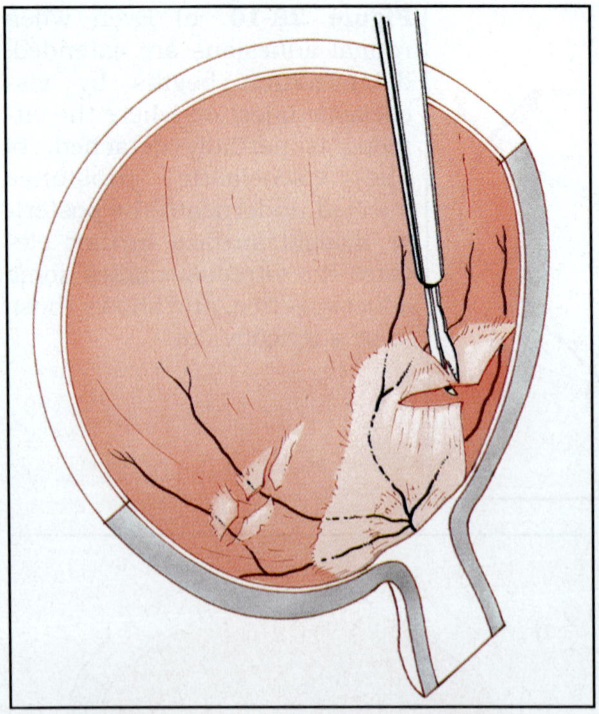

Figure 28-13. The most posterior fibrovascular membranes are lifted by viscoelastics where their adherence is weaker (bridges), and cut into pieces by vitreoretinal scissors cutting perpendicularly to retinal plane.

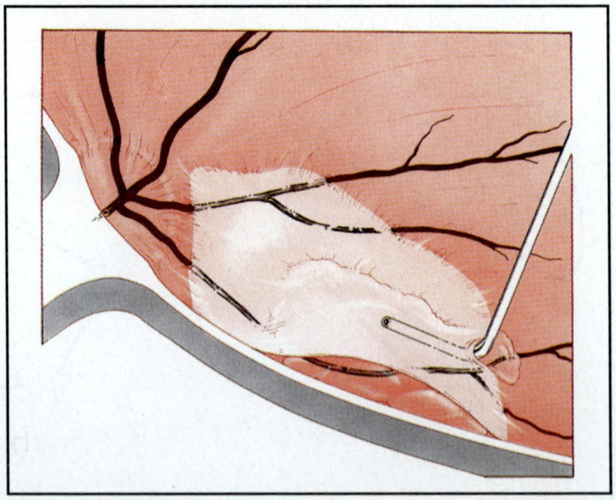

Figure 28-14. The angled tip of the viscoelastic cannula is introduced when the border of the fibrovascular membrane is separated from the retina. The injection of viscoelastic separates the proliferative tissue from the retina along the natural cleavage plane.

these must be as few as possible for the sake of surgical success.

Viscoelastic materials may play a central role in separating the fibrovascular epiretinal tissue from the underlying retina when diffuse and wide adhesions are present. Sodium hyaluronate (IAL or Healon®) is injected through the cannula with the flattened and bent tip described previously and placed between the epiretinal proliferative tissue and the more internal retina. While the viscoelastic is being injected, the fibrovascular membrane is lifted with the bent tip of the cannula at a point where it barely separates from the retina (Figure 28-14). The tip of the cannula is directed forward in the cleavage plane as the viscoelastic is injected and both tissues separate. The force of dissection exerted by the viscoelastic separates the tissues along the natural anatomic plane. This splitting is produced by the pressure exerted in all directions by the viscoelastic, and exposes the connections of the proliferative membrane with the underlying retina (Figure 28-14).

In this phase, the elasticity of the product chosen is important: it must compress when encountering tough adhesions and expand in the presence of less-resistant adhesions. The surgeon can then distinguish fibrovascular adhesions amenable to viscodissection from those requiring excision with vitreous scissors (Figure 28-15). Poor elasticity would lead to the laceration of tough adhesions, with a consequent increase in bleeding and a high risk of retinal tears. The risk of tears is present even when a product with high viscosity at rest (Healon® GV) is being used. The viscoelastic, which is very transparent in itself, also creates excellent mechanical hemostasis, thus increasing the visibility of the adhesion that it subjects to tension. Sites of bleeding can be identified and treated with diathermy or photocoagulation (Figure 28-16). The injection of viscoelastic is resumed after the surgeon cuts each tough adhesion with scissors, and dissection continues.

Fibrovascular membranes often originate along the retinal veins with the largest caliber. The vitreoretinal traction formerly present can cause the veins to lift, which may also occur during viscodissection

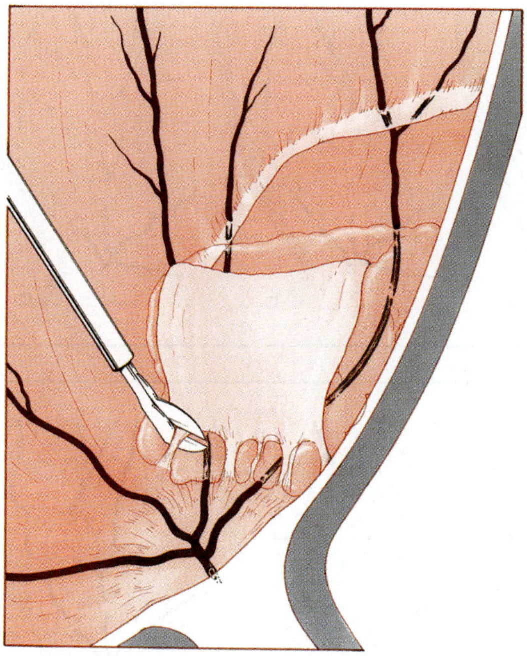

Figure 28-15. The viscoelastic allows identification of the connections between the membrane and the underlying retina, and creates the space where surgical cutting instruments can be introduced to cut stiffer adhesions.

of the membrane. The viscoelastic tends to immobilize such adhesions while permitting the surgeon to evaluate them accurately. Partially removed vessels must be respected during removal of the fibrovascular membrane (Figure 28-17) and treated surgically later. Careful dissection with scissors or the vitrector around these vascular adhesions is necessary to prevent damage related to vessel breakage.

At the end of viscodissection with membrane segmentation, most of the retina should remain free, with as few islets of proliferative tissue as possible, corresponding to fibrovascular adhesions that could not be excised without irreparable retinal damage (Figure 28-18).

The complications associated with the en bloc technique are also possible during segmentation, but with higher risk of bleeding, as this procedure is always used in eyes with marked fibrovascular adhesions. The viscoelastic material injected must be removed completely when the surgeon wishes to insert silicone oil. However, it can be left in place in whole or in part when the surgeon can foresee no need for internal tamponade, or when the procedure is performed with gas.

RETROHYALOID PREMACULAR HEMORRHAGE

Retrohyaloid premacular hemorrhage is a particular type of vitreoretinal pathology in diabetic patients that may also occur also in eyes treated with extended Argon laser photocoagulation. The hemorrhage typically expands between the internal limiting membrane and the posterior vitreous surface, often without posterior vitreous detachment. If not treated, the bleeding tends to reabsorb very slowly, leaving stimulus and time for vitreoretinal proliferation. This is why performing a vitrectomy is advised within 4 weeks of its diagnosis.

Surgical treatment of this premacular bleeding may consist of simple drainage, as the retina can be treated with photocoagulation to prevent proliferative retinopathy. After preparing the standard vitrectomy openings, the central portion of the vitreous is removed, enabling the surgeon to approach the area occupied by bleeding. The posterior vitreous cortex is incised with a sharp needle or vitrector to create access to the hemorrhage. At the beginning, blood is drained using Charles' blunt needle with a silicone tip. As removal of the hemorrhage continues, hyaluronate with low molecular weight (IAL) is injected into the bag containing the hemorrhage. Hyaluronate moves and collects the blood, thus easing the extraction of even small amounts. It also expands the bag containing the bleeding, improving its access and control; exposes possible membranes, previously formed or in the early phase; maintains excellent visibility; and, owing to its biocompatibility, can be left in site at the end of surgery (Figure 28-19).

NONDIABETIC EPIRETINAL MEMBRANES

Epiretinal membranes normally encountered outside diabetic retinopathy have particular characteristics. Because they are less adherent to the underlying retina, except in isolated areas, complete splitting is often possible. These membranes

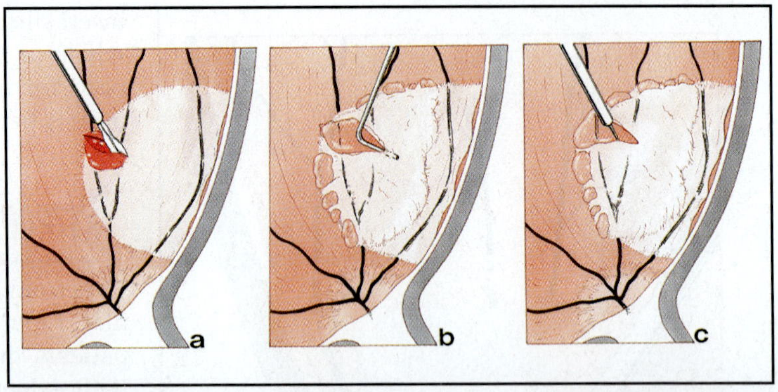

Figure 28-16. a) It is easy to observe minor hemorrhages during segmentation and removal of membranes, especially at the posterior pole. b) Viscoelastic substances, and particularly sodium hyaluronate, possess hemostatic properties that limit bleeding. c) The transparency of the viscoelastic that removes blood allows identification and treatment of the bleeding site.

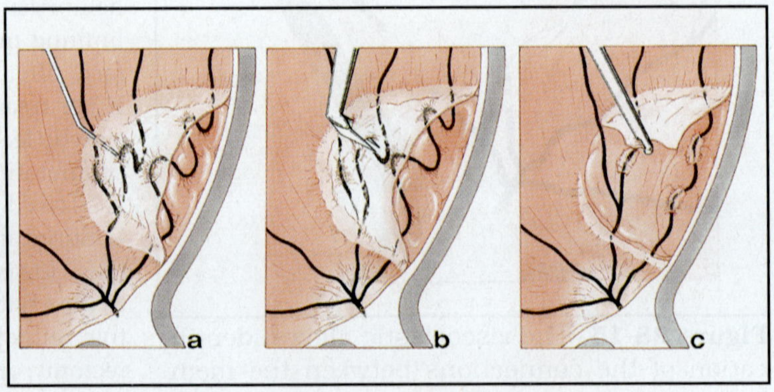

Figure 28-17. a) Traction by contracting fibrovascular tissue can induce lifting and partial avulsion of retinal veins. The proliferative tissue can be lifted and blocked by sodium hyaluronate. (The vessels are blocked.) b) The mechanical action and the transparency of viscoelastics make it easy to cut adhesions near vessels. Vessel integrity can be respected. c) The isolated fibrovascular tissue can be removed by vitrectomy.

are also very seldom vascularized. The most common location of nondiabetic epiretinal membranes is the macular region, where the cells creating them—often starting from the pigment epithelium—gather during night rest. When the membranes are associated with retinal detachment, whether they have already been treated or not, they can also be present in an extramacular area, generally the lower hemiretina.

Surgical removal of these membranes during vitrectomy must be as complete as possible owing to the risk that their fragments may become reattached to the macular retina, causing further retraction and decreased visual function. Fragments of premature membranes left inside the eye may also begin new proliferation, which will require another intervention.

Before the common use of viscoelastics, operation to remove epiretinal membranes—such as macular pucker, for example—involved first performing a pars plana vitrectomy. The surgeon then searched for a flap of the membrane that could be lifted with a special hook, peeled it away with the hook or a posterior segment forceps, and extracted the membrane from the eyeball, ideally as a whole, but more often in fragments.

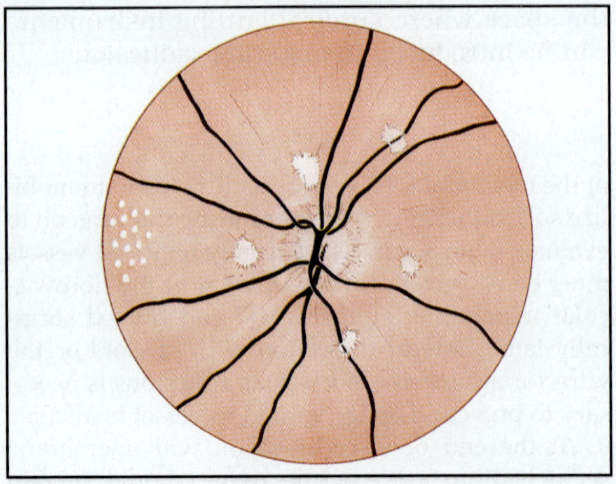

Figure 28-18. Once the removal of fibrovascular epiretinal membranes in diabetic retinopathy is completed, some islands of proliferative tissue usually remain and are not completely removable.

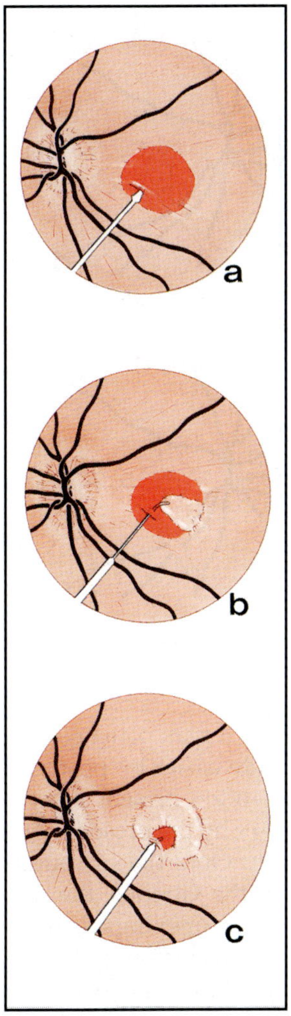

Figure 28-19. Treatment of premacular retrohyaloid hemorrhage. a) The first step is the incision of the posterior hyaloid membrane, to gain access to the space occupied by blood. b) Once the blood is partially removed, a viscoelastic substance (usually sodium hyaluronate at low or medium molecular weight) is injected into the retrohyaloid space to help complete removal. c) As soon as the last of the blood is removed, the viscoelastic substance allows the detection of any membranes and helps their removal.

Although this is not a difficult technique, it presents some risks that could reduce the effectiveness of the results. First, there is the possibility that the instruments used could cause retinal damage with bleeding or occasionally even laceration. This is especially likely to occur when the underlying retina is lifted and mobile. Therefore, most surgeons now prefer to stabilize the retina with liquid perfluorocarbon or a viscoelastic. There is also the possibility that the surgeon will cause a retinal tear of the same membrane by excessive stretching. It is not always easy to control the margins of the membrane while retracting it to detach it from the retina. It is therefore easy to pull it too hard and tear the retinal tissue, particularly when the tissue is detached or thinned from previous surgery. Again, the membrane may tear some of the vessels it was adhering to, causing marked bleeding. This is a rare complication, but must be considered.

Removing epiretinal membranes with viscoelastics prevents many of these surgical complications and difficulties, allowing for better resolution of cases that have had previous surgery and for application to cases with a previously poor prognosis. The viscoelastic planned for use must have excellent biocompatibility, transparency, and pseudoplasticity. The various preparations of sodium hyaluronate seem to best meet the requirements of this surgery. A product with low viscosity at rest, such as IAL, is less appropriate, as it is not able to overcome the force of a membrane's adhesion to the underlying retina. A product with medium viscosity at rest, such as Healon®, is able to split tissues and keep them separated without exerting too much force. A viscoelastic with high viscosity at rest, such as Healon® GV, can be used successfully when handled by experienced surgeons, but may cause retinal damage in certain cases. It is also more difficult to remove.

Dyed viscoelastics, such as Healon® Yellow, provide a distinct advantage. They can be easily detected inside the eyeball and therefore injected with precision into the site in the correct amount. At the end of surgery, when complete removal is required, they can be accurately extracted. Moreover, a dyed viscoelastic is more easily detected when out of place; for instance, when sliding under the retina through a laceration. Studies tested a range of colors, but identified fluorescein as the dye of choice for viscoelastics. They noted in particular that blue-colored product obscured the details of the retina, making surgery difficult to perform.

The method of injecting viscoelastic is the same as that used in the treatment of diabetic membranes. The surgeon uses a 30-G cannula bent at the tip, mounted on a 20-G body, the standard thickness for vitrectomy instruments. Although they change from case to case, basic surgical practices are consistent, which we describe in detail in the following.

EPIRETINAL MEMBRANES ON ATTACHED RETINA

The typical example of epiretinal membranes on attached retina is the retraction of epimacular vitre-

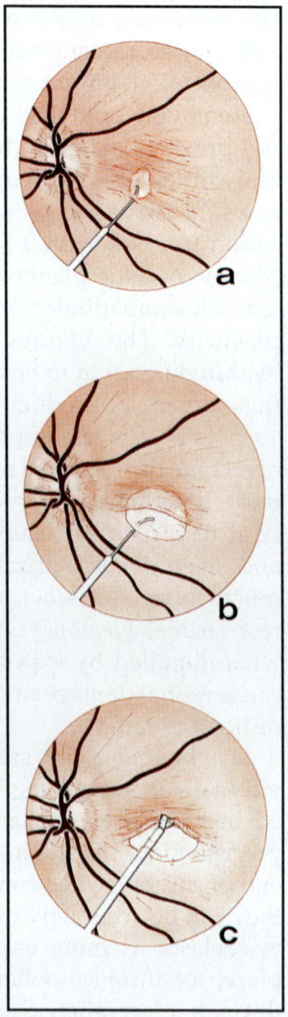

Figure 28-20. Viscodissection of macular epiretinal membranes. a) Viscodissection of an epiretinal membrane on an attached retina begins by injecting viscoelastic under the membrane. This is done through an existing aperture or through a hole produced by a bent needle in a location where the membrane is clearly identified. b) Viscoelastic injection lifts the membrane, makes it thoroughly visible, makes weaker adhesions free, controls small bleeding, stabilizes the retina without surgical instruments. c) Stronger adhesions are controlled and released by vitreous forceps while the retina is kept in position by the viscoelastic.

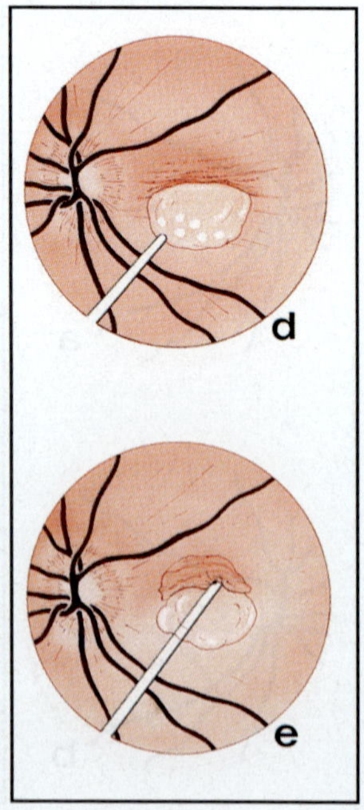

Figure 28-21. Viscodissection of macular epiretinal membranes (continued). d) Laser treatment, if needed, can be performed through the viscoelastic substance. The viscoelastic has to be transparent. Diathermy is more difficult in presence of viscoelastic substances, that are bad conductors of heath and electricity. e) Once made free, the membrane is removed by vitrectome or by forceps.

ous cortex. This tends to roll up the retina to which it adheres, severely altering visual acuity, first through metamorphopsia and then with decreased vision. The intervention to remove the membrane is not difficult in standard cases, but must be performed carefully owing to the risk of complications and the excellent visual recovery that potentially follows success. Many surgeons perform the intervention without viscoelastics, which are very useful in increasing safety and limiting mistakes when narrow field observation systems are used, such as Landers' lenses. Membranes often extend toward the retinal periphery beyond the observable field, and undesirable effects may follow from exerting traction with a forceps on a membrane still adherent to the retina.

The intervention starts with a pars plana central vitrectomy. Vitrectomy is made easier by posterior detachment of the vitreous—often present in eyes with epiretinal membranes—or by the presence of a large posterior vitreous cavity. Once the surrounding area has been freed from the vitreous, the surgeon inspects the membrane for openings. If there is no suitable opening for viscoelastic injection, a small hole is made in the membrane, possibly at a point where it is lifted from the retina, with a needle bent like a hook or with scissors (Figure 28-20a). The viscoelastic (sodium hyaluronate with a low molecular weight, such as IAL) can thus be injected under the membrane, lifting it progressively as the injection continues. Lifting the membrane in this way is atraumatic and the risk of retinal damage is minimal, as the retina is kept separated from the operating area by the viscoelastic. The bolus of viscoelastic lifting the membrane also allows the surgeon to see its whole extension, lacerating less-resistant adhesions while exposing those requiring more careful detachment (Figure 28-20b).

One advantage of viscoelastic materials is that they provide for great stability of both living and nonliving tissues involved in surgery. It is impossible for partly detached membranes to reattach (which would result in a less-precise assessment) or to lie flat again against the retina. Inadvertently

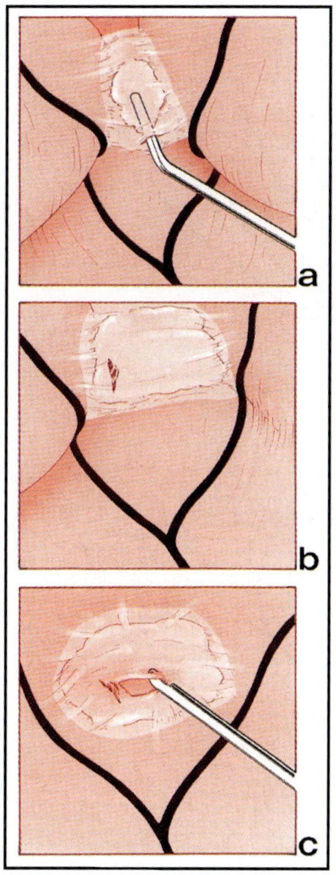

Figure 28-22. Viscodelamination of epiretinal membranes on a detached retina. a) The viscoelastic is injected under the membrane, the tip of the cannula is directly in the retinal fold (determined by the traction star.) Adherences are never firm inside the fold and the thin cannula can be introduced with relative safety. b) Tissue distension induced by the viscoelastic can start membrane delamination where adhesions to the retina are weaker. Progressive retinal distension may reveal hidden retinal lacerations. c) The viscoelastic acts as a cushion protecting the retina while the membrane is removed by the vitrectome.

detached fragments of membrane can no longer float in the vitreous chamber following the stream of the irrigating solution, but remain near the place of origin, thus permitting their removal. The retina itself is also kept in place by the bolus of viscoelastic, with less risk of damage (Figure 28-20c). In case of lacerated small vessels on the retinal surface, viscoelastics act mechanically to stop bleeding and permit the intervention to continue with consistently clear visibility. Any additional bleeding can be stopped by injecting more viscoelastic and by lifting the infusion bottle to increase pressure in the vitreous chamber. In special cases it may be better to perform endodiathermy, a practice that is far less necessary in these cases than for diabetic retinopathy membranes. When necessary, laser treatment can be applied through the viscoelastic with no difficulty (Figure 28-21d).

Release of the membrane lifted by the viscoelastic is continued by gently pulling the forceps near the remaining sites of adhesion to the underlying retina. Traction must always be exerted in such a way that no vector is produced perpendicular to the retina in the site of adhesion. Further injections of viscoelastic are useful to expose the position of the membrane at any phase of surgery, because at each step unsuspected tractions may lead to potentially severe complications. After the whole of the membrane or the necessary part of it is released, it can be removed with a forceps or vitrector (Figure 28-21e).

At the end of "peeling," the viscoelastic can be extracted or left in place, depending on the case. In simpler situations—for instance, after macular pucker in phakic eyes—a small amount of even dyed viscoelastic left in the vitreous chamber causes no complications. Conversely, it may not be beneficial to leave large amounts of viscoelastic material in the vitreous chamber, particularly products with high viscosity at rest, owing to the risk of postoperative ocular hypertension. In aphakic eyes, removing the viscoelastic product should be more complete, as the risk of hypertension in the following days is much higher. The viscoelastic should be completely removed when a nonexpandable internal tamponading means such as silicone oil is required, to avoid altering postoperative subdivisions inside the eye.

EPIRETINAL MEMBRANES ON DETACHED RETINA

Some epiretinal proliferation is almost always present in retinal detachments treated with vitrectomy, as this is the main indication for this type of intervention. Surgical problems due to the presence of epiretinal membranes on detached retina are slightly different from those previously described, mostly because the surgeon is often confronted with more adherent membranes and a more fragile retina due to the period of detachment. The peripheral retina is also less thick and adherent to the pigment epithelium than the more central retina.

After central vitrectomy, the intervention is continued as previously described, by searching for a space in the membrane through which to begin injecting the viscoelastic. Usually, a traction star lifts the retina, passing over both zones, even when these are relatively far apart. While adhering, these form a retinal fold that creates a recess where the viscoelastic can be injected (Figure 28-22a). The

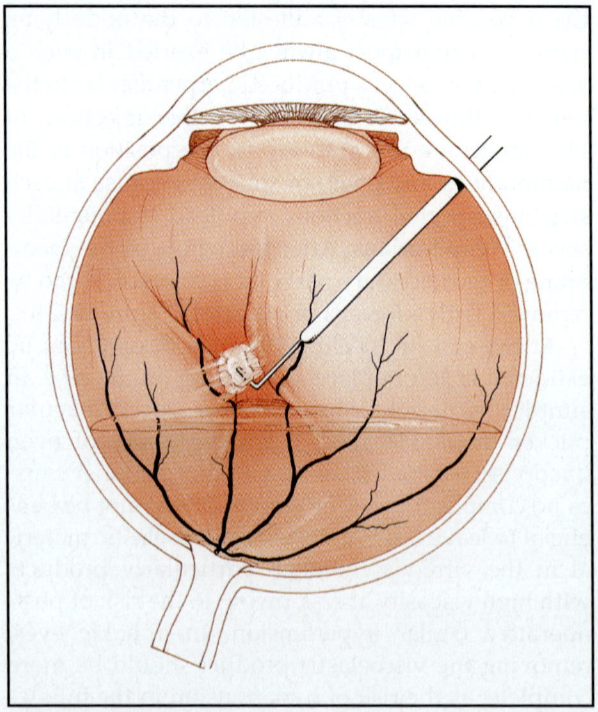

Figure 28-23. Liquid perfluorocarbon can be used to stabilize the posterior retina while delaminating (by viscoelastic) the anteriorly-located residual membranes.

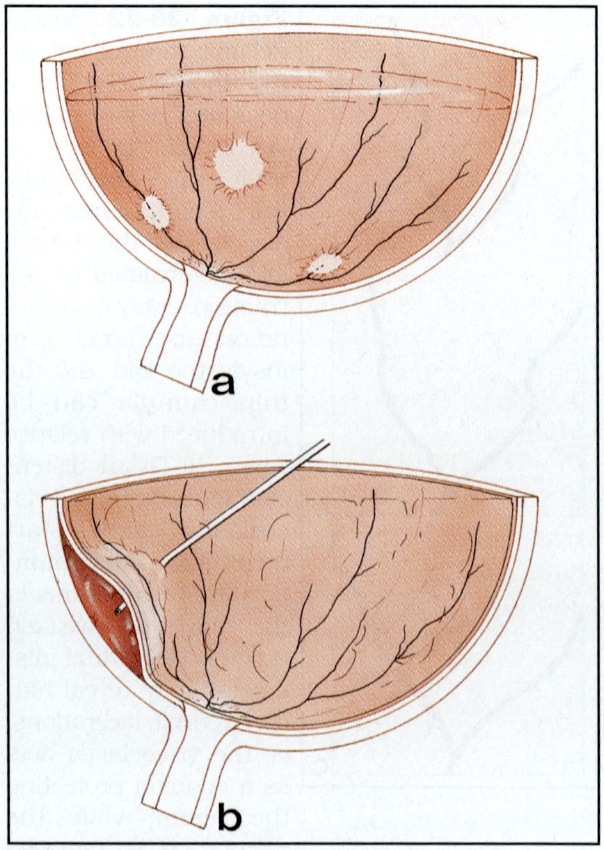

Figure 28-24. a) Liquid perfluorocarbon flattens the retina, but makes it difficult to identify and remove epiretinal membranes, especially those less evident. b) If some viscoelastic goes under the retina, it can be removed by Charles' cannula as if it were subretinal fluid. A viscoelastic with high viscosity at rest can be difficult to remove from the subretinal space through a narrow retinal hole.

product injected (IAL or Healon®) keeps the retina and membrane apart, creating the space required for surgical procedures and improving visibility, owing to its transparency. It exposes possible tears in the retina formerly hidden by folds or by epiretinal proliferation without tending to pass easily in the subretinal space (Figure 28-22b). The viscoelastic material is also able to resolve mild adhesions and allows the surgeon to assess those that need to be released with greater care. It stabilizes both the membrane to be removed and the detached retina while remaining in the site of injection. Thus, the surgeon can see the whole extent of the proliferation, with lower risk of iatrogenic retinal damage. In addition, during removal of the proliferation with the vitrector, the viscoelastic acts like a cushion, dampening microtractions that may occur on the retina (Figure 28-22c).

The best viscoelastics for these procedures are those with high viscosity at rest and high pseudoplasticity, like Healon® GV. Many researchers have achieved excellent results with this material, judged to be better than those achieved with Healon®. De Molfetta reported that based on his experience, in 80% of cases, separating the epiretinal membranes was more easily performed with this material than with Healon®, with more comfortable repositioning of the retina and better control of bleeding. In all cases the denser material provided consistent advantages without creating appreciable difficulties. In the postoperative period, increase in pressure appeared to be limited and easy to control, especially considering that the viscoelastic had been removed at the end of surgery. The transparency of the vitreous and degree of postoperative inflammation were not negatively affected.

After completing viscodissection of the epiretinal membrane and removing it from the area involved, the surgeon can look for another area of proliferation to treat to completely release the detached retina. Once released, the more posterior retina can be stabilized by liquid perfluorocarbon, whose weight enables it to stretch the retina, making it adhere to the pigment epithelium, and shift the subretinal fluid to the periphery. Viscodissection of more peripheral membranes can continue without difficulty as the two products cannot mix, always remaining separate inside the vitreous chamber (Figure 28-23). As release of the retina continues, further perfluorocarbon can stabilize the zones already mobilized.

Comparing the retinal stabilization achieved with viscoelastics and that provided by liquid perfluorocarbons, we must note that the greater weight of perfluorocarbons seems to make the posterior retina more adherent. On the other hand, perfluorocarbons also compress epiretinal membranes, making their removal more difficult, and sometimes can hide light residual tractions that become evident after surgery (Figure 28-24). Proliferation may redevelop from such residual membranes, even thin ones. In addition, heavy materials are not viscoelastic and cannot remain in the site of injection, so they tend to get placed in the most sloping portion of the space available. They are therefore almost useless as tissue separators. Liquid perfluorocarbons must also be used with the utmost caution when a posterior retinal break is present, owing to the risk of their shifting under the retina. Although the superficial tension of the material tends to prevent passage through small retinal breaks, it may not do so with larger breaks. This is obviously also true for viscoelastics, but these are much less toxic than liquid perfluorocarbons, and can be removed or washed more easily even from a subretinal position. Liquid perfluorocarbons must also be completely removed, whereas viscoelastic removal can be less complete.

For all these reasons, we believe that liquid perfluorocarbons and viscoelastics are complementary rather than alternative surgical means for interventions on epiretinal membranes performed by retinal detachment. The assistance provided by perfluorocarbons is important, but they cannot be used in certain surgical situations where viscoelastics prove to be most helpful.

EPIRETINAL MEMBRANES IN EYES WITH SILICONE OIL

In eyes internally tamponaded with silicone oil, epiretinal membranes may have different features from those generally present in eyes with retinal detachment and epiretinal proliferation. The main differences are their site and histologic composition. The site is macular but mostly in the inferior portion, as proliferative cells are moved there by the silicone oil. Their histologic composition makes them rather fragile early on, yet very tough and adherent to the retina over time. The retina is also thinner and more fragile in eyes with silicone oil. As a result, removing these epiretinal membranes requires special attention; they often create a localized retinal detachment, which, when not rhegmatogenous, must not be treated specifically.

Removing membranes in eyes with silicone oil is usually performed under the same silicone or BSS. One possible technique is to fill the space available behind the bubble of silicone oil with viscoelastic, reducing the volume of the internal tamponading device. Epiretinal membranes can be lifted with the viscoelastic product as described previously, then detached and extracted. Care must be taken to cause no retinal breaks, which can occur when old membranes are strongly adherent to the retina. For this reason we consider IAL to be suitable. Viscoelastics with higher viscosity at rest must be avoided, as they exert greater pressure on a circumscribed area of the retina, encouraging laceration (Figure 28-25).

When the retinal detachment backed by recurrent proliferation under silicone is rhegmatogenous, surgical treatment may become rather complicated. Retinal breaks are often associated with subretinal proliferation, which must be specifically treated. Although often not used, viscoelastics can stabilize tissues with retinal breaks, even those that extend onto the posterior pole. It is often necessary to remove the tamponade completely during the procedure, replacing it at the end of surgery.

SUBRETINAL MEMBRANES

The presence of subretinal membranes is characterized by long-lasting retinal detachments. The

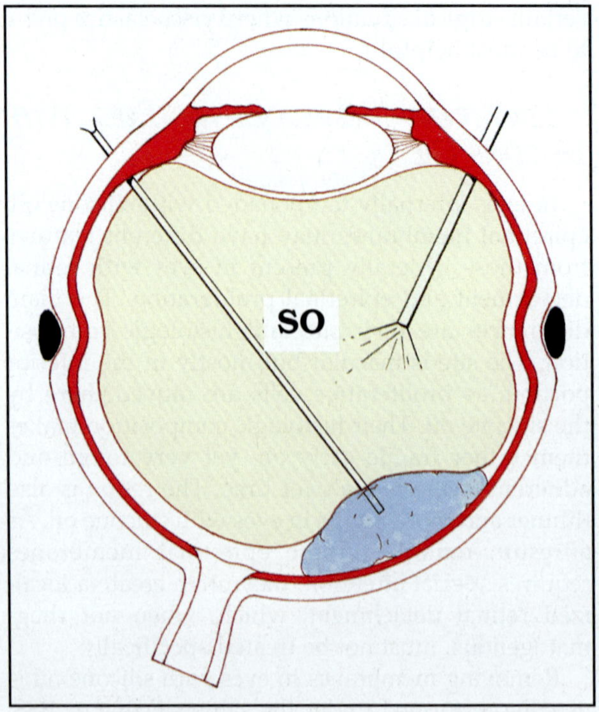

Figure 28-25. Epiretinal membrane proliferation in eyes with silicone oil can be treated by viscoelastic without removing of the oil, as it does not mix with aqueous solutions.

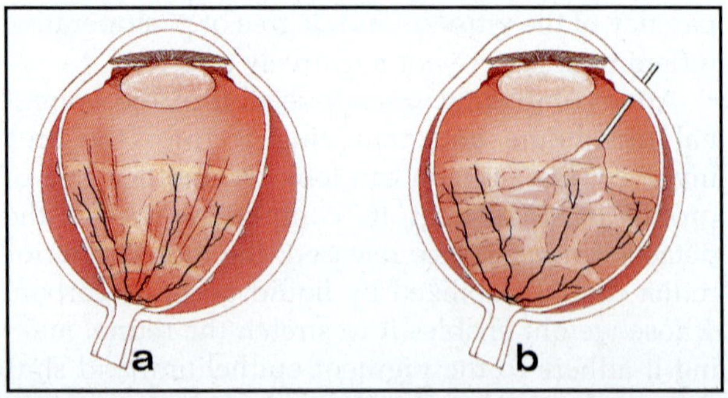

Figure 28-26. a) The presence of subretinal membranes is almost the rule in old retinal detachments. Often the proliferation appears as a ring surrounding the optic nerve head. b) After vitrectomy and removal of the epiretinal membranes, some viscoelastic injected over the posterior pole can expand the retina without compressing it against the choroid. Visualization of subretinal space is improved and subretinal membranes can be identified.

membranes appear as long whitish cords, often extended, or dendritic plaques. A peripapillary ring is frequently present, which gives the retina a funnel-shaped form directed toward the optic disk. Surgical extraction of subretinal membranes is not always necessary. The surgeon must assess this on a case by case basis, before or during the intervention. Subretinal membranes that do not involve the macular region and do not hinder reattachment of the retina may remain in place. Those causing a reduction in vision or hindering retinal reattachment must always be removed. Generally, the attachments between subretinal membranes and the retina are limited, and less than the internal cohesion of the membrane itself. Consequently, removing them with vitreous forceps entered through a retinal break or retinotomy is usually easy. Before the advent of viscoelastics, this was a very delicate procedure, with unavoidable retinal damage leading to widening of the retinal tear or the retinotomy, causing excessive damage.

The procedure to remove subretinal membranes assisted by viscoelastics begins by locating a retinal break near the membrane to be removed, or locating sites for retinotomy, as close as possible and as superior as possible to the equator to allow for the subsequent tamponade. The vitreous cavity, which must be free from vitreous, is filled with sodium hyaluronate with low molecular weight (IAL), up to a level just below the retinal openings (Figure 28-26). The viscoelastic properties of sodium hyaluronate tend to keep the retina stretched, but not flattened against the choroid as liquid perfluorocarbons do, and maintain the subretinal space required. The transparency of the viscoelastic ensures that the visibility of membranes is not affected.

At this point, one or more retinotomies are performed, according to need. The retina can be opened with diathermy, vitreous scissors, or a 30-G or 33-G needle suitably shaped for the purpose. The stretching of the retinal tissue achieved by the overlying viscoelastic allows the surgeon to open the retina at exactly the point overlying the membranes and then introduce a small amount of IAL under the retina itself. A small transparent bolus of viscoelastic is formed under the retina at the site of opening, which allows the surgeon to manipulate both scissors and vitreous forceps relatively safely to grasp, cut, and remove subretinal tissue (Figure 28-27).

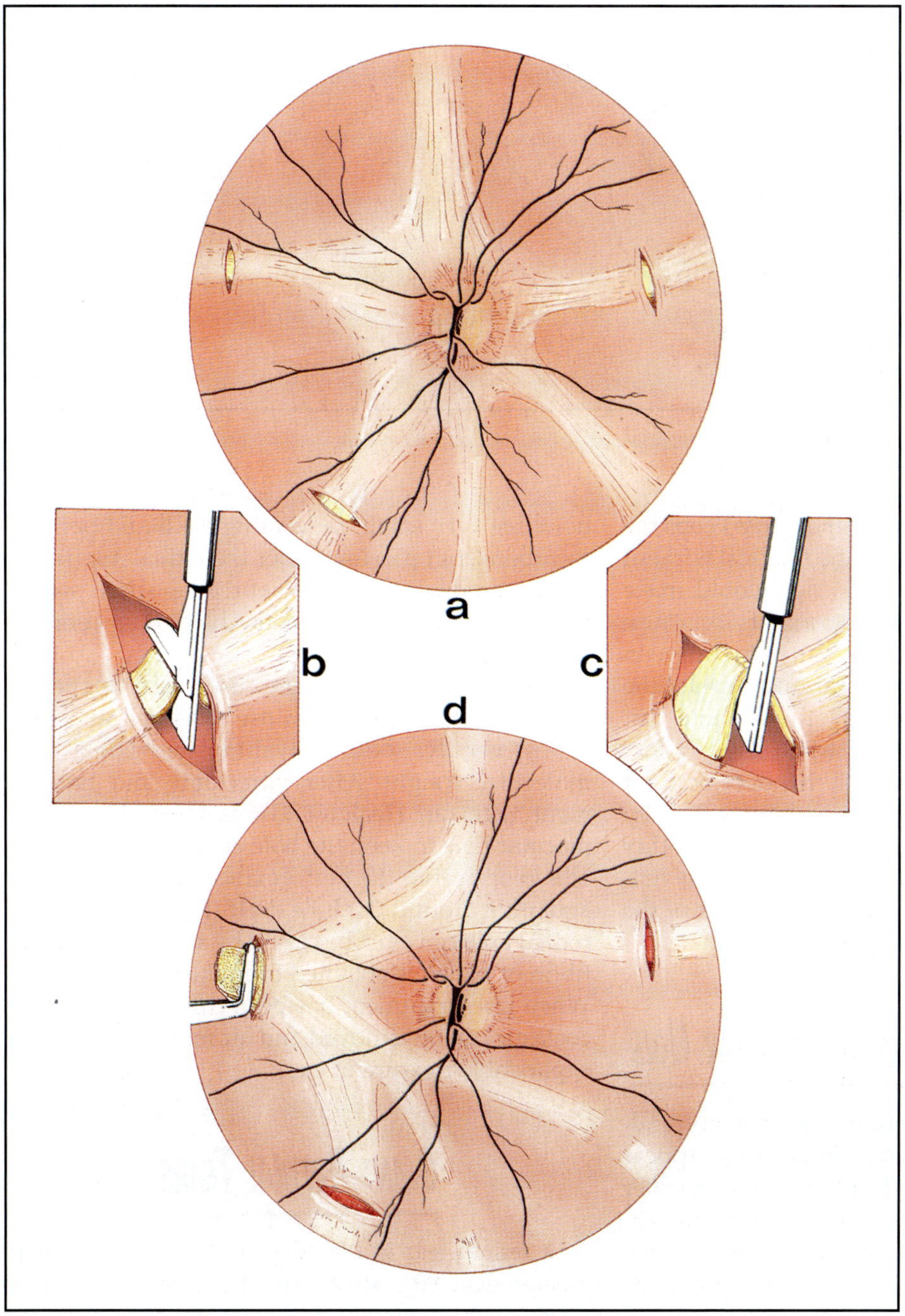

Figure 28-27. a) To remove subretinal membranes, some small retinotomies are produced in suitable locations. They are kept open by little amounts of viscoelastic. b) 90° degree vitreous scissors are employed to cut the tissue to be removed. c) The same scissors can lift the tissue before cutting. d) Once it is free from any adherences, the subretinal tissue is grasped with forceps and removed through a retinotomy.

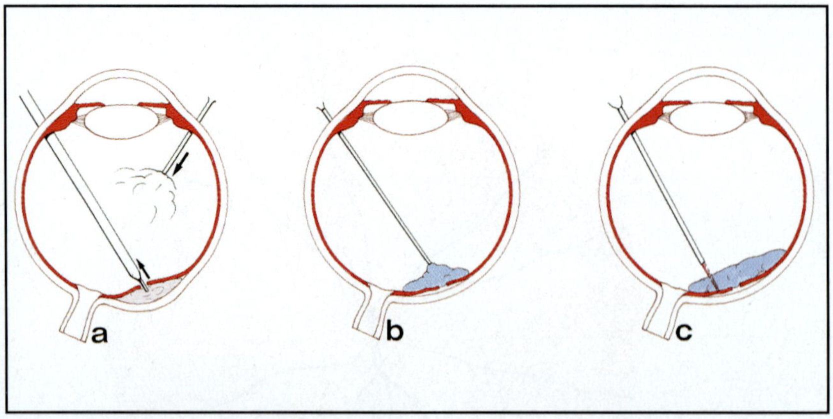

Figure 28-28. a) Treatment by viscoelastic of retinal detachment due to macular hole begins with central and premacular vitrectomy. Internal air tamponade and drainage of subretinal fluid through the hole follow. b) The viscoelastic substance, is applied above the hole to help flatten the retina. c) If needed, laser photocoagulation around the hole can be performed through the viscoelastic.

The viscoelastic present over the retina keeps the retina stretched during membrane removal without the pressure of a heavy fluid, which would make the retina collapse on the instruments or cause widening of the retinal opening. When the surgeon prefers not to inject sodium hyaluronate under the retina, the viscoelastic is unlikely to slide into that space through the retinotomy when the product used has high viscosity at rest. If this does occur, it causes limited difficulty, and is easily remedied by removing the product that has shifted. On the other hand, liquid perfluorocarbon sliding under the retina is more problematic, as the heavy weight of the material drops it rapidly under the macula.

Retinal Detachment Due to Macular Hole

Retinal detachment due to macular hole typically occurs in highly myopic eyes, but can also appear in cases of severe vitreous traction in the macular region. The treatment often requires complete vitrectomy from the site of vitreous adherent to the rims of the hole, which must be performed with the utmost care.

To make the retina adhere to the choroidal space, Charles' needle is used to evacuate all the subretinal fluid through the hole while the retina is pushed in place by the air being pumped in the vitreous chamber. Once the retina has been reattached, liquid perfluorocarbon is injected to compress the retina in its site, discharging the residual subretinal fluid through the heavy liquid. However, this procedure can be accomplished only when macular holes are very small, preventing the liquid perfluorocarbon from passing under the retina. Aspiration of the product from the subretinal space would cause further widening of the hole, thus compromising functional recovery.

An alternative technique, used less frequently now than in the past, is to use a viscoelastic product—generally, sodium hyaluronate with a high molecular weight. After vitrectomy and replacement with air, Healon® GV is injected over the macular hole to keep the hole closed and the retina adherent during the performance of laser photocoagulation around the hole itself (Figure 28-28). The retinal hole can even be closed by a small amount of fibrin or platelets obtained from the patient's blood. When laser treatment has been completed, the viscoelastic can be removed and air replaced by a nonexpandable mixture of gas.

Giant Retinal Tears

A retinal tear is regarded as "giant" when it is greater than 90°. Most giant tears occur in highly myopic eyes, even when rhegmatogenous lesions are present. The main pathogenic factor causing the onset of giant tears is thickening of the vitreous base. Vitreoretinal traction develops with time and may extend over a large surface area, evident as areas of "white without pressure," sometimes limited posteriorly by a whitish crest. When vitreous traction exceeds the internal cohesion of a retina that is already weak due to myopic thinning, the giant tear occurs, sometimes extending beyond 180°.

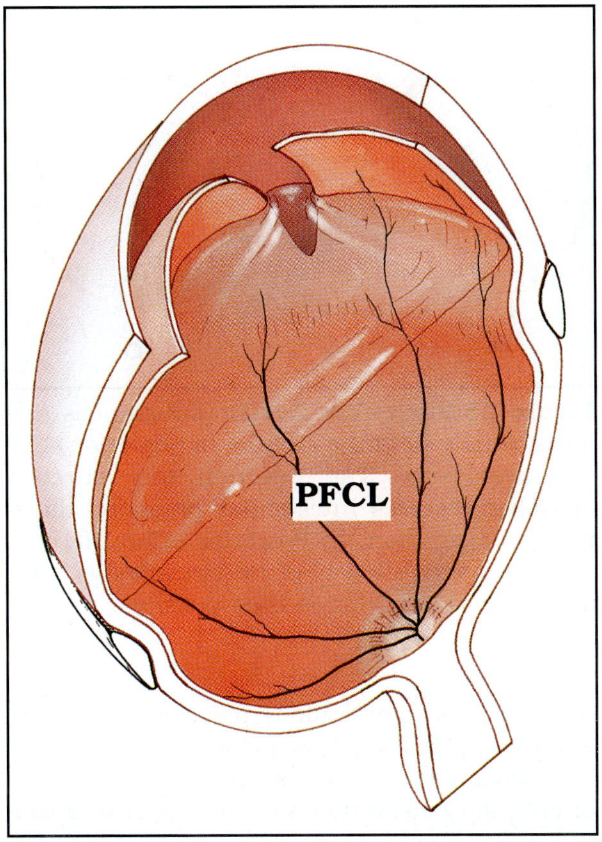

Figure 28-29. With giant retinal tears, especially if the tear extends posteriorly, liquid perfluorocarbons easily pass under the retina if excessive amounts are used, or if the eye is moved incautiously.

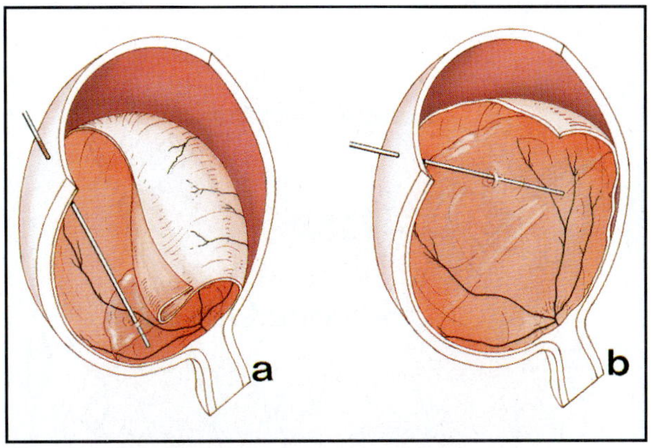

Figure 28-30. a) After completing central vitrectomy, viscoelastic injection starts the unrolling of the large retinal flap formed by the giant tear. It is better to use a product with low viscosity at rest, as low molecular weight sodium hyaluronate, that can be completely removed at the end of surgery. b) The viscoelastic allows complete unrolling of the flap without the risks connected with liquid perfluorocarbons.

Vitreoretinal proliferation follows, causing coarctation and wrinkling of the detached retinal flap, which tends to roll up and shrink toward the posterior pole. The large surface of pigment epithelium uncovered by the retinal tear aggravates proliferation.

Before vitrectomy was widely performed, the success rate of surgery to treat giant tears was low. Surgical possibilities have now greatly improved, but the success rate is still lower than that of other retinal detachments, particularly due to frequent recurrence. The intervention begins with a complete vitrectomy, which must be very accurate and careful, particularly at the detached and redundant retinal margin. Liquid perfluorocarbon is generally used to stabilize the posterior retina during treatment of the detached flap, even though it can be dangerous in its tendency to pass under the retina in the presence of a posterior radial extension of the laceration (Figure 28-29). In these conditions, using a viscoelastic, alone or preferably together with the perfluorocarbon, does not flatten the retina in place as much, but is less likely to pass under it. If this does occur, it is less dangerous. As the rim of the laceration is released from adhesions, the surgeon can continue to inject sodium hyaluronate, achieving better positioning of the redundant retinal flap (Figure 28-30).

The amount of viscoelastic injected is usually very large, up to 3 mL in the study by Brown. A viscoelastic with high molecular weight is a bit heavier than water, so it exerts a limited force in the posterior–anterior direction. This plus its internal cohesion allows the surgeon to unroll the retinal flap and detect residual membranes to dissect. When the lifted retina has been completely mobilized, the portion most proximal to the rim, which appears to shrunken and unstretchable, is usually removed with scissors or vitrector after diathermy, which prevents bleeding.

It is best to remove viscoelastic material having high molecular weight before internal tamponade with silicone oil. A less-dense viscoelastic can be

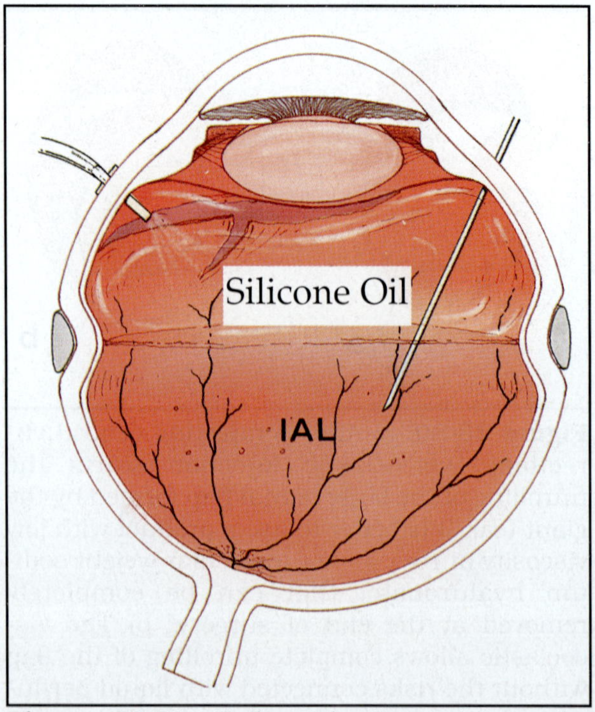

Figure 28-31. Sodium hyaluronate can be replaced by silicone oil for long-term internal tamponade once the flap has been repositioned against the eye wall.

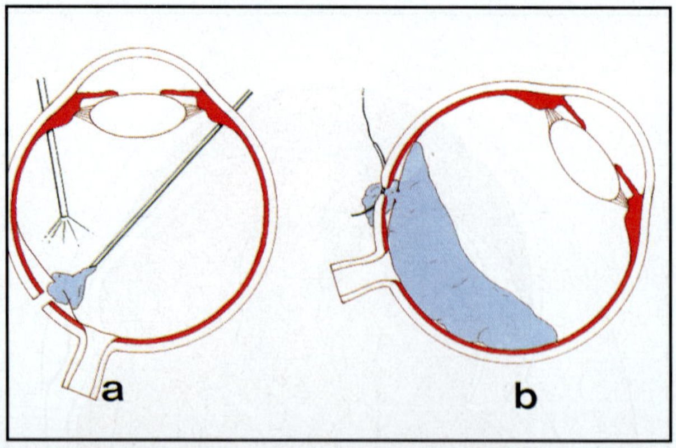

Figure 28-32. a) Viscoelastic substances can efficaciously help the closure of posterior scleral lacerations. The injection into vitreous chamber restores intraocular pressure allowing globe rotation. b) Posterior scleral lacerations are identified also by viscoelastic leakage. Precise suturing is thus possible.

removed by means of the tamponade itself. While silicone oil is being introduced, the superficial tension of the oil bubble versus the aqueous forms a small meniscus of peripheral fluid that allows the surgeon to reattach the retina despite the giant tear (Figure 28-31). Charles' cannula, placed as far under the detached retinal flap as possible, is used to evacuate the fluid from the vitreous cavity.

Once the retina has been repositioned, the cannula is shifted to the posterior pole to discharge the liquid or the residual perfluorocarbon until it has been completely replaced with silicone oil. Laser retinopexy completes the intervention.

Posterior Segment Trauma

Posterior segment trauma is a separate area of vitreoretinal surgical pathology. Owing to its complexity, it often escapes schematization, with the exception of the primary illustrations included here. For details of surgical treatment and a thorough study of complications, prevention, and therapy, please refer to specific publications.

When faced with a trauma involving the posterior pole, the general rule is to limit the first reparative intervention—that is, the one accomplished in emergency conditions. The surgeon repairs only the visible bulbar wounds, then reconstructs the anterior segment as much as possible, removing foreign bodies outside the vitreous. The characteristics of the foreign body may require a different approach, due to the risk of infection (wood) or strong reaction (copper). During this first operation, all measures possible must be taken that will facilitate the following more complete repair intervention. This usually takes place from 7 to 14 days after trauma, when posterior detachment of the vitreous has become as complete as possible, but before posttraumatic proliferative processes have begun. This lapse of time is the so-called "surgical window" where it is convenient to operate. In many cases of posterior perforating wounds and retention of foreign bodies, the anterior segment appears to be untouched, with a still-transparent lens. These are optimal conditions for the visibility of intraocular structures, even though the absence of anterior trauma may not be relevant to the anatomic and functional outcome of the wounded eyeball.

In posterior segment trauma, the role of viscoelastics is certainly less important than in anteri-

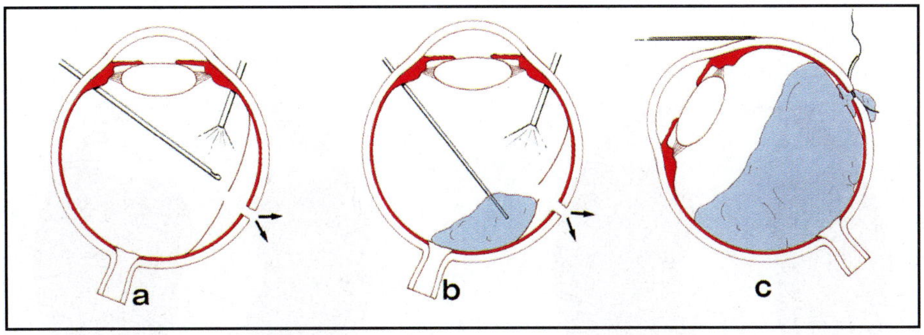

Figure 28-33. A posterior scleral laceration identified during vitrectomy (a) can be initially sealed by viscoelastic (b) and then sutured (c).

or segment trauma. Their use in initial repair procedures is limited by the frequent need to perform the least surgery possible in that area. Viscoelastics are often unnecessary for the correct performance of the surgical procedure in the main vitrectomy intervention. Nevertheless, they can be useful, especially in place of liquid perfluorocarbons when the surgeon is not certain that these can be completely removed.

POSTERIOR SCLERAL LACERATIONS

When posterior scleral lacerations are present, intraocular contents seep out through the wound, with continuous fluid leakage during the intervention. Difficulties thus arise in dissecting the tissues surrounding the wound, which are increased by marked bulbar hypotony. The assistance of viscoelastics is fundamental in this situation, as they provide a simple and effective solution to the problem. During the first intervention (the one not assisted by vitrectomy) sodium hyaluronate with a medium or low molecular weight (Healon®, IAL) can be injected in the vitreous chamber via the pars plana until bulbar consistency is restored (Figure 28-32a). The presence in the vitreous chamber of blood, air, or foreign bodies seems not to contraindicate this procedure, which allows the surgeon to complete the scleral suture in much better conditions than by relying on simple intraocular irrigation through a vitrectomy cannula. A highly pseudoplastic material such as IAL must be used, which can be injected through a 30-G needle inserted in pars plana 3.5 mm from the limbus.

Ophthalmoscopic examination of the needle's position before starting the injection is useful but not always possible in these traumatized eyes. Occasionally the injected viscoelastic leaks out through the scleral wound, revealing its precise extension and site, which is particularly useful when it is hardly visible owing to hemorrhages and tissue chemosis (Figure 28-32b). Inside the vitreous chamber, the viscoelastic acts as a temporary vitreous substitute and contributes to retinal tamponade, even though its action is short-lived. It is also likely to prevent or limit intravitreal or subretinal membranes. Its biocompatibility allows the surgeon to leave it in place, in most cases without problems, once the bulbar wall has been sutured. Possible postoperative increase of IOP promotes a better outcome.

In other situations a previously undiagnosed scleral wound may cause hypotony of the eyeball during vitrectomy. In this event, vitrectomy is interrupted, and sodium hyaluronate injected in the vitreous chamber. It will be possible to inject the viscoelastic through the infusion cannula with a syringe handled by the assistant surgeon or a with specially designed pump. The material tamponades lacerations internally, so that the outer surface of the wound can be identified and sutured without scleral collapse or large amounts of fluid leaking out through the wound, limiting visibility (Figure 28-33).

CHOROIDAL HEMORRHAGE

Both perforating and contusive traumas may cause severe choroidal hemorrhage, which does not allow ophthalmoscopic assessment of the conditions of the posterior segment. Most echographic investigations show the presence of choroidal hemorrhage, which can and must be treated without waiting for spontaneous healing unless healing begins immediately. The AC usually appears to be shallow, whereas bleeding in the AC or lens subluxation is less typical. IOP is generally normal

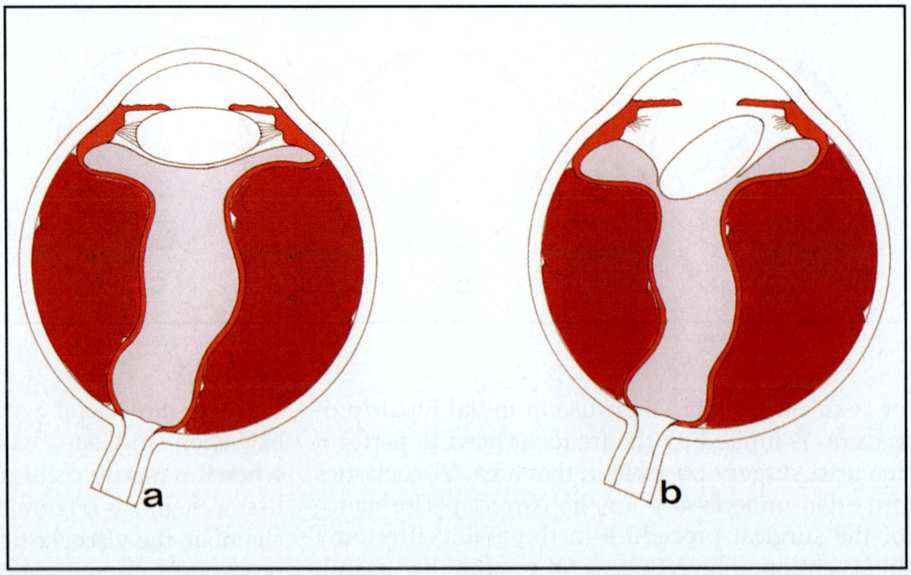

Figure 28-34. Massive choroidal hemorrhages always induce an important constriction of the vitreous cavity (a). The same lens is sometimes luxated due to the original trauma.

or increased, except in cases of scleral rupture (Figure 28-34).

The aim of repair surgery is first to drain the blood present in the AC and then to be able to drain the blood under the retina. For this purpose it is preferable to use heavy liquids, such as liquid perfluorocarbon. Injected in the vitreous chamber, these gather at the posterior pole, pushing blood into the anterior portion and allowing it to drain through a peripheral sclerotomy. The drawback of this technique is that it must be followed by complete vitrectomy, with accurate and complete removal of the perfluorocarbon.

A technique using viscoelastics, prescribed by Michels and Stirpe before the introduction of heavy liquids, begins by injecting sodium hyaluronate through the limbus in order to express blood from the AC (Figure 28-35). With the improved visibility of the posterior segment, a scleral buckle is placed to promote evacuation of blood and support retino–choroidal adhesion to the bulbar wall in the postoperative period. One or more sclerotomies of 1.5 to 2 mm are made in the pre-equatorial area, used to drain blood from under the choroid. At the same time, sodium hyaluronate with a low molecular weight is injected via the pars plana into the vitreous chamber (Figure 28-36). The viscoelastic pushes the retino–choroidal plane gently in place, also exerting the pressure needed to evacuate partially coagulated blood. The viscoelastic properties of the product are crucial, as while compressing and dilating it must avoid exerting too much localized pressure on the retina–choroid. At this point, the surgeon can see the aspect of the choroidal detachment ophthalmoscopically through the pupil, due to the high transparency of the viscoelastic. Occasionally, other sclerotomies are required, whereas in some cases all the blood can be evacuated without problems through the posterior scleral wounds.

At the end of surgery it is best to leave the viscoelastic in place, as an increase in internal pressure after the operation prevents the choroidal detachment from recurring. The presence of the viscoelastic also allows exploration of the ocular fundus in the days following, and requires no particular positioning of the patient's head.

In aphakic eyes, the technique is slightly different, as hyaluronate can be injected directly through the cornea. In these eyes, at least some viscoelastic should be removed at the end of surgery to avoid excessive increase in postoperative pressure. A limited injection of air can make up for the tamponade provided postoperatively by the viscoelastic, especially when the patient is then opportunely positioned. Unfortunately, the visibility of the retina through the ophthalmoscope is adversely affected (Figure 28-37).

INTRAVITREOUS FOREIGN OBJECTS

Following a perforating injury, a foreign object can be trapped inside the vitreous chamber due to

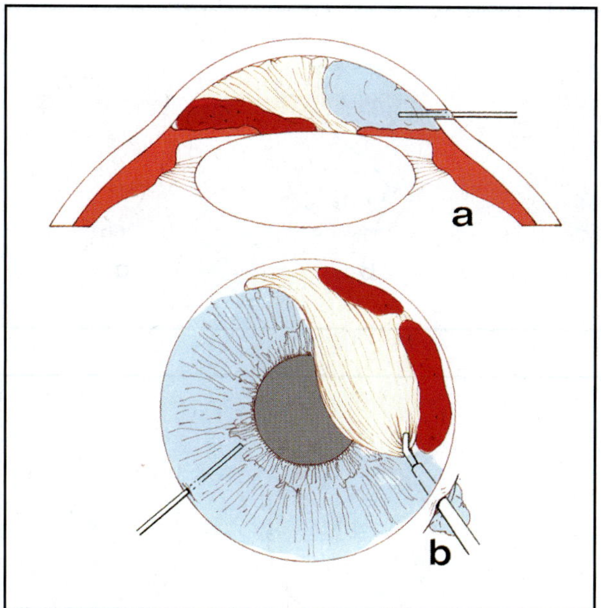

Figure 28-35. Blood or fibrin cloths are often present in the AC. Viscoelastic injection allows to separate these cloths from iris tissue (a), to mobilize and extract them (b).

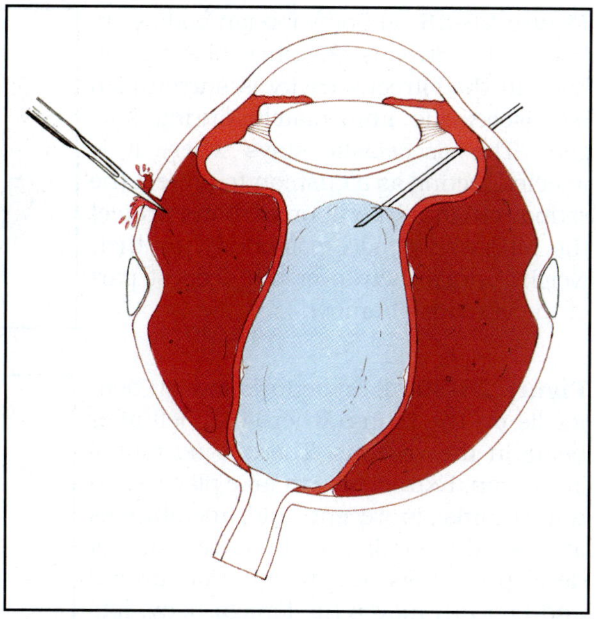

Figure 28-36. Choroidal hemorrhage drainage through scleral incision is combined with viscoelastic injection into the vitreous cavity. Retina and choroid repositioning is obtained without hypotony, that can cause new bleeding as well as other surgical inconveniences.

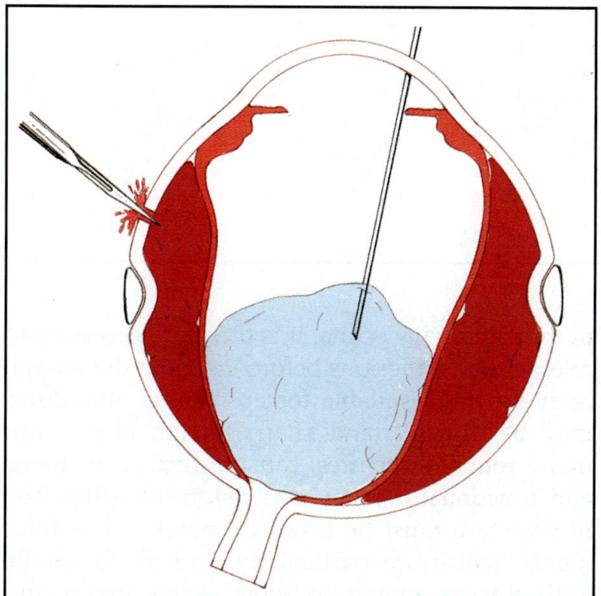

Figure 28-37. In aphakic eyes viscoelastic injection can be performed through the cornea. In these eyes there is a high risk of post-operative hypertension.

the diminution of its kinetic force on the moment of penetration or, more frequently, after rebounding on the posterior retina without enough energy to perforate it or remain fixed inside the retina itself. In this case, removal of the object may not require complete vitrectomy, but simply removal of the vitreous surrounding the foreign body to mobilize it and permit its extraction in the most atraumatic way possible. It is then important to protect the retina from possible contact with the object, which is encouraged by partial removal of the vitreous and is especially likely during removal procedures.

Viscoelastic materials, particularly adhesive ones, are able to surround the foreign object, making a viscous "cushion" that still allows it to move when grasped by a forceps or attracted by a magnet. The viscous layer partly absorbs the movements of the surrounding vitreous and helps to protect the retina in case the object slips from the forceps holding it. The most suitable viscoelastic seems to be Viscoat, which provides fair pseudoplasticity and high viscosity at rest and is able to

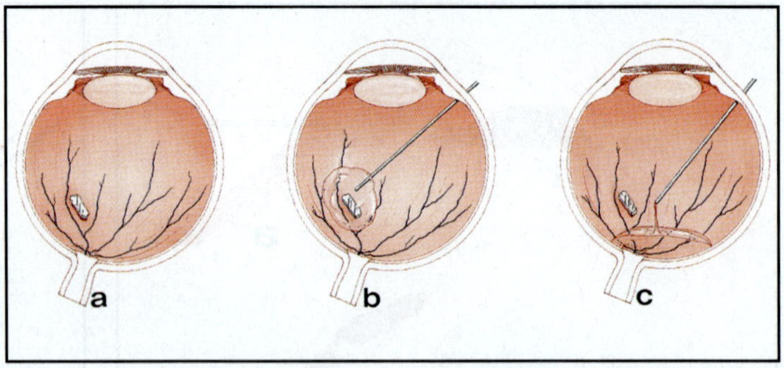

Figure 28-38. a) Some foreign bodies are free in the vitreous chamber. b) A foreign body in the vitreous cavity is surrounded by viscoelastic immediately during surgery. The viscoelastic stays where it is injected, acting as a cushion to protect the retina. c) Liquid perfluorocarbons protect the retina only more posteriorly, as their weight brings them over the deepest part of the vitreous chamber.

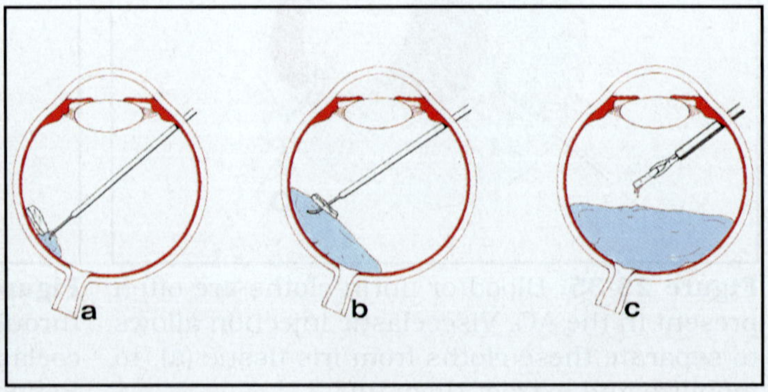

Figure 28-39. a) Sometimes foreign bodies lie on the retina, where they fell after being in the vitreous. There is no retinal laceration. Extraction can take place when the trauma is recent and membranes around the foreign body have not yet developed. b) Viscoelastic injection around and beneath moves the foreign body, lifts it and keeps it separate from the underlying retina. c) The foreign body can be grasped with forceps and extracted.

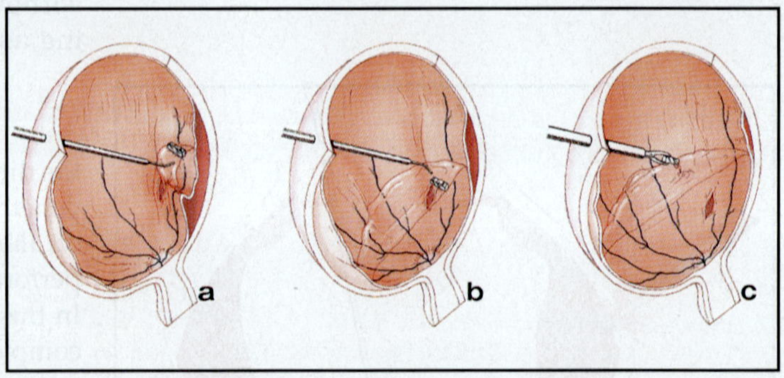

Figure 28-40. a) An initial retinal detachment can be already present at foreign body removal. b) Viscoelastic substance injected around the foreign body during or after vitrectomy helps retinal flattening. Some viscoelastic can pass under the retina through the hole, especially when low-cohesive products are employed. c) The foreign body can be grasped and removed while the viscoelastic separates and protects the other ocular structures.

slow down the movement of even the heaviest foreign objects, such as metal fragments (Figure 28-38). The same protection cannot be achieved with liquid perfluorocarbons, which do not remain where they have been injected but due to their weight tend to move toward the most inclined portion of the vitreous chamber. The use of heavy liquids seems not to be necessary in case of attached retina, and moreover requires a far more complete vitrectomy for their complete removal from the vitreous chamber.

Foreign Objects Laying on the Retina

Foreign objects laying on the retina are usually surrounded by fibrous tissue that causes adhesion to the underlying retina. It is therefore necessary to release such adhesions before grasping the foreign body with the suitable forceps. These procedures may be difficult, and sharp foreign objects can injure retinal structures, causing further anatomic and functional damage and risk of bleeding. The utmost care must be taken to remove glass fragments, which are particularly difficult to handle with forceps owing to their sharp angles and smooth surfaces. Sodium hyaluronate with medium molecular weight (such as Healon®) is injected through a thin cannula with bent tip between the foreign object and the retinal surface, so that it is lifted on the retinal plane prior to extraction (Figure 28-39). The viscoelastic material stabilizes the for-

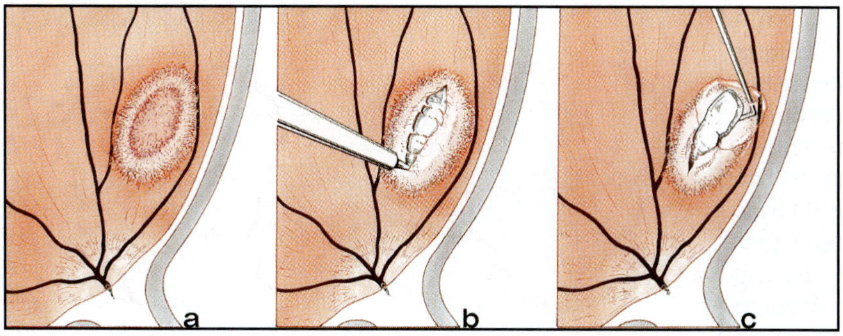

Figure 28-41. a) A foreign body on the retina is encapsulated by new fibrous tissue. Its removal begins with a wide vitrectomy. b) The fibrous capsule is opened by microvitreoretinal blade or by diathermy. c) A viscoelastic product is used to mobilize and lift the foreign body. When present, fragments can be identified and immobilized before removal by forceps.

eign body, exposes adhesions to the underlying retina, opposes any microbleeding that may develop, and protects the retina when the foreign object starts moving in the direction desired for its extraction. If the object falls inside the eyeball during removal, the viscoelastic continues to protect the retina, preventing or greatly limiting consequent trauma. At the end of surgery, the viscoelastic can remain in place, particularly in phakic eyes, where the risk of postoperative hypertension is lower.

When the retina is detached, the anatomic condition is more delicate, and the viscoelastic must also stabilize the retina during the vitrectomy and foreign object removal. The frequent presence of retinal tears near the foreign object very often prohibits the use of liquid perfluorocarbons, which may slide under the retina and greatly complicate the intervention (Figure 28-40). The lack of viscoelastic properties in liquid perfluorocarbon makes this material unsuitable for any manipulation of tissues except for retinal reattachment with no concurrent posterior retinal breaks. After the surgeon extracts the foreign object, surgical procedures to correct retinal detachment continue as required. The viscoelastic is completely or partly removed according to the case.

FOREIGN OBJECTS INCARCERATED IN THE RETINA

Foreign objects incarcerated in the retina are quickly surrounded by inflammatory or fibrous tissue. Those located in the periphery are more easily surrounded by a large amount of vascularized tissue, whereas those more posterior usually have a thinner and less vascularized capsule around them. Those in posterior locations require the most delicate treatment because of the greater importance of possible posterior retinal damage to ocular anatomy and visual function. Opening the capsule may cause bleeding, which also occurs due to breakage of vessels lying under the foreign object. Traction on the object is likely to cause laceration of the surrounding retina.

The most effective technique to remove foreign objects incarcerated in the retina while minimizing damage to this delicate tissue is that prescribed by Michels and Stirpe. Vitreous gel and any tissue strand surrounding the posterior foreign body are removed, to create access to the portion of retina involved. The capsule covering the foreign body is incised by a needle connected to a device for diathermy, so that the incised fibrovascular tissue can be cauterized at the same time (Figure 28-41). The foreign object thus can be partly released without exerting any pressure on the choroid, with lower risk of bleeding in that area. At this point, the bent tip of the 30-G cannula linked to the syringe with viscoelastic is inserted under the released portion of the foreign object, and injection begins. The viscoelastic, usually a sodium hyaluronate with medium molecular weight such as Healon®, lifts the object without exerting traction on the retina, instead pushing the retina into its natural position. Once the object has been completely released from adhesions and is floating in the viscoelastic, the surgeon can grasp it with the forceps and extract it.

LARGE FOREIGN OBJECTS

Large foreign objects are usually removed through the corneoscleral wound, after placement of a metal ring to prevent the sclera from collapsing. The intervention starts with lens removal, per-

Figure 28-42. a) When the foreign body is large, filling of the vitreous cavity by viscoelastic allows the retina to stabilize during extraction maneuvers. The viscoelastic must be transparent and easily removed due to the risk of subretinal penetration. b) Once vitrectomy is completed, the viscoelastic avoids globe collapse during extraction maneuvers. Large foreign bodies should be extracted through the AC after lens removal.

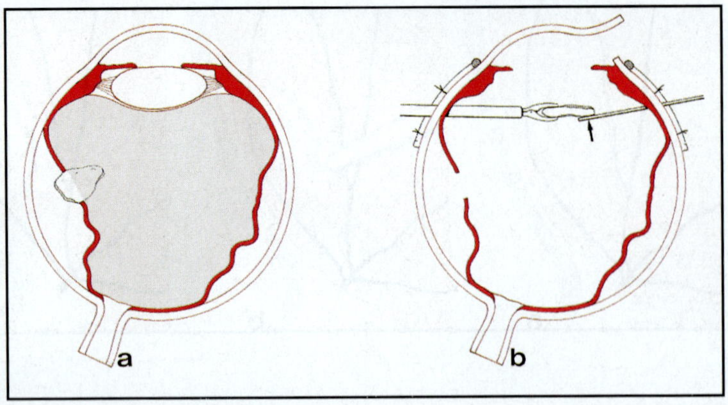

Figure 28-43. a) A large foreign body on the retina hidden by retinal folds can be located and removed by repeated viscoelastic injections. b) The viscoelastic substance injected into the vitreous distends the retina and gives the globe the pressure needed for foreign body removal. c) Once the vitreous chamber is filled, the foreign body can be grasped and removed through the AC angle.

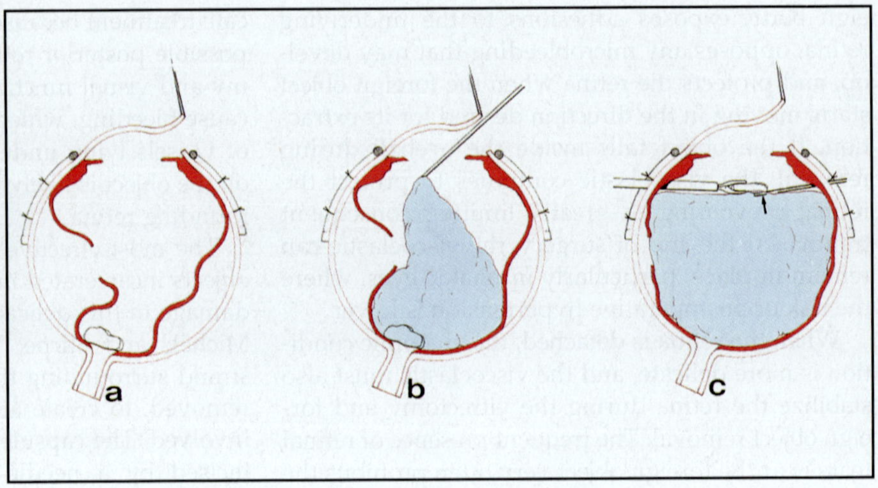

formed by phacoemulsification with a 3.2-mm beveled incision, which is sutured at the end of the procedure. The vitreous gel is removed, including the posterior vitreous cortex. When the foreign object is adherent to the detached retina, the detachment usually becomes more visible during the foreign body removal (Figure 28-42). A fair amount of sodium hyaluronate with medium molecular weight injected in the vitreous cavity keeps the retina stretched even when it is detached, and limits bleeding from the rim of the laceration in the retina caused by the object. In contrast to heavy liquids, the use of viscoelastics is not contraindicated when retinal laceration, even medium-sized, is present.

At this point the limbus is opened to extract the foreign object, which is grasped with a forceps and lifted. If the object falls inside the vitreous chamber during removal, the viscoelastic acts as a cushion protecting the retina. Further injection of the material keeps the retina stable while the foreign object is grasped again and extracted (Figure 28-43, a and b). The intervention usually continues with repair of the retinal detachment, which is usually associated with scleral buckling. Eventually, the contents of the vitreous chamber are replaced with a form of tamponade selected by the surgeon, generally silicone oil in cases complicated by late vitreoretinal proliferation.

Foreign Objects Under the Retina

It is unusual for foreign objects to be located under the retina, but they may slide there after perforating the retina. Objects can also escape control during removal procedures, sliding underneath the nonlacerated retina. One particular type of subretinal foreign object requiring removal is small bubbles of heavy fluids that may slide under retinal beaks during vitrectomy.

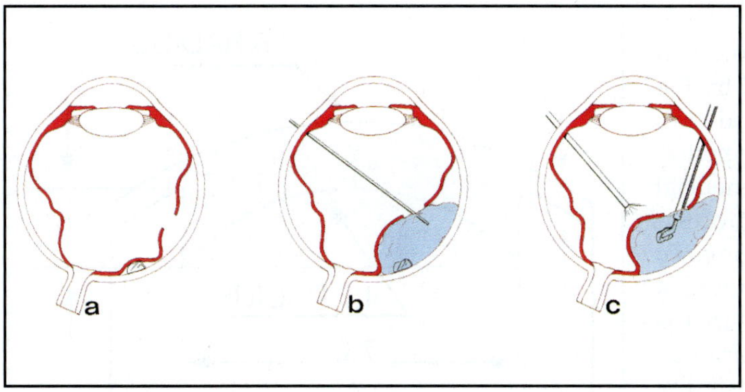

Figure 28-44. a) Sometimes foreign bodies, especially heavy ones, are located under the retina and far away from the retinal tear. b) A viscoelastic injected through the retinal opening lifts the retina and gives access to the subretinal space. c) The foreign body is grasped and removed by forceps through the retinal laceration. In some cases it is possible to move the foreign body by viscoelastic to help grasping.

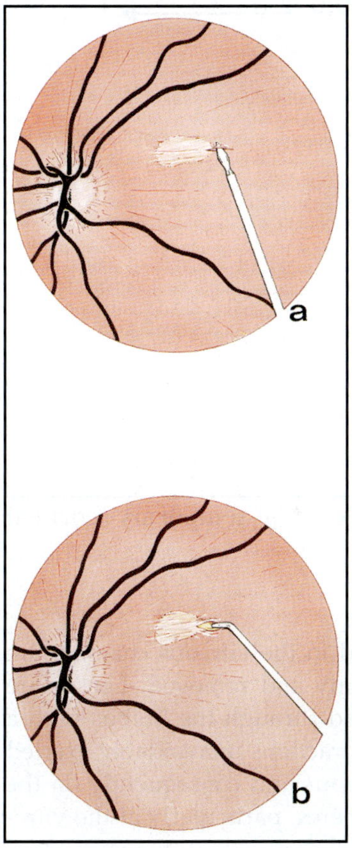

Figure 28-45. a) The removal of a subretinal neovascular membrane starts with the incision of the retina temporal to the macula by a suitable blade with very thin edge. b) The access to the subretinal space obtained allows enough room to introduce a thin forceps to removes the subretinal membrane. A very little amount of viscoelastic can be used to maintain the retinotomy open and to control bleeding.

In all these cases it is useful to perform subretinal injection of a highly biocompatible viscoelastic able to lift the retina. The procedure allows the retina to stretch, increasing the visibility of the foreign object lying under it, and creates a space underneath that can be used to extract the foreign body (Figure 28-44, a and b). The most suitable material seems to be sodium hyaluronate with low molecular weight (IAL), as its limited viscosity at rest means it is unlikely to extend retinal detachment beyond the amount required or widen the retinal tear. In special cases the foreign object can be shifted by the viscomaterial, but more often it must be grasped with bent forceps suitable for subretinal surgery. Heavy liquids in the subretinal space can be aspirated with a bent cannula (Figure 28-44).

All these procedures risk widening the retinal tear, even when it is kept open by the viscoelastic, as well as bleeding, which the viscoelastic helps to control. In case of subretinal hemorrhage where the presence of a foreign object is suspected, injecting sodium hyaluronate with low molecular weight under the retina improves visibility and controls recurrent bleeding. At the end of subretinal procedures, the viscoelastic can be removed without great difficulty from the subretinal space when internal cohesion is sufficient. Viscoadherent products are not appropriate for this use.

Foreign objects consisting of subretinal vascular membranes are now often treated surgically through incision of the retina and subsequent extraction with subretinal forceps. Recent advances in this type of surgery have meant that the retina can be pierced rather than incised, and the membrane removed with specially designed ultra-thin forceps. There is thus little need for viscoelastics (Figure 28-45). Subretinal hemorrhages not complicated by the presence of a foreign object are now treated with tissue plasminogen activators injected in the site, with no attempt at removal.

ANTERIOR/POSTERIOR PERFORATING TRAUMA

Severe ocular trauma involving both the anterior and the posterior segment presents particular visibility problems. Once the globe wall has been repaired, and the necessary emergency surgical procedures have been performed, the ensuing repair intervention is prevented or greatly hindered by the presence of corneal opacities caused by the trauma. Corneal transplantation, almost always necessary in these cases, imposes a waiting period before vitreoretinal surgery, which is not beneficial and may result in intraocular proliferative processes and an adverse effect on the surgical outcome. To overcome this inconvenience, Eckardt studied a temporary corneal prosthesis (Figure 28-46) that is inserted during vitrectomy to replace the original damaged cornea, thus providing suitable visibility of the retina (Figure 28-47). The dioptric power of the keratoprosthesis permits the surgeon to observe the retina directly with no need of further lenses, and allows vitrectomy to be performed in the best way and time.

When posterior segment intervention has been completed, the vitreous chamber is filled with liquid perfluorocarbon, provided that it is not contraindicated, while a viscoelastic is injected in the AC through a 30-G needle inserted in the corneal periphery or through a sclerotomy. The infusion of fluid is temporarily suspended once the vitreous cavity has been filled with perfluorocarbon underneath and with viscoelastic above, and the surgeon can remove the keratoprosthesis and suture the corneal graft. Lesnoni et al prefer using sodium hyaluronate and leave it in place as long as flap suturing is performed; it is removed later, together with the perfluorocarbon, in the following phases of surgery. The permanent tamponading device suitable to these severely damaged eyes is silicone oil, which fills the whole vitreous chamber, leaving the viscoelastic the task of keeping the AC deep in the hours following surgery.

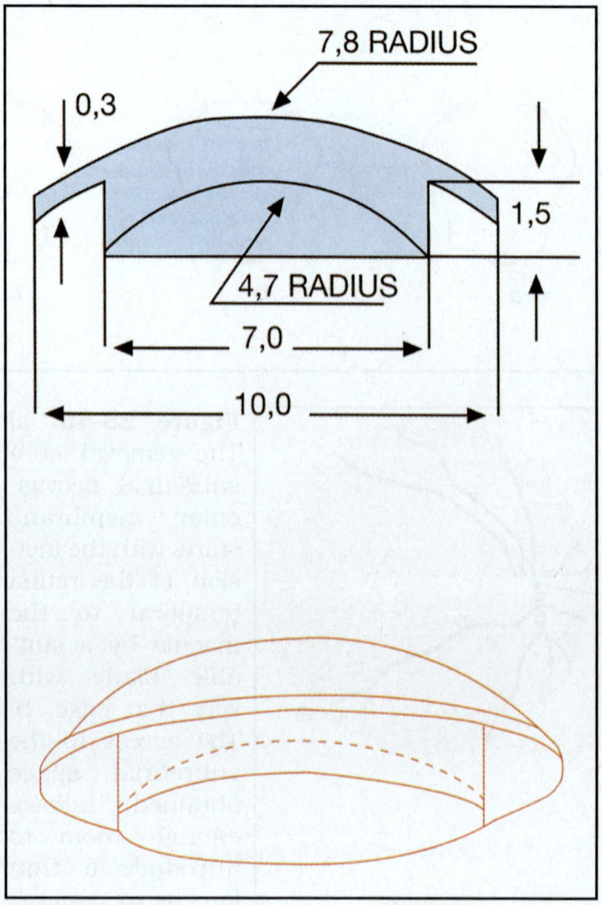

Figure 28-46. Eckardt's temporary corneal prosthesis.

INTRAOCULAR LENS LUXATED IN THE VITREOUS

Owing to modern cataract surgery techniques, luxation of an IOL into the vitreous chamber is now rare. Nevertheless, it sometimes happens that an IOL seemingly well-laid on capsular residues during surgery slides back in the first days following, or more rarely, some time afterward. In other cases a traumatic event may cause luxation, more frequently as a consequence of closed traumas rather than perforating or explosive wounds. All IOLs even partially luxated in the vitreous chamber are treated with vitrectomy and removed. Lenses are almost never extracted through the limbus with a forceps owing to the tractions unavoidably exerted on the posterior vitreous and consequently on the retina to which it adheres, particularly at the vitreous base.

In these circumstances, viscoelastic products are indispensable, assisting surgical interventions that could not otherwise be performed. The intervention starts with a pars plana vitrectomy, which gives the surgeon access to the misplaced IOL and releases it from adhesions to the surrounding vitreous (Figure 28-48a). Frequent inflammatory phenomena, although minor, thicken the vitreous around the implant, which when not dealt with during surgery causes tractions and retinal tears at the moment of

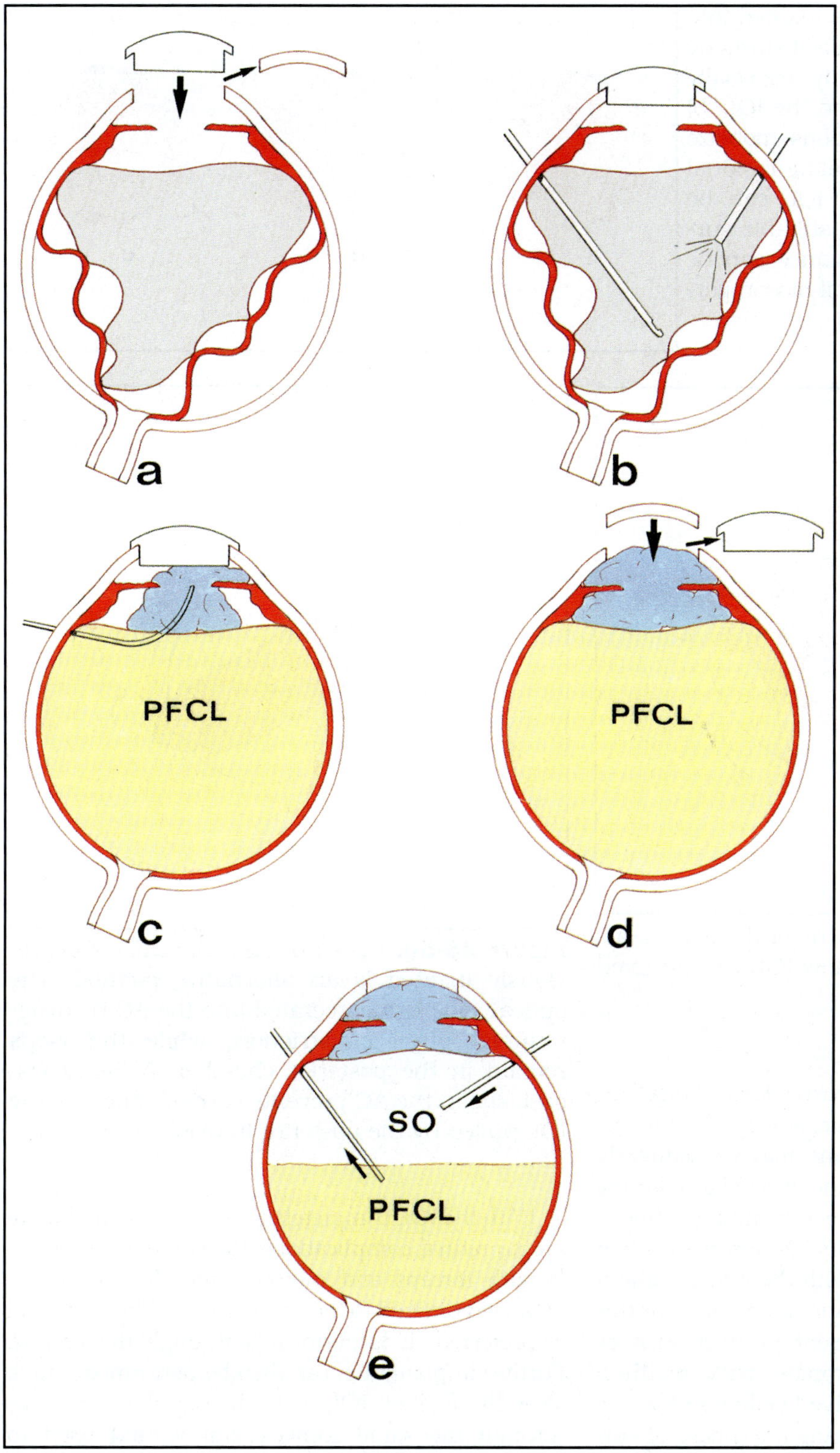

Figure 28-47. Vitrectomy in a case of corneal trauma. a) Removal of the damaged cornea and positioning of the keratoprosthesis. b) Vitreoretinal surgery. c) Viscoelastic helps maintaining anatomy in the anterior segment, while often liquid perfluorocarbons are used in the posterior segment. d) Keratoprosthesis removal and corneal transplantation. e) Silicone oil is used for long-term tamponade.

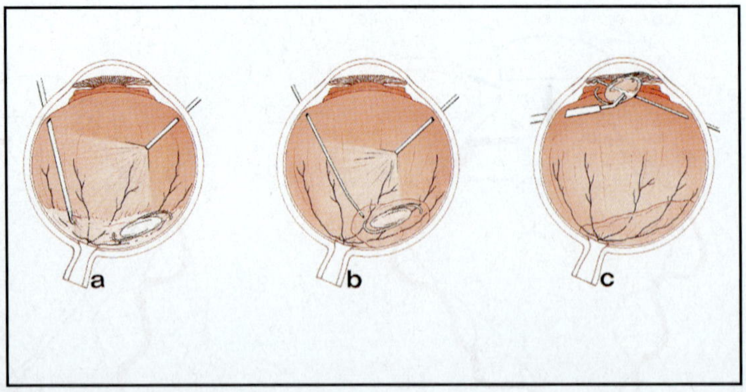

Figure 28-48. a) An IOL is luxated into the vitreous cavity. The removal starts by complete posterior vitrectomy, especially removing adherences around the IOL. b) Repeated viscoelastic injections mobilize and lift the IOL, while revealing residual vitreal adherences. c) The IOL can be removed or repositioned by suitable surgery. The viscoelastic substance can be left in the vitreous chamber if biocompatible.

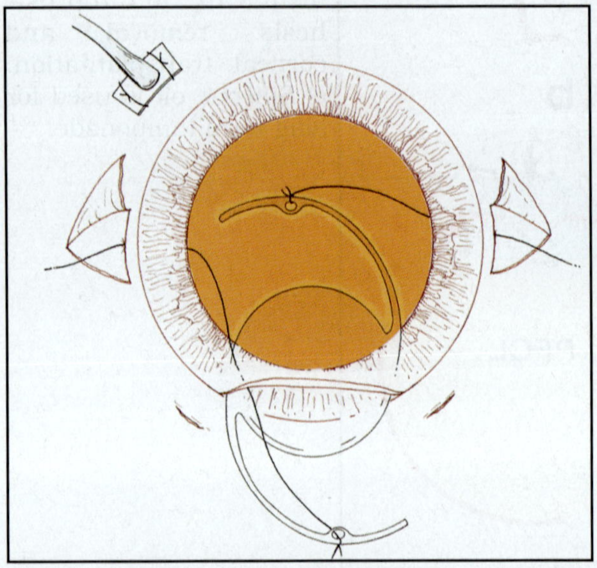

Figure 28-49. After removing of the IOL luxated into the vitreous, the new IOL can be fixed to the sclera.

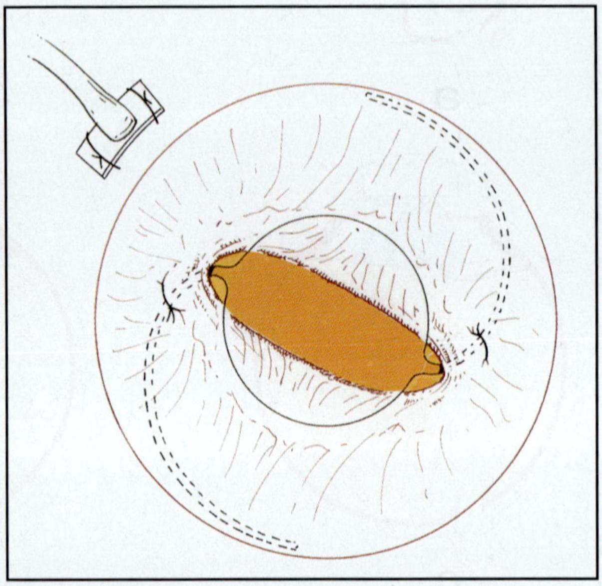

Figure 28-50. Iris suturing of the same IOL previously luxated is an alternative method. The optical zone is incarcerated into the AC by drug-induced pupil constriction, while the loops remain in the posterior chamber. A heavy viscoelastic in the AC prevents corneal touch by the IOL pulled by the posterior infusion.

extraction. Such tears are particularly dangerous because they may occur in areas very close to the retina involved in surgery, and may consequently escape detection. A viscoelastic injected around the IOL during removal of the surrounding vitreous helps stabilize the retina, reducing movements that may lead to direct contact with the retina without altering the visibility of the operating field. For this use we prefer a viscoadherent product such as Viscoat or sodium hyaluronate with medium molecular weight, possibly dyed yellow so that the surgeon can see it easily during any phase of surgery. The product is injected underneath the lens in particular, to lift and move it as far as possible from the retina (Figure 28-48b).

With the IOL completely released, provided there are no retinal complications, the surgeon can grasp it with forceps and move it into the AC, to be extracted or fixed to the iris or sclera. When removal is preferred, it is performed through the limbus. Further implantation can then be performed with a sclerally fixated IOL, introducing the new lens through the same corneoscleral wound used to extract the previous one (Figure 28-49). Replacing the lens is more invasive, even though it avoids creating a large opening like the one required to extract

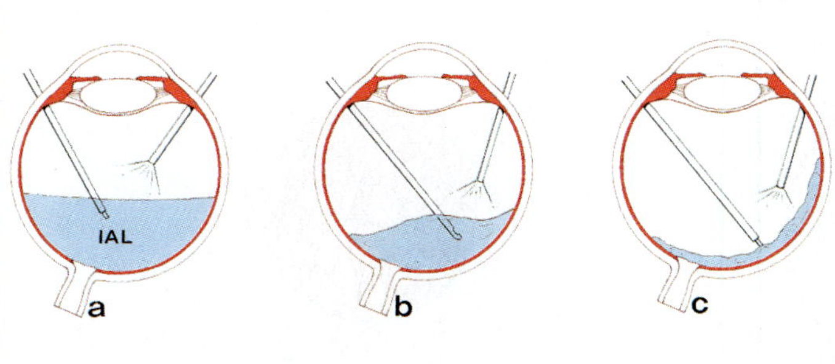

Figure 28-51. Viscoelastic removal from vitreous chamber. a) The removal of a cohesive viscoelastic with low viscosity at rest can be made with the simple Charles' cannula even during gas or oil injection. b) High molecular weight sodium hyaluronate can require vitrectomy and active suction to be removed. c) It can be impossible to remove a viscoadherent product completely.

and implant a lens with 6.5- or 7-mm optics. Some techniques of scleral fixation extract the loops through sclerotomies and attach them to the prolene thread, enabling later fixation to the sclera. These seem particularly suitable when the IOL has a large diameter suitable for the ciliary sulcus.

Another technique is to affix the IOL to the iris, which limits trauma to sclero–ciliary structures and seems particularly suitable for phacoemulsification lenses with 5- or 5.5-mm optics and radial origin of the loops (Figure 28-50). The AC must be filled with viscoelastic of high molecular weight and the pupil kept poorly dilated—not a difficult task in eyes so weakened by surgery. This way, it is possible to situate the optic zone of the lens in the AC, with the loops remaining in the posterior chamber so surgery can be completed.

With the IOL fixed in the desired position, the surgeon explores the posterior segment again for any retinal complications, treating them when it is most opportune to do so. The sodium hyaluronate is then removed as accurately as possible, as there is no barrier between the posterior and the anterior segment, and sclerotomies are closed.

SILICONE OIL TAMPONADING AND REMOVAL OF VISCOELASTICS

The presence of viscoelastic products inside the eyeball prevents complete filling with silicone oil. Completely removing the viscoelastic is then mandatory. This can be accomplished through various methods, depending on the viscoelastic used and retinal conditions.

Removing sodium hyaluronate is the easiest, owing to the features of the material. When the preparation has low molecular weight (IAL), it can be extracted with a Charles' needle during silicone oil replacement (Figure 28-51a). Poorly viscous hyaluronate penetrates easily with mild pressure in the silicone cannula of the blunt needle; its relatively high internal cohesion facilitates the procedure. If the hyaluronate has medium molecular weight, greater pressure is required to encourage it to come out of the eyeball. Sometimes it may be best to first lift the viscoelastic from the retina with liquid perfluorocarbon. The heavy liquid keeps the retina in place, allowing the surgeon to remove the viscoelastic in a completely safe zone, far from delicate ocular structures. Dyed viscoelastic is more easily detected and completely removed. Despite its viscoelasticity, sodium hyaluronate with high molecular weight should be removed with aspiration rather than by pressure from the inside, and always from a safe region (Figure 28-51b).

Removing other types of viscoelastics from the inside of the globe follows different procedures, which may consist of simple dilution with infusion solution or precise detection and removal by air or fluid exchange. Occasionally, complete removal may turn out to be impossible (Figure 28-51c).

LUXATION OF THE NUCLEUS OR WHOLE LENS IN THE VITREOUS

Viscoelastics are better than liquid perfluorocarbons to manipulate an IOL luxated in the vitreous, as they better stabilize the lens during procedures for removal and, being less toxic, do not require a subsequent total vitrectomy followed by complete removal. They can be dyed with fluorescein, enabling the surgeon to differentiate them from the

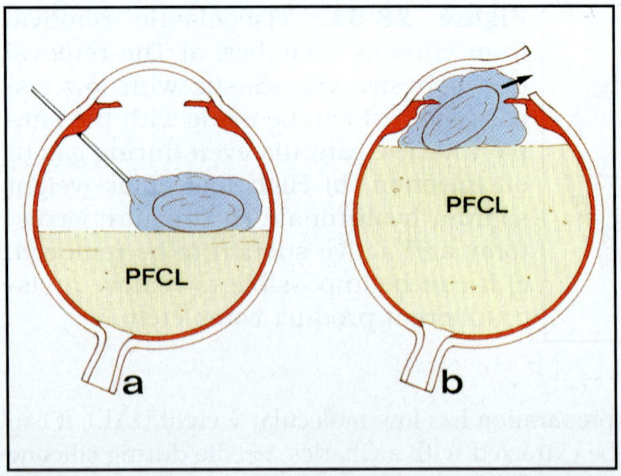

Figure 28-52. a) The liquid perfluorocarbon lifts the nucleus after vitrectomy. The viscoelastic substance stabilizes it, reducing movements caused by infusion streams. b) The viscoelastic protects the structures of the anterior segment during nucleus removal.

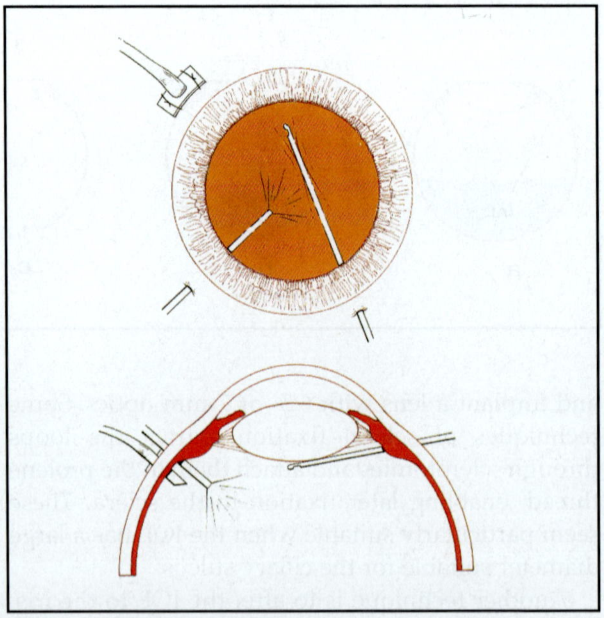

Figure 28-53. During anterior vitreous vitrectomy it is easy to indent and to damage the lens with the vitrector probe.

vitreous and the infusion fluid. These considerations are not applicable when either the lens nucleus or the lens itself are luxated in the vitreous chamber, as they cannot be removed through simple movements with an intraocular forceps.

Heavy liquids are the best means to direct the nucleus or the lens toward the AC, from which they can be extracted through the limbus. In this type of surgery, the crucial role of viscoelastics is to protect the corneal endothelium during the procedure. Once the limbus has been opened, a large amount of scleral infusion fluid streams from the posterior to the AC, which risks grazing the lens, which is often hard and sharp, along the corneal endothelium (Figure 28-52). Here, the most suitable viscoelastic to protect the anterior segment structures is a viscoadherent material, which will remain unaffected by the flow of liquid and will not transmit the abrasive force exerted by the passage of the lens. A mixture of chondroitin sulfate and sodium hyaluronate (Viscoat) is the best product for this use.

Removal of Retrolental Membranes

During vitrectomy performed in phakic eyes, it is often necessary to remove the portion of vitreous immediately behind the lens still adhering to it despite coarctation and posterior detachment. In many cases this part of the vitreous becomes opaque, owing to the presence of retractions or membranes in the vitreous gel, or is filled with blood that tends not to move posteriorly. Direct excision of this tissue inevitably leads to lens lesions, even when accomplished with the utmost care using both sclerotomies, right for the optic fiber and left for the vitrector and reversed. Instruments used for vitrectomy tend to touch the lens at 6 o'clock in particular, despite their indentation (Figure 28-53). Although lesions of the lens capsule are rare, even simple touching may cause postoperative increase of lens opacity, already encouraged by the intervention itself.

Applying viscoelastic materials can solve such surgical difficulty. Sodium hyaluronate, preferably dyed yellow, can be used to separate the membranes or the opaque vitreous from the posterior surface of the lens before removal by vitrector. The most common technique is to introduce the vitrectomy probe via the pars plana into the retrolental space, placing it in a safe position immediately underneath the membrane or the retrolental vitre-

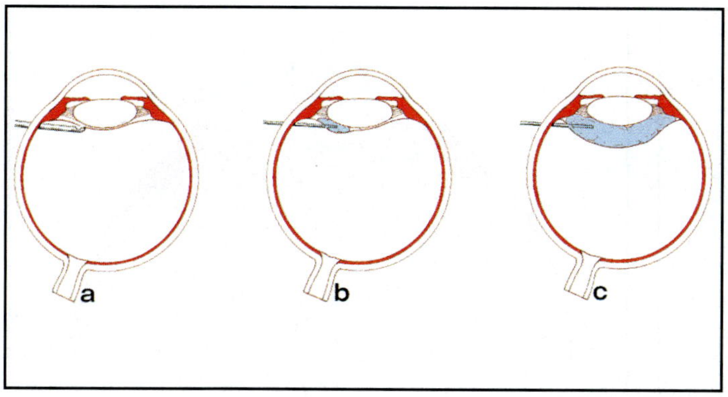

Figure 28-54. a) A strong suction without cutting keeps the anterior hyaloid adherent to the vitrector tip. The cut subsequently makes an opening in the anterior hyaloid without damaging the lens or the zonule. b) The tip of the cannula injecting viscoelastic is introduced into the retrolental space through the opening. c) The retrolental space is dilated by the viscoelastic allowing safe removal of all the anterior cortical vitreous.

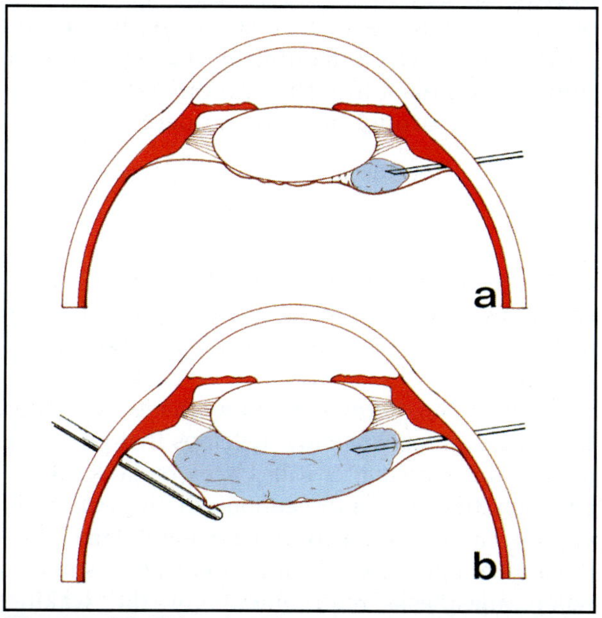

Figure 28-55. a) When a retrolental membrane is present, the viscoelastic can be injected in a space above the membrane under the zonule. The membrane is progressively separated from the lens. b) The membrane is removed without risk of lens damage.

ous portion to be removed. The tip of the vitrector should reach about halfway between the posterior pole of the lens and the equator, longitudinal to the sclerotomy for access (Figure 28-54). With the aspiration port turned upward, strong suction aspirates and keeps the portion of membrane or vitreous immediately overlying it adhered to the vitrector. At this point, the surgeon makes a cut with the vitrector that creates a hole in the anterior vitreous cortex. The vitrector is then retracted, and the smoothed tip of a curved cannula is placed inside the vitreous canal formed for viscoelastic injection.

The following injection of viscoelastic—preferably yellow-dyed sodium hyaluronate with medium molecular weight (Healon® Yellow*)—separates the vitreous membranes or the anterior vitreous cortex from the posterior surface of the lens. When the membrane is completely separated from the lens, the vitrector is reintroduced and the membrane dissected and extracted in total safety. The same procedure is performed on the opposite side to remove the retrolental vitreous completely, without passing the vitrector probe under the posterior pole of the lens and the consequent risk of touching it. When the portion of anterior vitreous to be removed does not adhere over 360° to the lens posterior capsule, the viscoelastic can be injected directly in Vogt's space in front of the hyaloid, if present. The injection can be accomplished through a very thin needle introduced via the pars plana, possibly bent for this purpose, which pierces the vitreous membranes to remove and progressively dilate the retrolental space while lowering the vitrectomy plane (Figure 28-55).

ANTERIOR CHAMBER RECONSTRUCTION DURING AND AFTER VITRECTOMY

Vitrectomy interventions often cause reduced corneal transparency, frequently due to epithelial edema, which can be solved by removing the epithelium. Sometimes the problem is decreased AC depth caused by leakage of aqueous humor

**Healon® Yellow is no longer being manufactured.*

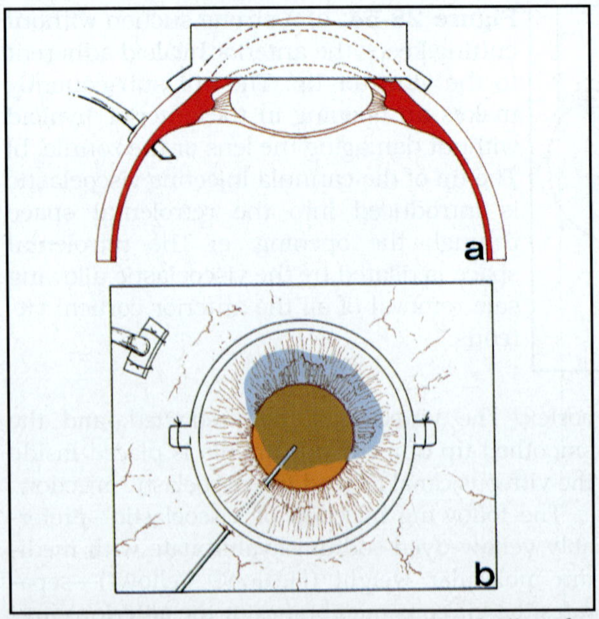

Figure 28-56. a) The AC can become shallow for various reasons during vitrectomy. b) The injection of a very transparent viscoelastic with high viscosity at rest, performed through the cornea by a 30 G needle, restores AC depth and transparency, also helping mydriasis.

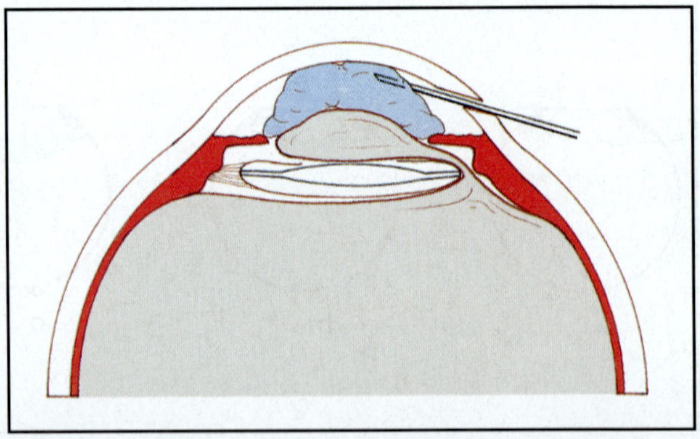

Figure 28-57. In pseudophakic eyes silicone oil can herniate into the AC through a damaged zonule. The injection of viscoelastic can push the oil back into the vitreous chamber, or evacuate it through a corneal opening.

through a small limbal wound used to extract a cataract via phacoemulsification that was too hard to be removed via the pars plana. This complication mostly occurs in eyes with an intact iris–capsular diaphragm, whereas in aphakic eyes the anterior passage of the infusion fluid usually ensures good visibility of the vitreous cavity. At times the aqueous humor clouds due to the presence of blood or other foreign material—for instance, silicone oil—and must be removed to continue surgery.

In such cases viscoelastic materials are indispensable to ensure visibility, and are universally used. They are injected in the AC until it is completely filled (Figure 28-56a). The best products for this application are the most transparent ones: various preparations of sodium hyaluronate. A product with high viscosity at rest, such as Healon® or Healon® GV, is also necessary. It will not leak out of the eyeball through the same wound and prevents the aqueous humor from doing the same. Any viscoelastic losses can be compensated for by further injections. Possible consequences on IOP must be prevented by removing the product after the intervention is completed, or by replacing it with another having a lower risk of hypertension (IAL or methylcellulose) when there is a risk of postoperative hypotony.

Because the permanent tamponade is lighter than water, a force usually develops that pushes it toward the cornea after it has been replaced at the end of vitrectomy interventions. If the patient is appropriately positioned, this force will later push the retina into place. Immediately after surgery, when anesthesia requirements or the waking patient's movements hinder maintaining a prone position, there is a risk of the AC becoming shallow, and the occasional danger that the tamponade may move in front of the iris–capsule diaphragm. This may require reintervention soon after surgery.

Viscoelastics can prevent such complications and assist in the correct restoration of aqueous flow. In phakic, pseudophakic, and aphakic eyes, it is important to re-form the AC with viscoelastic at the end of surgery.

In phakic eyes, reconstructing the AC with a viscoelastic that is unlikely to cause intraocular hypertension opposes the pressure exerted by the posterior tamponade when the patient is supine. The risk of angle closure glaucoma caused by forward shifting of the iris–lens diaphragm is greatly reduced, as is the risk that part of the tamponade will penetrate the AC through a break in the same diaphragm (Figure 28-57). Sodium hyaluronate with medium

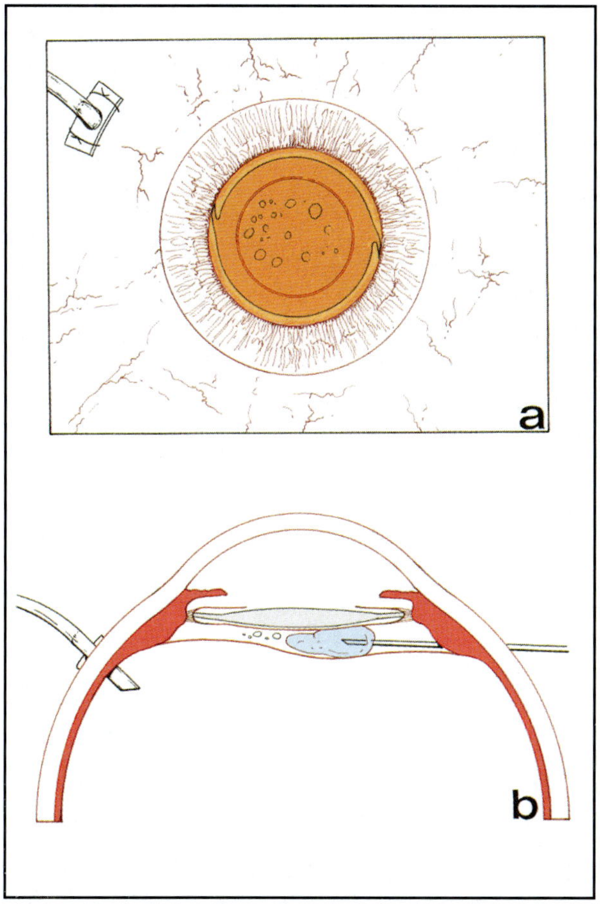

Figure 28-58. a) Some droplets of silicone, of other fluid or of air can remain adherent to the posterior surface of silicone IOLs during surgical maneuvers, thus reducing visibility. b) A thin layer of viscoelastic injected on the posterior IOL surface removes the droplets, and is kept in position by the posterior pressure exerted by oil or air.

or high molecular weight (Healon®, Healon® GV) is not suitable for this use; hyaluronate with low molecular weight (IAL) is preferable. More adhesive viscoelastics, such as chondroitin sulfate/hyaluronate (Viscoat) or methylcellulose (Hymecel), also appear to be appropriate.

PMMA IOLs present few problems during vitrectomy and during the exchange of liquid and tamponade. The same is not true for other lens materials such as silicone, which are less suitable for vitrectomy. In particular, it has been observed that bubbles tend to form on the posterior surface of silicone lenses during the liquid–air exchange. These are quickly removed by a layer of sodium hyaluronate adherent to the posterior lens surface. The internal cohesion of hyaluronate and the upward push of the gas keep the viscoelastic in place, thus allowing procedures to continue with unchanged visibility (Figure 28-58).

The usefulness of viscoelastics is even more marked in aphakic eyes. They can occupy the AC, thus forming a barrier against penetration of the tamponade, which otherwise would occur almost immediately even during the exchange. A material with high viscosity at rest, such as sodium hyaluronate with medium or high viscosity, is able to void the AC from any silicone oil that penetrated at the beginning of the replacement, while remaining in place as long as the vitreous cavity is filled. The viscoelastic is assisted in this task by its internal cohesion and by the pressure exerted by the oil bubble. The same considerations are true for air, although volumes are less when gas is used instead of silicone oil. Perfect transparency of the viscoelastic also assists the endovitreous exchange, and its physicochemical properties enable it to keep the AC and the overlying cornea stretched, without the formation of any stromal folds that might threaten transparency.

Chapter Twenty-Nine

Use of Viscoelastics in Strabismus Surgery

During and after strabismus surgery, inflammatory response, which can be extensive, often results from manipulation of and trauma to the conjunctiva, Tenon's capsule, and muscle sheaths. The particular characteristics of the patient typically treated surgically for strabismus, usually a child, intensify this reaction, which can be only partially remedied by anti-inflammatory medication. Consequently, in the first hours after surgery, connective adhesions of variable extent and severity may form. Sometimes they are so tough and large that they jeopardize the relationships of muscle and episcleral structures, and therefore the final outcome of the intervention. This why in recent years surgeons have avoided using postoperative bandages to stimulate quick recovery of ocular motility in the first hours after surgery. Continuous movement of muscle sheaths against the episclera and capsule avoids prolonged juxtaposition of the inflamed tissues and is therefore likely to prevent the formation of adhesions.

Based on properties of the natural lubricants in the joints of many animals, including man, hyaluronate was naturally a good candidate to assist in strabismus surgery. The theory supporting the early use of Healon® in this type of surgery was that it reduced the amount of postoperative cicatrization through improved reciprocal sliding of tissues and provided the anti-inflammatory effect of sodium hyaluronate. Later in this chapter, we will see how experimental and clinical studies confirmed this hypothesis.

Viscoelastic Requirements in Strabismus Surgery

Viscosity at Rest

Viscoelastic material used in strabismus surgery should act as a biologic envelope around the muscle sheath, maintaining space around the muscle for some days postoperatively. Viscosity at rest must therefore be the highest possible, to reduce the risk that the product may move far from the site where it has been placed through small outflow pathways or that it may be diluted and removed from the liquid transudate due to inflammation. According to publications on the subject, viscosity at rest similar to that of Healon® is sufficient.

Pseudoplasticity

High pseudoplasticity is of no benefit in a viscoelastic to be used in extraocular muscle surgery. The material can be injected through large cannulas with no difficulty. For example, an instrument the size of a strabismus hook is considered appropriate to move over and under the oculomotor muscle, even when the muscle has been sectioned and newly sutured. Pseudoplasticity can be a drawback of the viscoelastic in this case, as there are no problems of application. In strabismus surgery attempts has also been made to wrap the operated muscles in a wide variety of materials, which are not always reabsorbable.

ADHESIVENESS

A viscoelastic with fair adhesiveness is beneficial in attempts to prevent postsurgical adhesions after recession or resection of an oculomotor muscle. Whereas other features are similar, adhesiveness enables the material to remain longer in site, thus allowing better reciprocal movement of the biologic structures involved in surgery. However, no studies have been published on the subject, as the authors who have used viscoelastics in strabismus surgery, both experimentally and otherwise, have focused their attention on sodium hyaluronate.

BIOCOMPATIBILITY

Biocompatibility of the viscoelastic used in strabismus surgery must be very good to prevent even the least amount of inflammation from altering the outcome in the absence of inflammation and adhesions. No other problem is as delicate as the contact of the product with the retina or the corneal endothelium; the need to avoid any unnecessary complications suggests the use of a highly biocompatible product.

OTHER FEATURES

Other features generally influencing the choice of viscoelastic material in intraocular surgery are not as relevant in strabismus surgery. For instance, it is not necessary for the viscoelastic surrounding the oculomotor muscles to be transparent, whereas a greater hemostatic effect is important. Reduced bleeding is a very desirable element, as it reduces inflammation and the formation of fibrin in places where it has strong negative effects and also limits the need for cauterization. However, the hemostatic properties of hyaluronate preparations are in practice based on the compression of small vessels, which does not occur in a dilatable space such as that under the conjunctiva.

EXPERIMENTAL STUDIES

Early investigations into the usefulness of viscoelastics in strabismus surgery were performed in the mid-1980s. In a group of rabbits submitted to resection of an oculomotor muscle, Maselli injected amounts of Healon® ranging from 0.1 to 0.4 mL between the bulbar sheet of the muscle sheath and the parietal wall of the capsule, into Tenon's space, and outside it toward the intermuscular septi and the conjunctiva. The results of the anatomopathologic study performed postoperatively at various intervals showed a reduced activation of collagen production and fibrosis compared with the controls, with persistence of hyaluronate around the resected muscle for several days.

The data reported by Maselli in 1986 were confirmed in 1992, always with rabbit eyes. Yaacoby found fewer cicatricial adhesions around the operated muscles when they had been surrounded with sodium hyaluronate compared with controls in which BSS or activated cellulose sheath were used. Oh and Lee found that sodium hyaluronate was better than subconjunctivally injected triamcinolone in preventing adhesions following strabismus surgery. Dissenting opinions were also published by Searl in 1987 and by Faur in 1991. These researchers did not find anatomic differences between rabbits treated with Healon® and those not treated for postoperative cicatrization.

A different experimental approach was used by Searl, whose aim was to check the reduction of the forces necessary to make the eye move after surgery. Investigations performed with a dynamometer showed that 2 weeks after surgery, a much smaller force was required to move the eyes treated with Healon® compared with control eyes receiving equally induced movement. Although the differences disappeared later in the postoperative period, the finding is important because it confirms the general impression that ocular movement is enhanced by the use of viscoelastics in the immediate postoperative period.

SURGICAL TECHNIQUE

INTERVENTIONS WITH FIXED SUTURES

In extraocular muscle surgery interventions accomplished with viscoelastic materials, the early phases are performed as usual. The conjunctiva is opened next to the muscle planned for resection or recession, at the limbus or more posteriorly, according to the surgeon's preference. It seldom happens

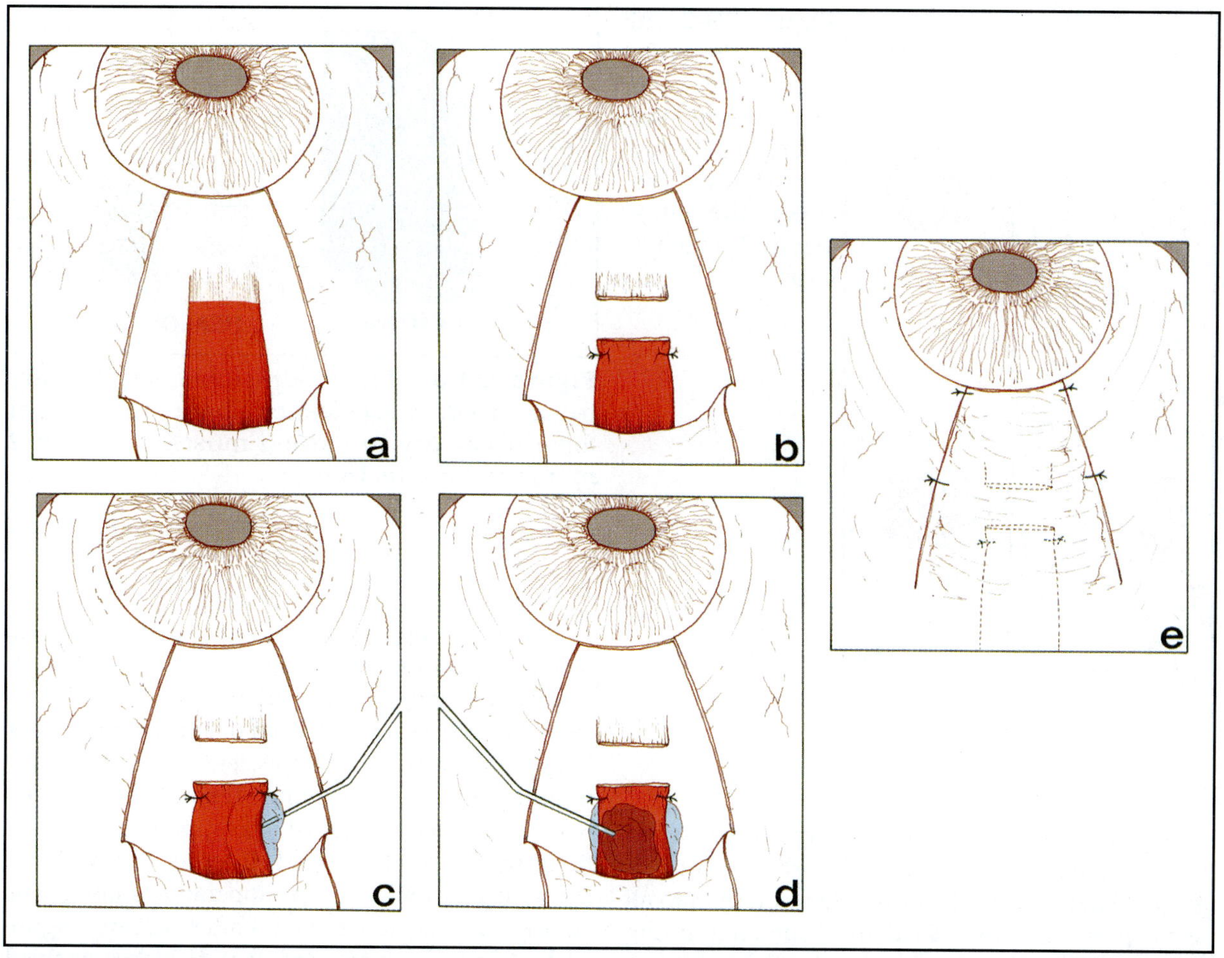

Figure 29-1. (a) The muscle to be recessed is released without the help of a viscoelastic. (b) Muscle recession is accomplished with the usual technique. (c) At the end of muscle–scleral suturing, a viscoelastic is applied under the muscle plane, between the cut tendon and sclera. (d) More viscoelastic is applied over the muscle, and closed under the conjunctiva. (e) At the end of surgery, the viscous product is left under the conjunctiva.

that a viscoelastic is necessary in conjunctival dissection, even when the conjunctiva has already been submitted to intervention, as the thickness of globe fasciae is rather high in younger patients, as in those usually undergoing strabismus surgery (Figure 29-1a). The muscle is isolated from its fasciae, released from ligaments, and resected or recessed according to need (Figure 29-1b). The viscoelastic is applied at the end of the muscle–scleral suture. Healon® is injected in the space between the muscle sheath and the scleral plane as well as over the muscle toward the conjunctival plane (Figure 29-1, c and d). This prevents the viscoelastic from leaking (Figure 29-1e).

Results achieved using sodium hyaluronate in strabismus surgery with fixed sutures were judged as positive, despite few publications on the subject. The difficult decision of best results in a type of surgery typically exposed to a large number of variables is a likely reason for the higher number of experimental studies compared with clinical investigations.

INTERVENTIONS WITH ADJUSTABLE SUTURES

Adjustable muscle sutures offer further control in strabismus surgery. Various versions have been pro-

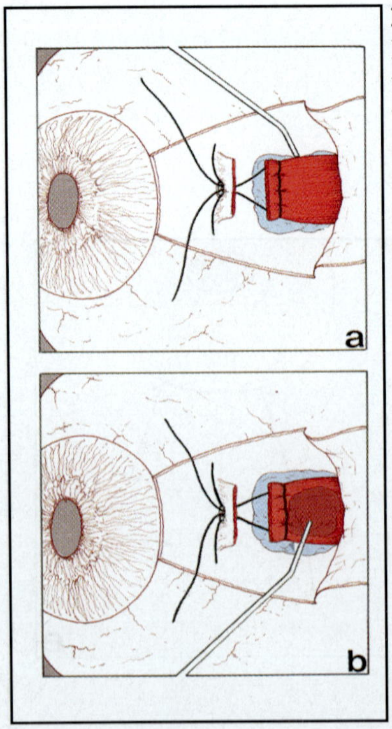

Figure 29-2. (a) Healon is positioned between the muscle and sclera. (b) Healon is positioned between the muscle and Tenon's capsule.

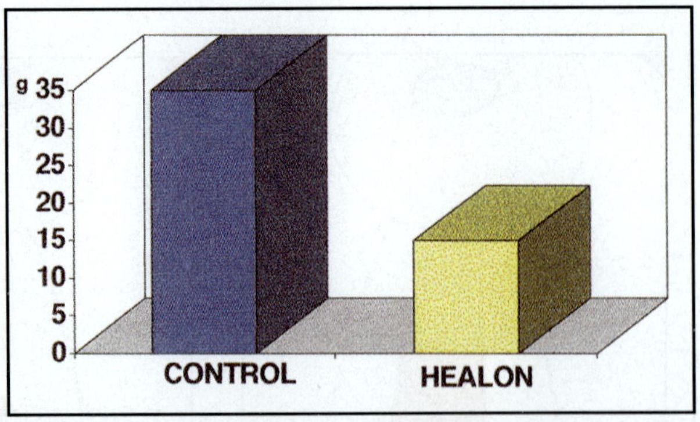

Figure 29-3. When adjustable sutures are being used, viscoelastics lower the weight force necessary to move a muscle insertion 2 mm from 36 g to 15 g.

posed, which mostly concern the type of knot used to tie the adjustable suture as well as the kind of conjunctival suture to make. A problem common to all techniques is the tissue friction encountered during final adjustment of the suture, which depends on the natural tissue adhesion occurring during cicatrization. The phenomenon occurs within 24 hours after surgery, the period during which sutures are usually adjusted. Getting the operated muscle to slide into its permanent place may then become difficult. In cases where the muscle has to be pushed further forward, tissue friction can usually be overcome by direct traction on the adjustable suture, although significant force is required.

In contrast, in cases where the muscle must be recessed further, the surgeon must rely on the force exerted by the muscle itself, which contracts during ocular movements made by the patient on suggestion. However, this force may be insufficient and adjustment impossible. Consequently, many surgeons intentionally operate their patients in such a way that postoperative adjustment will necessarily involve traction on the suture.

The first application of viscoelastic aimed to facilitate postoperative adjustment of sutures in strabismus surgery was reported by Clorfeine in 1987. The procedure consisted of applying Healon® between the muscle and episclera and between the muscle and the overlying Tenon's fascia. The researcher advised against also applying viscoelastic in the place of the knot, in order to avoid any possibility of undesired postoperative sliding. The suture was adjusted 24 hours after surgery (Figure 29-2). Clorfeine concluded that Healon® enabled the operated muscle to move more easily and smoothly, also permitting very minor adjustments equal to only two prism diopters. The procedure is simpler to accomplish and more comfortable for the young patient. Recessions could also be performed without difficulty.

A study by Granet et al confirmed the usefulness of viscoelastic in facilitating postoperative suture adjustment and indirectly confirmed the value of Healon® in strabismus surgery. Researchers measured the force necessary to move an oculomotor muscle postoperatively. Fifteen muscles receiving Healon® required an average force of 15 g to be moved 2 mm, whereas 36 g was required to move 13 control muscles that were not treated with viscoelastic material (Figure 29-3). The difference was clinically and statistically significant. The results of the study confirm Paris and Saya's findings published in 1990.

CONCLUSIONS

The mechanical ability of viscoelastics to maintain space and allow reciprocal sliding of tissues without trauma is evident in strabismus surgery. The ability to reduce inflammation and postoperative cicatrization depends on the inhibition of chemotaxis versus the chemical and cell agents peculiar to inflammation and tissue reparation, probably due to the separation of operated anatomic structures, which come in contact with each other far later than without viscoelastics.

CHAPTER THIRTY

Use of Viscoelastics in Ocular Adnexal Surgery

Vincenzo Pucci, MD

In recent years, viscoelastic materials have proved to be of great use in surgery involving eyelids and tear ducts. This short chapter provides some examples of how viscoelastics are used in adnexal surgery.

LACRIMAL DUCT SURGERY

Surgeons who perform tear duct surgery know the difficulties of interventions such as dacryocystorhinostomy. Previous malformations and inflammatory cicatricial adhesions, caused by numerous dacryocysts and canaliculites, make it hard to localize and recognize the canalicular lumen and the lacrimal sac. The use of special probes and tear duct dilators is often complicated by the creation of false ducts or even by the breakage of canaliculi or the sac, with consequent bleeding in the operating field. Difficulties are increased by substantial bleeding intensified by the anatomy of the area, as well as by hyperemia due to chronic inflammation.

Various researchers have studied the use of viscoelastics in this kind of surgery. In 1991, Shiwa and Tazawa described the results of a technique already developed by Hurwitz in 1984 to detect the lacrimal sac lumen with the help of viscoelastic materials during dacryocystorhinostomy. The most delicate phase of this intervention is the localization of the sac, which must be opened with a full-thickness incision to pair the nasal mucosa with that of the sac. This is often difficult because of hypertrophic sacs or the narrow lumen of the sac; in these cases, the intervention may be complicated by incorrectly made incisions or significant hemorrhage. After preparing the operating field and localizing the lacrimal sac, the researchers injected Healon® inside the lacrimal sac through a lacrimal punctum and the canaliculus, with slight pressure (Figure 30-1). Once Healon® had stretched the lacrimal sac from the inside, the surgeon incised the sac with a full-thickness anteromedial incision. The presence of Healon® provided good mechanical hemostasis and easy location of the sac's mucosa, which then fit well with the nasal mucosa.

The viscoelastic required for this procedure must have high viscosity at rest so it is able to remain in the sac without leaking, even when the sac is manipulated during surgical procedures. On the other hand, the viscoelastic must also be very pseudoplastic, so it can be injected through a thin cannula such as those used for lacrimal ducts. Adhesiveness and transparency are not relevant features, and the biocompatibility requirement is minimal. Healon®, the product used by Shiwa and Tazawa, seems very suitable for its pseudoplasticity, but Healon® GV can probably better stretch the lacrimal sac and keep it stretched. To our knowledge, no attempts have been made to dye Healon® on the spot with methylene blue, a coloring widely used in lacrimal duct surgery. When the viscoelastic has performed its tracing and stabilizing function, it can be removed easily with antibiotic and physiologic solution.

Using the technique described, Shiwa and Tazawa performed 52 interventions of dacryocystorhinostomy. In 20 cases, the sac appeared hypertrophic, whereas in 32 cases the lumen of the lacrimal sac was very narrow. The presence of the viscoelastic material allowed the surgeon to make a full-thickness incision in all the cases treated. Lerner and Boyton also used sodium hyaluronate injection to detect the lumen of the sac, but did not report on their results with this technique. Seiff and Ahn used Healon® to find the medial opening of the sac in cases of canalicular lacerations. Healon® proved to be useful in this kind of surgery as it creates space and permits the surgeon to perform more comfortable procedures such as intubation. It also does not infiltrate tissue, produces fair hemostasis, and is easily removed from the surgical field. Hurwitz has published an interesting use of Healon® with fluorescein to define operating spaces; Healon® Yellow* could also be used for this purpose. As for the application of sodium hyaluronate, no reports have emerged from the literature concerning cases of intolerance or inflammatory tissue response.

Lacrimal Duct Trauma

When they are full thickness, traumatic wounds of the eyelids often affect the lacrimal canaliculi. Such wounds are treated with great care when attempting to re-form the tear ducts. An incorrect suture or inflammation could cause cicatricial closure of the canaliculus, resulting in poor tear drainage, followed by epiphora and discomfort to the patient.

To preserve the integrity of the lacrimal duct and to prevent cicatricial adhesions, the surgeon inserts 1-mm silicone probes through the lacrimal punctum and tries to push them along the duct to reach the opposite punctum. In this type of reconstructive intervention, the surgeon can be greatly assisted by a surgical microscope and viscoelastics.

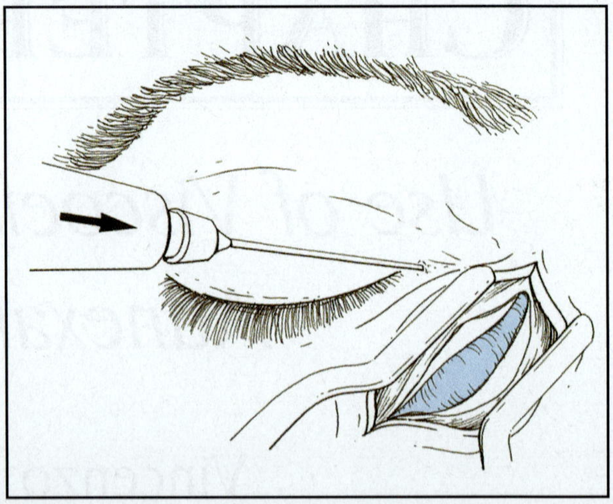

Figure 30-1. Injecting viscoelastic into the lacrimal sac through the duct widens the sac itself, allowing the surgeon to see the sac clearly and easing surgical maneuvers.

The features of viscoelastics used in these cases are biocompatibility, peculiar to hyaluronate products with limited inflammatory reaction; the ability to create space through tissues; and especially good hemostasis.

In 1988, Villa-Coro commented on the action of lubricants containing hyaluronate in expanding the lacrimal ducts and facilitating the passage of silicone probes. Researchers injected Healon® through a lacrimal punctum. Once it created space, a silicone probe was introduced and directed along the whole lacerated canaliculus. The hyaluronate assisted in hemostasis of lacerated tissues and was easily washed away by the irrigating solution after the procedure, although leaving it in place would not have caused inflammation. In 1990, Villa-Coro reported a new case where the use of hyaluronate allowed repositioning of a silicone tube in a 7-year-old patient. The small tube was repositioned after dilating the lacrimal duct and then gently pushing the cannula up to the nasal fossa. The position of the small tube was confirmed postoperatively by echographic examination.

Healon® Yellow is no longer being manufactured.

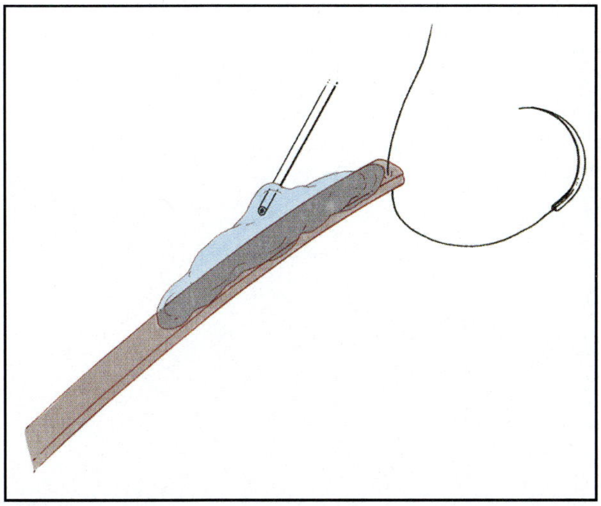

Figure 30-2. A viscoelastic product can be used to lubricate the strip of fascia lata used in palpebral ptosis surgery. A viscoadherent product such as methylcellulose seems most appropriate.

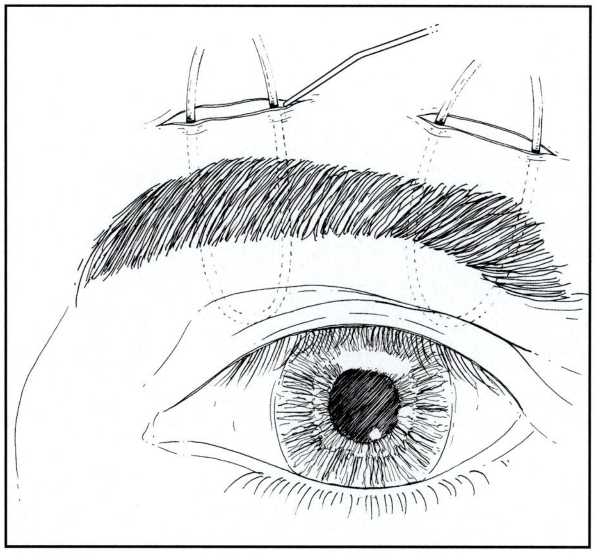

Figure 30-3. During the intervention to suspend the eyelid from the frontal muscle, the viscoelastic assists the passage of the fascia lata strip. Silicone strips require no lubrication.

PTOSIS SURGERY

Ptosis can be repaired by a range of techniques, chosen depending on the function of the levator palpebrae superioris. When the functionality of the levator complex is poor or absent, the eyelid is suspended from the frontalis muscle. This technique can be performed after levator resection or aponeurosis repair have failed.

The technical difficulty of suspending the tarsus palpebrae from the frontalis muscle lies in the construction of a subcutaneous tunnel that ends with the tarsus on one side and the frontalis muscle in the superciliary region on the other. The bands consist of fascia lata, autogenous fascia temporalis, preserved fascia lata, or silicone bands.

The use of viscoelastics in this type of surgery is poorly documented. In 1991, Law and McNeer published an article describing a technique for frontalis muscle suspension using preserved fascia lata and sodium hyaluronate as lubricating materials. According to the researchers, using preserved fascia lata strips is complicated by breakage and crumbling. The cause of such inconvenience is friction of the fascia with the subcutaneous layer while passing through the tunnel, and stretching done by the surgeon to attach it to the tarsus and the frontalis muscle. The researchers solved such problems by injecting sodium hyaluronate (Healon®), through a 27-G cannula on the main end of the strip and inside the subcutaneous tunnel (Figures 30-2 and 30-3). The presence of viscoelastic eased the passage of the fascia lata inside the tunnel, eliminating friction. The method was used successfully to treat 30 cases of palpebral ptosis. Despite the successful results achieved by Healon®, viscoadherent products such as Viscoat or methylcellulose now seem more appropriate for this purpose, as they adhere to the fascia lata and are unmoved by the tangent forces that develop when the strip enters the tunnel in the tissue.

Chapter Thirty-One

Use of Viscoelastics in Ocular Diagnostics and Treatment

Simonetta Morselli, MD

Ocular Diagnostics

Viscoelastics have been used as an interface between the cornea and diagnostic lenses for many years. They permit surgeons to apply diagnostic lenses or lenses for laser therapy onto the cornea, promoting perfect adhesion and perfect shifting during adjustments of any corneal unevenness. When movable devices are used, such as Goldmann's lens, the viscoelastic fills the meniscus between the lens and the cornea or sclera, allowing the surgeon to move the lens eccentrically without decreasing adhesion or visibility (Figure 31-1). The viscoelastic preserves perfect corneal transparency at all phases of the intervention and assists in heat dispersion during laser treatment.

Viscoelastics are also useful for ocular tonometry in the case of corneal diseases causing surface irregularity. The viscoelastic fills the empty spaces and smoothes the corneal surface, allowing the surgeon to take tonometric measurements.

Ophthalmic echography requires viscoelastic materials with good adhesiveness owing to the particular features of ultrasounds that pass through fluids rather than through air. Viscosity at rest, biocompatibility, and pseudoplasticity are irrelevant for this use; hence, HPMC is the most suitable material for the purpose.

Viscoelastic Requirements in Ocular Diagnostics and Treatment

Viscosity at Rest

Ocular diagnostics do not require particularly viscous products. In fact, it is necessary to place a thin layer of viscoelastic between the cornea and the contact lens, enabling the lens to shift without causing corneal abrasion during the examination. Low cost makes HPMC the most appropriate viscoelastic for this use.

Pseudoplasticity

Pseudoplasticity is not relevant in this application. The viscoelastic is applied directly onto the concave portion of the contact lens, squeezed from plastic containers through large holes. In this case the only consideration is that the viscoelastic does create air bubbles that may jeopardize good visibility. The container must therefore be kept upside down while squeezing the product out very slowly.

Adhesiveness

A viscoelastic with good adhesiveness is usefully applied on diagnostic lenses, as it must remain in site and form a homogenous layer that spreads over the concave surface of the lens. The material must also fill the gap between the curvature of the cornea and that of the contact lens, thus ensuring optical coupling (ie, Goldmann's lens).

BIOCOMPATIBILITY

Biocompatibility is not particularly important in ocular diagnostics, as the time the viscoelastic remains on the corneal surface is limited.

TRANSPARENCY AND HOMOGENEITY

The transparency of the product is a basic requirement for diagnostic use, particularly when laser therapy is being performed. Although all the products currently available are good, sodium hyaluronate with low molecular weight seems preferable for its low cost and good internal cohesion. HPMC is also commonly used, but it often contains air bubbles and requires replacement. Different packages providing different dispensations could avoid the problem.

OTHER FEATURES

Considering its overwhelming and daily use for this application, the material must be reasonably priced, which is another reason HPMC is the most commonly used product.

EXPERIMENTAL STUDIES

In electroretinography, viscoelastics are used as agents assisting application of the corneal lens with electrodes, providing perfect adhesion of electrodes to cornea. This prevents trauma to the corneal epithelium both during the examination and at the moment when the electrode is disconnected. In this case the viscoelastic also promotes electric conductivity, enhancing the width and clarity of the signal. Viscoelastic materials such as 0.4% HPMC have been used for this purpose since 1984, but they cause alterations to the electrodes owing to their density.

In 1991, Rispoli et al studied the application of hyaluronate contained in an agent available on the market (Hyalistil) to electroretinography, with decidedly better results than in the controls.

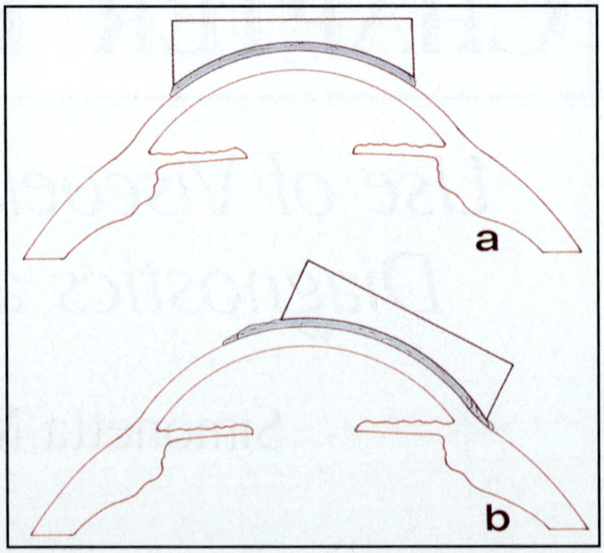

Figure 31-1. The use of a good viscoelastic allows the surgeon to move the contact lens without decreased adhesion or losses in optical continuity with the cornea.

OPHTHALMIC THERAPY

PROTECTION AGAINST PHYSICAL AGENTS

The effectiveness of viscoelastics in protecting ocular tissue from physical agents has been well established. Certain physical characteristics are especially important, such as adhesion to the corneal endothelium and ability to disperse the heat following laser treatment. The viscoelastic is able to form an effective barrier against the physical agents acting on ocular tissues. The material is applied onto the corneal epithelium either topically or through intraocular injection.

VISCOSITY AT REST

Viscosity at rest must be rather high, particularly when the viscoelastic is applied outside the eye. High viscosity prevents the material from shifting due to gravity or pressure exerted by lenses. The viscosity of Healon® makes it most appropriate for this use.

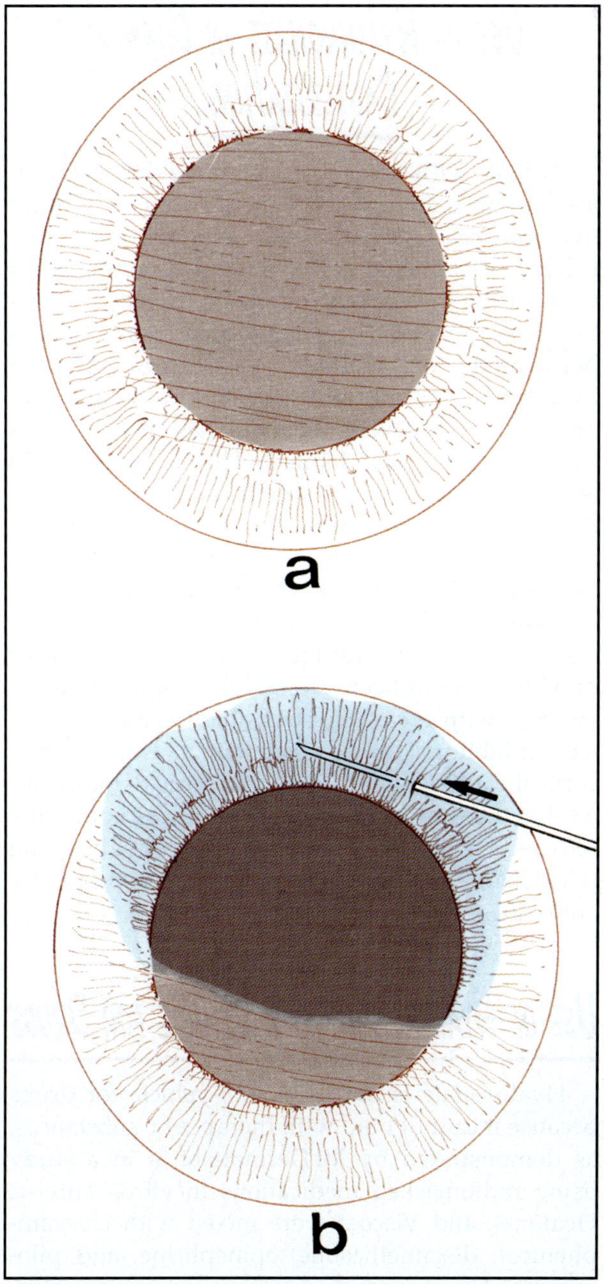

Figure 31-2. (a) Folds on Descemet's membrane hinder intraocular laser treatment. (b) Injecting a viscoelastic in the AC stretches the folds and protects the endothelium from the energy delivered.

PSEUDOPLASTICITY

High pseudoplasticity is required only when the viscoelastic is injected into the AC to protect the corneal endothelium from physical trauma, as it must pass through very thin needles (30-G). When the viscoelastic is applied to protect the epithelium, this aspect is far less important.

ADHESIVENESS

Adhesiveness is advantageous for this purpose, as an adhesive viscoelastic tends to stay in the site of application and therefore is likely to protect the underlying tissue from physical damage for longer periods.

AFFINITY WITH WATER AND LIPIDS

Features such as hydrosolubility and liposolubility are relevant when the viscoelastic comes in contact with the lacrimal film. Viscoelastic materials are made of hydrosoluble molecules, which mix with the water in the lacrimal film and become further diluted. Theoretically a very adhesive or highly viscous product remains in the conjunctival sac longer, but there have been no studies confirming this.

BIOCOMPATIBILITY

Biocompatibility must be very high in case of AC injection so the viscoelastic does not cause an inflammatory reaction of tissues already submitted to mechanical or physical stress. It is far less relevant when the material is used as a barrier for the corneal epithelium.

EXPERIMENTAL STUDIES

The use of sodium hyaluronate has been described for corneal endothelial protection during Nd:YAG laser anterior capsulotomy in patients with endotheliopathy. Alpar published a study involving patients with endotheliopathy who were scheduled for extracapsular cataract extraction with IOL implantation. Researchers performed Nd:YAG laser anterior capsulotomy after injecting Healon® in the AC (Figure 31-2). Compared with the control group, the researchers reported easier surgery with less postoperative endothelial cell loss.

Alpar published another study of patients who had previously undergone cataract extraction who had endotheliopathy and required Nd:YAG laser treatment for vitreous incarceration. The procedure here consisted of filling the AC completely with 1% sodium hyaluronate before laser treatment. Postoperative corneal complications were far more limited in the group receiving sodium hyaluronate than in those who did not.

ALTERED LACRIMAL SECRETION

Ocular surface pathologies caused by qualitative and quantitative deficiency of the lacrimal film greatly benefit from the therapeutic application of viscoelastic materials.

VISCOSITY AND PSEUDOPLASTICITY

The ability of sodium hyaluronate to remain on the corneal surface is due to the fact that the product presents non–Newtonian features at zero shear rate. Because of its high viscosity, it is retained in the precorneal film for a long period. High pseudoplasticity is not relevant because hyaluronate dilution ranges from 0.1 to 1%; thus it presents no problems of application, even through narrow passages.

In contrast, adhesiveness is very important, as it allows the viscoelastic to remain in place as long as possible. Diluted preparations of carboxymethylcellulose are also widely used as tear substitutes.

EXPERIMENTAL STUDIES

These characteristics of viscoelastics, particularly hyaluronate, were demonstrated by Snibson et al in 1990 in the performance of gamma scintigraphy. Mengher et al assessed the effect of 0.1% hyaluronate on tear film break-up time. Patients treated with hyaluronate experienced a much longer break-up but a marked reduction in "dry eye" symptoms. The effect of sodium hyaluronate contained in eye drops used on the lacrimal film during arborization tests was also assessed; results were that patients treated tended to normalize.

USE OF HYALURONATE IN CORNEAL CAUTERIZATION

Patients with severe corneal burns due to chemical agents can greatly benefit from a sodium hyaluronate agent (IAL 0.5%), which promotes the healing of epithelial defects. The therapeutic effect results from mechanical protection from eyelid friction and a real pharmacologic effect. Some studies performed on rabbits demonstrated that hyaluronate is naturally present in tissues, but greatly increases when the tissue has been mechanically or chemically injured. The useful physical features for this type of application are similar to those of products used to treat dry eyes. The only exception is that its concentration must be higher, as the material must achieve a greater barrier effect.

Sodium hyaluronate (IAL 0.5%) has been used to treat severe corneal cauterization caused by sulfur dioxide, and has been successfully applied in combination with cycloplegics, antibiotics, and collagenase inhibitors. In the treatment of experimental corneal cauterizations, Reim and Saric demonstrated that the time of re-epithelization was noticeably reduced in corneas treated with hyaluronate (Healon®) compared with those receiving only antibiotics.

USE OF HYALURONATE AS A VEHICLE FOR DRUGS

Hyaluronate is not used as a vehicle for drugs because it cannot bind with therapeutic substances, as demonstrated by McDermott et al in a study using radiomarked medications in vitro. Amvisc, Healon®, and Viscoat were mixed with chloramphenicol, dexamethasone, epinephrine, and pilocarpine. All were marked and placed in a semipermeable membrane for 24 hours. Researchers found that the bond of these materials with the hyaluronate ranged between 0 and 1.5%. They concluded that no interaction occurs between medications used intraoperatively and viscoelastics.

CHAPTER THIRTY-TWO

Viscocanalostomy

Robert Stegmann, MD, and Roberto Carassa, MD

Viscocanalostomy is a new surgical procedure for glaucoma therapy which has been made possible by the development of viscoelastic substances. In fact, the atraumatic dilation of Schlemm's canal, the maintenance of filtering spaces, and the inhibition of bleeding and fibrin clot formation in the surgical site have all been made possible by the use of these substances.

The procedure is nonpenetrating and independent from external filtration, thus having many important potential advantages over standard trabeculectomy. The avoidance of AC opening leads to reduced risk of infection, cataract, hypotony, and flat AC. The absence of external filtration prevents bleb formation and related discomfort, minimizes the risk of late infections, and, most important, makes the success of the procedure independent from conjunctival and episcleral scarring, which is the leading cause of failure in trabeculectomy. The procedure was first proposed in the late 1980s by one of us who mainly treats glaucoma in the African population. He was forced to develop a surgical alternative to MMC trabeculectomy, which is contraindicated in areas with poor hygienic standards owing to a greater incidence of endophthalmitis.

Viscocanalostomy allows the aqueous to leave the eye through Schlemm's canal and the episcleral veins, thus restoring the natural outflow pathway. The rationale of the technique is the evidence that the site of greater aqueous outflow resistance in open angle glaucoma is the trabecular meshwork. The procedure creates a bypass by which aqueous humor can reach Schlemm's canal while skipping the trabecular meshwork. This is obtained by producing a "chamber" inside the sclera in direct communication with Schlemm's canal. Such a chamber also communicates with the AC through the intact Descemet's membrane, which forms a "window" just anterior to the trabecular meshwork. The aqueous enters the chamber by percolating through the membrane and leaves it via Schlemm's canal.

Viscoelastics play such an important role in the procedure that they deserve mention. In fact, viscocanalostomy literally means "opening of the canal by means of viscoelastic substance." The substance of choice should have high pseudoplasticity to allow injection into Schlemm's canal through a very small needle, and a very high viscosity at a shear rate of zero to maintain the spaces as long as possible. Healon® GV is the viscoelastic that best meets these criteria and is of choice for viscocanalostomy. Recently, Healon®5 (Pharmacia & Upjohn) has also been successfully tested for use in the procedure.

SURGICAL TECHNIQUE

The use of a specific surgical set for viscocanalostomy (such as the one by Grieshaber; Switzerland) is advisable. This consists of a 0.5-mm diamond knife, a 1-mm round steel bevel-up blade, and a 165-μm blunt needle to cannulate Schlemm's

Since the completion of this book, viscoadaptive Healon®5 has been made available. Healon®5 is 2 1/2 times more viscous than Healon®GV and is an even better choice for viscocanalostomy.

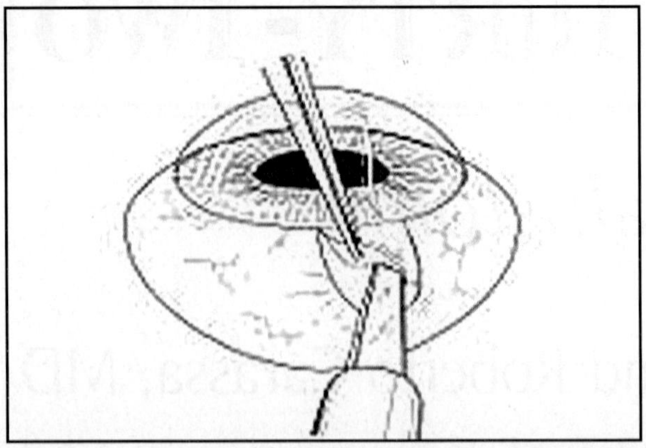

Figure 32-1. After choosing the correct plane of cut, the flap is dissected by advancing the incision with the bevel-up spatula, which allows easier following of the plane.

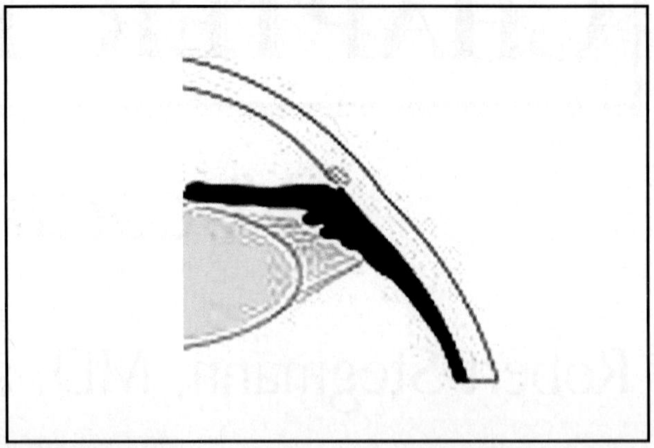

Figure 32-2. After choosing the correct plane of cut, the flap is dissected by advancing the incision with the bevel-up spatula, which allows easier following of the plane.

canal. Considering the need for precise flap dissections and accurate opening of Schlemm's canal together with its atraumatic cannulation, the use of generic instrumentation would make the surgery more difficult.

Viscocanalostomy is performed under retrobulbar or peribulbar anesthesia and usually requires 25 to 35 minutes depending on bleeding control. To avoid damage to outflow channels (eg, Schlemm's canal, aqueous veins, collector channels), cautery is used as little as possible, and bleeding is reduced by frequent irrigation of the surgical area with vasoconstrictive solutions such as ornipressin (POR 8; Sandoz, Switzerland). To provide optimal visualization of the surgical site, a bridle suture should be passed either on the superior rectus or in clear cornea.

The surgical technique can be divided into nine steps:

- Conjunctival flap dissection—Unlike all other filtering procedures, viscocanalostomy does not require any specific accuracy in the dissection of the conjunctival flap. After retrobulbar anesthesia, the procedure can be performed in any quadrant, although the upper and temporal ones are the most common choices owing to their easier access. The surgical field is prepared by creating a fornix-based conjunctival flap, using as little wet field cautery as possible.
- Outer scleral flap dissection—The outer scleral flap will form the roof of the intrascleral chamber. A 5 x 5 mm parabolic cut approximately 200 µm deep is made using the diamond knife (the incision can be outlined using a calibrated diamond knife to assure a constant depth of cut). After choosing the correct plane of cut, the flap is dissected by advancing the incision with the bevel-up spatula, which allows easier following of the plane (Figures 32-1, 32-2, and 32-3). Alternative flap shapes, such as rectangular or triangular, can be used. Using Colibri forceps and the 1-mm beveled spatula, the flap is dissected anteriorly until clear cornea is reached.
- Inner scleral flap dissection—The inner scleral flap provides access to Schlemm's canal and its removal leaves space for the intrascleral chamber. A 4 x 4 mm parabolic cut parallel to the outer incision is made beneath the outer flap. The choroidal plane must be almost reached, and this is revealed by the observation of a dark reflex at the bottom of the cut. Using the specific beveled spatula, a precise dissection is advanced until Schlemm's canal is reached and deroofed (Figure 32-4), leaving two patent openings on the lateral edges of the cut. To maintain the same plane of dissection and provide sharp lateral edges, progressive deepening of the lateral cuts is often needed.
- Paracentesis—To decrease IOP, make incannulation of Schlemm's canal easier, and reduce

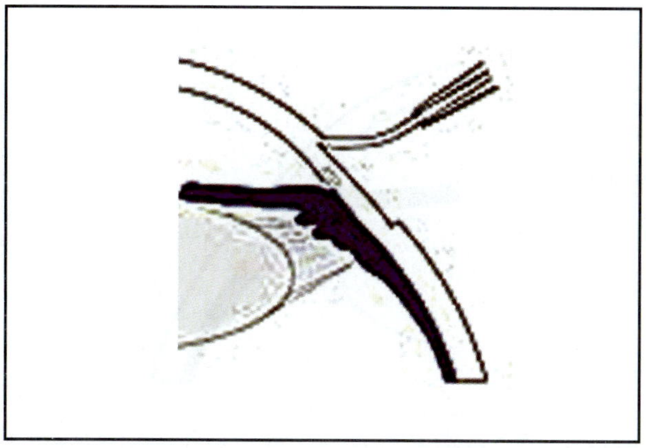

Figure 32-3. After choosing the correct plane of cut, the flap is dissected by advancing the incision with the bevel-up spatula, which allows easier following of the plane.

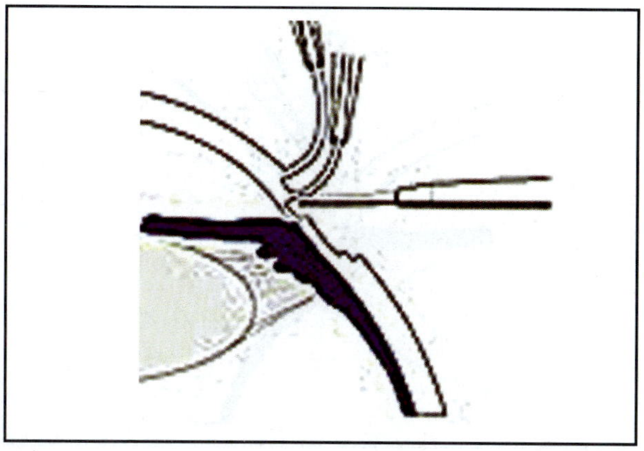

Figure 32-4. Using the specific beveled spatula, a precise dissection is advanced until Schlemm's canal is reached and deroofed, leaving two patent openings on the lateral edges of the cut.

bulging of Descemet's membrane during its cleavage from the corneal stroma, which increases the risk of tear formation, a paracentesis is made. This can be followed by aqueous drainage with an empty syringe and an AC cannula. For the same reasons and to avoid external pressure on the eye, the traction on the bridle suture is removed.

- Cannulation of Schlemm's canal—Using the specific 165-mm cannula, Healon® GV is slowly injected into Schlemm's canal by cannulating the two ostia at the lateral edges of the inner flap. To avoid damage to the canal endothelium, the insertion of the cannula should not exceed 1 to 1.5 mm from the ostia. The injection of a viscoelastic substance allows progressive atraumatic dilatation of Schlemm's canal up to 1 to 2 clock hours from the ostia. Moreover, its hemostatic properties prevent bleeding and fibrin clot formation, thus limiting healing processes and scarring of Schlemm's canal openings.
- Creation of Descemet's window—The alternative route by which aqueous humor bypasses the trabecular meshwork and reaches Schlemm's canal is a window created in the right anterior to the canal and closed by the intact Descemet's membrane, which, being permeable to aqueous, llows slow percolation. The window is realized by gently pulling the inner scleral flap upward and delicately depressing the floor of the canal and Descemet's membrane with the tip of a cotton swab (Figure 32-5). By delicately repeating the procedure, the membrane is progressively cleaved from the scleral flap. The flap itself is then advanced in the clear cornea for approximately 1 mm by a careful deepening of the lateral cuts with the tip of the diamond knife.
- Inner scleral flap excision—As soon as the window is completed, the inner scleral flap is excised using very sharp Vannas' scissors in order to avoid damage to Descemet's membrane.
- Outer scleral flap suture—The intrascleral chamber must be tightly sealed by the outer scleral flap (Figure 32-6). This is obtained by suturing it back in place with six or seven 10-0 nylon stitches. The different size of the two flaps creates a step which allows a better apposition of the external flap. Finally, Healon® GV is injected underneath the flap to temporarily fill the intrascleral lake. This controls possible bleeding and prevents collapsing and scarring of the chamber in the postoperative period.
- Closure of the conjunctiva—The procedure ends by repositioning the conjunctiva with two lateral stitches and by giving a subconjunctival injection of steroids and antibiotics.

An intrascleral chamber has thus been created. Its floor is made posteriorly by the thin scleral layer

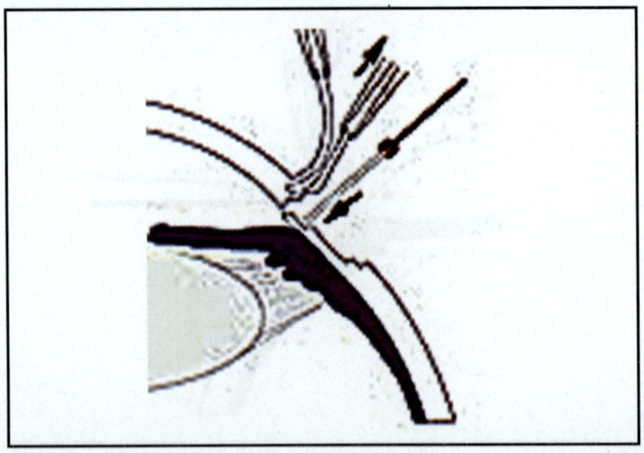

Figure 32-5. The window is realized by gently pulling the inner scleral flap upward and delicately depressing the floor of the canal and Descemet's membrane with the tip of a cotton swab.

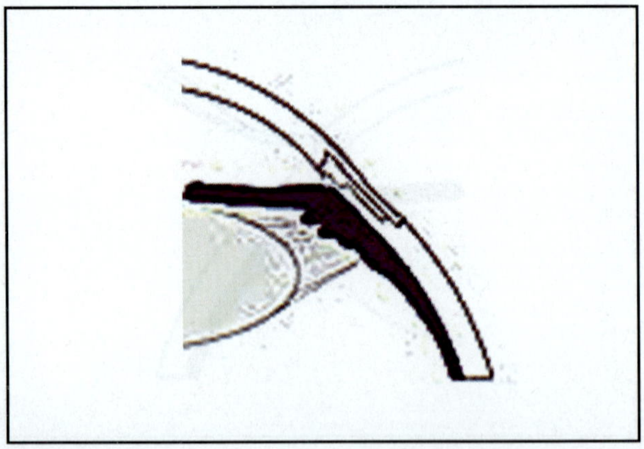

Figure 32-6. The intrascleral chamber must be tightly sealed by the outer scleral flap.

overlying the choroid, centrally by the deroofed Schlemm's canal, and anteriorly by the Descemetic window over the AC. The roof of the chamber is formed by the tightly sutured outer flap, and two openings existing in Schlemm's canal ostia are present in the lateral walls.

The aqueous humor will bypass the functionally impaired trabecular meshwork by percolating through Descemet's membrane into the intrascleral chamber. From there it will leave the eye through Schlemm's canal ostia without need of external filtration. Considering the low postoperative IOP and the anatomic configuration of the intrascleral chamber, it is likely that part of the aqueous will leave the chamber through the thin scleral layer and reach the suprachoroidal space.

Results

Although the procedure is still under investigation, preliminary reports are promising. In South Africa, one of us reported on a total of 214 eyes, with a success rate (IOP < 22 mmHg) of 82.7% without therapy and 89% with the addition of a beta blocker, over a mean follow-up of 35 months. In Italy, the procedure, performed on 33 eyes with a maximum follow-up of 10 months, allowed an IOP below 21 mmHg in 75.7% of the cases and below 16 mmHg in 69.7%, all without medications. Mean final pressure in the successful eye group was 11.8 mmHg. The procedure was graded as difficult, requiring a learning curve. Complications were minor. Twenty percent of the cases had a tear in Descemet's membrane, which caused iris to plug into the window in two eyes. One day postoperatively, a 2-mm hyphema, secondary to blood reflux in the AC, was present in 11% of the cases.

Conclusions

Viscocanalostomy appears to be a promising surgery for lowering IOP in glaucomatous eyes. It has several advantages over trabeculectomy, particularly the absence of external filtration and thus independence from conjunctival and episcleral scarring. The success rate in a limited number of cases seems high, with low final IOPs and minor complications. This procedure was made possible by the introduction of viscoelastic substances and is currently the only kind of glaucoma surgery that can be considered a true viscosurgical technique.

Chapter Thirty-Three

New Concept in Viscosurgery: Viscoadaptive Substance

Eugenio Leite, MD, PhD

Viscoelastic materials are useful and long-lived tools in ophthalmologic microsurgery. In 1937, Meyer and Palmer isolated hyaluronic acid from the cortical vitreous (concentration: 100 to 400 mg/mL). In 1958, Balazs suggested the use of hyaluronic acid as a possible substitute for the vitreous. In 1972, Balazs performed the first intravenous injection of hyaluronic acid, and during a video symposium on ocular surgery 7 years later, he presented the patent of a viscoelastic material with high molecular weight, consisting of purified hyaluronic acid, which was used in an IOL implantation.

At the same video symposium, a new terminology—viscosurgery—was born, also coined by Balazs. The use of viscoelastic became increasingly popular, allowing an advantage for a number of different steps of cataract techniques—namely, capsulorhexis, viscoexpression, small incision techniques, and foldable IOL implantation.

However, viscosurgery procedures are not limited to cataract surgery. They are now routinely used in antiglaucoma filtering surgery, combined surgical interventions, keratoplasty, and anterior vitrectomy.

Viscoelastics have a wide range of features with rheologic-related properties—namely, viscosity, elasticity, pseudoplasticity, and cohesiveness—and chemical characteristics (Table 33-1). Although the properties exist independently, they act synergistically. The same viscoelastic can be used as different tools according to specific needs, such as to separate or join tissues, maintain space, or protect surfaces (ie, corneal endothelium, lens capsule, or anterior hyaloid) from mechanical shocks or infusion fluids (Table 33-2). Sodium hyaluronate (Healon®) is now the most widely used viscoelastic in ophthalmic surgery and has become the gold standard against which all other viscoelastics are compared.

The production and use of viscoelastics require ongoing research regarding the evaluation of biocompatibility, purity, and ocular structure protection. In vivo studies have proven that the molecular and chemical structure of the material is ideal, and interactions between molecules and receptor tissues and inflammatory and immunogenic reactions have also been extensively studied.

All these issues could be summarized in a simple but very strong and fundamental statement: "ophthalmic surgery has become safer.

The development of new surgical techniques and consequently of IOLs—specifically, phacoemulsification and foldable IOLs—led to the development of new forms of viscoelastics. In 1992, a new standard viscoelastic, Healon® GV, was introduced to fulfill the needs of new techniques, such as phacoemulsification.

The main characteristics of viscoelastics include:

- Cohesiveness—The extent to which a material can stick to itself, this is a function of molecular weight and concentration, proportional to viscosity at zero shear rate. Basically, viscoelastic substances with high molecular weight tend to have high cohesiveness and those with low molecular weight have low cohesiveness. Another important feature is that viscoelastic substances with high cohesiveness will tend to be easily removed from the eye as a mass and those with low cohesiveness tend to fragment and become dispersive.
- Viscosity—The resistance to flow. Dynamic viscosity becomes apparent when shear is applied.

Table 33-1.
VISCOELASTICS FEATURES

General	Molecular
Transparency	Concentration
Purity/degree of biocompatibility	Viscosity
Nontoxicity/degree of softness	Elasticity
Inertia	Pseudoplasticity
pH	Cohesiveness

Table 33-2.
USEFULNESS OF VISCOELASTIC MATERIALS

Need	Solution
Creation of volume	Provide AC depth Stretch capsular bag
Space maintenance	Stabilize mydriasis Facilitate IOL implantation Act as vitreous counterpressure
Facilitated manipulation	Capsulorhexis Phacoemulsification Solving synechiae
Tissue protection	Corneal endothelium Iris Blood/aqueous barrier

It is indicated by an h and the units are centipoise. Viscosity is dependent on molecular weight (length of the chain, size of the molecule), concentration of the material, temperature, and solvent used. High viscosity can be obtained in two ways: increasing the concentration of a molecule or increasing the length of the molecule chain without affecting its concentration.

- Pseudoplasticity—The capacity to pass from a high to a low value of viscosity. The viscosity of a viscoelastic is determined by its shear rate. Pseudoplasticity is the basic feature of viscoelastic material. Changing its rheologic state allows the surgeon to use it as a surgical tool. Because pseudoplasticity is a function of viscosity at low and high shear rates, Healon® GV has the highest degree of pseudoplasticity among the current viscoelastics.
- Elasticity—The ability of the polymer of the viscoelastics to regain its original shape after being compressed, deformed, or elongated. Elasticity allows the molecule to absorb the energy of impact rather than passing that energy on to the tissue and causing damage. Basically, viscoelastics with long molecular chains are more elastic than those with short molecular chains, such as Healon® GV.

The different rheologic properties of the viscoelastic substance will determine its functions and applications during surgery.

Table 33-3.
CORRELATION BETWEEN VISCOELASTICS SUBSTANCES (VES) AND SURGICAL STEPS

Surgical Steps	Cohesive Type of VES	Dispersive Type of VES
Injection/AC filling	Bolus or small amount No bubbles No cleavage surfaces Transparent Create space—good	Chains (not bolus) Bubbles Cleavage surfaces (VES–BSS) Not transparent Create space—poor
Capsulorhexis	Spatula effect Soft Permanent	Spatula effect Not soft/mechanical Transient
Phaco/AC maneuvers	Leak from AC (++) No bubbles Cleavage surfaces (–)	Bubbles Cleavage surfaces (+)
Filling the bag /IOL implantation	+/Easy	–/Difficult (risk of overfilling AC)
Removal	Easy (mass)	Difficult (fractures)
Complications		
PC rupture	+/Better	–/Worse

Based on physical and chemical properties, viscoelastic substances can be divided into two groups: cohesive viscoelastic substances, which have high molecular weight; and dispersive viscoelastic substances, which have low molecular weight. These two groups are divided essentially by molecular weight and have specific surgical targets.

Viscoelastics that are very cohesive with high viscosity (Healon® GV, Healon®, Provisc, Amvisc Plus, Amvisc, and Biolon) are useful for creating space and stabilizing the tissues. Viscoelastics that are very dispersive with low viscosity and lower cohesiveness (Viscoat, Vitrax, and the methylcellulose products) will break very easily when injected into the eye and will disperse in fragments. They have a tendency to form a layer that will adhere to and coat different structures of the eye.

There is no agreement within the surgical community as to which viscoelastic type better protects the corneal endothelium. Some surgeons and researchers believe dispersive viscoelastic substances are better. However, others consider cohesive viscoelastic substances a better option as they form chemical bonds with the cornea or iris and protect the ocular structures against the release of free radicals during phacoemulsification. Chemical bonds are a better basis for protection than is mechanical protection (Table 33-3).

The ideal substance should be able to combine characteristics from both types and fulfill additional requirements (Table 33-4). At this stage, one product in particular is close to achieving these criteria. A new product, Healon®5, was presented during the 1998 European Society of Cataract and Refractive Surgery (ESCRS) meeting held in Nice, France. This product is a departure from the traditional viscoelastic concept and marks the introduction of a new one—the viscoadaptives. This product, besides having the function of the viscoelastics products, also adapts to environmental changes during the different types of anterior segment surgery.

During low flow or low turbulence, Healon®5 becomes highly viscous and acts as a cohesive device, thus maintaining chamber space better than a viscoelastic. Healon®5 remains in the AC during phacoemulsification as a retentive shield maintaining space and protecting the cornea. This effect is obtained by a high degree of molecular entangle-

Table 33-4.
IDEAL PRODUCT REQUIREMENTS OR CHARACTERISTICS

1. Easy to inject
2. Good space maintenance
3. Ocular structure protection (corneal endothelium, blood/aqueous barrier)
4. Ocular structure coatability
5. Ocular structure mechanical protection (impact)
6. Ocular structure chemical protection (free radical scavenger)
7. Allowing tissue manipulation (synechiae, posterior chamber rupture)
8. Easy to remove (transient IOP up)

ment. Because it has very high viscosity, it creates space, absorbs shock, and protects the eye from trauma during phacoemulsification, intraocular maneuvers, and IOL implantation. During the 1998 ESCRS symposium, Dr. S. Arshinoff stated that Healon®5 is a very viscous retentive soft surgical tool, the first of new generation of viscoadaptives. The viscosity at rest (ie, at 0 shear rate) is 7 million centipoise, a viscosity higher than any other viscoelastic product. During the same symposium, Arshinoff concluded with a sentence that defines the advantages of this new viscoadaptive: "this high viscosity, cohesive viscoadaptive—Healon®5—represents a far more responsive soft surgical tool at different shear rates than hitherto seemed available." These properties are likely to increase security during phaco and facilitate other stages of cataract surgery when compared to currently available viscoelastics.

USEFULNESS OF THE VISCOADAPTIVES

Table 33-5 summarizes the different steps of surgery in which a viscoelastic product is needed. In the following, we explain how this new viscoadaptive will affect each step of the surgical procedure.

ANTERIOR CHAMBER—FILLING AND MAINTENANCE

To optimize results throughout the phacoemulsification procedure, it is important that the viscoadaptive maintain a good, deep AC so the surgeon can perform all the surgical maneuvers. The viscoelastic product should be easy to inject, keep a deep AC, protect the ocular structures, and be transparent. This means having a high viscosity with 0 shear rate, high pseudoplasticity, and high transparency. This combination was achieved in a better blend with Healon®5 when compared with Viscoat, assuming one is the standard for phacoemulsification (Table 33-5, item 1).

CAPSULORHEXIS

One of the essential steps of phacoemulsification is performing a proper continuous curvilinear capsulorhexis, which requires four basic elements of the viscoelastic: 1) high molecular weight and high viscosity with 0 shear rate; 2) transparency; 3) ability to act as a soft permanent spatula; and 4) high pseudoplasticity and elasticity.

Healon® GV was considered the ideal substance for performing both filling and maintaining of the AC and capsulorhexis; however, Healon®5, in a qualitative five-degree scale, showed a very high performance rate (Table 33-5, items 1 and 2).

HYDRODISSECTION/HYDRODELINIATION

Two main points should be kept in mind by the surgeon at this step of phacoemulsification. First, the injected fluid wave should be able to circulate freely, not exercising excessive pressure on the posterior capsule or the zonules. Second, the viscoelastic product should protect these ocular structures from the turbulence of the fluids and the surgeon's maneuvers. The ideal product should have high viscosity at a low shear rate, be highly cohesive, and be highly pseudoplastic. One essential adjust-

Table 33-5.
SURGERY STEPS WHEN A VISCOELASTIC PRODUCT IS NEEDED

1. AC—filling and maintenance
2. Capsulorhexis
3. Hydrodissection/hydrodeliniation
4. Phacoemulsification
5. Irrigation and aspiration procedure
6. Capsular bag filling/IOL implantation

ment in surgical technique while performing this surgical step is to take care not to overfill the AC. If one uses a slow and steady injection force, he or she can feel the fullness of the AC through the syringe. Owing to the characteristics of this viscoadaptive, it is sufficient to fill the AC by covering and coating the ocular structures; this will create and maintain the shape of the AC. Proper filling of the AC will leave enough space for the previously described surgical maneuvers. This viscoadaptive productís dispersive–cohesive characteristics will allow for a good performance of all intraocular maneuvers, including the following step—phacoemulsification.

PHACOEMULSIFICATION

During this step, there will be a certain number of nuclear fragments floating in the AC, air bubbles through cavitation, and a high degree of fluid turbulence and exchange, regardless of which technique is chosen by the surgeon. The viscoelastic product should protect not only the corneal endothelium but also the other ocular structures. It should absorb free radicals generated by the emulsification, maintain space in the AC, and not leave the AC in an uncontrolled manner. The viscoadaptives have several properties that fulfill these requirements; specifically, they are supercohesive, with a high degree of elasticity to absorb the mechanical vibrations. They are also pseudoplastic and easily removed.

Another important issue at this stage is the maintenance of a deep AC. This is influenced by the machine settings, bottle height, flow rate, vacuum setting (based on the type of pump), and phaco power. Healon®5 protects the ocular structures as it deepens the AC.

IRRIGATION AND ASPIRATION

The viscoelastic product should have the same behavior as described in phacoemulsification. It should allow removal of the remaining cortex while maintaining the AC. This should be completed while providing protection of the ocular structures.

CAPSULAR BAG FILLING/IOL IMPLANTATION

For this step, the viscoadaptive should be easily injected in the bag, reinflate the capsular bag, have good visibility, and allow for safe implantation of the IOL. The properties that allow Healon®5 to accomplish this are its high viscosity, pseudoplasticity, and cohesiveness. Healon®5 should be injected gently into the capsular bag. Because Healon®5 has remained in the AC, not as much will be needed when the capsular bag is reinflated.

Another important feature of this new generation of viscoadaptives is related to elastic property. The viscoadaptives provide protection to the ocular structures as the IOL unfolds. Because of its high molecular weight, Healon®5 acts as a buffer for ocular tissues as it absorbs the force of the unfolding IOL.

REMOVAL OF VISCOADAPTIVES

With this new generation of viscoadaptives, it is essential to remove them completely to prevent one of the most common complications—ocular hypertension. Owing to their supercohesive features, the surgeon should be completely educated on different removal techniques. Our experience shows that there are two ways to remove Healon®5 successfully. The first technique is a variation of the rock and roll technique. With proper machine settings, the Healon®5 is removed from the AC. Then, the irrigation and aspiration handpiece is placed on the optic as it is rocked back and forth, allowing the viscoadaptive to flow from behind the bag to the AC where it can be removed. Sweeping the irrigation and aspiration handpiece around the AC is important to remove all the viscoadaptive from the AC angle. A second technique is used to ensure complete removal of the viscoadaptive from behind the IOL. This is achieved by going behind the IOL with the irrigation and aspiration tip into the capsular bag immediately after IOL implantation without starting the flow of irrigation fluid. One can easily view the Healon®5 moving out from behind the optic. With the irrigation and aspiration still running, the surgeon can move the tip on top of the optic and finish removal at the iris plane. Sweeping the irrigation and aspiration handpiece around the AC is important to remove all the viscoadaptive from the AC angle.

The Portuguese Experience with Healon®5—University of Coimbra

Study Rationale

A study was performed to compare the new viscoadaptive agent (Healon®5) with a commercially available viscoelastic (Viscoat). The study was conducted on an open, randomized, parallel-group, single-center, phase III basis. Six different variables were evaluated, together with an overall assessment of the performance of the two products during phacoemulsification with IOL implantation.

Objectives

Primary Efficacy Endpoint

An overall assessment of Healon®5 in comparison with Viscoat, using a five-graded scale.

Secondary Efficacy Endpoints

Assess the following six secondary endpoints on the same basis:

- Ease of injection of the viscoelastic solutions
- Maintenance capacity of AC depth during continuous curvilinear capsulorhexis
- Ability of both products to stay in the eye during phacoemulsification
- Facilitation of IOL implantation
- Ease of removing the products at the end of surgery
- IOP development throughout the study

The final results of this study are scheduled to be published. Experience gained during this study and years of surgical experience are the basis for this chapter.

Blood/Aqueous Barrier Breakdown Evaluation

A pilot study involving 20 patients was performed to evaluate the breakdown of the blood/aqueous barrier in patients submitted to phacoemulsification with IOL implantation. There were two groups of 10 patients. Healon®5 was used in Group A and Viscoat in Group B.

All patients were submitted to a blood/aqueous barrier breakdown evaluation through anterior segment fluorometry before surgery and 1 month after surgery. No statistical analysis was performed because of the small sample, but there was a trend in favor of Healon®5, showing more suitable protection of the blood/aqueous barrier.

Comments

Based on the Portuguese study that evaluated safety, efficacy, and blood/aqueous barrier, we conclude the following with regard to viscoadaptives.

First, with respect to cases of increased IOP, research has shown that there is clearly a learning curve in the management of this new product. Complete removal of any viscoelastic/viscoadaptive is important to minimize postoperative IOP rises. Results in the second group of patients demonstrate that this issue is irrelevant as long as the surgeon keeps it in mind and adjusts his or her removal technique to the specific product. With experience, this new removal technique will not result in an increase in surgical time.

Second, with respect to efficacy, even on a qualitative scale, the advantages of using viscoadaptives are evident throughout the main steps of phacoemulsification. It is as if they are two different products combined—one with dispersive properties and a second with cohesive properties. The first viscoadaptive showed several major advantages; namely, it creates space between tissues, allows complete control of surgical instruments, and provides unsurpassed corneal endothelium cell protection.

Third, with respect to blood/aqueous barrier breakdown, despite a small number of patients, a trend was shown in favor of the viscoadaptive in reducing blood/aqueous barrier breakdown. Further randomized, double-blind studies are needed.

At the viscosurgery session of the 1998 ESCRS meeting, it was made clear that "Healon®5, as the first member of the viscoadaptives, clearly represents an evolutionary step in contributing toward improving the quality of the ocular surgery that we perform."

Chapter Thirty-Four

The Dispersive–Cohesive Viscoelastic Soft Shell Technique

Steve A. Arshinoff, MD, FRCSC

This chapter was written before the development of Healon®5 and the discussion therefore does not refer to it. The reader is referred to Chapter 35 for a discussion of that viscoelastic. The advent of Healon®5 does not make the soft shell technique obsolete. It divides ophthalmologists into two groups based on their preference for a universal, generally applicable viscoelastic system. The first group will be the "soft shell group," which wants the benefits of using two classes of viscoelastics with disparate properties together to obtain the maximum rheologic potential from each group simultaneously. The second group will include the ophthalmologists who feel most comfortable working in a high-viscosity environment and have generally preferred highly viscous, cohesive viscoelastics. However, the advent of the soft shell technique has made this group aware of the deficiencies of viscous, cohesive viscoelastics, and even more aware of the tremendous benefits these devices have to offer. This group will be the first to recognize the unique potential of the viscoadaptive Healon®5, and will gravitate toward that option.

Recognizing that the two groups are very different leads to an awareness of their individual advantages and drawbacks. My advice to the reader is to study and understand both approaches to viscosurgery and learn to use both techniques. As in all other surgeries, every surgeon will eventually come across a situation in which one of these two choices is clearly superior to the other in managing a unique surgical problem. Even if that never happens, an understanding of both approaches will provide a working knowledge of the options available with the wide variety of viscoelastics on the market, and the surgeon will better use whatever viscoelastic is chosen, having gained that knowledge. The discussion to follow will not include Healon®5, because a discussion of a competitive strategy while trying to explain the soft shell technique would make explanations unreasonably complicated. The reader is again referred to the chapter on Healon®5—Chapter 35—for that discussion.

There was a large variety of ophthalmic viscoelastics available for use in cataract and intraocular surgery (Table 34-1) even before the advent of Healon®5, each possessing differing chemical and physical rheologic properties. The question of which is the best viscoelastic for cataract surgery has led the chapter author to a 15-year investigation of the rheologic properties of viscoelastics that are most important in anterior segment surgery.

This chapter is reprinted with permission from the Journal of Cataract and Refractive Surgery. A paper upon which the chapter was based was presented in part by the author at the annual meeting of the American Society of Cataract and Refractive Surgery; Seattle, Washington; June 3, 1996. This study was supported in part by The Toronto Eye Foundation, Toronto, Canada.

Table 34-1.

OPHTHALMIC VISCOELASTICS: CONTENT, MOLECULAR WEIGHT & ZERO-SHEAR VISCOSITY

HIGHER VISCOSITY-COHESIVE VISCOELASTICS

Viscoelastic	Content	MW(D)	V0(mPs)
Super Viscous-Cohesive Viscoelastics (V0 > 1M):			
MicroVisc (iVisc) Plus	1.4% NaHa	7.9M	4.8M
Healon® GV	1.4% NaHa	5.0M	2.0M
Viscous-Cohesive Viscoelastics (1M>V0 > 100K):			
MicroVisc (iVisc)	1.4% NaHa	6.1M	1.0M
Allervisc (Viscorneal)Plus	1.4% NaHa	5.1M	500K
Provisc	1.0% NaHa	2.0M	280K
Healon®	1.0% NaHa	4.0M	230K
Biolon	1.0% NaHa	3.0M	215K
Allervisc (Viscorneal)	1.0% NaHa	5.1M	200K
Amvisc	1.2% NaHa	1.0M	100K
Amvisc Plus	1.6% NaHa	1.0M	100K

MW(D) = molecular weight (Daltons)
V_0(mPs) = 0 shear viscosity (milli Pascal-seconds)
M = million, K = thousand

LOWER VISCOSITY-DISPERSIVE VISCOELASTICS

Viscoelastic	Content	MW(D)	V0(mPs)
Medium Viscosity Dispersive Viscoelastics (100K>V0 > 10K):			
Viscoat	3.0% NaHa 4.0% CDS	500K 25K	50K
Cellugel	2.0% chemically modified HPMC	100K	40K
Vitrax	3.0% Ha	500K	25K
Very Low Viscosity Dispersive Viscoelastics (10K>V0 > 1K):			
i-Cell	2.0% HPMC	90K	6.0K
Ocuvis	2.0% HPMC	90K	4.3K
Occucoat	2.0% HPMC	86K	4K
Hymecel	2.0% HPMC	86K	4K
Adatocel	2.0% HPMC	86K	4K
Visilon	2.0% HPMC	86K	4K

NaHa = sodium hyaluronate
HPMC = hydroxypropylmethylcellulose
CDS = chondroitin sulfate

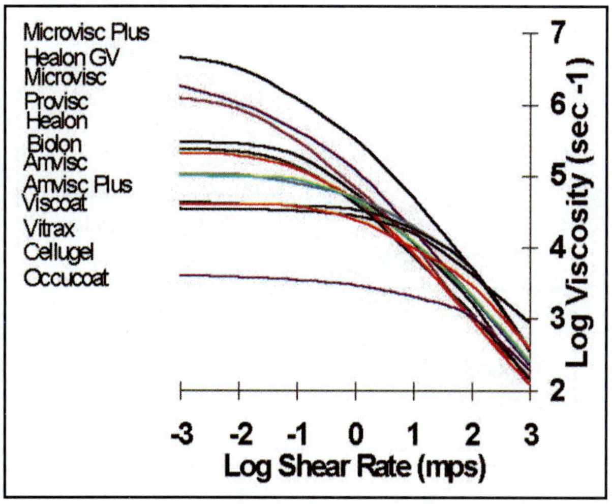

Figure 34-1. Pseudoplasticity curves of common commercial ophthalmic viscoelastics. These curves are usually plotted as shown here with log dynamic viscosity (milliPascal-seconds) versus log shear rate (seconds^{-1}). The zero shear or stationary viscosity is the level at the far left of each curve, and is indicative of the ability of the viscoelastic to maintain space when stationary. The viscosity level in the mid shear rate ranges (10^{-1} to 10^{1}) represents the resistance offered by the viscoelastic to the normal rate of movement of surgical instruments through the eye during surgery. The viscosity at high rates of shear (about 10^{3}) is indicative of the resistance offered by the viscoelastic to flow through a small cannula. Different laboratories report these data with significant variation. It is therefore wise to consider differences of less than 10% in any given point as equivalent.

Despite this effort and a lengthy competitive dialogue among ophthalmologists and pharmaceutical companies, no general consensus on the "ideal viscoelastic" has emerged, as demonstrated by the essentially unchanged market share distribution of vastly different viscoelastics over the last decade. Healon®5 now claims to be viscoadaptive, and undoubtedly is more suited than anything before to lay claim to the title of "ideal viscoelastic"; however, experience is needed to validate that claim. The lack of consensus on what is best suggests that different viscoelastic properties may be useful to ophthalmic surgeons in different surgical situations, frequently during the same surgical operation. Therefore, instead of looking for the best viscoelastic, the author aimed to analyze their differing properties to develop a new surgical approach, using cohesive and dispersive viscoelastics sequentially, avoiding mixing, which fully takes advantage of the positive attributes of each type of viscoelastic while minimizing the drawbacks.

CLASSIFICATION OF OPHTHALMIC VISCOELASTICS

Given the chemical constraints that a viscoelastic preparation intended for intraocular use must be an isotonic, pH balanced, aqueous solution, the acceptable ranges of physical properties are governed by the molecular nature, chain length, and concentration of the rheologically active polymer constituent in a given viscoelastic. Concentration of the rheologically active agent affects viscosity primarily in the middle range of shear rates, and not at 0 shear (or stationary) viscosity. To devise a simple, surgically useful classification system for ophthalmic viscoelastics, it is essential to identify, as criteria, the rheologic parameters that best apply to the viscoelastic in terms of its behavior in surgery. Currently, the two most useful parameters for such a classification are 0 shear viscosity and cohesive or dispersive behavior (relative degree of cohesion).

Zero shear viscosity correlates with the molecular weight of the rheologically active viscoelastic component and can be used to establish a ranking of ophthalmic viscoelastics for the purpose of classification (Table 34-1, Figure 34-1). Long-chain ophthalmic viscoelastic molecules tend to entangle in solution, causing them to aggregate, and are therefore referred to as cohesive. As 0 shear viscosity declines below 100,000 mPs (milliPascal–seconds, previously centipoise [cps], with 1 mPs = 1 cp, the dynamic viscosity of water), molecular chain entanglement becomes a far less significant factor. Consequently, less viscous viscoelastics tend to be easily broken up, and are accordingly referred to as dispersive. Because cohesion of all currently marketed viscoelastics correlates with 0 shear viscosity and with molecular weight of the rheologically active constituent (but not in a simple, linear relationship), degree of cohesion falls neatly into the

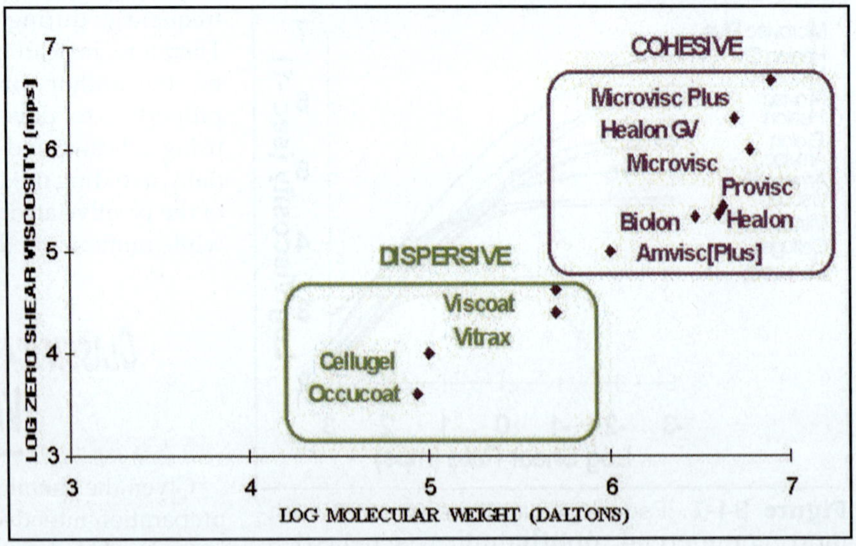

Figure 34-2. Cohesive and dispersive viscoelastics. Relative cohesion of ophthalmic viscoelastics correlates with zero shear viscosity and molecular weight. When viscoelastics are plotted on a graph where log zero shear viscosity is on the ordinate, and log molecular weight on the abscissa, cohesive and dispersive viscoelastics cluster in their respective groups.

same classification with 0 shear viscosity (Figure 34-2). Future viscoelastics may be manufactured with viscosity and cohesion somewhat dissociated from each other, consequently not correlating as well, and therefore one of these parameters alone is insufficient for classification. The tasks for which ophthalmic viscoelastics are used in surgery are generally facilitated by higher 0 shear viscosity, but in some cases a dispersive nature may be preferable to cohesion (eg, if one wants to retain a thick layer of viscoelastic adjacent to the corneal endothelium during vigorous irrigation of the AC with a phacoemulsifier or an irrigation and aspiration handpiece). Therefore, it is very useful when assessing for surgical utility to classify ophthalmic viscoelastics based on 0 shear viscosity as well as cohesive or dispersive nature.

Higher Viscosity—Cohesive Viscoelastics

All current ophthalmic viscoelastics in this category possess, as their active rheologic agent, various concentrations and chain lengths of non crosslinked, long-chain hyaluronic acid, and have zero shear dynamic viscosities greater than 100,000 mPs. Super viscous cohesive viscoelastics, a subcategory that includes MicroVisc (iVisc in Canada) Plus and Healon® GV, have zero shear viscosities exceeding 1,000,000 mPs. Viscous cohesive viscoelastics—including, among others, MicroVisc, Allervisc (Viscorneal) Plus, Provisc, Healon®, Biolon, Allervisc (Viscorneal), Amvisc, and Amvisc Plus (Table 34-1)—possess 0 shear viscosities between 100,000 and 1,000,000 mPs. Clinical trials have shown that various members of each of these subcategories share similar physical properties, behave in a similar fashion intraoperatively, and lead to comparable surgical results, except that the super viscous cohesive viscoelastics appear to have an advantage over the regular viscous cohesive viscoelastics in facilitating surgical maneuvers, ease of removal, and endothelial protection.

Zero shear viscosity also correlates well with elasticity. Highly viscous cohesive viscoelastics are best at creating space with their viscosity, preserving it by being elastic and displacing and stabilizing tissues in the surgical environment. IOP can only be induced in an unsealed eye with an elastic substance and consequently only the highly viscous cohesive elastic viscoelastics are capable of neutralizing positive posterior pressure, which is always present to some extent in cases of topical or intracameral anesthesia (because the extraocular muscles are not paralyzed), by pressurizing the AC to a degree equal to the posterior pressure. I have termed this viscoelastic pressure neutralized situation "pressure equalized cataract surgery," which can only be accomplished with viscous cohesive and super viscous cohesive viscoelastics. A pressure equalized AC stabilizes the lens during capsulorhexis by flattening out the anterior lens capsule, thus reducing the risk of errant tears, facilitating

Table34-2.
BEST SURGICAL USES FOR VISCOELASTIC GROUPS

HIGHER VISCOSITY-COHESIVE	LOWER VISCOSITY-DISPERSIVE
To create and stabilize spaces	*To selectively isolate and partition spaces*
To deepen the AC in hyperopic eyes to insert phaco	To protect corneas with Fuchs' Endothelial Dystrophy
To stabilize a difficult capsulorhexis	To isolate a piece of frayed iris from aspiration by the phaco tip
To enlarge small pupils	To isolate an area of disinseted zonules
To dissect adhesions	To isolate vitreous behind a small hole in the posterior capsule
To implant foldable intraocular lenses	To partition the AC

soft lens implantation, stabilizing the viscoelastic expanded capsular bag, and preventing it from developing folds in the posterior capsule as the IOL is being inserted and unfolded.

The high cohesion of viscous cohesive and super viscous cohesive viscoelastics results in the ease of removal by irrigation and aspiration at the end of the surgical procedure. However, owing to the cohesive behavior, cohesive viscoelastics leave the AC rapidly during phaco, except for a thin layer of hyaluronate, which remains bound to the endothelial cell membrane specific binding sites. This permits a clear, unobstructed view of the posterior capsule. Sometimes the early disappearance of cohesive viscoelastics from the AC during phaco can lead to suboptimal corneal endothelial protection during the turbulence of phacoemulsification. Furthermore, cohesive viscoelastics are unable to partition fluid spaces in the AC. In other words, using a cohesive viscoelastic renders it impossible to envelop a structure on one side of the AC and then go back in with either the irrigation and aspiration tip or phaco to work on the other side of the AC. Doing so would result in dragging the viscoelastic back into the aspiration port, along with the tissue the surgeon wanted sequestered.

Consequently, the higher viscosity cohesive viscoelastics are best used to create space and stability where it is otherwise inadequate. This may include expanding a shallow AC in a hyperopic patient to facilitate the insertion of a phacoemulsification tip, creating a pressure-equalized environment to facilitate a difficult capsulorhexis, enlarging small pupils, dissecting adhesions, and implanting foldable IOLs (Table 34-2).

LOWER VISCOSITY DISPERSIVE VISCOELASTICS

Lower viscosity dispersive viscoelastics may be defined as those with a 0 shear viscosity of less than 100,000 mPs (to date, all have zero shear viscosities less than 50,000 mPs). In viscoelastics that have zero-shear viscosities below this level, molecular chain entanglement becomes far less important and cohesion tends to be significantly weaker, resulting in a tendency for them to disperse when injected into the AC. The medium viscosity dispersive viscoelastics, the first subgroup of this group, possess 0 shear viscosities between 10,000 and 100,000 mPs, and include Viscoat, Cellugel, and Vitrax. The second subgroup—the very low viscosity dispersive viscoelastics, consisting of all the unmodified HPMCs—includes iCell, Ocuvis, Occucoat, Adatocel, Hymecel, Visilon, Celoftal, and many others (Table 34-1).

Surgically, the most useful properties of dispersive viscoelastics are their resistance to aspiration and their ability to partition spaces. Their dispersive nature is one of the factors, along with negative electrical charge and the presence of hyaluronic acid to bind to specific binding sites, that improves the retention of viscoelastics in the AC, adjacent to the corneal endothelium, throughout phacoemulsification and irrigation/aspiration. Dispersive viscoelastics are also extremely useful in situations when it may be necessary to move or isolate a single structure in the AC selectively (eg, holding back vitreous at an area of zonule disinsertion). They are capable of partitioning the AC into a viscoelastic-occupied space and a surgical zone in which phaco or irrigation and aspiration can be continued, without the two areas mixing.

The major drawback of lower viscosity dispersive viscoelastics is that their relatively low viscosity and elasticity do not allow them to maintain or stabilize spaces as well as higher viscosity cohesive viscoelastics (eg, in the performance of a capsulorhexis or implantation of a foldable IOL). In other words, their decreased cohesion can be used to the advantage of the surgeon, but their lower viscosity and elasticity is a definite drawback. In addition, lower viscosity dispersive viscoelastics tend to be aspirated in small fragments during phaco and irrigation and aspiration, leading to an irregular viscoelastic/aqueous interface that partially obscures the surgeon's view of the posterior capsule during phacoemulsification. The microbubbles that form during phacoemulsification tend to become trapped in this irregular interface, further obscuring the surgeon's view of the posterior capsule and rendering surgical maneuvers in the posterior chamber more difficult.

Lower viscosity dispersive viscoelastics, because of their low cohesion, are more difficult to remove at the end of the surgical procedure. Assia et al demonstrated, in a controlled in vitro study, that lower viscosity dispersive viscoelastics such as Viscoat, Occucoat, and Orcolon may take more than seven times longer to remove than highly viscous cohesive viscoelastics such as Healon® and Healon® GV. The additional manipulation and aspiration required to remove dispersive viscoelastics completely may actually increase the likelihood of complications, such as endothelial damage or puncturing of the posterior capsule.

Lower viscosity dispersive viscoelastics are most advantageous when dealing with problematic cases such as zonule disinsertions, small holes in the posterior capsule, a frayed piece of the iris, and Fuch's endothelial dystrophy, the latter being a situation in which the surgeon specifically wants to isolate the corneal endothelial cells from the phaco procedure's turbulent flow (Table 34-2).

The Dispersive–Cohesive Soft Shell Technique

The dispersive–cohesive viscoelastic soft-shell technique is a method that uses dispersive and cohesive viscoelastics sequentially to derive the benefits of both viscoelastic types and eliminate the drawbacks of each. If optimal results are to be achieved, the viscoelastics should not mix in the eye, but should occupy adjacent spaces within the AC.

The technique relies on three principles:

- A pressurized elastic device (eg, a cohesive viscoelastic) in a confined space will transmit pressure through adjacent fluids within the confined space to pressurize the entire space.
- A dispersive viscoelastic will maintain its dispersive characteristics when subjected to moderate pressure from an adjacent cohesive fluid.
- Two rheologically dissimilar but both transparent viscoelastics can be placed in adjacent spaces within the AC without mixing and without blurring the surgeon's view, to take maximum advantage of the unique properties of each viscoelastic, in the exact location where it is most needed.

Method

At the commencement of the surgical cataract procedure, a lower viscosity dispersive viscoelastic, such as Viscoat, is injected into the AC first, and a mound is formed on the anterior surface of the lens (Figure 34-3). A high viscosity cohesive viscoelastic, such as Provisc or Healon® GV, is then injected into the posterior center of the lower viscosity dispersive viscoelastic mound, such that the incoming viscous cohesive viscoelastic fills the center of the eye and pushes the lower viscosity dispersive viscoelastic up and out, eventually forming a smooth, even, pressurized layer adjacent to the corneal endothelium. The high viscosity cohesive viscoelas-

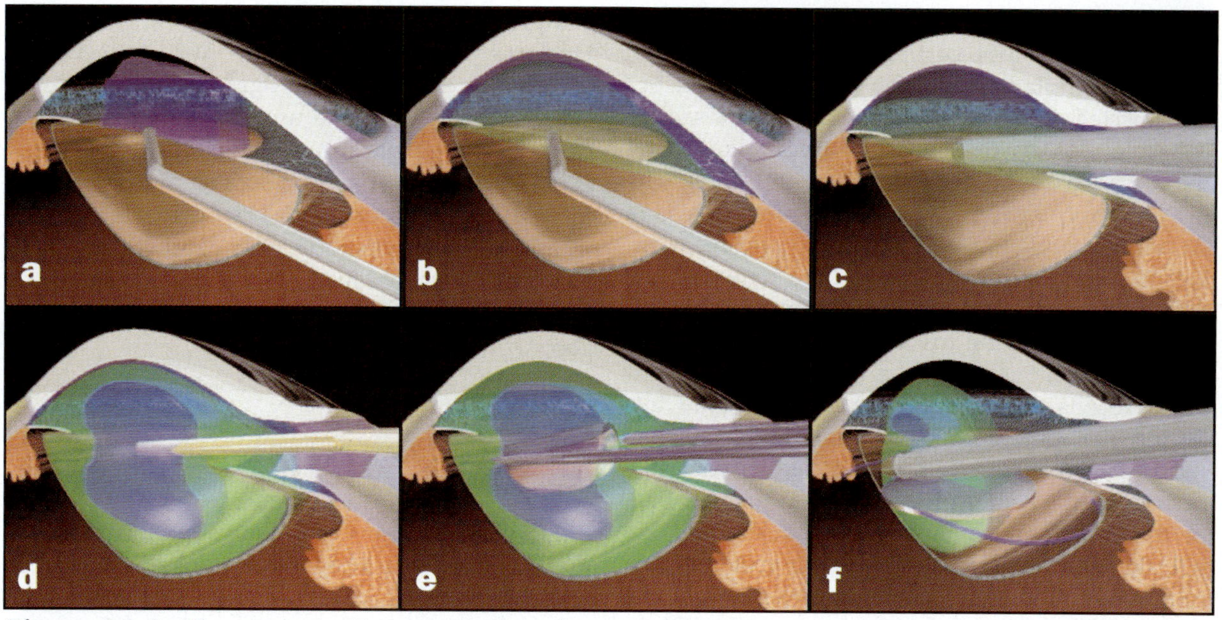

Figure 34-3. The viscoelastic soft-shell technique. (a) The lower viscosity dispersive viscoelastic (violet) is injected first to form a mound on the surface of the center of the cataractous lens. (b) The higher viscosity cohesive viscoelastic (green) is injected into the posterior center of the lower viscosity dispersive viscoelastic, such that continued injection pushes the lower viscosity dispersive viscoelastic upward and outward, finally pressurizing it into a smooth layer against the corneal endothelial cells. (c) After performance of the capsulorhexis, when the phaco is begun, the higher viscosity cohesive viscoelastic (green) rapidly leaves the eye, leaving behind the smooth layer of lower viscosity dispersive viscoelastic (violet) ironed out against the corneal endothelial cells, which remains largely intact throughout the phaco and irrigation and aspiration procedures. (d) After completion of removal of the nucleus and cortex, the viscoelastics are injected in reverse order. The higher viscosity cohesive viscoelastic (green) is injected first to stabilize the iris, capsule, and AC. The lower viscosity dispersive viscoelastic (violet) is then injected into its center, placing the cannula tip approximately in the geographic center of the capsulorhexis. (e) The presence of the lower viscosity dispersive viscoelastic (violet) in the center of the higher viscosity cohesive viscoelastic mass (green) allows freer movement of the incoming IOL with better stabilization of the surrounding iris and capsular bag. (f) Because the lower viscosity dispersive viscoelastic (violet) is enveloped within the higher viscosity cohesive viscoelastic (green), both are easily aspirated out of the eye together at the end of the procedure, as if only a higher viscosity cohesive viscoelastic had been present.

tic permits creation of space and pressurization of the AC, to deepen the AC, stabilize it, and facilitate capsulorhexis in a manner that could not be achieved with a lower viscosity dispersive alone. The lower viscosity dispersive is fashioned into a smooth, even protective layer adjacent to the corneal endothelial cells, where it will remain throughout the turbulence of the surgical procedure, whereas the high viscosity cohesive viscoelastic will be aspirated out of the eye more rapidly.

A CCC is then performed and followed by hydrodissection. As the phaco is begun, the high viscosity cohesive viscoelastic is aspirated out, leaving a smooth, ironed out layer of lower viscosity dispersive viscoelastic adjacent to the corneal endothelial cells, having been smoothed out by the higher viscosity cohesive viscoelastic, without irregular fracture boundaries, allowing for clearer visualization of the posterior capsule while protecting the delicate endothelial cells against fluid turbulence.

After the lens has been emulsified and irrigation and aspiration of the cortical remnants completed, but before implantation of the IOL, the viscoelastics are injected in reverse order: the high viscosity cohesive viscoelastic is injected first, followed by the lower viscosity dispersive into its center. The high viscosity cohesive viscoelastic pressurizes the AC and expands the capsular bag to prevent wrinkles in the posterior capsule and facilitate foldable lens implantation. Its presence in the periphery of the AC stabilizes the iris and lens capsule so that they do not move when the IOL is introduced. It also protects the delicate structures of the eye against the sometimes rapid unfolding of silicone IOLs. The low viscosity dispersive viscoelastic, occupying the center of the AC and capsular bag, permits easier movement of instruments and the IOL through the viscoelastic. Because of the concentric partitioning of the AC into two different viscoelastic filled spaces, the unfolding of the IOL in the central lower viscosity dispersive filled space transmits far less force into the surrounding high viscosity cohesive viscoelastic filled space than would occur with either type of viscoelastic alone. Consequently, IOL implantation is achieved through a much better stabilized AC, and the tendency for a haptic to catch on the iris or posterior capsular folds, or to be reluctant to drop into the capsular bag, is greatly reduced. Furthermore, the AC, iris, and capsular bag are all more stable during IOL implantation.

The incision is enlarged to the appropriate size to allow implantation of the selected IOL after both viscoelastics have been injected. Once the lens has been implanted, the viscoelastics are aspirated from the eye. Because the lower viscosity dispersive viscoelastic is enveloped by the high viscosity cohesive viscoelastic, removal of both viscoelastics is quick and easy, similar to the experience of removing a high viscosity cohesive viscoelastic alone.

Using the Soft-Shell Technique

I have been using this soft-shell technique to manage difficult phacoemulsification cases and complications for about 10 years, using Healon® or Healon® GV in combination with Viscoat. Earlier, the cost of using two syringes of viscoelastic for each case precluded the use of soft shell for every case. However, the recent availability of Duovisc from Alcon, consisting of a smaller syringe each of Provisc and Viscoat, has allowed me to use this technique more generally with excellent results. It is a bit tedious, because of the extra step involved with the extra viscoelastic syringe, but advantageous, especially in difficult cases.

Summary

Despite the claims of unique superiority of each marketed viscoelastic by its manufacturer, the relatively unchanged market share of dispersive and cohesive viscoelastics over many years is indicative of the fact that ophthalmologists have recognized unique advantages and disadvantages of both types of viscoelastics. This issue has led me to study, over the last 15 years, the rheologic properties of viscoelastics. We now know enough about viscoelastic rheology to be able to classify ophthalmic viscoelastic devices into the surgically applicable categories of high viscosity cohesive viscoelastics and lower viscosity dispersive viscoelastics.

I developed the viscoelastic soft shell technique in the 1980s to assist in dealing with some of the complications of cataract surgery, but there was little interest in viscoelastic surgical techniques at the time, probably because viscoelastic rheology was not understood well enough to explain why this method works. The more recent development of viscoelastic measurement methods, along with better understanding of the importance of cohesion in ophthalmic surgery, now permits logical explanation of this technique. The viscoelastic soft-shell technique greatly facilitates cataract surgery by taking advantage of the best properties of both high viscosity cohesive viscoelastics and lower viscosity dispersive viscoelastics while eliminating the drawbacks of both classes.

Chapter Thirty-Five

Healon®5

Steve A. Arshinoff, MD, FRCSC

Healon®5, the first "viscoadaptive," is the first viscoelastic to be designed rheologically, as a result of a project that began in September 1996. The desired rheologic parameters were determined based on what was thought to be optimal for modern phacoemulsification surgery, and rheologic knowledge of hyaluronic acid solutions was used to engineer about 20 "candidate formulations," which were then extensively tested in masked trials of simulated phacoemulsification before the final version was chosen. The purpose of the exercise was to make a highly viscous viscoelastic that possessed the best properties of Healon® GV but was also highly retentive in the AC throughout all the steps of phacoemulsification, at least as much as the best of the dispersive viscoelastics, thus conforming to the current concept of an ideal viscoelastic (Table 35-1, Figure 35-1). Healon®5 was launched at the September 1998 meeting of the European Society of Cataract and Refractive Surgery.

A general idea of how viscous ophthalmic viscoelastics compare with items in daily experience can be obtained from Figure 35-2, which shows the viscosities of common items.

It can be seen from Table 35-2 that Healon®5 has the highest 0 shear viscosity (7 million milliPascal seconds) of any viscoelastic yet marketed. Similar to Healon® GV and Healon®, Healon®5 is also very pseudoplastic (Figure 35-3), making injection into the AC through a 25-G or 27-G cannula similar to Healon® GV with respect to required force and feedback sensation. Its molecular weight average is 4 million daltons, similar to Healon®, but its concentration is 2.3%, compared with Healon® at 1.0% and Healon® GV at 1.4%. It is the increased concentration of hyaluronic acid at this high molecular weight that allows Healon®5 to display its unique characteristics (Figure 35-4). The graph, however, explains only the effect on zero shear viscosity. Another important factor is that, given constant molecular mass, ophthalmic viscoelastics will appear to the surgeon to be more dispersive as concentration is increased.

The rheologic issue in the design of Healon®5 was the fact that all preceding viscous–cohesive ophthalmic viscoelastics were effective in space creation and maintenance, but in long or complicated surgical cases tended to emerge from the eye in a bolus too early in the procedure.

Viscous–cohesive viscoelastics have been helpful in deepening the AC in hyperopic patients, where space was previously nonexistent; in stabilizing the AC for the performance of pressure-equalized capsulorhexis; and in implanting IOLs, especially foldable, while the viscoelastic stabilizes the capsular bag. Viscous–cohesive viscoelastics are optimal for creating space and stability in the surgical microenvironment. They are also easily removed at the end of surgery by irrigation and aspiration because they are cohesive and therefore tend to move as a mass. The only drawback of viscous–cohesive viscoelastics is that they are unable to partition spaces and sometimes leave the AC too soon in surgery.

Lower viscosity–dispersive viscoelastics have their best advantages in performance of the surgical tasks for which viscous–cohesives come up short. Their retention in the AC on the corneal endothelial cell surface is superior and they can selectively move and isolate tissues, whereas viscous–cohesive viscoelastics move everything at once. Dispersive

Table 35-1.
VISCOELASTIC CLASSIFICATION

Viscoelastic Product	Company	Other Names
HIGHER VISCOSITY COHESIVES		
Super viscous cohesive viscoadaptive (0 shear viscosity >5 M mPaS)		
Healon®5	Pharmacia & Upjohn	
Super viscous cohesives (0 shear viscosity >1 M mPaS)		
MicroVisc Plus	Bohus Biotech	iVisc Plus, Hyvisc Plus
Healon® GV	Pharmacia & Upjohn	
Viscous cohesives (100 K mPaS < 0 shear viscosity < 1 M mPaS)		
Microvisc	Bohus Biotech	iVisc, Hyvisc
Healon®	Pharmacia & Upjohn	
Provisc	Alcon Laboratories	
Biolon	BTG (Ophthopharma Canada)	
Amvisc Plus	IOLab Corporation (B&L Surgical)	
Amvisc	IOLab Corporation (B&L Surgical)	
Viscorneal Plus	Corneal	Allervisc Plus
Viscorneal	Corneal	Allervisc
Biocorneal	Corneal	
Ophthalin	Ciba	
Ophthalin Plus	Ciba	
LOWER VISCOSITY DISPERSIVES		
Medium viscosity dispersives (10 K mPaS < 0 shear viscosity < 100 K mPaS)		
Viscoat	Alcon Laboratories	
Vitrax	Allergan Inc.	
Optimize	Mentor Ophthalmics	
Ocumax	CIMA Technology	
Cellugel	Vision Biology (Alcon)	
Lower viscosity dispersives (0 shear viscosity <10 K mPaS)		
Occucoat	Storz (B&L Surgical)	
iGel	International medical Devices	
Ocuvis	CIMA Technology Inc.	
Visilon	Shah & Shah	
Viscomet	Milmet Oftho Laboratories	
iCell	I Med Pharma	
Celoftal	Alcon Laboratories	

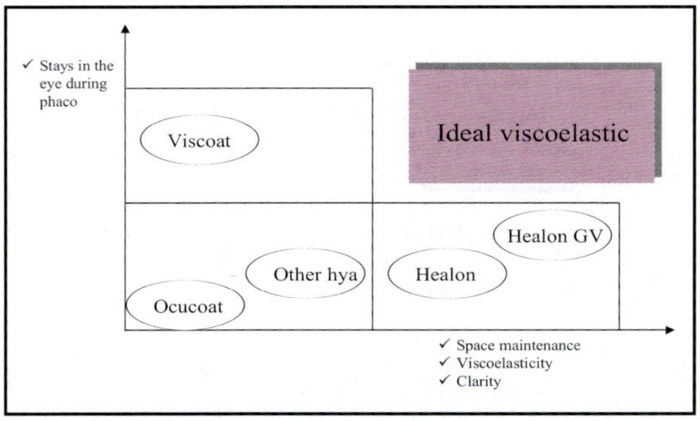

Figure 35-1. The theoretically ideal ophthalmic viscoelastic should: possess high viscosity and elasticity, thus making it capable of excellent space maintenance; be optically clear; and be retained well in the AC during phacoemulsification. Before the development of Healon®5, no single viscoelastic possessed all of these attributes.

Table 35-2.
COMPARATIVE PROPERTIES OF HEALON®5

	HPMC	Viscoat	Healon®	Healon® GV	Healon®5
Molecular mass (million)	0.08	0.05+0.5	4	5	4
Concentration (mg/mL)	20	70	1 0	14	23
Viscosity (shear 0) in mPaS	4000	50,000	200,000	2,000,000	7,000,000

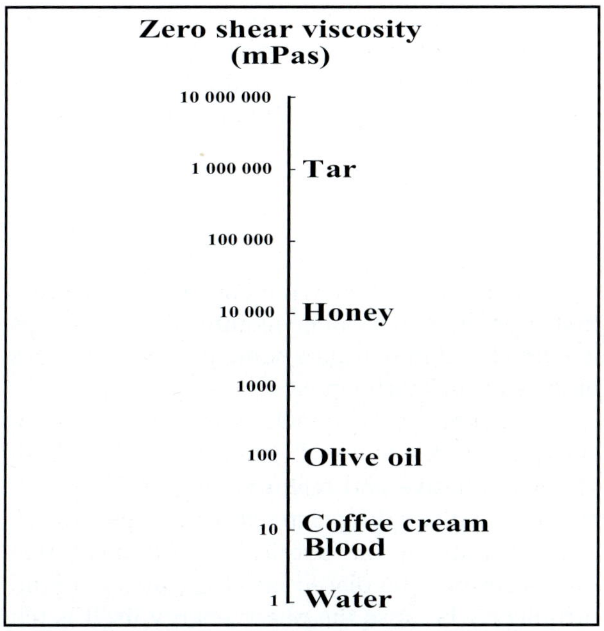

Figure 35-2. The viscosities of substances in common daily usage reveal that at 0 shear, when stationary, ophthalmic viscoelastics are much more viscous than objects that we commonly experience, and are in the range of tar.

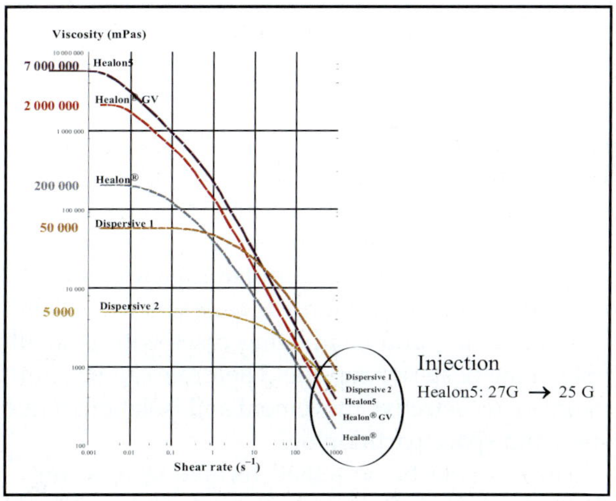

Figure 35-3. Healon®5 is seen to be three times more viscous at zero shear than Healon® GV, but is very pseudoplastic, such that it can easily be injected through a 25- or even 27-G cannula.

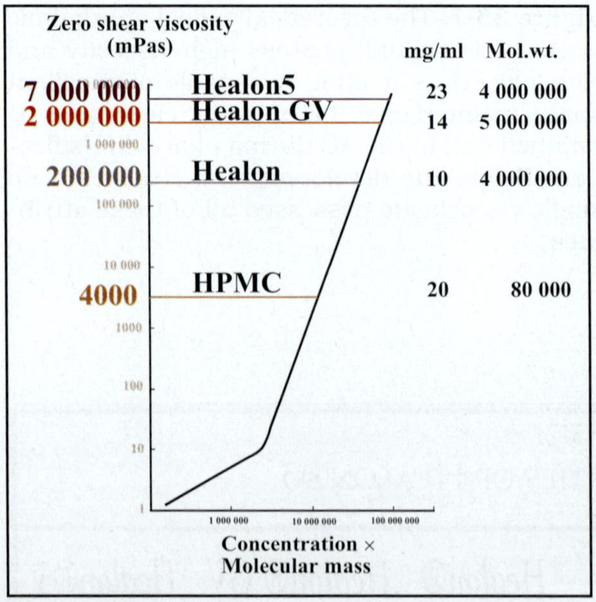

Figure 35-4. The graph demonstrates how zero shear viscosity of common ophthalmic viscoelastics is a function of both the molecular mass and concentration of the rheologically significant component. This, however, is only one aspect of the complex behavior of viscoelastics in ophthalmic surgery.

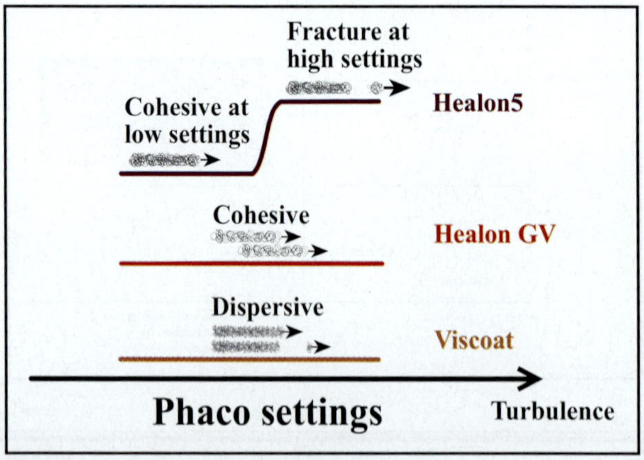

Figure 35-5. Dispersive viscoelastics—for example, Viscoat—behave as dispersives over all the common ranges of turbulence experienced in phacoemulsification surgery. Similarly, cohesives—for example, Healon® GV—behave as cohesives throughout the range of turbulence commonly experienced. Viscoadaptives, like Healon®5, are unique in that at low turbulence they behave like super viscous cohesive viscoelastics, but as the flow rate increases above 20 cc/min, they begin to fracture, allowing them to mimic, in some respects, the behavior of dispersive viscoelastics. This is shown graphically by having the step in viscoelastic behavior characteristics occur in the middle of common phaco settings (representing flow and therefore turbulence).

viscoelastics can be used to partition the AC into a viscoelastic-filled space and a BSS-filled space, where surgery can take place while the viscoelastic-filled space remains relatively undisturbed. Consequently, they are best suited for cases of inadvertently frayed iris, traumatic cataracts with disinserted zonules, and completing cases with a small hole in the posterior capsule. Their role can be summarized as "selective movement and isolation of tissues, and space partitioning".

The viscoelastic soft shell technique was introduced by Arshinoff to avoid the detriments of both classes of viscoelastics by using one viscoelastic from each of the two classes sequentially, in a logical system that takes advantage of the best properties of each type of viscoelastic while avoiding the problems associated with each when used alone. The disadvantage of the viscoelastic soft shell technique is that it requires the use of two separate syringes of viscoelastics that must be used sequentially instead of a single viscoelastic syringe, increasing cost and inconvenience. In addition, there is the risk that the wrong one may be injected first, a problem that can be require additional steps to correct and may negate some of the advantages of the soft shell technique.

The essence of Healon®5 is its rheologic idiosyncrasy, which makes it unique by being both viscous–cohesive and retentive. Figure 35-5 illustrates the outstanding characteristic of Healon®5. The attribute of the surgical environment that causes stress to be placed on viscoelastics is fluid turbulence. Because the phaco energy itself is felt only a very small distance from the phaco tip, the viscoelastic present remote from the immediate vicinity of the phaco tip remains unaffected by the power used. Fluid turbulence, however, as well as being an important factor in potential endothelial damage, is constant throughout the AC during

Table 35-3.
EXPLANATION OF VISCOADAPTIVITY

A viscoadaptive viscoelastic is one which spontaneously adapts its rheologic behavior to the fluid environment created by the surgeon. The viscoadaptive "knows" whether to behave as a cohesive or dispersive device based upon a predetermined clue signalled by the surgeon. The clue chosen is one that is appropriate to the task at hand: the fluid turbulence in the environment of the viscoadaptive. Therefore, during capsulorhexis, when there is no turbulence, the viscoadaptive acts as a super viscous-cohesive, whereas during phacoemulsification, the viscoadaptive adopts more dispersive properties, due to it's fracturability.

phaco, except when the phaco or irrigation and aspiration tip is kept within the capsular bag behind an intact capsulorhexis. Lower viscosity dispersive viscoelastics behave as dispersives over the entire range of fluid turbulence normally encountered in the AC during cataract surgery. Similarly, viscous cohesive viscoelastics behave as viscous devices over the entire range of turbulence encountered. Both of these classes are therefore appropriately named, because their behavior is consistent under the conditions to which we expose them. Healon®5 is referred to as viscoadaptive because under conditions of low turbulence it behaves just like a viscous cohesive device, whereas when the turbulence is increased, Healon®5 fractures into smaller pieces and therefore somewhat mimics the behavior of dispersive viscoelastics, but in a different way.

As viscoelastics are made ever more viscous and cohesive—from, for instance, Viscoat to Healon® to Healon® GV to Healon®5—they begin to approach the properties of solids somewhat, and start to become brittle or fracturable. This is analogous to what happens to viscous chocolate pudding when it is placed in the refrigerator for varying periods of time. If tested after different periods of cooling, the pudding will become more and more viscous until it reaches a point when it appears to be almost solid, but a spoon inserted into it can very easily fracture it into pieces. The unique fracturable quality of Healon®5 is what makes it viscoadaptive (Table 35-3). It allows Healon®5 to be used throughout surgery as a viscous–cohesive viscoelastic, somewhat like Healon® GV, but when removal is desired, one need only turn up the flow rate to fracture the viscoelastic matrix and use high vacuum to aspirate the viscous pieces. Similarly, Healon®5 can be broken at the iris plane and the cataract procedure can be carried out in the capsular bag, while the AC, exposed to low flow and protected from turbulence by an intact capsular bag, can remain full of Healon®5, yielding superlative protection of the endothelial cells. Furthermore, the fracturable characteristic of Healon®5 allows it to be used in cases of traumatic subluxated cataracts, frayed iris, small holes in the posterior capsule, and other circumstances where tissue isolation and protection is desired, unlike other viscous–cohesive viscoelastics. Healon®5 can therefore compete with the viscoelastic soft shell technique in that it can be adapted to any intraocular surgical circumstance.

The author acted as a consultant to Pharmacia & Upjohn for the development of Healon®5. During the process of development, we wanted to see if this type of viscoadaptive device actually was superior to conventional viscous–cohesive and lower viscosity–dispersive viscoelastics during all phases of cataract surgery. Preeminent cataract surgeons were asked to take part in masked handling tests on eye bank eyes in simulated phaco surgery, using Miyake type preparation. The cumulative results of these tests are shown in Figure 35-6. It can be seen from the Figure that although Healon®5 was not judged as absolutely the best at every stage of phacoemulsification, it was judged either best or insignificantly different from the best at each and every stage of phaco surgery, whereas a review of Figure 35-3 clearly shows that cohesive and dispersive viscoelastic groups both had decidedly weak performance in some aspects of phaco surgery. In fact, Healon®5 is unique in having been judged as excellent for every surgical task.

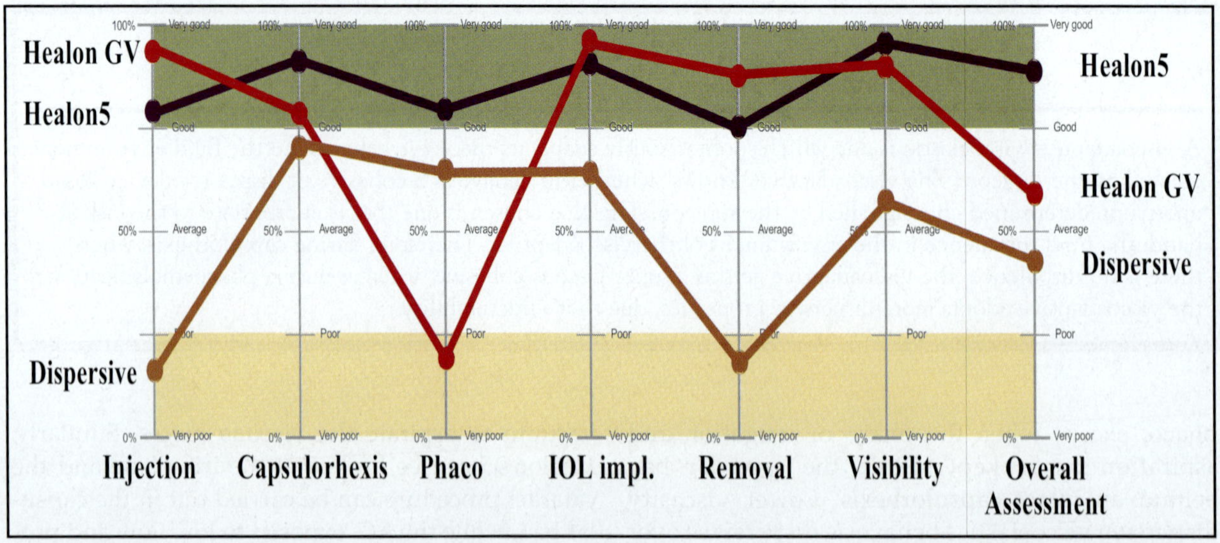

Figure 35-6. Handling tests of Healon®5, performed by experienced phaco surgeons in Miyake-prepared eye bank eyes, with the surgeons being blinded to the viscoelastic being tested, revealed that the behavior of Healon®5 was judged to be superior or close to the best in every aspect of phaco surgery. Cohesive viscoelastics, like Healon® GV, were found to excel in space maintenance and cohesion dependent roles (eg, IOL insertion and viscoelastic removal), whereas dispersives were found to be retained well during phacoemulsification. Overall, only Healon®5 was judged as excellent in all phases of phacoemulsification.

Removal of Healon®5

As in all innovations, the work with Healon®5 has taught us an important lesson. Like all viscoelastics, Healon®5 must be removed as completely as possible from the eye at the end of the surgical procedure to avoid unacceptable postoperative elevations of IOP. Here too, we performed a number of studies in the Miyake laboratory to ascertain what removal technique was necessary. I had previously reported that the "rock 'n' roll" technique of viscoelastic removal was the best way to remove all viscoelastics consistently, this having been confirmed by a comparative study of different techniques by Auffarth et al in 1994. Healon®5 is best removed using the rock 'n' roll technique with settings causing sufficient turbulence to achieve easy fracturing of the Healon®5 matrix, as follows (Table 35-3).

The aspiration flow rate is set at 25–30 cc/min. The vacuum is set at 350–500 mmHg. The bottle height is at 70 cm above the patient's eye, and a 0.3-mm irrigation and aspiration tip aspiration port size is used. The irrigation and aspiration tip is placed on the surface of the IOL and the surgeon's foot fully depresses the pedal. The irrigation and aspiration tip is now rolled back and forth across the surface of the IOL so that the fluid wave emitted from the irrigation ports carves a break through the matrix of the Healon®5, allowing aspiration of the pieces. At the same time there is slight posterior pressure from the irrigation and aspiration tip on the surface of the lens so that as the irrigation and aspiration tip is rolled, the IOL is gently rocked from side to side with each side of the IOL alternately tilting forward for easier aspiration of the viscoelastic mass from behind the IOL. This procedure maintains the IOL between the irrigation and aspiration tip and posterior capsule, thus protecting the posterior capsule from contact with the aspiration port. The vacuum level is set very high, allowing sufficient turbulence to fracture the Healon®5, and sufficient vacuum to aspirate the very viscous Healon®5. This technique takes about 30 seconds with Healon®5, but as with all viscoelastics, the endpoint is complete removal and not any specific time period. The time estimate is only a general guide. The rock 'n' roll technique has been shown to be the most efficient and effective

Table 35-4.
ROCK AND ROLL REMOVAL TECHNIQUE FOR HEALON®5

- Vacuum 350–500 mmHg
- Flow rate 25–30 mL/min
- Bottle height 60–70 cm
- Irrigation and aspiration tip port size 0.3

An effective technique to remove Healon®5 must create sufficient turbulence to make Healon®5 fracture into pieces.

method for viscoelastic removal with all types of viscoelastics.

SUMMARY

Healon®5 is the first viscoadaptive to reach the marketplace. It possesses the unique property of being fracturable when exposed to high turbulence, making it the most viscous cohesive viscoelastic yet marketed. It exhibits all the best properties of viscous cohesive viscoelastics while being highly retentive in the AC during the more turbulent phases of phaco. By allowing fracturing of the viscoelastic mass at the iris plane, the viscoelastic can be retained in the AC while phacoemulsification is carried out in the capsular bag. Similar strategies of viscoelastic fracturing can be used in other examples of desired partitioning of the AC into a viscoelastic-filled space and an operative zone (eg, broken zonules, Fuchs' endothelial dystrophy, a piece of frayed iris, a small hole in the posterior capsule). Healon®5 is the first viscoelastic to be judged as excellent in blind trials by experienced phaco surgeons in all aspects of phacoemulsification surgery.

CHAPTER THIRTY-SIX

Healon®5: Clinical Performance and Special Removal Technique (TCT)

Manfred R. Tetz, MD, and Mike P. Holzer, MS

Healon®5 is the first of a new group of products called viscoadaptive substances. Whereas in the past viscoelastic agents were classified according to their main physical behavior as dispersive or cohesive, intraoperatively these substances maintained their properties and always behaved as either dispersive or cohesive. Viscoadaptive substances may change the physical behavior according to the operative situation which is influenced by irrigation and aspiration flow characteristics, phaco settings etc.

Viscoadaptives are supposed to adapt to the surgical situation as the name supposes.

Healon®5 has the highest viscosity of all currently commercially available viscoelastic substances, which exceeds that of Healon® GV by 3.5 times (Table 36-1). The substance is cohesive at slow to moderate drag. At fast drag the molecule becomes brittle and behaves "pseudodispersive", ie the forces created by the entanglement of the molecules exceed chemical binding forces and the substance is separated into several pieces.

The increased versatility of Healon®5 allows for better surgery. Some features include better endothelial cell protection during phacoemulsification, controlled viscodilation of small pupils, superior space maintaining capacity during capsulorhexis, more controlled unfolding of foldable lenses, and more controlled management of complicated cases such as capsulorhexis in hypermature cataracts without dispersion of emulsified lens matter in the AC. In normal unselected eyes an open randomized single center parallel groups study was performed. Viscoelastic performance was assessed by three surgeons in routine phacosurgery using a 5-point scale and from a subjective assessment of the ease of injection, maintenance capacity during continuous circular capsulotomy (CCC), remaining capacity during phacoemulsification, facilitation of the IOL implantation, removal from the eye, transparency, and overall performance throughout the operation. The two substances used included Healon®5 and Viscoat, two substances that will remain in the AC during phaco to a significant extent but have different characteristics—dispersive versus adaptive. The percentage of good or very good performance during surgery as judged by the surgeons is shown in Table 36-2. In addition to phacoemulsification procedures possible applications and advantages in keratoplasty, viscocanalostomy and anterior segment trauma are just being recognized.

In order to avoid postoperative intraocular pressure (IOP) peaks complete removal of any viscoelastic agent used during cataract surgery is important. Also viscoelastic capture behind the IOL optic can only be prevented by thorough removal of the viscoelastic agent from the capsular bag. Several techniques to safely and completely remove viscoelastics from the anterior segment have been described in the literature. One of the techniques widely applied is the rock and roll technique as described by Arshinoff.

Table 36-1.
OVERVIEW OF COHESIVE VISCOELASTICS.

SUPER VISCOUS-COHESIVE		VISCOUS-COHESIVE	
Viscoelastic	*Vo (mPas)*	*Viscoelastic*	*Vo (mPas)*
Healon®5	7.0 M	Micro Visc	1.0 M
MicroVisc Plus	4.8 M	Allervisc Plus	500 K
Healon® GV	2.0 M	Provisc	255 K
		Healon®	230 K
		Biolon	215 K
		Allervisc	200 K
		Amvisc	100 K
		Amvisc Plus	100 K

Table 36-2.
PERCENT OF PATIENTS WITH GOOD OR VERY GOOD SCORES FROM SUBJECTIVE ASSESSMENT OF HEALON®5 AND VISCOAT DURING SURGERY

	Number (%) of patients	
Parameter	Healon®5 (n= 44)	Viscoat (n = 46)
Ease of injection	34 (77)*	27 (59)
Maintenance of AC	34 (77)*	31 (68)
Retention during phacoemulsification	36 (82)*	23 (50)
Facilitate IOL implantation	36 (82)*	20 (44)
Ease of removal	22 (50)*	0
Transparency	29 (66)*	13 (28)
Overall performance	34 (77)*	16 (35)

****p* < 0.05 *vs.* Viscoat**

Initially incorporating a learning curve Healon®5 was removed by the rock and roll technique. With this ease of removal was judged good or very good in only 50% (Table 36-2). A new technique which was then used in more than 250 consecutive eyes for safe removal of viscoelastics, especially viscoadaptive substances such as Healon®5 is described in the following. It takes full advantage of the viscoadaptive properties of Healon®5 and was named the Two Compartment Technique (TCT).

SURGICAL TECHNIQUE

Removal starts directly after IOL implantation while the AC is still is filled with the viscoadaptive

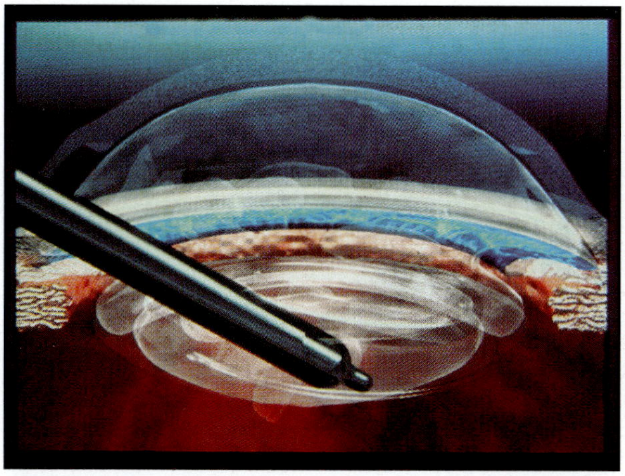

Figure 36-1. Schematic illustration of the first step of the TCT. The IA tip has been placed behind the IOL optic with the pseudophakos still slightly decentered (starting dry down under).

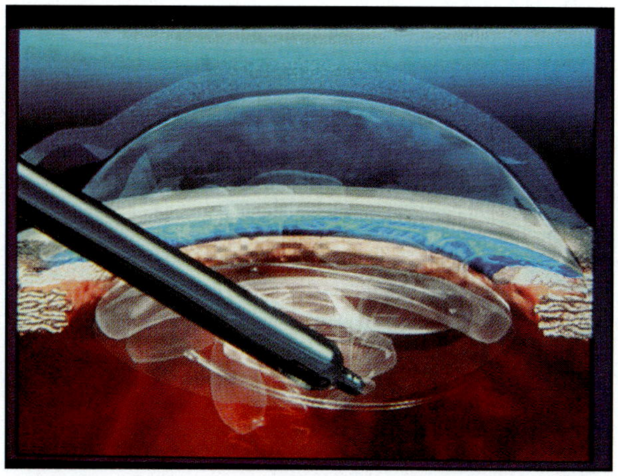

Figure 36-2. Schematic illustration TCT. Following positioning of the IA tip the flow is engaged. The capsular bag is emptied and the viscoadaptive removed while the AC remains filled and stabilized by Healon®5. The bag is inflated by the irrigation flow and the posterior capsule is held at distance.

agent and ideally before the IOL has been centered. The irrigation and aspiration port irrespective whether a one-hand or two-hand technique is used is facing the cornea and the handpiece is positioned behind the IOL optic without engaging flow. Irrigation and aspiration tips are essentially placed behind the IOL optic in a dry stage starting *dry* and *down under*. With a standard irrigation and aspiration port of 0.3 mm the effectual flow setting is normally kept at 20 to 25 ml per minute and vacuum setting is around 250 to 300 mmHg with a potential maximum setting at 500 mmHg. Bottle height should be around 60 to 70 cm above eye level. The flow of the irrigation and aspiration is not engaged until the tip has been positioned behind the IOL optic. Thus the tip is initially protected by the surrounding viscoelastic agent like any surgical instruments (Figure 36-1).

Only after the IOL optic rim has been arrested against the sleeve or irrigation chamber of the tip the flow is started. Thus the viscoadaptive agent is removed from the capsular bag first while the AC remains filled and the iris stabilized by Healon®5. The irrigation and aspiration flow takes place within the compartment of the capsular bag while the viscoadaptive substance maintains the AC and prevents fluids from coming forward (Figure 36-2). The posterior capsule is held at distance by the irrigation fluid that is continuously inflating the capsular bag and preventing the posterior capsule from coming forward. Thus, the risk of inadvertently aspirating the posterior capsule is avoided. After the viscoadaptive agent has been completely removed out of the capsular bag, which can be easily visualized due to the high refractive index of Healon®5, the tip is removed from behind the optic with a continuous flow and placed on top of the optic, irrigation port facing upwards.

The removal is continued by circling the irrigation and aspiration tip at the iris plane or on the optic surface and the viscoadaptive is visualized while removing (Figure 36-3). A final sweep may be made along the AC angle in order to remove any potential remainder of viscoadaptive agent. By performing this technique the removal time of viscoadaptive agents such as Healon®5 could be reduced from an average of 40 to 50 seconds for example by using the rock and roll technique to 10 to 20 seconds with TCT.

REMOVAL: CLINICAL PERFORMANCE

The authors have used this removal technique with Healon®5 over a period of five months now in more than 250 eyes and in none of these eyes a severe pressure spike or a posterior capsular rupture occurred. Ever since using this technique we also found it easy to remove any kind of viscoelastic such as Methylcellulose, Healon® and Viscoat because it takes the additional advantage of having some viscoelastic agent in the AC while cleaning out the capsular bag. However, the technique works best with a viscoadaptive agent because due to the high space maintaining capacity, the AC remains filled until the bag is completely freed from the viscoadaptive substance.

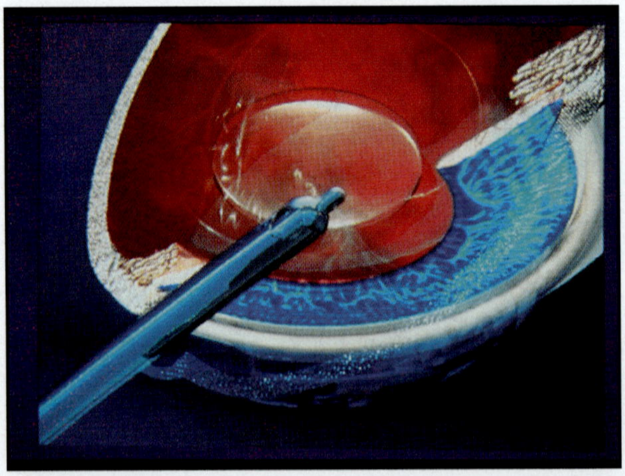

Figure 36-3. Schematic illustration TCT. In the second step the viscoadaptive is removed from the AC.

SUMMARY

The use of viscoelastic agents in cataract surgery is very important for making the operation safe and more controlled. However, some viscoelastic-induced complications after surgery may occur. Important among these are intraocular pressure peaks during the first 24 hours postoperatively and capsular bag distension syndromes.

To minimize these complications a complete, safe and fast removal of viscoelastic agents is required. New viscoadaptives, such as Healon®5 may be best removed by TCT, since this technique takes full advantage of its versatility. Superior space maintaining capacities of Healon®5 in the AC are utilized while removing substance from the capsular bag. In the second step the AC is cleansed.

As new viscoelastic substances are being introduced surgeons continue to adapt certain steps of their procedure to the new features of the substances. While it is still impossible to completely remove a dispersive viscoelastic agent from the eye the TCT allows fast and complete removal of viscoadaptive devices.

BIBLIOGRAPHY

Auffarth GU,Wesendahl TA, Solomon KD, Brown SJ, Apple DJ. Evaluation of different removal techniques of a highviscosity viscoelastic. J Cataract Refract Surg. 1994;Best papers of session:Suppl.30-32.

Apple. Removal of viscoelastic materials after experimental cataract surgery in vitro. *J Cataract Refract Surg.* 1992;18:3–6.

Assia EI, Apple DJ, Lim ES, Morgan RC, Tsai JC. Removal of viscoelastic materials after experimental cataract surgery in vitro. *J Cataract Refract Surg.* 1992;18:36.

Arshinoff SA. Comparative physical properties of ophthalmic viscoelastic materials. *Ophthalmic Practice.* 1989;7(1):16–36.

Arshinoff SA. The physical properties of ophthalmic viscoelastics in cataract surgery. *Ophthalmic Practice.* 1991;9(2):1–7.

Arshinoff SA. Dispersive and cohesive viscoelastic materials in phacoemulsification. *Ophthalmic Practice.* 1995;13(3):98–104.

Arshinoff SA. The dispersive/cohesive viscoelastic soft-shell technique for compromised corneas and anterior chamber compartmentalization. Presented at the *American Society of Cataract and Refractive Surgery Film Festival;* Seattle, Wash; June 1–5, 1996.

Arshinoff SA. Rock 'n' roll removal of Healon® GV (video). Presented at the *American Society of Cataract and Refractive Surgery Film Festival;* Seattle, Wash; June 1–5, 1996.

Arshinoff SA. Rock 'n' roll removal of Healon® GV. In: Arshinoff SA, ed. Proceedings of the 7th annual *National Ophthalmic Speakers Program;* Ottawa, Canada; June 1996.

Arshinoff SA, Hofinann I. Prospective, randomized trial of Microvisc and Healon® in routine phacoemulsification. *J Cataract Refract Surg.* 1997;23:761–765.

Arshinoff SA. Presented at the *European Society of Cataract and Refractive Surgery;* 1998 symposium.

Arshinoff SA, Hofinann I. A prospective, randomized trial comparing Microvisc Plus to Healon® GV and superviscous cohesive viscoelastics to viscous cohesive viscoelastics in routine phacoemulsification. *J Cataract Refract Surg.* 1998.

Arshinoff SA. The dispersive-cohesive viscoelastic soft shell technique. *J Cataract Refract Surg.* February 1999;25(2):167-173.

Assia EL, Apple DJ, Lim ES, et al. Removal of viscoelastic materials after experimental cataract surgery in vitro. *J Cataract Refract Surg.* 1992;18:3–6.

Beesley et al. The effects of prolonged phacoemulsification time on the corneal endothelium. *Ann Ophthalmol.* 1986.

Caporossi A, Baiocchi S, Sforzi C, Frezzotti R. Healon® GV vs Healon® in demanding cataract surgery. *J Cataract Refract Surg.* 1995;21(7):10–13.

Carassa RG, Bettin P, Brancato R. Viscocanalostomy: preliminary report. *Eur J Ophthalmol.* 1998;8:57–61.

Cobo et al. Advance in therapy: Vitrax in anterior segment surgery—a review and clinical study. 1990;7.

Colin. Presented at the annual meeting of the *European Society of Cataract and Refractive Surgery;* Innsbruck; September 1993.

Craig et al. Air bubble endothelium damage during phaco in human eye bank eyes: the protective effect of Healon® and Viscoat. *J Cataract Refract Surg.* 1990.

Dick B, Schwenn O. *Viskoelastika Eine Ubersicht.* New York, NY: Springer; 1998;l9,73-77.

Frucht-Perey. Presented at the annual meeting of the *European Society of Cataract and Refractive Surgery;* Innsbruck; September 1993.

Fry et al. Postoperative intraocular pressure rises: a comparison of Healon®, Amvisc and Viscoat. *J Cataract Refract Surg.* 1989.

Fry et al. Healon® GV in ECCE with intraocular lens implantation. *J Cataract Refract Surg.* 1993.

Glasser. Protective effects of viscous solutions in phacoemulsification and traumatic lens implantation. *Arch Ophthalmol.* 1989.

Glasser. Endothelium protection and viscoelastic retention during phacoemulsification and intraocular lens implantation. *Arch Ophthalmol.* 1991.

Hammer. Viscous corneal protection by sodium hyaluronate, condroitin sulfate and methylcellulose. *Invest Ophthalmol Vis Sci.*

Hazariwala et al. Comparison of 2% hydroxypropylmethylcellulose and 1% sodium hyaluronate in implant surgery. *Can J Ophthalmol.* 1988.

Keats et al. *Ophthalmic Surg.* 1987;18:693–697.

Kohnen T von Ehr M, Schutte E. Postoperative intraocular pressure in the first days after intraocular administration of hyaluronic acid solution with different viscosities. *Klin Monatsbl Augenheilkd.* 1995;207:29-36.

Kohnen T von Ehr M, Schutte E, Koch DD. Evaluation of intraocular pressure with Healon® and Healon® GV in sutureless cataract surgery with foldable lens implantation. *J Cataract Refract Surg.* 1996;22:227-37.

Lane et al. Prospective comparison of the effects of Occucoat, Viscoat and Healon® in intraocular pressure and endothelial cell loss. *J Cataract Refract Surg*. 1991.

Lehmann R, Brint S, Stewart R, et al. Clinical comparison of Provisc and Healon® in cataract surgery. *J Cataract Refract Surg*. 1995;21:543–547.

Madsen K, Stenevi U, Apple D, Harfstrand A. I-Estochen-úcal and receptor binding sites of hyaluronic acid and hyaluronic acid binding sites on the corneal endothelium. *Ophthalmic Practice*. 1989;7(3):2–8.

McCulley. *Invest Ophthalmol Vis Sci*. 1989;30.

Miyake K, Ota I, Ichihashi S, Miyake S, Tanaka Y, Terasaki H. New classification of capsular block syndrome. J Cataract Refract Surg. 1998;24:1230-4.

Pedersen. Comparison of the protective effects of methylcellulose and sodium hyaluronate on corneal swelling following phacoemulsification of senile cataracts. *J Cataract Refract Surg*. 1990.

Probst. Corneal endothelium and intraocular pressure after phacoemulsification with Amvisc Plus and Viscoat. *J Cataract Refract Surg*. 1993.

Poyer JF, Chan KY, Arshinoff SA. A new method to measure the retention of viscoelastics on a rabbit corneal endothelial cell line after irrigation and aspiration. *J Cataract Refract Surg*. 1998;24:84–90.

Rafuse. Effects of Healon® versus Viscoat on endothelial cell count and morphology after phacoemulsification and posterior chamber lens implantation. *Can J Ophthalmol*. 1992.

Rappazzo. *Ophthalmic Surg*. 1984;15.

Stegmann R, Pienaar A, Miller D. Viscocanalostomy for open-angle glaucoma in black African patients. *J Cataract Refract Surg*. 1999.

Molander
Molander et al 1993
Nichols
Nishida 1991
Oh and Lee
Osher
Packer 1985
Pallikaris
Paris and Saya 1990
Pedersen. Comparison of the protective effects of methylcellulose and sodium hyaluronate on corneal swelling following phacoemulsification of senile cataracts. *J Cataract Refract Surg*. 1990.
Pfeiffer
Probst. Corneal endothelium and intraocular pressure after phacoemulsification with Amvisc Plus and Viscoat. *J Cataract Refract Surg*. 1993.
Polack 1982
Poyer JF, Chan KY, Arshinoff SA. A new method to measure the retention of viscoelastics on a rabbit corneal endothelial cell line after irrigation and aspiration. *J Cataract Refract Surg*. 1998;24:84–90.
Rafuse. Effects of Healon® versus Viscoat on endothelial cell count and morphology after phacoemulsification and posterior chamber lens implantation. *Can J Ophthalmol*. 1992.
Rappazzo. *Ophthalmic Surg*. 1984;15.
Reed et al
Reiboldi et al 1992
Reim and Saric
Rispoli et al 1991
Rispoli et al 1993
Riss et al
Romeo et al
Ruiz
Ryan
Searl 1987
Seiff and Ahn
Shimizu 1991
Shimmura
Shiwa and Tazawa 1991
Singer
Singh
Smedsrod 1984
Snibson et al
Snibson et al 1990
Stark
Stegmann and Miller
Stegmann 1979
Stegmann R, Pienaar A, Miller D. Viscocanalostomy for open-angle glaucoma in black African patients. *J Cataract Refract Surg*. 1999.
Stenevi
Stirpe et al 1992
Strampelli
Tan
Toda et al 1993
Tomazzoli et al
Uram
Verstraeten et al
Vidaurri-Leal et al 1984
Vieira et al 1985
Villa-Coro 1988
Villa-Coro 1990
Volker-Dieben and Balestrazzi
Wand
Wilson
Wirt 1992
Wong
Yaacoby

Index

For your information...

This book and many others on numerous different topics are available from SLACK Incorporated. For further information or a copy of our latest catalog, contact us at:

Professional Book Division
SLACK Incorporated
6900 Grove Road
Thorofare, NJ 08086 USA
Telephone: 1-856-848-1000
1-800-257-8290
Fax: 1-856-853-5991
E-mail: orders@slackinc.com
WWW: http://www.slackinc.com

We accept most major credit cards and checks or money orders in US dollars drawn on a US bank. Most orders are shipped within 72 hours.

Contact us for information on recent releases, forthcoming titles, and bestsellers. If you have a comment about this title or see a need for a new book, direct your correspondence to the Editorial Director at the above address.

If you are an instructor, we can be reached at the address listed above or on the Internet at educomps@slackinc.com for specific needs.

Thank you for your interest and we hope you found this work beneficial.